D O N A T E D   T O

Morriston Hospital

X-ray Department Library

BY

NYGAARD (U.K.) LIMITED

D1333431

Myelography

MYELOGRAPHY

ROBERT SHAPIRO, M.D.

Chairman, Department of Radiology, Hospital of St. Raphael
Clinical Professor of Radiology
Yale University School of Medicine, New Haven, Connecticut

FOURTH EDITION

YEAR BOOK MEDICAL PUBLISHERS, INC.

CHICAGO

Library of Congress Cataloging in Publication Data
Shapiro, Robert.
  Myelography.
  Includes index.
  1. Myelography. I. Title. [DNLM: 1. Myelography. WL
405 S529m]
RC402.2.M94S53   1984   616.7'3'07572   83-21577
ISBN 0-8151-7668-6

Sponsoring editor: Daniel J. Doody
Editing supervisor: Frances M. Perveiler
Copyeditor: Lois M. Smit
Production project manager: Sharon W. Pepping
Proofroom supervisor: Shirley E. Taylor

To the many students and residents who offer living testimony to the abiding wisdom of Rabbi Judah the Prince. "Much have I learned from my teachers, more from my colleagues, but most of all from my pupils" (Talmud: Taanit, 7a).

Contributors

RICHARD A. BAKER, M.D.
Lahey Clinic Hospital
Burlington, Massachusetts

RENE DJINDJIAN, M.D. (DECEASED)
University of Paris
Paris, France

H. PAUL HATTEN, JR., M.D.
Presbyterian Hospital
Charlotte, North Carolina

VICTOR M. HAUGHTON, M.D.
Medical College of Wisconsin
Milwaukee, Wisconsin

E. LEON KIER, M.D.
Yale University School of Medicine
New Haven, Connecticut

ARTHUR E. ROSENBAUM, M.D.
Johns Hopkins Medical School
Baltimore, Maryland

MILAN ROTH, M.D., C.Sc.
Medical Faculty Hospital
J. Ev. Purkyne's University
Brno, Czechoslovakia

CHATRACHI VIRAPONGSE, M.D.
Yale University School of Medicine
New Haven, Connecticut

Preface to the Fourth Edition

THE INTRODUCTION of metrizamide and high-resolution CT scanning has dramatically changed the complexion of myelography as we have classically known it. In the seven years since publication of the third edition, significant new knowledge has also been acquired in a number of areas, i.e., congenital lesions, spinal trauma, low back pain–sciatic syndrome, etc. The obvious need for a new edition has provided an opportunity for major revisions in other portions of the book.

I have been very fortunate in enlisting the cooperation of a group of highly talented colleagues to participate in this enterprise. Their special skills and expertise have resulted in a number of illuminating new chapters. The chapter on trauma has been rewritten by Drs. Chat Virapongse and E. Leon Kier based on their experience at the Yale spinal cord trauma center. A new chapter on pneumomyelography has been prepared by Dr. Arthur E. Rosenbaum and Dr. Richard A. Baker. Dr. H. Paul Hatten has contributed a chapter on epidurography. Dr. Milan Roth has distilled his uniquely singular concepts on neurovertebral relationships into a new chapter. Finally, Dr. Victor M. Haughton has written an authoritative overview of the role of CT in the diagnosis of spinal lesions.

As previously, some of my friends and colleagues have graciously shared their material with me. In this regard, I am especially indebted to Dr. E. Leon Kier, Dr. Robert M. Quencer, Dr. John C. Stears, and Dr. Maer B. Ozonoff for their unstinting generosity.

I am happy to acknowledge the expert photography of Ovidio Gallo and Doris Barclay and the artistry of Virginia Simon, Patrick Lynch, and Veronica Vigliotti. I owe a special debt of gratitude to my secretary, Angela Brunetti, for her unflagging patience in typing and retyping the manuscript and her invaluable assistance with the many details associated with this revision. Finally, this work would not have been possible without the understanding, encouragement, and forbearance of my wife, Pearl.

ROBERT SHAPIRO

Preface to the First Edition

ALTHOUGH myelography has become an important method of examining the spinal canal and its contents, no comprehensive treatise dealing with the subject is available. This hiatus is painfully evident when one is concerned with training residents. The purpose of this book is to help correct the deficiency by describing in some detail the technique of examination, the anatomic basis of the normal myelogram and the findings in various pathologic states.

The bulk of the material has been drawn from personal experience at The Hospital of St. Raphael and The Grace-New Haven Community Hospital, augmented by original studies in the postmortem and anatomic laboratories. However, when my personal files were meager, I have not hesitated to borrow freely from many generous colleagues, to whom I am greatly indebted. In this regard, I would be remiss if I failed to acknowledge a special indebtedness to Drs. William German, Robert M. Lowman, Franklin Robinson, and Charles M. D'Alessio. I am also happy to express my appreciation to that masterful myelographer, Dr. H. O. Peterson, for teaching me his technique, to Harry Assadurian and Tom McCarthy for the photography, to Drs. Orlando F. Gabriele and Franklin Robinson for reading portions of the manuscript, and to my secretary, Angela Brunetti, for her invaluable assistance, including the typing of the manuscript. Last but not least, I wish to express my gratitude to Mrs. Franklin Robinson for her excellent illustrations.

ROBERT SHAPIRO

Contents

1

History

THE BIRTH OF MYELOGRAPHY was presaged by Dandy's classic description of pneu-moencephalography in 1919. In this paper, he prophetically remarked, "It seems probable that we shall be able to localize spinal cord tumors by means of intraspi-nous injections of air. In one of our cases, the spinal cord and the surrounding air-filled space are sharply outlined." However, Dandy did not actually publish his experience with myelography until 1925, when he reported a series of 10 spinal cord tumors that he localized with this technique. Meanwhile, in 1921, Jacobeus in Sweden described the successful use of pneumomyelography to localize intraspinal tumors in three patients. The same author noted that Josephson had presented a patient with a spinal cord tumor diagnosed by this technique earlier that year to the Medical Congress in Helsinki. Also in 1921, Wideröe in Norway unsuccessfully attempted pneumomyelography on a patient with a spinal cord tumor.

Further impetus was given to myelography in 1922 through a striking example of serendipity. While treating a patient with sciatica by the extradural injection of iodized poppy seed oil (Lipiodol), Sicard and Forestier accidentally introduced some of the oil into the subarachnoid space. Noting that the subarachnoid oil moved freely, they decided to use it for the localization of spinal cord tumors. Before long, Lipiodol supplanted air as the myelographic medium of choice. Even-tually, myelography achieved widespread popularity, largely due to Mixter and Barr's publication in 1934 on the syndrome of the herniated intervertebral disk.

The universal acceptance of Lipiodol myelography brought to light a number of its disadvantages. The relatively high viscosity of the oil and its nonmiscibility with spinal fluid frequently produced large, irregularly distributed globules, which made interpretation and removal difficult. Moreover, Lipiodol proved to be irritating to the pia-arachnoid. These drawbacks soon spurred efforts to find a more satisfactory contrast medium, a search that proceeded in several directions.

THOROTRAST MYELOGRAPHY.—In 1932, Radovici and Meller in France injected colloidal thorium dioxide (Thorotrast) into the cisterna magna, but the alarming severity of the reaction soon prompted them to abandon this medium. Capua in Italy and Löhr and Jacobi, as well as Wüstman, in Germany had similar experi-ences. In an effort to reduce this toxicity, Nosik and Mortensen introduced forced spinal drainage to remove the Thorotrast after completion of the study. Even with this technique, 10%–15% of the Thorotrast remained in the subarachnoid space to produce varying degrees of meningeal irritation. This undesirable consequence eventually led to the abandonment of Thorotrast for myelography.

PANTOPAQUE MYELOGRAPHY.—In 1940, the University of Rochester group introduced Pantopaque, an oily medium considerably less viscid and less irritating to the meninges than Lipiodol. Before long, Pantopaque became the myelographic medium of choice in most instances in the United States.

PNEUMOMYELOGRAPHY.—Gas myelography continues to play a role in the examination of the spinal canal in a few specific instances. The present technique, which involves tomography, represents the culmination of a number of contributors in the past—Young and Scott in the United States, Lindgren in Sweden, and Jirout and Roth in Czechoslovakia.

WATER-SOLUBLE MEDIA.—In 1931, Arnell and Lidström first employed Abrodil (Skiodan), a water-soluble organic iodine compound, for myelography. Arnell's experimental studies, carried out in collaboration with a German chemist, were interrupted by World War II. Nevertheless, he continued to use Abrodil in a small group of patients during this period, summarizing his experience before the Swedish Society for Radiology in 1944. In the meantime, Felström published a brief communication on Abrodil myelography in Norway in 1942. Since that time, numerous reports dealing with Abrodil myelography appeared in the continental literature, climaxed by Arnell's classic monograph in 1948. Although Abrodil was widely used for lumbar myelography in the Scandinavian countries, it never achieved popularity in the United States because of its irritating effect on the spinal cord and meninges.

In the late 1960s, and early '70s, water-soluble myelography was revitalized on the Continent with the introduction of two new compounds, Conray-60 and Dimer-X. Again, the disadvantages associated with the toxicity of these agents prevented their general acceptance in the United States. During the past few years, however, the picture has changed dramatically because of the availability of metrizamide, a new, less toxic, nonionic, aqueous medium.

BIBLIOGRAPHY

Arnell S., Lidström F.: Myelography with Skiodan (Abrodil). *Acta Radiol.* 12:287, 1931.
Capua A.: Encephalomyelography with subarachnoid injections of Thorotrast. Clinical and experimental study. *Radiol. Med.* 20:1376, 1933.
Dandy W.E.: Ventriculography following the injection of air into the cerebral ventricles. *Ann. Surg.* 68:5, 1918.
Dandy W.E.: Roentgenography of the brain after the injection of air into the spinal canal. *Ann. Surg.* 70:397, 1919.
Dandy W.E.: Diagnosis and localization of spinal cord tumors. *Bull. Johns Hopkins Hosp.* 33:190, 1922.
Felström E.: On myelography with Abrodil. *Nord. Med.* 14:1653, 1942.
Jacobeus H.C.: On insufflation of air into the spinal canal for diagnostic purposes in cases of tumors in the spinal cord. *Acta Med. Scandinav.* 21:555, 1921.
Jirout J.: Pneumomyelographic examination of the cervical spine. *Acta Radiol.* 50:221, 1958.
Lindgren E.: Myelographie mit Luft. *Nervenarzt* 12:57, 1939.
Löhr W., Jacobi W.: Die Darstellung der peripheren Nerven im Röntgenbild. *Arch. Klin. Chir.* 171:538, 1932.
Mixter W.J., Barr J.S.: Rupture of the intervertebral disc with involvement of the spinal canal. *N. Engl. J. Med.* 211:210, 1934.

Nosik W.A., Mortensen O.: Myelography with Thorotrast and subsequent removal by forced drainage, experimental study: Preliminary report. *Am. J. Roentgenol.* 39:727, 1938.

Radovici A., Meller O.: Encéphalographie liquidienne par le thorotrast sousarachnoidien. *Rev. Neurol.* 1:479, 1932.

Ramsey G.H.S., Strain W.E.: Pantopaque: New contrast medium for myelography. *Radiol. & Clin. Photog.* 20:25, 1944.

Roth M.: Gas myelography by the lumbar route. *Acta Radiol.* [*Diag.*] 1:53, 1963.

Sicard J.A., Forestier J.: Méthode générale d'exploration radiólogique par l'huile iodée (Lipiodol). *Bull. et Mém. Soc. Méd. Hôp. Paris* 46:463, 1922.

Wideröe S.: Über die diagnostische Bedeutung der intraspinalen Luftinjektionen bei Rückenmarksleiden besonders bei Geschwülsten. *Zentralbl. Chir.* 48:394, 1921.

Wideröe S.: Diagnosis of spinal cord tumors. *Norsk Mag. Laegevidensk.* 82:491, 1921.

Wüstman O.: Experimentelle Untersuchungen über die Reliefdarstellung (Umrisszeichnung) des Zentralnervensystems in Röntgenbild durch Thoriumkontrastmittel. *Dtsch Z. Chir.* 238:529, 1933.

Young B.R., Scott M.: Air myelography, substitution of air for Lipiodol in roentgen visualization of tumors and their structures in spinal canal. *Am. J. Roentgenol.* 39:187, 1938.

2

Contrast Media

THE IDEAL MYELOGRAPHIC MEDIUM has not as yet been discovered. Such a medium should (1) have a low viscosity and be thoroughly miscible with CSF, (2) be rapidly excreted, (3) be nonionic and iso-osmolar with CSF at concentrations necessary for satisfactory radiopacity, (4) be highly hydrophobic with minimal or no local and systemic toxicity. There is a direct relationship between the hydrophobic characteristics of a contrast medium and a lesser propensity to interfere with an organism's macromolecular structure. This chapter will review the various substances that have been utilized for myelography.

AIR AND OTHER GASES

Air, the original myelographic agent, may still be the medium of choice in a few situations. Occasionally, other gases (particularly oxygen) are used because of their greater diffusibility and more rapid elimination. From the diagnostic point of view, however, air is equally satisfactory. In general, gases are the least irritating of all the known contrast media. Save for a transient slight pleocytosis and increase in spinal fluid protein, they are essentially nontoxic. Furthermore, they are completely resorbed in a relatively short period of time. Consequently, there are no absolute contraindications to gas myelography except increased intracranial pressure.

There are, however, a number of disadvantages associated with pneumomyelography. Because gases do not mix with cerebrospinal fluid, the fluid must be drained off and replaced by the gas. This makes the examination uncomfortable and trying for the patient, particularly when it is necessary to study the entire spinal subarachnoid space. In such cases, postmyelographic headache may be quite severe and last for several days.

Most of the other problems associated with pneumomyelography are functions of the modest contrast produced by gases in the spinal canal, which can be overcome by meticulous radiographic technique and body section radiography. However, since gases do not freely permeate the subarachnoid space along the nerve roots, the latter are not visualized. Thus, sacral root cysts, nerve root avulsions, and small lateral-lying disk protrusions may be completely missed. Furthermore, various non-obstructive lesions such as arachnoiditis and vascular malformations may not be recognized as such. On the other hand, pneumomyelography is superior to positive contrast techniques in demonstrating the cystic nature of some intramedullary lesions, atrophy of the spinal cord, and various congenital lesions.

AQUEOUS SUSPENSIONS

Thorotrast

Thorotrast is a stable, aqueous colloidal sol containing 25% thorium dioxide by volume suspended in a tapioca-dextrin medium. A preservative of 0.15% methyl p-hydroxybenzoate is added to the sol. Thorium is a potent alpha emitter with a half-life of 1.4×10^{10} years. Because of its prolonged retention within the body, the surrounding tissues are continuously bombarded by alpha particles with a penetration range of 30–50 microns. Of all the media employed for myelography, Thorotrast is the most irritating to the pia-arachnoid. It produces not only an alarming systemic reaction accompanied by high fever but also local inflammatory changes resulting in intense arachnoiditis, which may culminate in a disabling cauda equina syndrome. In this regard, Maltby described three patients with a slowly progressive cauda equina syndrome that manifested itself approximately 8 years following Thorotrast myelography. In addition, various benign and malignant tumors have been reported as late sequelae. For these reasons, there is no present justification for using Thorotrast for myelography.

SH-617L

In 1963, Zeitler reported on the use of SH-617L as a myelographic contrast medium. This substance is a 20% crystalline suspension of β-(3-dimethylaminomethylenamino-2,4,6-tri-iodophenyl) propionic acid ethyl ester in 5.5% glucose. The same year, Vogler and Walcher published their investigations in rabbits and dogs as well as in a clinical series of 160 myelograms. The compound contains 60.45% iodine, all organically bound. The material is hyperbaric, requires no preliminary anesthesia, is absorbed almost completely in 6–8 weeks (50% absorbed in 3–4 weeks), and may be instilled by either cisternal or lumbar puncture. Its lower viscosity results in coating of the nerve roots and cord, permitting visualization of the latter in both the frontal and lateral projections. The original enthusiasm expressed by Vogler and Walcher was followed by a number of critical reports culminating in Lindgren and Törnell's paper, which clearly demonstrated that SH-617L produces parenchymatous degeneration of the spinal cord as well as severe leptomeningeal irritation. This substance, therefore, has been abandoned for myelography.

Lipiodol

Lipiodol is a viscid, halogenated, poppy seed oil containing 40% iodine (w/v) in organic combination. Normally, it has a light yellow color that turns dark brown on long standing or exposure to light due, to the liberation of free iodine. In the latter circumstance, the material should be discarded.

Because of its oily nature, it is not miscible with cerebrospinal fluid. It is also irritating to the leptomeninges, as evidenced by a prompt, significant increase in cell count and spinal fluid protein after injection. Furthermore, it is absorbed extremely slowly (if at all), and has a distinct tendency to become encysted and produce varying degrees of late arachnoiditis. The relatively high viscosity not only makes complete removal difficult but also favors fragmentation and the formation of large, irregular globules. Because of these disadvantages, Lipiodol should no longer be used as a myelographic medium.

Pantopaque

Originally introduced by Strain and his co-workers at the University of Rochester in 1940, Pantopaque is a mixture of ethyl esters of isomeric iodophenylundecylic acids containing 30.5% of firmly bound organic iodine. Normally clear or pale yellow in color, it tends to become discolored when exposed to sunlight and should not be used in the latter state. Pantopaque has a specific gravity of 1.260 at 20 C and is, therefore, much less viscous than Lipiodol ($\frac{1}{22}$ as viscous at 20 C and $\frac{1}{17}$ as viscous at body temperature).

Like all oily media, Pantopaque is not miscible with CSF and forms globules in seeking a shape with the lowest surface tension. Pantopaque flows more freely, has a lesser tendency to form large irregular globules, and can be more readily removed from the spinal canal than Lipiodol. Because of its viscosity and immiscibility with CSF, Pantopaque has difficulty in entering the nerve root sheaths. On the other hand, the immiscibility and insolubility in CSF are responsible for its remarkable lack of acute neurotoxicity.

When injected into the subarachnoid space, Pantopaque produces a modest lymphocytosis and a prolonged elevation of total CSF protein and gamma globulin (Ferry et al.). These authors point out that elevated CSF gamma globulin and total protein and a normal or slightly elevated beta globulin fraction differentiate the postmyelographic inflammatory response from multiple sclerosis, which usually is associated with normal total protein values, low or normal beta globulin values, and a decreased beta-gamma globulin ratio. Uncommonly, the spinal fluid changes may be associated with mild fever, headache, and malaise (Schnitker and Booth, Ford and Key, Tarlov).

Rarely, more severe reactions have been described in the literature. Erickson and Van Baaren reported a patient who exhibited acute meningeal irritation after a Pantopaque myelogram for a dorsal angioma (6 ml). Four months thereafter, persistent headache developed, followed a year later by disorientation, meningismus, headache, and vomiting. Ventriculography revealed a cerebrospinal fluid protein level of 650 mg, intracerebral Pantopaque, and hydrocephalus associated with obstruction of the fourth ventricle. A suboccipital craniotomy with lysis of adhesions of the fourth ventricle led to death on the second postoperative day.

Taren also described a patient who had a lumbar myelogram (9 ml of Pantopaque were used but only 4 ml were removed). Nineteen hours after myelography, the patient complained of severe headache with a temperature of 103 F. Thirty hours postmyelography, the patient became irritable and irrational, with marked rigidity and a white blood cell count of 22,000/cu mm. At this point, he was given penicillin and intravenous sulfadiazine. Because of acute increased intracranial pressure and multiple cranial nerve palsies, the patient was trephined and a ventriculogram was made. The ventricular fluid was cloudy and oily, under markedly increased pressure, with 5,800 WBC/cu mm. No organisms were recovered. Roentgenograms revealed large amounts of Pantopaque throughout the ventricles and the cisternae. The patient eventually recovered with minimal neurologic residua after prolonged massive antibiotic and steroid therapy. It is difficult to be certain whether this reaction was an infectious meningitis due to a break in technique or a rare hypersensitivity phenomenon.

Mason and Raaf reported an unusual reaction in a 31-year-old truck driver. Following uneventful lumbar puncture at L2-3, 9 ml of Pantopaque were injected into the lumbar subarachnoid space and spot films taken during fluoroscopy. While waiting for the films to be processed, the patient had an urge to defecate, complained of pain in the coccyx, and became agitated. The needle was removed and the patient placed on a bedpan. The needle was reinserted and aspiration of the Pantopaque begun. However, the procedure had to be discontinued because the patient became violent. In all, four aspirations were attempted that day and it was estimated that 5 of the 9 ml of Pantopaque had been removed. Films made at this time demonstrated marked swelling of the lumbosacral roots. The Pantopaque remained fixed in this position, as evidenced by an upright radiograph 19 days later. Immediately after myelography, the patient complained of headache, backache, and leg pain. Ten days later, he noted difficulty in voiding and weakness of the lower extremities. Radiographs of the skull 3 weeks following myelography demonstrated Pantopaque intracranially. An electroencephalogram at the same time showed diffuse, markedly abnormal activity. Lumbar puncture was again attempted unsuccessfully. The patient remained afebrile during this period. He was started on steroids and vitamins, but these drugs were discontinued because of no improvement. Four weeks postmyelography, the patient was almost totally unresponsive, areflexic, and, at times, catatonic. There were bilaterally dilated pupils, paralysis of cranial nerve VI, and papilledema on the left. Another lumbar puncture (6 weeks postmyelography) produced a small amount of thick yellow fluid that clotted. The fluid was negative for bacteria and fungi. Cisternal puncture was performed a week later with the removal of 85 ml of clear fluid, which was replaced by air. Radiographs at this time demonstrated marked hydrocephalus. The ventricular fluid contained no cells and a protein level of 10 mg/100 ml. Varidase was placed in the cisterna magna and a ventriculopleural shunt carried out. The papilledema subsided. Lumbar puncture was attempted 5 months postmyelography, but no fluid could be obtained. A month later, the patient was able to respond to some verbal commands. There was little change in the patient's condition until his sudden demise 7 months after myelography. Necropsy revealed complete obliteration of the cerebrospinal subarachnoid space with the formation of a dense fibrous membrane, which completely encircled the cord. There were adhesions between the nerve roots and the meninges in the region of the cauda equina. Because of the absence of bacterial meningitis and the fact that three other myelograms had been carried out uneventfully that day with packs prepared by the same nurse, Mason and Raaf concluded that the patient had developed a diffuse aseptic leptomeningitis due to a hypersensitivity to Pantopaque.

Luce et al. reported two cases of a rare form of delayed Pantopaque meningitis apparently due to hypersensitivity. Both patients had seasonal hay fever due to ragweed. Both had a preliminary negative intradermal test to Pantopaque and an uneventful myelogram. In each instance, a small amount of Pantopaque was left in the subarachnoid space following removal of most of the dye. Nine days postmyelography in one patient and 30 days postmyelography in the other, a flare-up was observed at the site of the skin test. More or less coincident with the skin reaction, signs of an acute aseptic meningitis occurred and rapidly subsided, followed by somewhat slower disappearance of the skin reaction. Smith and Ross demonstrated a meningeal inflammatory reaction to Pantopaque in rabbits and guinea pigs that could be suppressed by the daily administration of cortisone.

Several cases of aseptic eosinophilic meningitis following Pantopaque myelography have been reported in the literature. All of the patients had uneventful myelograms followed by the onset of a sterile meningitis approximately 10 to 30 days after the initial study. The percentage of eosinophils in the CSF ranged from 25 to 90. The symptoms subsided spontaneously or after the administration of prednisone after varying intervals of time. A Gram stain cannot be used to differentiate eosinophils from neutrophils. Therefore, a Wright's stain differential cell count should also be done on CSF specimens with elevated cell counts after myelography.

Newmark et al. reported two cases of esotropia that developed 8 and 7 days after Pantopaque myelography and pneumoencephalography, respectively. Presumably, this extremely rare complication was secondary to the CSF fluid leak following the lumbar puncture. The diminished CSF pressure in the lumbar region results in a caudal shift of the brain stem, with stretching of the cranial nerves. Since the abducens nerve has the longest intracranial course, it is usually the first to be affected.

When left behind in the subarachnoid space, Pantopaque is absorbed slowly. (Ramsey et al. estimate that the rate of absorption is approximately 1 ml per year, although, in my experience, this is quite variable.) It also has a tendency to become encysted and produce local arachnoiditis (Tarlov). In spite of the practice in England of leaving the Pantopaque in the spinal canal, in my opinion it should be removed as completely as possible unless there is a block or a need for restudying the patient. It is important to remember that serum protein-bound iodine levels may remain elevated for many years following Pantopaque myelography. This may produce confusion in diagnosis, possibly increase the incidence of thyrotoxicosis in patients with nodular goiter, and promote the occurrence of congenital goiter in infants whose mothers had undergone Pantopaque myelography (where the oil was not completely removed).

In an effort to overcome the excessive radiopacity of Pantopaque, Bleasel suggested the use of an emulsified Pantopaque. He punctured the lumbar theca with a 20-gauge spinal needle and withdrew 14 ml of cerebrospinal fluid into a 20-ml glass syringe containing 6 ml of Pantopaque and a bubble of air. A hypodermic needle was fitted to the syringe to prevent spillage, and the syringe shaken vigorously for at least a minute to suspend the Pantopaque in fine globules. The syringe was then held with the needle upright so that the Pantopaque suspension settled out. According to Bleasel, this suspension moves slowly in the subarachnoid space because of its decreased specific gravity but offers no problem in visualization of the lumbar and lower thoracic segments. Unfortunately, there are untoward reactions associated with this technique, such as headache, nausea, and fever. For this reason, emulsified Pantopaque should not be used.

In 1966, Heinz et al. studied less dense forms of Pantopaque, i.e., 15% and 22%, in the hope of providing better visualization of the spinal cord and nerve roots. These studies were repeated and amplified by Kieffer et al. in 1970. The 15% Pantopaque proved to be disappointing because it flowed too slowly and failed to give a clear-cut interface between the intraspinal structures and the surrounding bone. On the other hand, 22% Pantopaque (sp. gr. 1.174) provided sharper delineation of the cervicothoracic cord and nerve roots than conventional 30% Pantopaque, although it flowed somewhat more slowly than the latter (yet more rapidly than the 15% oil). At present, the manufacturer does not appear to be interested in developing 22% Pantopaque for commercial use. To some degree, it is possible to circumvent the marked opacity of the available 30% Pantopaque by using higher KVP (i.e., 145), filtration, and sharp coning.

WATER-SOLUBLE CONTRAST MEDIA

Abrodil (Sodium Methiodal)

Abrodil, a Swedish trade name for sodium iodomethanesulfonate, is an aqueous, organic salt containing 52% iodine firmly bound. This material, originally introduced for myelography by Arnell and Lidström, should not be confused with Per-Abrodil (Diodrast, 3,5-diiodo-4-pyridone-N-acetic acid diethanolamine), which is extremely toxic when injected into the subarachnoid space. Because Abrodil has a number of desirable properties, it was widely employed in 20% concentration in the Scandinavian countries. These advantages include satisfactory radiopacity, miscibility with cerebrospinal fluid, and rapid, complete absorption into the bloodstream. The latter characteristic obviates the necessity for removal of the contrast material from the subarachnoid space. Its ready solubility permits clear visualization of the roots of the cauda equina, thus facilitating the diagnosis of small, laterally placed herniated disks. In this respect, it is definitely superior to Pantopaque.

On the other hand, there are serious disadvantages associated with Abrodil myelography. Because of its marked hypertonicity (sp. gr. of Abrodil 1.130 versus sp. gr. of spinal fluid 1.006–1.008), Abrodil is quite irritating to the pia-arachnoid and the enclosed neural elements. This is readily demonstrable by an initial fairly severe pleocytosis and increase in spinal fluid protein the day following Abrodil myelography. These changes usually subside in 5–7 days, so that lumbar puncture performed a week after the subarachnoid injection of Abrodil generally reveals a normal spinal fluid. The prompt leptomeningeal irritation is evidenced clinically by pain sufficiently severe to require the preliminary use of spinal anesthesia. Indeed, if the spinal anesthesia is inadequate or the Abrodil is permitted to drift above the anesthetic level, shock may occur in addition to excruciating pain. Occasionally, this technique may also be associated with severe spasm and leg cramps, and rarely with paraplegia, sphincteric disturbances, transverse myelitis, and death.

Since sciatic pain may be produced by lesions as high as the tenth thoracic vertebral level, the lower thoracic as well as the lumbar subarachnoid space should be routinely studied in patients with sciatica. Because the toxicity of Abrodil and other toxic aqueous media limits the examination to the lumbar and lumbosacral regions,

Abrodil myelography is not adequate for thorough investigation of these patients. I have seen several neoplasms of the lower thoracic cord mimicking a ruptured intervertebral disk that were missed by myelography terminated at the level of the first lumbar vertebra (Fig 2-1). Because of its toxicity and the availability of less toxic, nonionic, water-soluble contrast media, there is no present justification for using Abrodil for lumbar myelography.

Conray and Dimer-X

In 1936, Kodama and his co-workers reported that methylglucamine iothalamate had a relatively low toxicity when injected intrathecally into laboratory animals. The following year, Campbell et al. independently published their studies on the same compound in a series of 12 patients, as well as in rabbits and dogs. In the latter report, there was one fatality, a second patient with tonic spasm of the legs that lasted for several days, and a third patient with weakness of thigh flexion of several days' duration. In October of 1968, a group of physicians met in Paris to pool their experience with Conray in myelography. This collective series of 847 Conray myelograms included one death, one cauda equina syndrome (24 hours' duration), six serious meningeal reactions (four lasting 4 days), and 29 patients who experienced chronic contractions of the legs. In 1971, Gonsette reported three additional fatalities and four patients with medullary or cortical irritation.

Because of the neurotoxicity of Conray, Gonsette was led to evaluate Dimer-X, i.e., methylglucamine iocarmate. The latter compound is formed by linking two molecules of methylglucamine iothalamate with adipic acid. The principal physicochemical difference between Conray and Dimer-X in similar iodine concentrations (28%) is the lower osmolarity of the latter compound (Dimer-X 1040 mOsm/L vs. Conray 1570 mOsm/L). The physicians who participated in the cooperative study of Conray met again in Paris in 1970 to share their experience with Dimer-X. In a collective protocol of 630 Dimer-X myelograms, there was a substantial decrease in radicular irritation and there were no fatalities. However, meningeal irritation was more frequent (22% Dimer-X vs. 12% Conray). Hammer and Scherrer suggest that the dichotomy between meningeal and radicular irritation may be due to the slower absorption of Dimer-X, which necessitates a longer period of immobilization of the patient in the sitting position. Under these circumstances, cerebrospinal fluid and contrast medium drain off through the puncture site, perhaps thereby increasing local meningeal irritation. In 1971, Gonsette estimated that 3,000 Dimer-X myelograms had been performed uneventfully except for a "few rare cases" of myoclonia, which responded to diazepam (Valium). It is noteworthy that electromyographic studies demonstrate similar subclinical irritation of the spinal cord with both compounds. With respect to myoclonia, I know of two patients who developed severe myoclonia following an otherwise uneventful Dimer-X lumbar myelogram. Both patients suffered subcapital fractures of the femoral neck with subsequent aseptic necrosis, which required total hip replacement. Similar cases have been reported in the literature.

In addition, follow-up myelograms on patients who had undergone previous myelography with Conray or Dimer-X almost uniformly demonstrated evidence of arachnoiditis. Since the introduction of metrizamide, there is no justification for using Conray or Dimer-X for myelography.

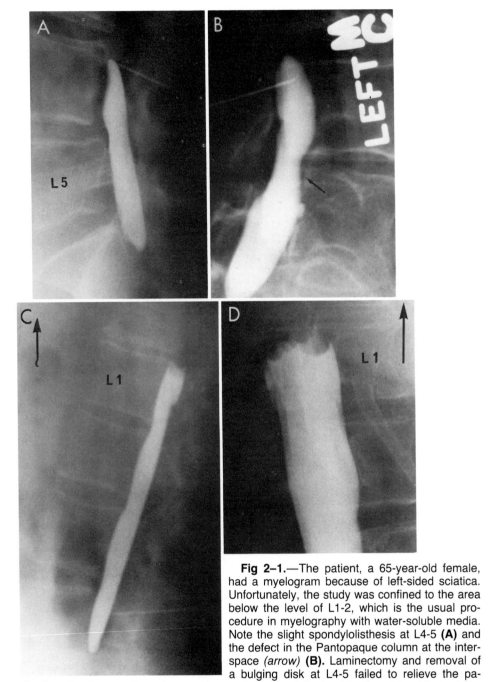

Fig 2–1.—The patient, a 65-year-old female, had a myelogram because of left-sided sciatica. Unfortunately, the study was confined to the area below the level of L1-2, which is the usual procedure in myelography with water-soluble media. Note the slight spondylolisthesis at L4-5 **(A)** and the defect in the Pantopaque column at the interspace *(arrow)* **(B).** Laminectomy and removal of a bulging disk at L4-5 failed to relieve the patient's pain. A second myelogram demonstrated an intradural lesion with a block at the level of T12-L1 **(C** and **D).** At operation, a cystic neurilemoma was removed; postoperatively, the patient's sciatica disappeared.

Metrizamide

In 1968, Almen suggested that a nonionic aqueous contrast medium could provide the same iodine concentration (i.e., radiopacity) as Conray or Dimer-X with a lower osmolality (i.e., diminished toxicity), because of the absence of ionic dissociation. After prolonged screening of more than 80 nonionic compounds, Nyegaard & Co. synthesized metrizamide (Amipaque) in their laboratories in Oslo.

Metrizamide (Amipaque) is a nonionic, water-soluble, tri-iodinated substituted amide with the following chemical structure:

2- (3-acetamido-5-N-methylacetamido-2,4,6 triiodobenzamido) -2- deoxy-D-glucose

Its physical properties are:

Molecular weight	789.1
Iodine content	48.2%
Melting point	230–240 C (decomp.)
Solubility in H_2O	80% w/v
Viscosity (cP)	5.01 (at 37 C, conc. 280 mg I per ml)
Specific gravity (at 37 C)	1.184 (sp. gr. CSF, 1.006–1.008)

Osmolality comparisons of metrizamide with other water-soluble contrast media are presented in Table 2-1.

The nonionic character of metrizamide accounts for its relatively low osmolality. A solution of 0.3 osmols/kg of metrizamide containing 170 mg I/ml is isotonic with CSF. Since the other water-soluble contrast media are salts, they dissociate into osmotically active particles with a much higher osmolality.

Absorption of metrizamide from the CSF into the blood occurs largely through the arachnoid villi and granulations adjacent to the site of injection. Some of the contrast medium ascends into the cerebral subarachnoid space where it is absorbed, usually within 24–72 hours. The biologic half-life of metrizamide in the CSF after

TABLE 2–1.—COMPARATIVE OSMOLALITY* OF VARIOUS
WATER-SOLUBLE CONTRAST MEDIA

MEDIUM	CONCENTRATION (mg I)	OSMOLALITY (mols/kg H_2O)
Human blood or CSF		0.301
Metrizamide	300	0.484
Metrizamide	280	0.456
Metrizamide (isotonic)	166	0.300
Meglumine iocarmate (Dimer-X)	280	1.040
Meglumine iothalamate (Conray)	280	1.470
Methiodal sodium (Abrodil)	104	1.570

*The osmotic concentration of a fluid expressed in osmols of solute per kilogram of water.

lumbar injection is approximately 4 hours. After absorption into the bloodstream, there is a rapid rise in the blood level within 1 hour. Maximal blood levels tend to occur between 1 and 6 hours, although there is considerable individual variation. The primary route of excretion is renal, but some excretion also occurs through the gut. The urinary-fecal excretion ratio is reported to be 26:1. Approximately 90% of the metrizamide can be recovered from the urine and 2%–4% from the feces within 48 hours. Little or no metrizamide is excreted in the form of other metabolites. Fecal metrizamide results from excretion of the contrast medium into the bile by active transport mechanisms. Most of the intrabiliary metrizamide is reabsorbed by the gut for ultimate excretion by the kidneys. However, a small amount (2%–4% of the injected dose) is not reabsorbed and is excreted into the feces. Small quantities of metrizamide are excreted in breast milk. This is unlikely to be hazardous to the infant unless the child is hypersensitive to the drug. Metrizamide does not bind to serum proteins.

Metrizamide is significantly less toxic than any of the other aqueous contrast media. However, the incidence of acute side effects is considerably greater with metrizamide than with Pantopaque, due to passage of the former into the intracranial space. Metrizamide produces a smaller reduction in myocardial conduction and contractility, and less vasodilatation than any of the diatrizoate, metrizoate, or iothalamate compounds, and minimal hepatic and renal toxicity. Also, metrizamide has significantly diminished neurotoxicity. The neurotoxic effects may be classified into three groups, depending on the segment of the nervous system irritated.

1. CEREBRAL CORTICAL IRRITATION.—Headache, epileptic or clonic convulsions, fibrillations or fasciculations, increased patellar reflexes, visual and auditory disturbances, confusion, dysphasia, and dysarthria are symptoms due probably to penetration of the metrizamide from the subarachnoid space into the cerebral cortex. The time it takes for the contrast medium to flow from the spinal to the cerebral subarachnoid space and to penetrate the cortical tissue varies considerably from patient to patient. The site of injection, the concentration and total quantity of iodine used, hydration, patient positioning, individual variations in spinal and cerebral CSF circulation, and local cerebral absorption conditions all play a role in influencing the degree and the time of onset of the reactions. Metrizamide has substantially less of an epileptogenic effect on the cerebral cortex than any of the other ionic contrast media. However, it can produce transient slow wave activity, paroxysmal delta waves, or spikes in the EEG. It can also produce epileptic sei-

zures and mild clonic convulsions of the legs. These effects are potentiated by phenothiazine derivatives and other drugs which lower the convulsion threshold, i.e., MAO inhibitors, tricyclic antidepressants, analeptics, antihistamines, CNS stimulants, some antifungal and antimycobacterial drugs. The cortical irritative effect of metrizamide can also be potentiated by disease processes which lower the seizure threshold.

2. RADICULAR IRRITATION.—Symptoms include hyperesthesia, hyperreflexia, pain in the buttocks and thighs, and urinary retention.

3. MENINGEAL IRRITATION.—Symptoms are headache, dizziness, nausea, vomiting, meningismus, mild elevation of temperature, with or without aseptic meningitis. Since similar symptoms occur after lumbar puncture, it is difficult to determine the relative roles of CSF leakage and the neurotoxic effect of the contrast medium in producing this type of reaction. Baker et al. reported a case of purulent aseptic meningitis following metrizamide myelography. The lumbar puncture revealed a grossly cloudy fluid with 100% neutrophils and a negative Gram stain. The peripheral white blood cell count was 21,000/cu mm with 22% eosinophils. The patient defervesced after the administration of multiple antibiotics but died several weeks later of metastatic adenocarcinoma.

Haughton and his co-workers have shown in animal experiments that large doses of metrizamide can cause arachnoiditis. Even in isotonic concentrations, metrizamide can produce mild arachnoiditis in the occasional animal. To be sure, the degree of arachnoiditis is significantly less than that produced by iocarmate. Unlike Pantopaque, metrizamide does not enhance the effect of blood in producing arachnoiditis.

A report on some 320,000 metrizamide myelograms in 1980 disclosed 58 (0.02%) major adverse reactions including aseptic and septic meningitis, mental disturbances, visual and auditory aberrations, convulsions, and neuropathy. The aseptic meningitis (20 cases) is similar to that described following spinal anesthesia and myelography with other iodinated contrast media. The patient classically presents with headache, meningismus, fever, nausea, and vomiting. Lumbar puncture reveals an elevated CSF protein (200–800 mg%) level, a low glucose (10–25 mg%) level, and an elevated WBC (10,000–40,000) count. Wright's stain should be used to determine the number of eosinophils. The syndrome has been attributed to hypersensitivity or meningeal irritation caused by the contrast medium. All of the patients recovered completely in 1–2 days, except one who required a shunting procedure 5 weeks later because of obstructive hydrocephalus. Three patients developed septic meningitis. In my opinion, this is usually due either to a break in sterility or to the presence of a disease process capable of producing a bacteremia.

A variety of transient mental disturbances were reported (10 patients), ranging from drowsiness and lack of concentration to serious anxiety, disorientation, hallucinations, and deep stupor. Visual or auditory abnormalities tend to be transient, delusional, and associated with severe mental disturbances or aseptic meningitis. However, there has been a single report of permanent cortical blindness. Convulsions occurred in nine patients. In approximately half of these cases, there were precipitating factors, i.e., previous epilepsy, excessive metrizamide, poor technique, or the use of drugs that lower the seizure threshold. The convulsions were mild, brief (1–3 episodes), and responded promptly to intravenous diazepam. No sequelae were noted. Metrizamide is derived from metrizoic acid and glucosamine. According to Bertoni, metrizamide is a competitive inhibitor of hexokinase at the first step in glycolysis. Impaired brain glucose metabolism with secondary anoxia may play an important role in the toxic cerebral reactions associated with metrizamide. Marder et al. have shown that metrizamide is an acetylcholinesterase inhibitor and an antagonist of cholinergic transmission in concentrations in the cerebral subarachnoid space likely to occur after myelography. Perhaps this mechanism plays a role in the etiology of postmetrizamide cerebral seizures, since topical cerebral application of other cholinergic agonists and antagonists and cholinesterase inhibitors produces convulsions. Perhaps also, postmetrizamide nausea and vomiting are due to irritation of the vomiting center in the medulla.

Five patients developed peripheral sensory or motor disturbances, which sometimes persisted for weeks. Paresis of the abducens nerve was reported in two patients, and paraplegia in one patient 2 days following an uneventful metrizamide myelogram. There were two deaths in the series. There have been several reports of patients who developed asterixis after metrizamide myelography.

Experimental studies in the dog by Dubois and his co-workers demonstrated penetration of metrizamide into the parenchyma of the spinal cord, presumably by diffusion. If a similar phenomenon occurs in man, it would explain the rare case of lower extremity myoclonus occurring several hours after lumbar myelography.

Paling et al. reported a case of spinal seizures with prolonged myoclonic spasms of the trunk in a patient with a complete block at T-8 due to an astrocytoma extending from T2-9. In addition, the lumbar sac below L-3 was obliterated. The authors suggest that it might be wise to remove the metrizamide in the presence of a block to prevent a high concentration of metrizamide from coming in contact with the spinal cord for a prolonged period of time.

A rare patient may have pruritus or hives. In this regard, it is interesting that Irstam performed uneventful metrizamide myelography in five patients with iodine hypersensitivity.

OTHER NONIONIC AQUEOUS CONTRAST MEDIA

Attempts have been, and are being, made to synthesize other aqueous contrast agents in the hope that the acute neurotoxicity associated with metrizamide can be reduced or eliminated. Such media fall into two major groups: (1) monoacid dimers, e.g., Iogloxate (Hexabrix) and (2) nonionic monomers, e.g., Iohexol, Iopamidol. Metrizamide is a member of this group of aqueous contrast media, whose physical properties are listed in Table 2-2.

The radiographic properties of these media are comparable to those of metriza-

TABLE 2–2.—PHYSICAL PROPERTIES OF NONIONIC AQUEOUS
CONTRAST MEDIA

	IODINE (mg/ml)	VISCOSITY	OSMOLALITY (mOsm/kg H_2O)	MOLECULAR WEIGHT
Metrizamide	280	5.0	430	789
Hexabrix	320	7.5	580	1,269
Iohexol	280	4.8	620	821
Iopamidol	280	3.8	570	777

mide, i.e., the subarachnoid space is well demonstrated. However, they are still experimental drugs which have not been in use long enough to permit firm conclusions. Preliminary experiments in primates by Haughton et al. suggest that Iohexol does not produce arachnoiditis. Presently available data also suggest that the incidence and the severity of minor side effects are less with Iohexol. Other distinct advantages of Iohexol include a significantly lower cost than metrizamide and stability in solution.

BIBLIOGRAPHY

Agnoli A., Kirchoff D., Eggert H.R.: Lumbar tomomyelography with water-soluble contrast medium. *Acta Radiol* (Suppl.) 347:419, 1976.

Ahlgren P.: Amipaque myelography. The side effects compared with Dimer X. *Neuroradiology* 9:197, 1975.

Ahlgren P.: Amipaque myelography without late adhesive arachnoid changes. *Neuroradiology* 14:231, 1978.

Allen W.E., III, VanGilder J.E., Collins W.F., III: Evaluation of the neurotoxicity of water-soluble myelographic contrast agents by electrophysiological monitors. *Radiology* 118:89, 1976.

Almen T.: Contrast agent design. Some aspects on the synthesis of water-soluble contrast agents of low osmolality. *J. Theor. Biol.* 24:216, 1969.

Amundsen P., et al.: Excretion of metrizamide (Amipaque) in humans following lumbar subarachnoid injection. *Acta Radiol. (Diagn.)* 20:401, 1979.

Arnell S.: Weitere Erfahrungen über Myelographie mit Abrodil. *Acta Radiol.* 25:408,1944.

Arnell S.: Myelography with water-soluble contrast. *Acta Radiol.* (Suppl.) 75, 1948.

Arnell S.: Myelography with Skiodan. *Am. J. Roentgenol.* 66:241, 1951.

Arnell S., Lidström F.: Myelography with Skiodan (Abrodil). *Acta Radiol.* 12:287, 1931.

Autio E., Suolanen J., Norrbäck S., Slätis P.: Adhesive arachnoiditis after lumbar myelography with meglumine iothalamate (Conray). *Acta Radiol. (Diagn.)* 12:17, 1972.

Baciocco A., Galluzzo A., Sassaroli S.: Experiences with SH-617L myelography. *Acta Radiol. (Diagn.)* 5:981, 1966.

Bagchi A.K.: Convulsions, subarachnoid haemorrhage and death following myelography with meglumine iothalamate 280. *Surg. Neurol.* 5:285, 1976.

Baker F.J., Gossen G., Bertoni J.M.: Aseptic meningitis complicating metrizamide myelography. *A.J.N.R.* 3:662, 1982.

Baker R.A., et al.: Sequelae of metrizamide myelography in 200 examinations. *A.J.R.* 130:499, 1978.

Bentson J.R.: Comparison of metrizamide with other myelographic agents. *Clin. Orthop.* 127:111, 1977.

Bergvall U., Brismar T., Lyng-Tunell U., Valdimarsson E.: Confusion, myoclonus and speech arrest: Epileptic manifestations after metrizamide myelography. *Acta Neurol. Scand.* 63:315, 1981.

Bering E.A., Jr.: Notes on retention of Pantopaque in subarachnoid space. *Am. J. Surg.* 80:455, 1950.

Bertoni J.M., Schwartzman R.J., Van Horn G., Partin J.: Asterixis and encephalopathy following metrizamide myelography: Investigations into possible mechanisms and review of the literature. *Ann. Neurol.* 9:366, 1981.

Bharuche E.P., Desai A.D.: Meningeal irritation following introduction of Pantopaque for myelography; case. *Indian J. Med. Sci.* 8:220, 1954.

Bleasel, K.: Nerve root radiography. *Br. J. Radiol.* 34:596, 1961.

Bonati F., Felder E., Tirone P.: Iopamidol: New preclinical and clinical data. *Invest. Radiol.* 15(suppl.):S310, 1980.

Bonneau R., Morris J.M.: Complications of water-soluble myelography. Review of the literature and case report. *Spine* 3:343, 1978.

Bories J., Bamberger-Boco C., Rosier J.: Mono-iodo-stearate d'ethyle et myelographie. *Acta Radiol. (Diagn.)* 9:686, 1969.

Boyd J.T., Langlands A.O., MacCabe A.J.: Long-term hazards of Thorotrast. *Br. Med. J.* 2:517, 1968.

Boyd W.R., Gardiner G.A., Jr.: Metrizamide myelography. *A.J.R.* 129:481, 1977.

Braband H., Wenker H., Groth W., et al.: Klinische Prüfung eines neuen wasserlöslichen Kontrastmittels zur lumbosakralen Myelographie (I. Mitteilung). *Fortschr. Geb. Röntgenstrahlen* 115:609, 1971.

Brandt M.: Cerebral deposits of iodized oil after myelography. *Fortschr. Geb. Röntgenstrahlen* 47:463, 1933.

Bruskin J., Popper N.: Experimental myeloencephalography on dogs. Influence of Iodipin and Lipiodol on spinal cord, brain and meninges. *Ztschr. Ges. Exper. Med.* 75:34, 1931.

Bucy P.C., Spiegel I.J.: Unusual complications of intraspinal use of iodized oil. *J.A.M.A.* 122:367, 1943.

Bull J.W.D.: Positive contrast ventriculography. *Acta Radiol.* 34:253, 1950.

Bunts A.T.: Surgical aspects of ruptured intervertebral disc with particular reference to Thorotrast myelography. *Radiology* 36:604, 1941.

Busch E.: Luftmyelographie zur Diagnose des lumbalen Discusprolapsus und der ligamentären Wurzelkompression. *Acta Radiol.* 22:556, 1941.

Camp J.D.: Contrast myelography. *Med. Clin. North Am.* 25:1067, 1941.

Campbell R.L., Campbell J.A., Heimburger R.F., et al.: Ventriculography and myelography with absorbable radiopaque medium. *Radiology* 82:286, 1964.

Chamberlain W.C., Young B.R.: Air myelography in diagnosis of intraspinal lesions producing low back and sciatic pain. *Radiology* 33:695, 1939.

Coe F.O., Otell L.S., Hedley O.F.: Thorotrast encephalography by cisternal puncture. Preliminary report of experimental studies. *Med. Ann. District of Columbia* 2:277, 1933.

Coggeshall H.C., von Storch T.J.C.: Diagnostic value of myelographic studies of caudal dural sac. *Arch. Neurol. Psychiatr.* 31:611, 1934.

Craig R.L.: Effect of iodized poppyseed oil in spinal cord and meninges. *Arch. Neurol. Psychiatr.* 48:799, 1942.

Craig W.McK.: Use and abuse of iodized oil in the diagnosis of lesions of the spinal cord. *Surg. Gynecol. Obstet.* 49:17, 1929.

Dandy W.E.: Diagnosis and localization of spinal cord tumors. *Ann. Surg.* 81:223, 1925.

Davies F.L.: Effect of unabsorbed radiographic contrast mediums on central nervous system. *Lancet* 2:747, 1956.

Davis F.M., Llewellyn R.C., Kirgis H.D.: Water soluble contrast myelography using meglumine iothalamate (Conray) with methyl prednisolone acetate (Depo-Medrol). *Radiology* 90:705, 1968.

Davis L., Haven H.A., Stone T.T.: The effect of injections of iodized oil in the spinal subarachnoid space. *J.A.M.A.* 94:772, 1939.

Denstad T.: Resorption of Abrodil (Skiodan, iodine preparation) in myelography. *Acta Radiol.* 32:428, 1949.

Dietz H., Zeitler E., Fontaine X.: Expérience clinique avec la suspension SH617(L) en myélographie. *Acta Radiol. (Diagn.)* 9:693, 1969.

Dubois P.J., Drayer B.P., Sage M., et al.: Intramedullary penetrance of metrizamide in the dog spinal cord. *A.J.N.R.* 2:313, 1981.

Dugstad G., Eldevik O.P.: Lumbar myelography. *Acta Radiol. (Suppl.)* 355:17, 1977.

Dullerud R., Mørland T.J.: Adhesive arachnoiditis after lumbar radiculography with Dimer-X and Depo-Medrol. *Radiology* 119:153, 1976.

Dürwald W., Schmidt R.M.: Complications of myelography. *Arztl. Wehnschr.* 9:932, 1954.

Eastwood J.B., Parker B., Reid B.R.: Bilateral central fracture-dislocation of hips after myelography with meglumine iocarmate (Dimer-X). *Br. Med. J.* 1:692, 1978.

Ebaugh F.G., Mella H.: Use of Lipiodol in localization of spinal lesions. *Am. J. Med. Sci.* 172:117, 1926.

Eldevik O.P., Haughton V.M.: Risk factors in complications of aqueous myelography. *Radiology* 128:415, 1978.

Eldevik O.P., Haughton V.M., Sasse E.A.: Elimination of aqueous contrast media from the subarachnoid space. *Invest. Radiol.* 15:260, 1980.

Eldevik O.P., Haughton V.M., Sasse E.A., Ho K.: Excretion of aqueous myelographic contrast media in animals undergoing a repeat myelogram. *Invest. Radiol.* 15:507, 1980.

Erickson T.C., Van Baaren H.H.: Late meningeal reaction to ethyl iodophenylundecylate, used in myelography. Report of a case that terminated fatally. *J.A.M.A.* 153:636, 1953.

Ferry D.W., Jr., Gooding R., Standefer J.C., Wiese G.M.: Effect of Pantopaque myelography on cerebrospinal fluid fractions. *J. Neurosurg.* 38:167, 1973.

Ford L.T., Key J.A.: An evaluation of myelography in the diagnosis of intervertebral disc lesions in the low back. *J. Bone Joint Surg.* 32A:257, 1950.

Frazier C.H., Glaser M.A.: Iodized rape-seed oil (Campiodol) for cerebrospinal visualization. *J.A.M.A.* 91:1609, 1928.

Freiberger R.H., Harvey P.J.: Myelography with water-soluble medium. *Semin. Radiol.* 7:224, 1972.

Fumarola G., Enderle C.: Dangers, disadvantages and injuries in myelography. *Radiol. Med.* 19:1271, 1932.

Fundquist B.: Cervical myelography with water-soluble contrast medium: Experimental study in dogs. *Acta Radiol.* 56:257, 1961.

Fundquist B., Obel N.: Tonic muscle spasms and blood pressure changes following the subarachnoid injection of contrast media. *Acta Radiol.* 53:337, 1960.

Garland L.H.: The effect of iodized oil on the meninges of the spinal cord and brain. *Radiology* 35:467, 1940.

Garland L.H., Morrissey E.J.: Intracranial collections of iodized oil following lumbar myelography. *Surg. Gynecol. Obstet.* 70:196, 1940.

Gelmers H.J.: Adverse side effects of metrizamide in myelography. *Neuroradiology* 18:119, 1979.

Gilbert G.J.: CSF eosinophilia following myelography (letter). *J.A.M.A.* 244:548, 1980.

Giminez M., Martinez F., Feijoo M.: Asterixis or myoclonus after metrizamide myelography (letter). *Arch. Neurol.* 38:472, 1981.

Gonsette R.: An experimental and clinical assessment of water-soluble contrast medium in neuroradiology. A new medium—Dimer-X. *Clin. Radiol.* 22:44, 1971.

Gonsette R.: Metrizamide as contrast medium for myelography and ventriculography. Preliminary clinical experiences. *Acta Radiol.* (suppl.) 346:51, 1975.

Gonsette R.: New applications of water-soluble contrast media in neuroradiology. *J. Belge Radiol.* 54:385, 1971.

Grainger R.G., Gumpert J., Sharpe D.M., Carson J.: Water-soluble lumbar radiculography. A clinical trial of Dimer-X—a new contrast medium. *Clin. Radiol.* 22:57, 1971.

Haguenau J.: Question of danger of subarachnoidal injection of Lipiodol in diagnosis. *Monde Méd. Paris* 46:825, 1936.

Halaburt H., Lester J.: Leptomeningeal changes following lumbar myelography with water-soluble contrast media (meglumine iothalamate and methiodal sodium). *Neuroradiology* 5:70, 1973.

Hamby W.B.: Misplaced Lipiodol, analysis of 104 Lipiodol spinograms. *Radiology* 37:343, 1941.

Hammer B., Lackner W.: Iopamidol, a new non-ionic hydrosoluble contrast medium for neuroradiology. *Neuroradiology* 19:119, 1980.

Hammer B., Scherrer H.: Choice of contrast medium in lumbosacral myelography. *Neuroradiology* 4:114, 1972.

Hansen E.B., Fahrenkrug M.D., Praestholm J.: Late meningeal effects of myelographic contrast media with special reference to metrizamide. *Br. J. Radiol.* 51:321, 1978.

Hauge O., Falkenberg H.: Neuropsychologic reactions and other side effects after metrizamide myelography. *A.J.N.R.* 3:229, 1982.

Haughton V.M., Eldevik O.P., Ho K., et al.: Arachnoiditis from experimental myelography with aqueous contrast media. *Spine* 3:65, 1978.

Haughton V.M., Ho K-C, Lipman B.T.: Experimental study of arachnoiditis from iohexol, an investigational nonionic aqueous contrast medium. *A.J.N.R.* 3:375, 1982.

Haughton V.M., Ho K., Unger G.F.: Arachnoiditis following myelography with water-soluble agents. The role of contrast medium osmolality. *Radiology* 125:731, 1977.

Haughton V.M., Ho K., Unger G.F., et al.: Seventy cases of postmyelographic arachnoiditis and concentration of meglumine iocarmata in primates. *A.J.R.* 130:313, 1978.

Heinz E.R., Brinker R.A., Taveras J.M.: Advantages of a less dense Pantopaque contrast material for myelography. *Acta Radiol. (Diagn.)* 5:1024, 1966.

Hesse R.: Incidents during myelography with Methiodal. *Beitr. Klin. Chir.* 188:368, 1954.

Hilal S.K., Dauth G.W., Hess K.H., Gilman S.: Development and evaluation of a new water-soluble iodinated myelographic contrast medium with markedly reduced convulsive effects. *Radiology* 126:417, 1978.

Hindmarsh T.: Elimination of water-soluble contrast media from the subarachnoid space. Investigation with computer tomography. *Acta Radiol.* (Suppl.) 346:45, 1975.

Hindmarsh T., Grepe A., Widén L.: Metrizamide-phenothiazine interaction. Report of a case with seizures following myelography. *Acta Radiol. (Diagn.)* 16:129, 1975.

Hirsch C., Rosencrantz M., Wickbom I.: Lumbar myelography with water-soluble contrast media with special reference to the appearances of root pockets. *Acta Radiol. (Diagn.)* 8:54, 1969.

Holley H.P., Jr., Al-Ibrahim M.S.: CSF eosinophilia following myelography. *J.A.M.A.* 242:2432, 1979.

Horwitz N.H.: Positive contrast ventriculography. A critical evaluation. *J. Neurosurg.* 13:300, 1956.

Hurteau E.F., Baird W.C., Sinclair E.: Arachnoiditis following the use of iodized oil. *J. Bone Joint Surg.* 36A:393, 1954.

Ilett K.F., Hackett L.P., Paterson J.W.: Excretion of metrizamide in milk (letter). *Br. J. Radiol.* 54:537, 1981.

Irstam L., Selldén U.: Side effects after lumbar myelography with dimeglumine iocarmate (Dimer-X). Further experiences. *Acta Radiol. (Diagn.)* 16:449, 1975.

Irstam L., Selldén U.: Adverse side effects of lumbar myelography with Amipaque and Dimer-X. *Acta Radiol. (Diagn.)* 17:145, 1976.

Jaeger R.: Irritating effect of iodized vegetable oils on the brain and spinal cord when divided into small particles. *Arch. Neurol. Psychiatr.* 64:715, 1950.

Jensen F., Reske-Nielson E., Ratjen E.: Obstructive hydrocephalus following Pantopaque myelography. *Neuroradiology* 18:139, 1979.

Jensen T.S.: Intraspinal arachnoiditis and hydrocephalus after lumbar myelography using methylglucamine iocarmate. *J. Neurol. Neurosurg. Psychiatry* 41:108, 1978.

Johansen A.H.: Death following myelography with Diodrast. *Nord. Med.* 17:163, 1943.

Johanson C.E.: Results of myelographies with water-soluble media. *Acta Chir. Scandinav.* 99:560, 1950.

Johnson A.J., Burrows E.H.: Thecal deformity after lumbar myelography with iophendylate (Myodil) and meglumine iothalamate (Conray 280). *Br. J. Radiol.* 51:196, 1978.

Kaada B.: Transient EEG abnormalities following lumbar myelography with metrizamide. *Acta Radiol.* (Suppl.) 335:380, 1973.

Karlén A.: Komplikationen bei intraduralen Per-abrodil myelographie. *Acta Chir. Scandinav.* 87:182, 1942.

Karlén A.: Death from bone marrow and fat embolism and uremia following intradural Diodrast myelography. *Acta Chir. Scandinav.* 87:497, 1942.

Kaufman P., Jeans W.D.: Reactions to iophendylate in relation to multiple sclerosis. *Lancet* 2:1000, 1976.

Kelley R.E., Daroff R.B., Sheremata W.A., McCormick J.R.: Unusual effects of metrizamide lumbar myelography. Constellation of aseptic meningitis, arachnoiditis, communicating hydrocephalus, and Guillaine-Barré syndrome. *Arch. Neurol.* 37:588, 1980.

Kendall B., Schneidau A., Stevens J., Harrison M.: Clinical trial of iohexol for lumbar myelography. *Br. J. Radiol.* 56:539, 1983.

Kieffer S.A., Peterson H.O., Gold L.H.A., Binet E.F.: Evaluation of dilute Pantopaque for large volume myelography. *Radiology* 96:69, 1970.

Klason T.: Myelography with Intron. *Nord. Med.* 27:1415, 1945.

Knutsson F.: Sedimentation of oil in myelography and its diagnostic significance. *Acta Radiol.* 20:537, 1939.

Koberg H.: Necessity of lumbar myelography with water-soluble contrast substance. *Fortschr. Geb. Röntgenstrahlen* 82:236, 1955.

Kodama J.K., Butler W.M., Tusing T.W., Hallett F.P.: Cited by Praestholm and Lester.

Kristiansen K.: Myelography using iodized oil (dangers). *Nord. Med.* 13:43, 1942.

Kruchen C.: Jodipin in den Lymphwegen nach Myelographie. *Fortschr. Geb. Röntgenstrahlen* 49:155, 1941.

Kühn G.: Myelography with methiodal in examination and localization of lumbar prolapse of disk. *Beitr. Klin. Chir.* 188:352, 1954.

Kyle R.H., Oler A., Lasser E.C., Rosomoff H.L.: Meningioma induced by thorium dioxide. *N. Engl. J. Med.* 268:80, 1963.

Lee B.C.P., Gomez D.G., Potts D.B., Pavese A.M.: Subacute reactions to intrathecal Amipaque (metrizamide), Conray and Dimer-X: A structural and ultrastructural study. *Neuroradiology* 20:229, 1980.

Lehtinen E., Seppänen S.: Side effects of Conray meglumin 282 and Dimer-X in lumbar myelography. *Acta Radiol (Diagn.)* 12:12, 1972.

Lindblom A.F.: On the effect of Lipiodol on the meninges. *Acta Radiol.* 5:129, 1926.

Lindblom A.F.: Effects of various iodized oils on meninges. *Acta Med. Scandinav.* 76:395, 1931.

Lindblom K.: Lumbar myelography by Abrodil. *Acta Radiol.* 27:1, 1946.

Lindgren E.: Myelography with air. *Acta Psychiatr. Neurol.* 14:385, 1939.

Lindgren E.: Myelographie mit Luft. *Nervenarzt* 12:57, 1939.

Lindgren E., Ribbing S.: Complications of myelography with contrast medium. *Nord. Med.* 42:1378, 1949.

Lindgren E., Törnell G.: Experiences with SH-617L. *Acta Radiol. (Diagn.)* 9:701, 1969.

Lönnerblad L.: Eine Komplikation bei Myelographie. *Acta Radiol.* 14:56, 1935.

Luce J.C., Leith W., Burrage W.C.: Pantopaque meningitis due to hypersensitivity. *Radiology* 57:878, 1951.

Lucherini T.: Radiomyelography with Thorotrast. *Riv. Osp.* 24:475, 1934.

Madrazo M.F.: Sequels of iodized oils used in myelography. *Cir. y Ciruyanos* 9:167, 1941.

Maltby G.L.: Progressive thorium dioxide myelopathy (caudia equina syndrome). *N. Engl. J. Med.* 270:490, 1964.

Marcovich A.W., Walker A.E., Jessico C.M.: Immediate and late effects of intrathecal injection of iodized oil. *J.A.M.A.* 116:2247, 1941.

Marder E., O'Neill M., Grossman R.I., et al.: Cholinergic actions of metrizamide. *A.J.N.R.* 4:61, 1983.

Mascher W., Okonek G.: Causes for extra-arachnoid storage of Iodipin (iodized oil) during myelography. *Nervenarzt* 19:272, 1948.

Mason M.S., Raaf J.: Complications of Pantopaque myelography. Case report and review. *J. Neurosurg.* 19:302, 1962.

McBeath A.A.: Eosinophilic meningitis following myelography. *J.A.M.A.* 243:2396, 1980.

McKee B.W., Ethier R., Vezina J.L., Melancon D.: The disappearance of a large intracranial deposit of Pantopaque twenty years after myelography. *Am. J. Roentgenol.* 107:612, 1969.

Mifka P.: Complications of myelography. *Wien. Klin. Wehnschr.* 59:700, 1947.

Mixter W.J.: Use of Lipiodol in tumor of the spinal cord. *Arch. Neurol. Psychiatr.* 14:35, 1925.

Moll H.H.: Observations on diagnosis of spinal block by means of Lipiodol. *J. Neurol. Psychopath.* 13:14, 1932.

Morrey B.F., O'Brien E.T.: Femoral neck fractures following water-soluble myelography-induced spinal seizures. *J. Bone Joint Surg.* 59A:1099, 1977.

Munro D., Elkins C.W.: Two-needle oxygen myelography, new technic for visualization of subarachnoidal space. *Surg. Gynecol. Obstet.* 75:729, 1942.

Newmark H., III, Levin N., Apt R.K.: Esotropia: An unusual complication of myelography and pneumoencephalography. *A.J.N.R.* 2:278, 1981.

Nichols B.H.: Thorotrast and the diagnosis of lesions involving the lower spinal canal. *Radiology* 38:679, 1942.

Nichols B.H., Nosik W.A.: Myelography with use of thorium dioxide solution (Thorotrast) as contrast medium. *Radiology* 35:459, 1940.

Norman A.: Comparison of reaction to Pantopaque myelography. *Bull. Hosp. Joint Dis.* 13:149, 1952.

Nosik W.A.: Clinical application of Thorotrast myelography and subsequent forced drainage (case report). *Cleveland Clin. Quart.* 5:262, 1938.

Nosik W.A.: Intraspinal Thorotrast. *Am. J. Roentgenol.* 49:214, 1943.

Nosik W.A.: Thorotrast Myelography, in Glasser O. (ed.): *Medical Physics* (Chicago: Year Book Medical Publishers, Inc., 1944), vol. 1, p. 1323.

Nosik W.A.: Contrast myelography with emulsified Pantopaque. *Am. J. Roentgenol.* 63:374, 1951.

Noto G.G.: Arachnoiditis following myelography with iodized oil in patient with hernia of lumbosacral disk. *Riv. Pat. Nerv.* 74:166, 1953.

Notter G.: Lumbar myelography with methiodal. *Fortschr. Geb. Röntgenstrahlen* 76:754, 1952.

Ødegaard H.: The absorption of Myelotrast (Abrodil) from the spinal canal. *Acta Radiol.* 30:464, 1948.

O'Malley B.P.: Some observations on non-oily myelographic media. *Clin. Radiol.* 16:405, 1965.

Paling M.R., Wuindlen E.A., CiChiro G.: Spinal seizures after metrizamide myelography in a patient with a spinal block. *A.J.R.* 135:1091, 1980.

Panter K.: Complications and danger in use of methiodal for myelography. *Deutsche Med. Wehnschr.* 78:937, 1953.

Panter K.: Spinal canal roentgenography with use of contrast substances. *Fortschr. Neurol., Psychiatr.* 23:173, 1955.

Peacher W.G., Robertson R.C.L.: Pantopaque myelography, results, comparison of contrast media and spinal fluid reaction. *J. Neurosurg.* 2:220, 1945.

Peacher W.G., Robertson R.C.L.: Absorption of Pantopaque following myelography. *Radiology* 47:186, 1946.

Perassi F.: Unusual complication of myelography with iodized oil. *Ann. Radiol. (Diagn.)* 27:206, 1954.

Perrigot M., Pierro-Deseilligny E., Bussel B., Held J.P.: Paralysis following Dimer-X radiculography. *Nouv. Press. Med.* 5:1120, 1976.

Petit-Dutaillis D., Feld M.: Aseptic cisternitis due to Lipiodol; dangers of headdown position during myelography with Lipiodol. *Rev. Neurol.* 84:288, 1951.

Praestholm J.: Experimental evaluation of water-soluble contrast media for myelography. *Neuroradiology* 13:25, 1977.

Praestholm J., Lester J.: Water-soluble contrast lumbar myelography with meglumine iothalamate (Conray). *Br. J. Radiol.* 43:303, 1970.

Praestholm J., Moller S.: Cardiovascular reactions to myelography with water-soluble contrast media. *Neuroradiology* 13:195, 1977.

Punto L., Suolanen J.: Testing of myelographic contrast media using the pig as an experimental animal. *Invest. Radiol.* 11:331, 1976.

Radovici A., Meller O.: La liquidographie chez l'homme (essai d'encéphalomyélographie par le thorium colloïdal). *Rev. Neurol.* 1:541, 1933.

Ramsey G.H., French J.D., Strain W.H.: Iodinated organic compounds as contrast media for radiographic diagnoses. IV. Pantopaque myelography, *Radiology* 43:236, 1944.

Ramsey G.H.S., French J.D., Strain W.H.: Myelography with ethyliodophenylundecylate (Pathopaque). *New York J. Med.* 45:1209, 1945.

Reinhardt K.: Actual problems in contrast myelography. *Fortschr. Geb. Röntgenstrahlen* 83:809, 1955.

Reiser E.: Theoretisches und kasuistiches zur Myelographie. *Fortschr. Geb. Röntgenstrahlen* 34:443, 1926.

Richert S., Sartor K., Holl B.: Subclinical organic psychosyndromes on intrathecal injection of metrizamide for lumbar myelography. *Neuroradiology* 18:177, 1979.

Rolfe E.B., Maguire P.D.: The incidence of headache following various techniques of metrizamide myelography. *Br. J. Radiol.* 53:840, 1980.

Ropper A.H., et al.: The effect of metrizamide on the EEG: A prospective study in 62 cases. *Trans Am. Neurol. Assoc.* 103:159, 1978.

Rubin B., Horowitz G., Katz R.I.: Asterixis following metrizamide myelography. *Arch. Neurol.* 37:522, 1980.

Russell D., Nyberg-Hansen R., Slettnes O., et al.: Complex partial status epilepticus following myelography with metrizamide. *Ann. Neurol.* 8:325, 1980.

Säker G.: Contrast substances in myelography. *Nervenarzt* 18:216, 1947.

Salberg D.J.: CSF eosinophilia following myelography (letter). *J.A.M.A.* 243:1806, 1980.

Schatzki R.: Myelography. Air versus iodized oil. *N. Engl. J. Med.* 224:1101, 1941.

Schmidt R.C.: Mental disorders after myelography with metrizamide and other water-soluble contrast media. *Neuroradiology* 19:153, 1980.

Schmidt R.C.: Remarks about the paper by H.J. Gelmers: Adverse side effects of metrizamide in myelography (letter). *Neuroradiology* 19:111, 1980.

Schnitker M.T., Booth G.T.: Pantopaque myelography for protruded discs of the lumbar spine. *Radiology* 45:370, 1945.

Sicard J.A., Forestier J.E.: Méthode radiographique d'exploration de la cavité epidurale par le Lipiodol. *Rev. Neurol.* 38:463, 1922.

Sicard J.A., Forestier J.: Roentgenologic exploration of the central nervous system with iodized oil (Lipiodol). *Arch. Neurol. Psychiatr.* 16:420, 1926.

Siebner M.: Hypertrophic cervical pachymeningitis and acute injury after myelography. *Chirurg.* 7:177, 1935.

Sikl H.: Question of harmful effects of iodized oil used in myelography. *Ztschr. Ges. Neurol. Psychiatr.* 171:615, 1941.

Skalpe I.O.: Myelography with metrizamide, meglumine iothalamate and meglumine iocarmate: An experimental investigation in cats. *Acta Radiol.* (Suppl.) 335:57, 1973.

Skalpe I.O.: Adhesive arachnoiditis following lumbar myelography. *Spine* 3:61, 1978.

Smith J.K., Ross L.: Steroid suppression of meningeal inflammation caused by Pantopaque. *Neurology* 9:48, 1959.

Söderberg L., Sjöberg S., Langleland P.: Neurological complications following myelography with water-soluble contrast media. *Acta Orthop. Scandinav.* 28:220, 1959.

Sovak M., Ranganathan R., Speck U.: Nonionic dimer: Development and initial testing of an intrathecal contrast agent. *Radiology* 142:115, 1982.

Steinhausen T.B., et al.: Iodinated organic compounds as contrast media for radiographic diagnoses: Experimental and clinical myelography with ethyliodophenylundecylate (Pantopaque). *Radiology* 43:230, 1944.

Stenström R.: Widening of the root defect in lumbar myelogram by Abrodil. *Acta Radiol.* 29:303, 1948.

Stenström R., Lindfors M.: Lumbar myelography in the water-soluble contrast medium in children. *Acta Radiol. (Diagn.)* 11:243, 1971.

Strain W.H., French J.D., Jones G.E.: Iodinated organic compounds as contrast media for diagnoses. V. Escape of Pantopaque from intracranial subarachnoid space of dogs. *Radiology* 47:47, 1946.

Summer K., Traugott U.: Eosinophil leucocytes in CSF after myelography. *J. Neurol.* 210:127, 1975.

Taminiau A.H., Sloff T.J.J.H.: Bilateral femoral neck fractures as a complication of myelography. *Acta Orthop. Scand.* 51:621, 1980.

Taren J.A.: Unusual complication following Pantopaque myelography. *J. Neurosurg.* 17:323, 1960.

Tarlov I.M.: Pantopaque meningitis disclosed at operation. *J.A.M.A.* 129:1014, 1945.

Teplick J.G., Haskin M.E., Skelley J.F.: Total myelography with radiopaque emulsions. *Radiology* 90:698, 1968.

Teplick J.G., Haskin M.E., Skelley, J.F., et al.: Experimental studies with a new radiopaque emulsion (Ethiodol). *Radiology* 82:478, 1964.

Themel K.: Harmful sequels after use of Iodipin (iodized oil) in myelography. *Zentralbl. Chir.* 77:1508, 1952.

Thurzo E.U., Nagy M.: Die Wirkung der pneumoencephalischen Lufteinblasungen auf Liquor und Liquorläsion. *Deutsche Ztschr. Nervenhlk.* 79:374, 1923.

Valk J.: Aseptic meningitis after use of Amipaque. *Nederl. Tijdschr. Geneesk.* 124:1788, 1980.

Van Der Werff J.T.: Myelography by resorbable contrast substances. *Acta Radiol.* 30:493, 1948.

Van Der Werff J.T., Prick J.J.G.: Fast resorbing contrast media in myelographic diagnoses of hernia of nucleus pulposus. *Nederl. Tijdschr. Geneesk.* 93:853, 1949.

Van Wagenen W.P.: Röntgenological localization of spinal subarachnoid block by use of air in subarachnoid space. *Ann. Surg.* 99:939, 1934.

Vogler E., Walcher W.: Investigations with a new contrast medium for subarachnoid myelography (Versuche mit einem neuen Kontrastmittel für die subarachnoidale Myelographie). *Fortschr. Geb. Röntgenstrahlen* 99:493, 1963.

Walsh M.N., Love J.G.: Meningeal response following subarachnoidal injection of iodized oil. *Proc. Staff Meet. Mayo Clin.* 13:792, 1938.

Weber R.J., Weingarden S.I.: Electromyographic abnormalities following myelography. *Arch. Neurol.* 36:588, 1979.

White A.G.: Prolonged elevation of serum protein-bound iodine following myelography with Myodil. *Br. J. Radiol.* 45:21, 1972.

Wild H., Lehmann L.: Experiences with ethyliodophenylundecylate in myelography. *Fortschr. Geb. Röntgenstrahlen* 73:213, 1950.

Wirell S.: Binding of metrizamide to human serum proteins. *Acta Radiol. (Diagn.)* 23:239, 1982.

Wollen D.G., Lamon C.B., Cawley A.J., Wortzman G.: The neurotoxic effect of water soluble contrast media in the spinal canal with emphasis on appropriate management. *J. Can. Assoc. Radiol.* 19:296, 1967.

Woringer E.: Myelography with reabsorbable contrast medium for diagnosis of hernia. *Arch. Neurochir.* 1:61, 1952.

Wyatt C.M., Spurling R.G.: Pantopaque. Absorption following myelography. *Surgery* 16:561, 1944.

Zeitler E., Dietz H.: Über den diagnostischen Wert der Myelographie mit Suspensionen. *Radiologe* 5:489, 1963.

Zsebok K.: Joduron (iodine preparation) myelography. *Fortschr. Geb. Röntgenstrahlen* 82:501, 1955.

3

Indications for Myelography

MYELOGRAPHY IS USED too freely by various enthusiasts and not often enough by the iconoclasts who underestimate its value. It is difficult to draw up a rigid set of indications for its use. However, it is definitely helpful in a number of situations.

1. To exclude an operable lesion when the clinical data are inconclusive and the working diagnosis is a degenerative disease. One should be as certain as possible that one is dealing with amyotrophic lateral sclerosis, for example, and not with a surgically remediable lesion masquerading as a degenerative process—i.e., benign tumor or Arnold-Chiari malformation.

2. To confirm or exclude an intraspinal lesion when other methods have failed to establish an unequivocal diagnosis.

3. To establish the general pathologic characteristics and extent of a known lesion.

4. To localize the level of a lesion accurately and determine its nature prior to operation. This is subject to the handicaps discussed in Chapters 11 and 20 dealing with diseases of the spinal cord and the limitations of myelography. It is well known, however, that the clinical localization of a lesion producing radicular pain is not always reliable. The neurologic findings may be identical regardless of whether a herniated disk is located at L3-4 or L4-5. Thus, Lansche and Ford, in a correlative review of the myelographic, clinical and operative findings in a series of 560 patients with herniated intervertebral disks, reported correct preoperative clinical localization in only 39.2%. I have personally seen several patients subjected to laminectomy for a herniated intervertebral disk without antecedent myelography whose symptoms were not relieved by removal of the protruding disk fragment. Persistent postoperative pain eventually prompted myelography, which then disclosed a tumor at a higher level.

5. To exclude multiple lesions. Approximately 4% of spinal neoplasms are multiple. Multiple ruptured disks likewise are not uncommon, although the exact incidence of multiple clinically significant herniated disks is difficult to determine (MacCarty and Lane 12.5%, Camp 18%). In a series of 583 patients with herniated disks, Lombardi and Passerini reported 82 (14%) multiple prolapses. In the same report dealing with 952 patients who were operated on for spinal cord disease, 100 (10.5%) had multiple lesions. Rarely, a herniated disk and a tumor may coexist.

The possibility of multiple lesions re-emphasizes the necessity for thorough, complete myelography.

6. To determine the cause of recurrent symptoms in a patient with a previous laminectomy. This may not be possible when the sole myelographic defect is located at the site of the previous operation. Under these circumstances, one may be unable to differentiate preoperatively between localized arachnoiditis or recurrent disk herniation. This technique is particularly useful when the myelographic defect is at a level different from the previous operative site.

7. Medicolegal purposes. It probably is in this category that myelography is most abused. Unfortunately, in some places, myelography has improperly achieved almost divine medicolegal status, largely due to pressures exerted by the legal profession. This should be resisted, and myelography should be utilized for strictly medical indications. It is important, therefore, to be familiar with the limitations of myelography.

It is wise to eschew the philosophy of extremists at both ends of the spectrum. Myelography is neither an absolute answer to all spinal diagnostic problems nor a technique to be avoided in favor of routine exploratory laminectomy. Myelography should always follow a careful clinical evaluation of the patient. Under these circumstances, its use frequently will result in more accurate evaluation of a diagnostic problem. Here, as in the case of other techniques, a great deal depends on the examiner. To paraphrase Falk's comments about encephalography, inadequate or ill-chosen myelography often discloses more information about the examiner than it does about the patient.

BIBLIOGRAPHY

Camp J.D.: Contrast myelography past and present. *Radiology* 54:477, 1950.

Falk B.: Encephalography in cases of intracranial tumor. *Acta Radiol.* 40:220, 1953.

Lansche W.E., Ford L.T.: Correlation of the myelogram with clinical and operative findings in lumbar disc lesions. *J. Bone Joint Surg.* 42:193, 1960.

Lombardi G., Passerini A.: *Spinal Cord Diseases. A Radiologic and Myelographic Analysis.* Baltimore, Williams & Wilkins Co., 1964.

MacCarty W.C., Jr., Lane F.W.: Pitfalls of myelography. *Radiology* 65:663, 1955.

Pugh D.G.: Present status of contrast myelography. *Am. J. Med. Sci.* 206:687, 1943.

Young H.H.: Non-neurological lesions simulating protruded intervertebral disk. *J.A.M.A.* 148:1101, 1952.

4

Technique

PANTOPAQUE MYELOGRAPHY

CONSISTENTLY SUCCESSFUL MYELOGRAPHY requires meticulous attention to a number of details. Careful regard for these details is rewarded by rich dividends. Conversely, disregard for an orderly, logical technique results in a significant incidence of unsatisfactory, indeterminate examinations. In my opinion, myelography often can be carried out quite satisfactorily on an ambulatory outpatient basis.

Previous Lumbar Puncture

Ideally, myelography should not be performed sooner than 2 weeks after a preceding lumbar puncture. This, of course, is not always feasible. However, whenever possible, diagnostic puncture should not be carried out prior to myelography. Review of a series of subdural and mixed subdural-subarachnoid injections disclosed an antecedent lumbar puncture within a week of attempted myelography in a surprisingly large percentage of cases. Presumably, cerebrospinal fluid leaks out through the original lumbar puncture hole into the subdural and extradural spaces, thereby creating a common subarachnoid-subdural fluid reservoir (Fig 4–1). Under these circumstances, a steady flow of spinal fluid at myelography does not necessarily indicate a purely subarachnoid position of the needle point. The point of the needle, and hence the Pantopaque, may be partly within the subdural-extradural space and partly within the subarachnoid space.

Hypersensitivity to Contrast Medium

The patient should be questioned about previous hypersensitivity. A documented, clear-cut, prior reaction to iodine should make gas the medium of choice whenever pneumomyelography can provide the necessary information. In those rare cases in which the latter can be obtained only by positive contrast myelography, I carefully balance the benefit to the patient against the possible increased risk (assuming that there is an increased risk). If there are compelling reasons for

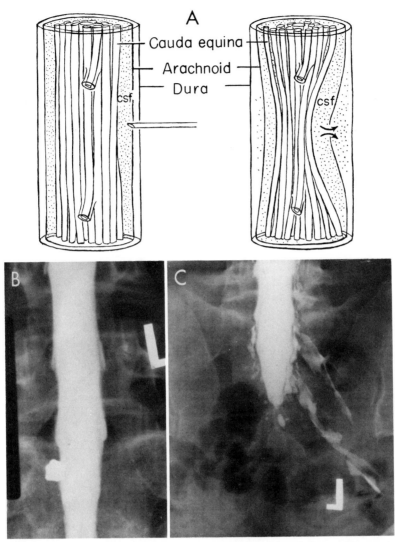

Fig 4–1.—A, diagram showing, **left,** normal relationship of the cauda equina, sub-arachnoid space, arachnoid, and dura; **right,** tear of the arachnoid following lumbar puncture resulting in a common subarachnoid–extra-arachnoid pool of cerebrospinal fluid; **B,** radiograph with the patient in the prone position following uncomplicated lumbar puncture at L5-S1 and the injection of 15 ml of Pantopaque; **C,** radiograph with the patient in the supine position immediately after removal of the lumbar puncture needle. Pantopaque promptly ran out at the site of the puncture into the extradural space along the nerve roots.

positive contrast myelography, I explain the problem to the patient and the referring physician and record this on the informed request slip. Under these circumstances, I would prepare the patient with corticosteroids, start an intravenous infusion, and have an anesthesiologist in attendance. I do not use the intradermal or any other test to determine possible sensitivity to iodine because the correlation with systemic hyperreactivity is poor.

Reassurance and Premedication

The procedure should be explained to the patient in simple, concise terms. The explanatory remarks should include assurance that the procedure is not painful. In addition, the patient should receive some sedation, such as 45-60 mg of secobarbital (Seconal) orally 1 hour before myelography. For high-strung patients with a low pain threshold, 50–75 mg of meperidine hydrochloride (Demerol) and 25 mg of promethazine hydrochloride (Phenergan) or 5–10 mg of diazepam (Valium) are helpful. The meal immediately preceding myelography should be omitted.

Puncture Site and Angle

The examination is best performed with the patient prone on a radiographic-fluoroscopic tilt table with a spot film device. Ideally, the table should tilt 90 degrees in one direction and at least 45 degrees in the other direction. It is possible to do myelography on a table with a 15-degree tilt by reversing the patient to direct the oil into the upper lumbar, thoracic, and cervical regions. A shoulder support or a harness is desirable for cervical and thoracic myelography. Preliminary films of the lumbar spine should be taken (if not already available) and studied to determine the number of lumbar vertebrae, the optimal puncture site and angle, and the presence or absence of bony lesions.

The puncture site depends on the presenting clinical problem and the local anatomical factors in the lumbar spine. Thus, if a herniated lumbar disk is suspected, the puncture should be performed at the L3-4 or L2-3 level if possible, since most herniated lumbar disks are found at the L4-5 and L5-S1 interspaces. It is unwise to puncture either of the latter two interspaces because of the possibility of introducing a confusing needle artifact. If the L3-4 interspace is anatomically unsatisfactory, the L2-3 interspace is selected instead. It is not always as easy, however, to remove the Pantopaque completely through a needle at the L2-3 level. Under these circumstances, after the radiographs are made, one should not hesitate to keep the L2-3 needle in place and make another puncture at L4-5 or L5-S1 to remove the Pantopaque. The L4-5 or L5-S1 interspace, therefore, is routinely marked on the skin, in addition to the interspace selected for introduction of the Pantopaque. Rarely, it may not be possible to obtain spinal fluid with the patient prone. Under these circumstances, the lumbar subarachnoid space can be distended by gravity with the patient in the sitting position and successful puncture accomplished.

The most suitable angle of puncture is determined by inspecting the interlaminar and the interspinous distances in the anteroposterior and lateral projections. These spaces may be wide or extremely narrow. In the former case, the needle should be directed toward the posterior surface of the vertebral body to avoid possible confusion in interpretation due to a needle artifact at the interspace (Fig 4–2). This also facilitates aspiration of the Pantopaque, since even the normal disk may bulge somewhat posteriorly and produce thinning of the oil column at the interspace. However, it may not always be possible to achieve the ideal angle, i.e., when the interspinous distance is so narrow that the course of the needle is predetermined. In this situation, a pillow (or two pillows) placed under the patient's abdomen and hips helps to increase the interspinous distance. Rarely, the pillow will compress

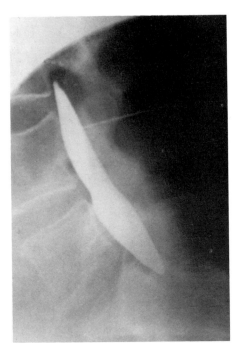

Fig 4–2.—Needle directed toward the upper third of the posterior surface of the fourth lumbar vertebra, thus eliminating the possibility of a factitious defect at the L3-4 interspace.

the inferior vena cava sufficiently to decrease venous return to the right side of the heart and produce a fall in systemic blood pressure. This complication should be watched for. The patient's spine should be absolutely straight, with the spinous processes perfectly centered. If the patient has a scoliosis, it should be corrected by elevating the corresponding hip with a pad; if the curvature of the spine is toward the right, the right hip should be elevated (Fig 4–3). A metallic marker is taped to the undersurface of the fluoroscopic screen to identify right and left sides.

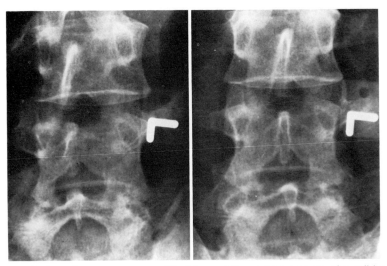

Fig 4–3.—**Left,** spinous processes tilted toward the right because of a mild scoliosis; **right,** scoliosis corrected by placing pad under the right hip.

Lumbar Puncture and Injection of Pantopaque

The puncture point is marked on the skin with a metal-tipped pen or pencil under fluoroscopic guidance (Fig 4–4). With the spine properly centered, a point is selected midway between the pedicles between the appropriate spinous processes. The skin is shaved if necessary and prepared with Betadine. The operator then dons sterile gloves and drapes the lower back with a sterile towel just below the lumbosacral interspace. The towel is fastened to the patient's skin on either side by adhesive tape. A sterile fenestrated sheet is then securely fastened to the patient's shoulders and thighs by strips of adhesive tape. A second sterile towel is taped to the undersurface of the fluoroscopic screen. Lidocaine 1% is used to infiltrate the skin, subcutaneous, and muscle tissues. A 20-gauge, sharp, short-beveled 3- or 3.5-inch-long spinal needle is then inserted (a 4-inch or longer needle should be used for very muscular or obese patients). Neither the tip nor the stylet of the needle should be handled, in order to avoid starch or talc contamination from the gloves. The bevel of the needle originally faces upward. After CSF is observed to flow from the needle hub, the bevel is rotated so that it faces downward. The position of the needle is checked under the fluoroscope to be certain that it is perfectly centered. The importance of this part of the examination cannot be overemphasized. A little extra time initially spent in obtaining a central puncture greatly facilitates complete removal of the Pantopaque. A lateral puncture tends to prolong the time necessary to remove the Pantopaque and frequently makes complete removal difficult or impossible. If a midline puncture is not feasible (e.g., thick midline laminectomy scar, close approximation of spinous processes), I use a posterolateral oblique approach. Under fluoroscopic control, a point is selected above and lateral to the spinous process of L-3 or L-4 and marked on the skin. The

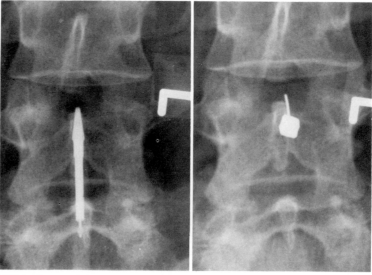

Fig 4–4.—Left, metal-tipped pencil marking the site of puncture on the skin midway between the pedicles, proximal to the spinous process of L4; **right,** lumbar puncture needle in midline position.

needle is angled medially as it passes through the ligamentum flavum. The object is to have the needle tip end up in the midline as it punctures the dura and arachnoid. A similar result can be achieved by placing the patient in a slightly oblique position with the left knee flexed and the left hip slightly elevated. The spinal needle is then directed ventrally and medially under fluoroscopic guidance through the interlaminar foramen into the center of the spinal canal. Some examiners use the posterolateral oblique approach routinely.

The spinal needle is introduced slowly. As soon as the dura is punctured, the needle is advanced slightly, i.e., 1–2 mm, and the stylet withdrawn. The needle is not advanced after the appearance of spinal fluid in patients with spinal stenosis. In these patients with altered CSF dynamics, the flow may be slow. An unobstructed free flow of fluid indicates that the needle is in the subarachnoid space. If the flow is feeble, a minor adjustment of the needle may be necessary, such as rotation of the hub of the needle and/or reinsertion and removal of the stylet. The head of the table is tilted 15–20 degrees caudad to facilitate a brisk flow of spinal fluid. A specimen is collected and sent to the laboratory for a cell count and protein determination. At this point, 0.5 ml of Pantopaque, warmed to body temperature, is carefully injected (Fig 4–5). The Pantopaque vials should be sterilized by autoclaving, since this does not adversely affect the oil. Fluoroscopy is utilized to confirm the subarachnoid location of the Pantopaque. Subarachnoid Pantopaque moves promptly and briskly in response to coughing, straining, or tilting of the table. Subdural Pantopaque, on the other hand, moves somewhat more sluggishly. After the subarachnoid position of the oil is established, the residual Pantopaque is injected with a dry syringe in a slow, steady stream. Rapid, jerky injection tends to promote globulation of the oil. To minimize radiation exposure, the injection should be made through sterile connecting polyethylene tubing. The stylet then is re-

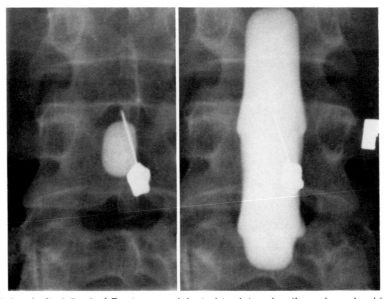

Fig 4–5.—**Left,** 0.5 ml of Pantopaque injected to determine the subarachnoid position of the needle tip; **right,** injection of the full amount of Pantopaque after fluoroscopic corroboration of the subarachnoid location of the oil.

placed, the needle hub covered with a sterile towel, and the fluoroscopic-radiographic portion of the examination carried out.

If difficulty is encountered in obtaining a free flow of spinal fluid after considerable effort, it is wise to terminate the examination and postpone it to a later date (for 2 weeks, if feasible). It is likely that the arachnoid has been punctured in several places, thereby greatly enhancing the possibility of an extra-arachnoid injection of Pantopaque.

Amount of Pantopaque

The amount of Pantopaque depends on the region to be examined, the clinical problems, and various anatomical factors. If too little Pantopaque is used, a lesion may be overlooked and artifactual defects created. On the other hand, routine use of the complete "full-column" technique may obscure a small lesion. One should use sufficient Pantopaque to do the required job. There is no relationship between the quantity of Pantopaque used and the incidence and severity of postmyelographic reactions.

In the cervical and thoracic regions, 18–36 ml suffice for the average myelogram, but as little as 2 ml may be sufficient in the presence of a complete block (Fig 4–6).

In the lumbar region, I prefer a modified "full-column" technique, which usually can be obtained with 18–24 ml. This is desirable to ensure adequate filling of the subarachnoid space in the oblique projections. With the patient prone and one side elevated, the oil accumulates on the dependent side. If insufficient Pantopaque is used, the nerve root pouches on the elevated side are not surrounded by oil. Consequently, deformities of these pouches may be missed (Fig 4–7).

If the lumbar subarachnoid space is unusually wide, larger quantities of Pantopaque may be necessary. Another significant anatomical factor in this regard is the shape of the posterior aspect of the lumbar vertebrae. When these surfaces are deeply concave, the intervertebral disk spaces cannot be studied until the posterior bony concavities are first filled (Fig 4–8).

Fluoroscopy and Films

Fluoroscopy is an integral part of Pantopaque myelography. A persistent slowing and localized thinning of the advancing Pantopaque column as it passes over a lumbar interspace may be the only sign of a small central disk herniation. Similarly, in other areas of the spine, a constant slight indentation of the Pantopaque column indicative of a lesion may be obscured on the radiographs by the density of the full column.

Lumbar Myelography

In the lumbar area, spot films are made to demonstrate each interspace in the anteroposterior and both oblique projections (Fig 4–9). This is accomplished by tilting the table gradually from the horizontal into the upright and Trendelenburg positions. Jerky movements of the table may cause the column of oil to break up. Additional anteroposterior spot films are made to show the opaque column up to the level of T-9 (Fig 4–10). Finally, lateral films with the horizontal beam are taken

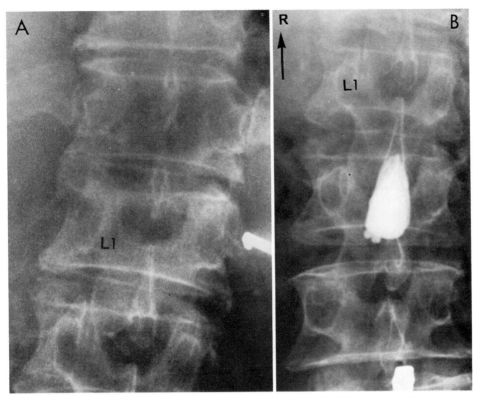

Fig 4–6.—Lumbar myelogram illustrating the use of 2 ml of Pantopaque in the presence of a complete block. **A,** the patient, a 57-year-old male, had an oat cell carcinoma of the R.L.L. bronchus with metastasis to the first lumbar vertebral body. Lumbar puncture at the time of myelography revealed xanthochromic spinal fluid. **B,** myelography, carried out with a small amount of Pantopaque, demonstrated a complete obstruction at the level of L1-2, with displacement of the oil column to the left. At operation, extradural spinal metastases were found extending from T-10 to L-2.

of the Pantopaque outlining the lowermost three or four lumbar interspaces. Since the Pantopaque fills the anterior portion of the subarachnoid space in the prone position, the relationship between the posterior aspect of the intervertebral disks and the anterior surface of the subarachnoid space is shown best in this projection. One of the lateral films is made using the horizontal beam, with the patient standing erect in the neutral position. Breig has demonstrated that the spinal canal elongates in flexion and shortens in extension (see Fig 17–50,*B*). The spinal dura accommodates to the shortened bony canal by forming transverse, accordion-like folds at the interspaces. This occurs in both the cervical and the lumbar regions. These folds, which bulge into the cord or equina, may produce anterior extradural defects at myelography that can simulate a herniated disk.

An optional projection, which may at times be helpful in studying the L5-S1 interspace in the presence of a short caudal sac, is a posteroanterior film with the tube angled 15–25 degrees caudad (Fig 4–11). Right and left lateral decubitus films made with the horizontal beam and a grid cassette may be helpful at times in evaluating failure of filling, or a minor defect of an axillary sleeve (Fig 4–12).

After the films are developed and inspected, the sterile towel is folded back and

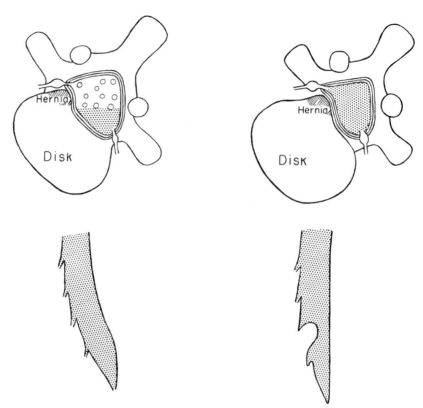

Fig 4–7.—Diagram of patient in the prone oblique position with a left lateral disk herniation. **Left,** insufficient Pantopaque (3 ml) in the subarachnoid space—defect not demonstrated; **right,** 12 ml of Pantopaque filling the subarachnoid space with clear delineation of the herniation.

the Pantopaque is removed through the original needle left in situ by gentle, steady traction on a 10-ml syringe plunger. If some difficulty is experienced and the needle is correctly placed, substitution of a 2-ml syringe may be helpful. To facilitate removal of the final droplets of oil under fluoroscopic control, a sterile, small-lumen polyethylene tube approximately 16 inches long may be used to connect the syringe to the needle. This also increases the radiation protection of the operator. Epstein has suggested siphonage for removal of the Pantopaque from the spinal canal, a technique which I have often found useful. The siphon action is created by removing the stylet, attaching the male end of a sterile polyethylene Venotube to the hub of the spinal needle, and applying gentle, steady suction to the female end of the Venotube with a syringe. The syringe end of the Venotube is placed below the level of the spinal canal. If the patient complains of sharp pain during the aspiration, a nerve root has probably been sucked against the needle point. Under these circumstances, aspiration should be temporarily discontinued and the needle hub slightly rotated to change the bevel, or a minor adjustment in the needle depth should be tried. If the radicular pain continues, it may be necessary to insert a second needle at a lower level. The table should be tilted until the oil is collected around the tip of the needle. An effort should be made to remove all of the Pantopaque with a minimum of spinal fluid. If a disproportionately large amount of

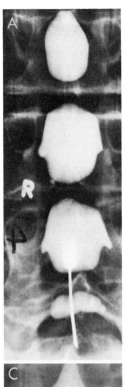

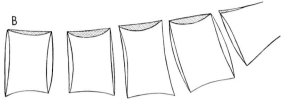

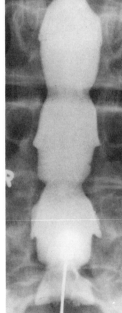

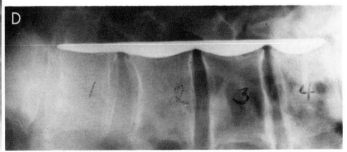

Fig 4–8.—Patient with deep concavities on the posterior aspect of the lumbar vertebral bodies. **A** and **B,** anteroposterior radiograph and corresponding lateral diagram show bizarre configuration of interrupted column of oil collected in the posterior concavities with no oil at the intervertebral disk spaces (12 ml of Pantopaque); **C** and **D,** anteroposterior and lateral radiographs show a continuous column of oil with visualization of the interspaces (30 ml of Pantopaque). (Courtesy of H. O. Peterson.)

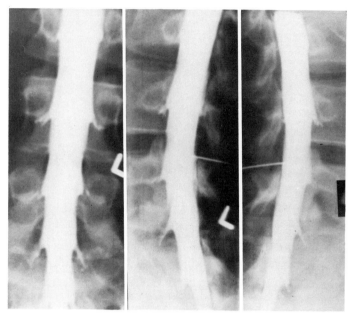

Fig 4–9.—Upright frontal and oblique spot films in routine lumbar myelography.

fluid is drawn off with the Pantopaque, the needle should be very slightly advanced into the principal Pantopaque column, which lies ventrally in the prone position because of its greater specific gravity. Should the oil column break up, it is helpful to run the globules down into the caudal sac and then slowly tilt the table craniad.

If the lumbar puncture is eccentric and the needle point is lateral to the midline,

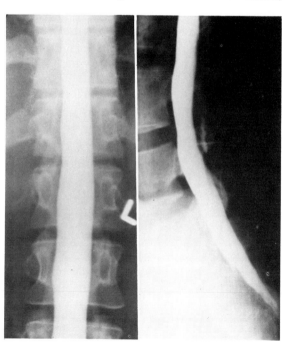

Fig 4–10.—**Left,** frontal spot film demonstrating the upper lumbar and lower thoracic subarachnoid spaces; **right,** lateral shoot-through radiograph with the horizontal beam demonstrating the lowermost three lumbar intervertebral disk spaces.

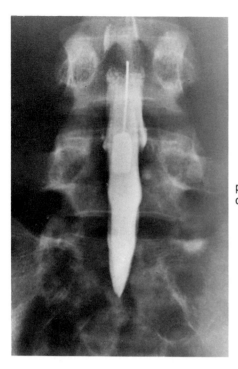

Fig 4–11.—Posteroanterior projection with the tube tilted 25 degrees caudad.

the patient should elevate the opposite side of the body. This tends to promote flow of the oil into a more favorable dependent position for removal. If there is difficulty in removing the Pantopaque through the needle at the original puncture site, there is no objection to making a second puncture at L5-S1. In most instances (95% of the time), the Pantopaque can be completely removed by alternate aspiration and fluoroscopy. After removal of the Pantopaque, the needle is withdrawn and a dry sterile dressing applied to the puncture site. In the presence of a complete block, it may be wiser not to remove the Pantopaque because of the possibility of increased cord compression due to the reduction in cerebrospinal fluid pressure below the obstruction. The oil may be removed later at operation, if desirable. It may be helpful to leave the Pantopaque in the subarachnoid space for 1–2 days to permit restudy if the examination is not definitive. It may also be helpful to leave the oil in place if one wishes to follow the progress of a tumor after radiation therapy. Erect films made 24–48 hours after the original examination may provide better visualization of a lesion not satisfactorily visualized previously or may delineate the lower border of a lesion producing a high-grade, incomplete obstruction. The Pantopaque may then be removed by a second lumbar puncture at the time of re-examination. When an obstruction is encountered, the table should be tilted craniad as far as possible (90 degrees if the table permits) and frontal and lateral radiographs (with the horizontal beam and a grid cassette) taken. Not infrequently, with the table tilted 90 degrees craniad, one can succeed in getting some of the oil above what appeared to be a complete block, thereby avoiding a C1-2 puncture. Only in this way can one be certain that the head of the Pantopaque column is arrested at the actual site of obstruction and not at a spurious lower level (Fig 4–13).

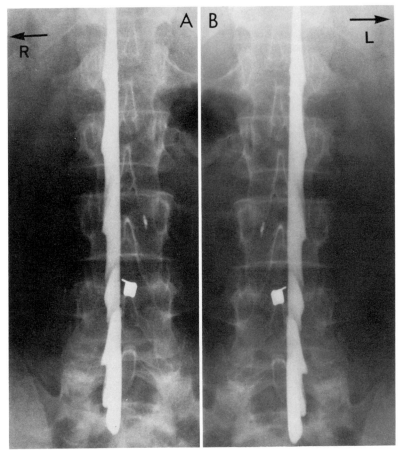

Fig 4–12.—Frontal projections made with the horizontal beam and the patient in the lateral decubitus position **A,** right side up; **B,** left side up.

Following the procedure, the patient should be instructed to lie recumbent without a pillow for several hours. The patient should also be advised to drink liberal quantities of fluid in an effort to decrease the incidence of postlumbar puncture headache. Furthermore, it is wise to forewarn the patient of the possibility of post-puncture headache, indicating its cause and usual response to continued recumbency, hydration, and analgesics.

Thoracic Myelography

Thirty-six or more ml of Pantopaque are recommended for the usual thoracic problem. In patients with severe scoliosis or kyphoscoliosis, Gold has pointed out the usefulness of large-volume myelography, i.e., up to 88 ml of Pantopaque. It is important to fill the subarachnoid space completely in the region of the curvature in order to be able to evaluate the spinal cord and dural sac at that site. It is also wise to use multiple metallic markers for accurate localization every two or three vertebrae from the cervical region to L-1. When any thoracic lesion is found, it is helpful to mark the level of the lesion on the patient's back. A permanent record is

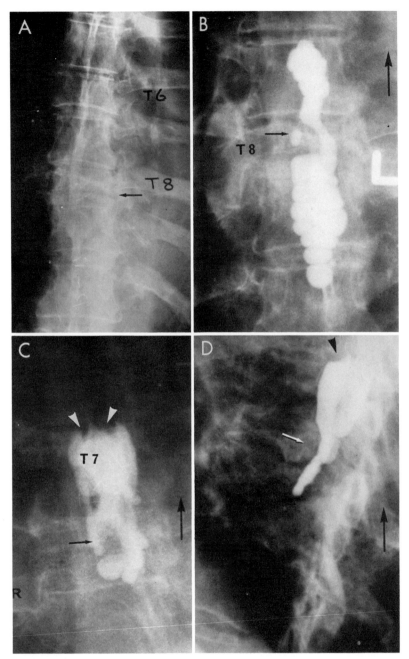

Fig 4–13.—The patient, a 74-year-old female, had a metastatic pathologic fracture of the eighth thoracic vertebra *(arrow)* from a primary carcinoma of the endometrium **(A). B,** at myelography, the resident reported a partial obstruction of the Pantopaque column at T-8, the site of the fracture *(arrow)*. The attending radiologist suggested tilting the table 90 degrees craniad. **C** and **D,** spot films made in this position show a complete block at T6-7 *(arrowheads)* with posterior and left lateral displacement of the oil column at T7-8 interspace *(thin arrow)*. At operation, a herniated disk was found at the latter interspace associated with the fracture. There was extensive extradural metastatic tumor at T6-7.

desirable, using a 7″ × 17″ or a 14″ × 17″ film in the frontal projection with the vertical tube. Thoracic myelography with Pantopaque is most successful when the oil is kept in a single compact column (Fig 4–14). In an effort to achieve this ideal, the table should be tilted slowly. As a rule, the Pantopaque column tends to break up in the lower midthoracic region (T8-9). At times, turning the patient into the oblique or lateral position while tilting the table may help to keep the oil in a column without fragmentation (Fig 4–15). This is also useful in cervical myelography in patients with severe spondylosis to facilitate craniad flow of the column of oil. Should these maneuvers fail, it may be helpful to run the oil up into the cervical region and study the thoracic subarachnoid space as the column of oil descends. Occasionally, it is possible to maintain a solid, elongated column of oil by having the patient perform a Valsalva maneuver at this point. The same effect can be achieved by jugular compression. A well-padded shoulder support should be available for the patient's comfort. When a 90–90-degree tilt table is unavailable, it may be necessary occasionally for the patient to assume the knee-chest position to facilitate passage of the oil into the high thoracic and cervical regions. When the contrast medium is in the cervical region, the patient's head should be hyperextended to prevent the oil from passing into the cranial cavity.

In addition to routine spot films covering the entire thoracic area, radiographs should be taken with the horizontal beam in the prone and right and left lateral decubitus positions. A single 7″ × 17″ or 14″ × 17″ film should also be taken in the frontal projection with the vertical beam in order to identify the levels of the metallic markers.

Herskowitz et al. have suggested the use of three appropriately placed foam rubber pads for supine myelograpy, i.e., under the buttocks, legs, and scapulae. Hinck utilizes a firm, polystyrene rectangular ring to accomplish the same result.* The

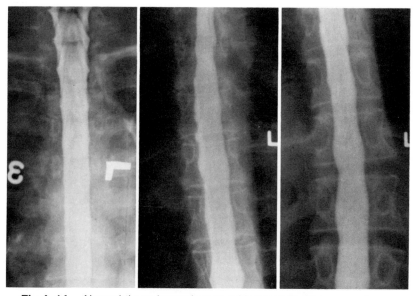

Fig 4–14.—Normal thoracic myelogram with intact Pantopaque column.

*Manufactured by Stanco Medical, Inc., Goleta, CA 93017.

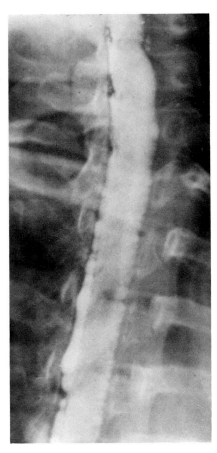

Fig 4–15.—Oblique position of patient resulting in an intact oil column in the thoracic region. The oil broke up into globules in the prone position.

needle hub is thereby maintained at a safe distance from the fluoroscopic screen, obviating the need for a second spinal puncture in those patients in whom supine myelography is desirable.

Cervical Myelography

Eighteen ml of Pantopaque are usually used to examine the cervical subarachnoid space. A shoulder support or preferably a canvas sling around the shoulders and waist is desirable. An alternate satisfactory method for cervical myelography utilizes a folded pillow taped to the footboard of the table. The patient is asked to flex the knees on the pillow and is taped to the table in that position. The table is then tilted to the horizontal position and the lumbar puncture performed. It is most important to keep the head in marked hyperextension to prevent the Pantopaque from rolling up into the cranial subarachnoid space. This can be facilitated by placing a small pad, sponge, or wooden block on the table under the patient's chin. For most cervical problems, particularly herniated disks, it is not necessary to run the Pantopaque higher than the C1-2 interspace. As in the lumbar area, anteroposterior, oblique, and lateral films (made with the horizontal beam) are desirable (Figs 4–16 and 4–17). Two lateral projections with the horizontal beam are made. The first film, with the shoulders dropped as low as possible, usually shows the Panto-

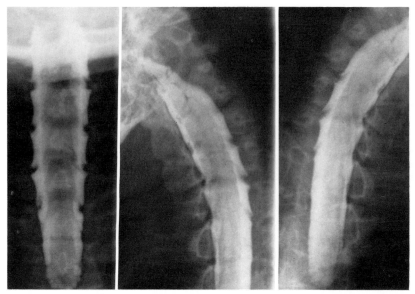

Fig 4–16.—Normal cervical myelogram; frontal and oblique projections.

paque column from C-2 to C-6 or C-7. Cooperative patients should be asked to place the palms of the hands on the table under each shoulder and roll the shoulders back. This frequently visualizes C-7 and makes it unnecessary to obtain a film in the swimmer's position. If this is not satisfactory or feasible, a second film is made in the swimmer's position, i.e., with the arm farther from the x-ray tube over the patient's head and the arm closer to the tube down at the patient's side. The

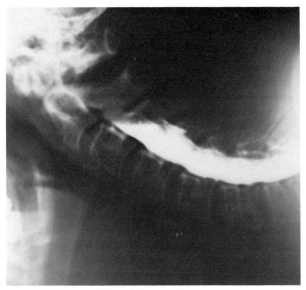

Fig 4–17.—Lateral film made with the patient prone, using the horizontal beam and a grid cassette. The lower four cervical intervertebral disk spaces are well demonstrated.

Pantopaque should be centered over the cervicothoracic junction by fluoroscopy. The central ray is angled craniad slightly above the shoulder farthest from the x-ray tube to avoid superimposition of the C6-7 and C7-T1 interspaces on the shoulder (Fig 4–18).

In patients with marked cervical spondylosis, the Pantopaque tends to break up into a series of interrupted collections due to the multiple bony spurs. Indeed, there may be difficulty in advancing the oil column above the lower cervical region, even with a greater craniad tilt of the table. This can be minimized by using large quantities of Pantopaque. Under these circumstances, the oil usually can be made to flow craniad past the pseudo-obstruction by turning the head obliquely and bringing the table back toward the horizontal position. A bona fide obstruction in the cervical region is constant and can be demonstrated by frontal and lateral films (made with the horizontal beam) in both the deep Trendelenburg and the horizontal positions.

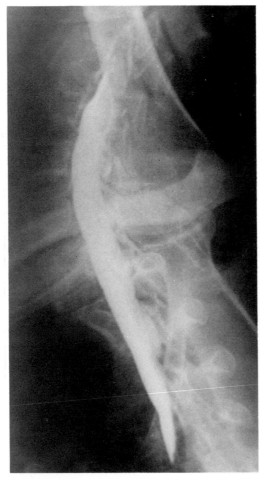

Fig 4–18.—Oblique lateral radiograph with the beam directed through the axilla. This view is particularly useful in patients with a short, stocky neck in whom the C5-6, C6-7, and C7-T1 disk spaces are usually obscured by the soft tissue shadows of the lower neck and shoulders.

Foramen Magnum and Posterior Fossa

When a high cervical or a posterior fossa lesion is suspected, it is essential that the oil pass up into the cisterna magna and/or cisterna pontis. Under these circumstances, it is important to explain to the patient prior to lumbar puncture that successful examination of the atlanto-occipital region depends on complete cooperation. The patient should be told that he must not move his head and neck in any direction by himself. All movements must be controlled by the examiner or an aide. Flexion and extension of the head and neck should be carefully demonstrated by the examiner and practiced with the patient. In order to facilitate ascent of the oil into the cervical region in an unbroken column, it is advisable to place one or two pillows under the patient's hips. This reduces the lumbodorsal angle, thereby permitting the oil to flow over the dorsal hump more readily. Once the oil column has collected in the cervical subarachnoid space, the table is tilted back as close to the horizontal plane as is feasible. With the head straight, the chin in marked hyperextension, and the oil pooled in the cervical subarachnoid space, the planes of the posterior margin of the upper cervical spine and the clivus approach a straight line and the slope of the clivus is maximal (Fig 4–19). The table then is slowly tilted craniad, and the oil can be seen to pass on either side of the dens and then onto the clivus. At this point, the motion of the table is stopped. Further interrupted slight craniad tilting of the table is carried out under constant fluoroscopic observation until the head of the Pantopaque column reaches a point below the level of the posterior cerebral arteries. It is important to remember that spilling of the oil through the tentorial notch into the middle fossa will not occur as long as the apex of the notch is higher than the advancing oil column. At this point, frontal spot films are made. In addition, a frontal radiograph with the vertical beam and a lateral radiograph with the horizontal beam and grid cassette are made. These films usually demonstrate the structures lying in the pontine cistern (Figs 4–20 and 4–21).

If it is desirable to study the posterior aspect of the foramen magnum, the needle is removed and the patient is carefully placed on his back with the head and neck

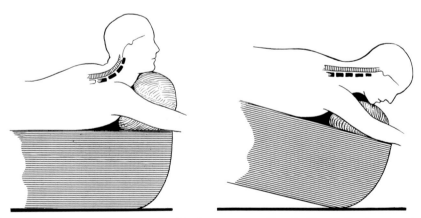

Fig 4–19.—Diagram showing patient in the prone position **(left)** with the head and neck extended and the table horizontal—the oil pools ventrally in the U-shaped cervical subarachnoid space; **right,** the clivus and the posterior surface of the vertebral bodies lie in a straight line so that the oil can run up the clivus with facility.

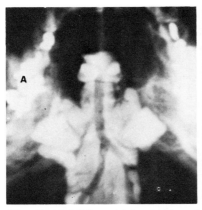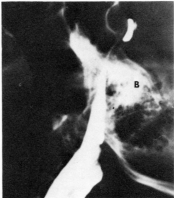

Fig 4–20.—Frontal **(A)** and lateral **(B)** radiographs of a normal Pantopaque study of the anterior aspect of the foramen magnum with the patient prone and the head properly hyperextended.

straight and in maximal flexion. A balsa wood block (2–3 inches square) is placed beneath the occiput. The table is again tilted craniad until the Pantopaque passes into the cisterna magna and the fourth ventricle. If the fourth ventricle does not fill spontaneously, slight extension of the head, gentle coughing, or shaking of the patient's head (by the examiner) may be helpful. When the cisterna magna and fourth ventricle are well filled, straight anteroposterior and lateral radiographs (with the horizontal beam and grid cassette) are taken (Fig 4–22). The table then is tilted caudad with the head in a neutral position and the Pantopaque collected in the lumbar region, where it is removed by a second lumbar puncture.

An alternate simple technique for studying the region of the foramen magnum has been suggested by Margolis. I have used this method for many years and have found it to be eminently satisfactory. With the contrast medium pooled on the clivus and the patient's head hyperextended, the table is tilted 10 degrees caudad. The head is turned laterally with the occiput slightly dependent and the nose elevated toward the ceiling. The right arm is placed at the patient's side, and the corresponding hip and the right side of the chest are slightly elevated. The table is then tilted 5–10 degrees craniad. The Pantopaque will be seen to flow around the dependent tonsil into the cisterna magna (Fig 4–23). Spot films are made, the patient's head is returned to a neutral position, and the table is returned to a 10-degree caudad tilt. The procedure is repeated for the left side.

Cerebellopontine Cisternography

Visualization of the cerebellopontine cisterns and the internal auditory canals is carried out with the same precautions and explanation to the patient as in posterior fossa myelography. The patient is placed in the prone position and secured with a shoulder strap or a harness. The head is maximally extended on the neck, and the head and trunk are rotated as a unit 45 degrees from the table top. The patient must understand that he cannot move once he is finally positioned. His discomfort can be minimized by supporting the elevated shoulder and trunk with a 45-degree-angle foam rubber pad. The table is gradually tilted craniad under constant fluoro-

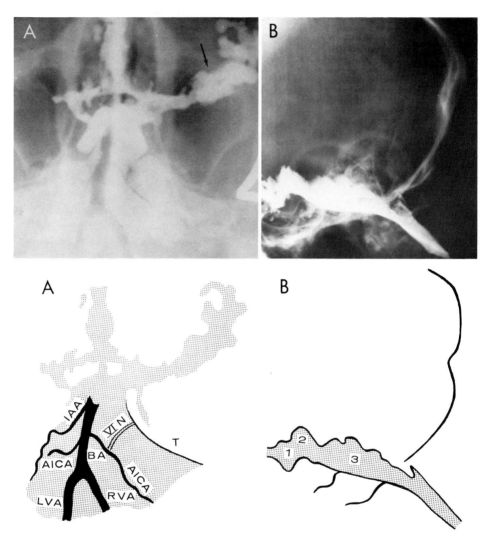

Fig 4–21.—A, prone frontal spot film and, **B,** lateral projection with the horizontal beam showing normal structures in the upper cervical subarachnoid space and pontine cistern. Note that the Pantopaque has spilled over the tentorium into the right sylvian fissure *(arrow)* because of flexion of the head.

scopic control until a slow flow of Pantopaque is noted on the clivus (this rarely requires more than a 35–45-degree tilt of the table). It cannot be emphasized too strongly that the radiologist must continually monitor the oil column to prevent spillage of Pantopaque through the tentorial notch into the middle fossa. With the table ideally angled, the oil flows from the clivus into the dependent cerebellopontine angle and internal auditory canal. The danger of spillage through the tentorial notch is minimized by returning the table to the horizontal position. Appropriate radiographs (spot and overhead films) are made and examined. The oil then is pooled in the upper cervical region by shaking the patient's head gently. The patient is repositioned for examination of the opposite side and similar films are made.

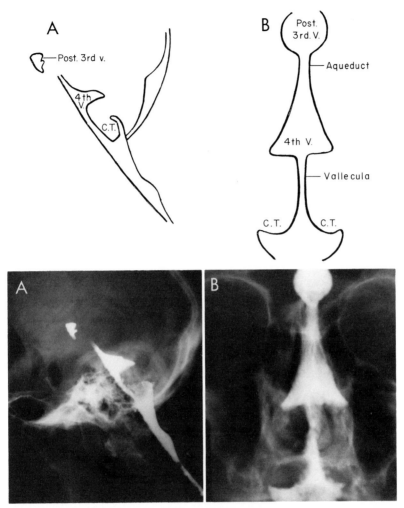

Fig 4–22.—Normal Pantopaque study of the posterior aspect of the cervical subarachnoid space and fourth ventricle in the **(A)** lateral and **(B)** frontal projections with the patient supine. The cisterna magna could not be filled because of arachnoiditis (proved at surgery).

The routine radiographs that I take are (1) spot film with the head obliqued 45 degrees (Fig 4–24, A), (2) submentovertical projection (using the horizontal beam) with the patient in the lateral decubitus position (Fig 4–24,B), (3) horizontal beam anteroposterior view projecting the internal auditory canal into the middle of the orbit, with the head in the lateral position, and (4) reverse Towne projection (35 degrees PA) (Fig 4–24,C). Before the last film, the patient is turned into the prone position and the head carefully flexed until the oil re-enters the cerebellopontine cisterns. This view is particularly helpful when there is nonfilling of one or both canals due to adhesions.

Hitselberger and House recommended the use of 1 ml of Pantopaque combined with polytomography for small tumors confined to the internal auditory canal. The oil is injected into the lumbar subarachnoid space with a 24-gauge spinal needle.

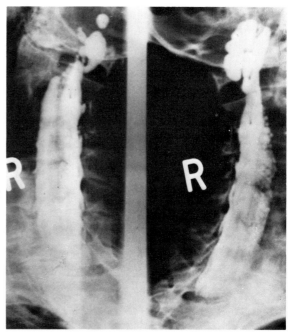

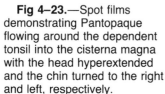

Fig 4–23.—Spot films demonstrating Pantopaque flowing around the dependent tonsil into the cisterna magna with the head hyperextended and the chin turned to the right and left, respectively.

The patient is placed in the lateral decubitus position with the involved side down and the shoulders firmly secured. The table is tilted craniad approximately 35 degrees to pool the oil in the dependent cerebellopontine angle and internal auditory canal. The tilt is maintained for approximately 3 minutes, after which the table is returned to the horizontal and the patient turned prone. A Stenvers view is taken, followed by a series of Polytome sections through the internal auditory canal. The patient's head then is hyperextended and rotated 135 degrees to transfer the oil to the opposite side. Identical films are taken of the second petrous pyramid. At the conclusion of the study, no effort is made to remove the Pantopaque. I have used a similar technique for many years without routine tomography, which is reserved for the unusual occasion where the issue is not clearly resolved by conventional radiography. I routinely take an AP film through the orbit and a submentovertical projection utilizing a horizontal beam (Fig 4–25). The small-volume technique is not suitable for larger tumors in the cerebellopontine (CP) angle. Thus Long et al. reported three large angle tumors with nonvisualization of the internal auditory canal that were missed with the 1-ml technique. They were diagnosed only by filling the CP angle with a large volume of Pantopaque, i.e., 6 ml. It is my practice to begin the examination with 1 ml if an intracanalicular tumor is suspected. If the internal auditory canal is not filled with oil, I inject an additional 5 ml of Pantopaque to visualize the CP angle.

The 1-ml Pantopaque myelogram has been replaced by air CT cisternography in many centers equipped with a high-resolution scanner (Fig 4–26). In my opinion, this technique will ultimately become the radiologic procedure of choice for the diagnosis or exclusion of intracanalicular neurinomas and small CP angle masses. The procedure is simple and can be rapidly performed. To utilize the CT scanner most efficiently, the lumbar puncture is carried out in an adjacent room with a tilt

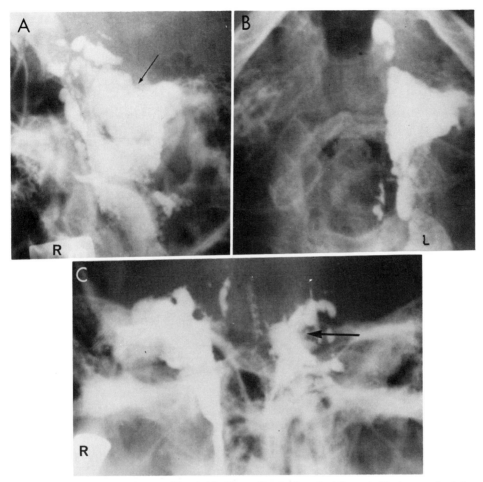

Fig 4–24.—A, frontal spot film (with the patient's head obliqued 45 degrees) of the right cerebellopontine angle showing normal neurovascular structures and filling of the internal auditory canal. Defect produced by the trigeminal nerve crossing the tentorium *(arrow)*. **B,** submentovertical view (with horizontal beam) of left cerebellopontine cistern with the patient on the left side and the head extended. **C,** reverse Towne projection (35 degrees PA). The right internal auditory canal is normal. Note the typical cup-shaped defect produced by the large acoustic neurinoma *(arrow)*.

table or stretcher. The patient lies in the lateral decubitus position with the side of interest uppermost. The head of the table is elevated 20 degrees with the patient's head turned 10 degrees toward the table. Approximately 4–5 ml of air are injected. The table is returned to the horizontal position with the head elevated 15–20 degrees and the face slightly turned toward the table. The patient is then transferred to the scanning table in the lateral decubitus position, and the head is turned directly forward. The gantry is aligned parallel to the interorbital plane to include both sides in the same slice. Scanning is first done with 5-mm contiguous slices to find the internal auditory canal. Then, two 1.5-mm slices are cut on either side of the canal.

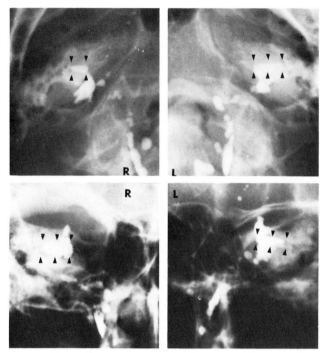

Fig 4–25.—Top, submentovertical view of the normal right and left internal auditory canals filled with Pantopaque *(arrowheads).* **Bottom,** transorbital anteroposterior view of the right and left internal auditory canals.

Cisternal Puncture

Injection of Pantopaque into the cisterna magna may be useful under the following circumstances: (1) to demarcate the superior margin of an obstructive lesion if this is deemed necessary, (2) to demonstrate a clinically suspected second lesion craniad to an obstructive lesion visualized by Pantopaque introduced by lumbar puncture, and (3) when lumbar puncture is technically impossible or contraindicated, e.g., because of infection.

The patient is preferably placed in the sitting position with the head slightly flexed. The hair is shaved from the external occipital protuberance to the midcervical region, and the skin is prepared with Betadine. Using sterile gloves, the operator infiltrates the skin with 1% lidocaine. A spinal needle is inserted in the midline between the external occipital protuberance and the upper margin of the spine of C-2 and directed slightly craniad (Fig 4–27). Before each advancement of the needle, gentle suction is applied with an empty syringe until CSF flows out. The cisterna magna usually lies at a depth of 4–6 cm from the skin surface. As the needle passes through the atlanto-occipital membrane and dura, there often is a distinct "giving" or "popping" sensation. If the needle strikes the basiocciput, it should be partially withdrawn and directed somewhat more caudally.

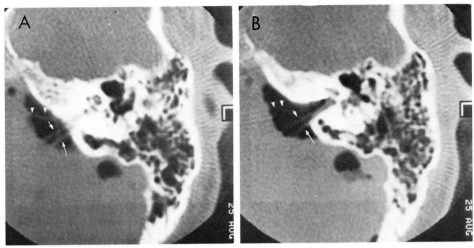

Fig 4–26.—Two sections at 1.5-mm increments of a CT air cisternogram of the left cerebellopontine (CP) angle in a patient with a sensorineural hearing loss. Note that the CP cistern, the internal auditory canal, the internal auditory artery *(arrowheads),* and the seventh and eighth nerves *(arrows)* are exquisitely outlined by air.

Lateral Cervical Puncture

Since the publication in 1968 by Kelly and Alexander of the lateral cervical approach, I no longer use cisternal puncture for myelography. The aforementioned authors point out that their technique is an application of the lateral cervical cordotomy approach described by both Mullan and Rosomoff. Under certain circum-

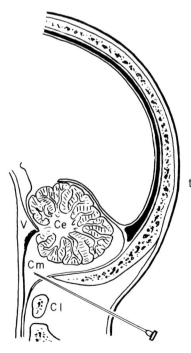

Fig 4–27.—Diagram illustrating the technique of cisternal puncture.

stances, it may not be possible to perform a successful lumbar puncture, i.e., in patients with extensive arachnoiditis, extensive involvement of the cauda equina or epidural space with tumor, an unusually narrow spinal canal, an antecedent recent lumbar puncture resulting in a lowered CSF hydrostatic pressure, or a complete obstruction. In these situations, the lateral cervical puncture is preferable to cisternal puncture because it is both easier and safer to do. Goodman has also commented on the advantage of this myelographic technique for patients with acute cervical cord injuries. In patients with a complete obstruction, the lateral cervical puncture is useful to demonstrate the upper extent of the lesion.

With the patient supine and the head and neck flexed by a pad under the occiput, the site of the puncture between the laminar pillars of C-1 and C-2 is marked under fluoroscopic control. The skin is prepared as for lumbar myelography and infiltrated with 1% lidocaine. The needle is directed toward the junction of the middle and posterior thirds of the bony spinal canal in order to avoid anomalous vertebral or posterior inferior cerebellar arteries that lie in the anterior half of the spinal canal. The bevel of the needle is directed cranially. Serial check radiographs may be necessary to ensure proper direction and position of the needle when biplane fluoroscopy is not available (Fig 4–28). Puncture of the cervical dura transmits the same sensation (i.e., a "pop") to the operator as in lumbar puncture. After dural puncture, the stylet is withdrawn, CSF removed for examination, and Pantopaque or metrizamide slowly injected. The fluoroscopic table is tilted caudad as much as necessary, depending on the clinical problem. After sufficient contrast medium has been directed to the desired area, the needle is removed and the appropriate radiographs taken.

C1-2 puncture can also be carried out with the patient prone or in the decubitus position.

METRIZAMIDE MYELOGRAPHY

General Comments and Contraindications

On the day of the examination, the patient should have a generous liquid diet until 2 hours prior to myelography. Solid foods should be withheld. Dehydration

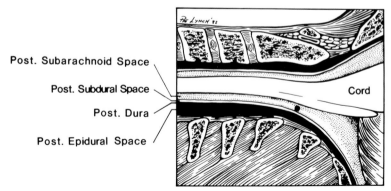

Fig 4–28.—Diagram showing position of needle for a C1-2 puncture with the patient supine.

should be avoided because headache, nausea, and vomiting are less frequent and less pronounced in patients who are well hydrated. If the patient cannot tolerate liquids orally, intravenous fluids should be given. I do not routinely use sedation. However, I do not hesitate to give 5–10 mg of diazepam (Valium) intramuscularly to the anxious patient before the examination.

Because metrizamide irritates the cerebral cortex, I prefer not to use it in patients with known seizure disorders, alcoholism, severe chronic obstructive lung disease, or chronic uremia. I also do not use it in patients who require (and cannot dispense with) neuroleptic analgesics or any other drugs that lower the seizure threshold. If these drugs can be temporarily discontinued 48 hours before myelography, I have no objection to using metrizamide. I would also consider using Pantopaque instead of metrizamide in patients with ventricular shunts and advanced cerebral arteriosclerosis.

PREPARATION AND INJECTION OF SOLUTION

The metrizamide solution is prepared to the predetermined concentration approximately 10 minutes before injection. The appropriate aliquot of buffered diluent is added to the lyophilized powder. The solution is *swirled gently* (not shaken) for several minutes until it becomes clear and is then *slowly* injected into the subarachnoid space through a 22-gauge needle. Theoretically, a small-gauge needle should produce less leakage of CSF and, therefore, less severe headache. However, there is a difference of opinion as to whether there is a decreased incidence of headache associated with a 22- versus a 20-gauge needle. In this regard, Tourtellotte et al. compared 18- and 20-gauge spinal needles and were unable to demonstrate a difference in the incidence of postlumbar puncture headache. Apparently, needles of 24–26 gauge are necessary to reduce the frequency of headache significantly. However, a 22-gauge needle is recommended because this is the smallest caliber that is practical for metrizamide injection.

The injection should be carried out over a period of 1–2 minutes. Rapid injection promotes turbulence of the contrast medium within the CSF with a resultant diminution in concentration and radiopacity. The needle is removed after completion of the injection. I do not use a preliminary test dose of metrizamide because the results are unreliable. Filming should be done without delay because radiocontrast gradually diminishes with time, due to spinal absorption and craniad ascent of the contrast medium. Movement of the patient should be minimized because motion also produces CSF turbulence with resulting dilution of the metrizamide. There is a definite loss of contrast at the end of 30 minutes. After 1 hour, the metrizamide is usually too dilute for satisfactory conventional radiography, although diagnostic images can still be obtained by tomography.

In a few situations (e.g., lumbar spinal stenosis, adhesive arachnoiditis), there may not be a free flow of CSF from the needle even though the latter is in the subarachnoid space. At best, a few drops of clear or xanthochromic CSF (depending on the degree of block) and, at worst, a dry tap, may be obtained. Although it is inappropriate to inject Pantopaque under these circumstances, Stovring et al. have shown that successful metrizamide lumbar myelography is feasible. The position of the needle tip should first be confirmed by frontal and lateral shoot-through radiographs. This is followed by injection of 1 ml of metrizamide under fluoroscopic guidance. The contrast may have an abnormal appearance, i.e., streaky in arachnoiditis and segmented in spinal stenosis. If there is still doubt concerning the subarachnoid position of the needle, frontal and lateral shoot-through radiographs should be repeated before continuing the injection. In these patients, there is frequently resistance to the injection of contrast medium because of crowding of the nerve roots and a reduced capacity of the spinal canal and/or subarachnoid space. Consequently, a smaller volume of metrizamide (10 ml of 170 mg I/ml) may be sufficient.

Dosages for various types of myelograms are given in the procedural descriptions in this chapter and are summarized in Table 4–1.

During the injection, the patient may complain of low back pain or pressure radiating to the lower extremities. Hence, the injection should be made slowly. If the patient has intolerable radicular pain when the needle is inserted, Stovring suggests the injection of 0.2–0.3 ml of 1% lidocaine. Larger amounts of lidocaine should not be used because of the risk of producing spinal anesthesia. Needless to say, a C1-2 puncture is an alternate possibility.

If the metrizamide is inadvertently injected into the epidural or subdural space, the examiner has two options. One can either perform a second puncture at a higher level and proceed with the myelogram or postpone it to a later date. There is no need for concern if the metrizamide inadvertently enters the vascular system because the contrast medium has proved to be safe for intravascular use.

Postmyelography

Ambulatory patients may walk about or sit in a chair for 6 hours and are then advised to lie flat in bed for the next 12–16 hours. Studies have shown no significant difference in the incidence of headache or leg or back pain in patients confined to bed for 24 hours, compared to those permitted to ambulate. However, there is definitely a decreased incidence of nausea and vomiting in the ambulatory group. If confined to bed, the patient is transported from the radiology department with the head and body elevated approximately 35–45 degrees. This position is maintained for approximately 8 hours until the metrizamide is resorbed. Thereafter, the patient should lie flat in bed for the next 12–16 hours to minimize CSF leakage. Approximately 35–40% of patients develop headache following metrizamide myelography. Most headaches are mild or moderate. The headaches can theoretically be divided into two types, although it is often difficult to distinguish between them: (1) early-onset headache due to leakage of CSF through the meningeal fistula, or

TABLE 4–1.—Metrizamide Dosage

PROCEDURE	CONCENTRATION OF SOLUTION (mg I/ml)	VOLUME (ml)	MAXIMUM DOSE (mg I)
Lumbar myelogram	170	12–14	2,380
Thoracic myelogram	220	12	2,640
Cervical myelogram			
Via lumbar puncture	250	10	2,500
Via C1-2 puncture	250	5–7	1,750

(2) later-onset headache due to the irritating effect of the contrast medium on the meninges and cortex. This is probably related to the concentration of metrizamide in the CSF and the length of time that the meninges are in contact with the contrast medium. The incidence of lumbar-puncture headache alone ranges from 9% to 40% in various reports. Tourtellotte et al. have reported the incidence of post-lumbar-puncture headache with a 22-gauge needle to be 36%. This type of headache is characteristically positional in character and usually responds to recumbency in bed for 24 hours. Rarely, however, a patient may be forced to lie flat in bed for as long as 1 week. The headache, due to the irritating effect of metrizamide upon the cervical nervous system, is minimized with the patient erect because the hyperbaric contrast medium remains in the distal lumbar sac for a longer period of time. Consequently, the metrizamide that ultimately enters the head is more dilute. On the other hand, the erect position theoretically enhances CSF leakage. There are conflicting reports about the efficacy of metrizamide aspiration upon adverse side effects, particularly headache. I do not routinely aspirate the metrizamide at the end of the study. I treat postmyelographic headache with various analgesic drugs, e.g., acetaminophen, aspirin, codeine sulfate. Rarely, in cases of severe headache, I administer meperidine hydrochloride (Demerol) orally or intramuscularly.

Nausea and vomiting rarely last longer than 24 hours and usually respond to trimethobenzamide (Tigan) or other antiemetic drugs. Keeping the patient well hydrated decreases the incidence and severity of nausea and vomiting. Hence, the patient should be encouraged to drink liberal quantities of fluid after the myelogram. If this is not feasible, intravenous fluids should be given.

Drugs that lower the seizure level are interdicted for 24 hours after myelography. Seizures can usually be controlled by a single intravenous injection of 10 mg of diazepam. Rarely, a second injection may be necessary because of the short anticonvulsive action of diazepam. In such cases, one should be aware of the fact that the sedative or depressant effects of repeated doses of diazepam tend to be cumulative. Consequently, it is important to be on the lookout for respiratory depression. Because of this, barbiturates or phenytoin should be considered for a more prolonged anticonvulsant effect in the rare case of repeated seizures. There is no evidence that intrathecal methylprednisolone is effective in preventing arachnoiditis in monkeys undergoing iocarmate myelography. Indeed, some arachnoiditis was found in control animals receiving intrathecal methylprednisolone per se. Hence, I do not use intrathecal corticosteroids in patients undergoing metrizamide myelography.

Metrizamide Myelography in Children

Young children should be immobilized on a U-shaped cushion under general anesthesia, as described by Harwood-Nash and Fitz. Some young children below the age of 5–6 years can be examined satisfactorily with appropriate sedation (IM cocktail 10–20 minutes prior to examination—Demerol 25 mg/ml, Largactil 6.25 mg/ml, Phenergan 6.25 mg/ml in a dose of 0.1 ml/kg up to a maximum of 2 ml). I study most children above the age of 10 years with preliminary sedation and local anesthesia.

I use a 22-gauge needle and perform the puncture at the L3-4 level with the patient prone, even in cases of spinal dysraphism. In the latter instance, I use an off-center puncture. Harwood-Nash and Fitz recommend a concentration of 210 mg/ml and a volume less than 0.5 ml/kg in the usual case. In children with large subarachnoid spaces, e.g., those with dysraphism, they use additional metrizamide up to one third of the original volume. I have employed their technique in a few cases and have found it to be safe.

As in adults, the metrizamide solution is injected slowly with a table tilted 15–25 degrees toward the feet. If a thoracic lesion is suspected, the table is not tilted caudad; the patient is slowly and carefully turned into the supine position with the needle in place, to minimize leakage. Appropriate films are taken, i.e., frontal, oblique, right and left lateral decubitus, and a cross-table lateral with the horizontal beam (if necessary). The examination is completed, as in the adult, with the table tilted 35 degrees toward the feet

Radiographic Principles in Metrizamide Myelography

Because metrizamide solutions used for myelography have considerably less radiopacity than Pantopaque, films are made at 60–75 kvp to take advantage of the K edge of iodine. At times, supplementary techniques such as tomography, subtraction, and direct geometric magnification may be helpful. Tomography is useful in salvaging a study when the contrast medium is too dilute to provide satisfactory contrast with conventional radiography (Fig 4–29). Subtraction can enhance definition of the cervical cord in the frontal projection when necessary. Magnification may also be used to advantage to improve detail in the cervical region and foramen magnum, whenever indicated.

Lumbar Myelography

Metrizamide is the contrast medium of choice for lumbar myelography for several reasons, but particularly because it clearly delineates the nerve roots and their sheaths. The patient is positioned prone with a pillow under the abdomen to reduce the normal lordotic curve. The skin is marked under fluoroscopy at L2-3 and L3-4, prepped, and draped with a sterile fenestration sheet. With the table tilted 25% caudad (i.e., head up) to facilitate flow of CSF, a midline puncture is made at L3-4, or L2-3 (if an L3-4 lesion is suspected clinically). Metrizamide solution in a concentration of 170 mg I/ml is slowly injected (12–14 ml, total iodine 2,040–2,380 mg), depending upon the capacity of the individual subarachnoid space. The needle is removed and the patient examined in the erect position, if possible. I take anteroposterior and two sets of right and left oblique spot films. The latter are made with the patient obliqued 20 degrees and 45 degrees (Fig 4–30,A). Thereafter, an upright radiograph is taken with the horizontal beam. The patient is placed prone with the table horizontal, and a second radiograph is made with the horizontal beam (Fig 4–30,B). Spot films of the upper lumbar area are made under fluoroscopic control in the anteroposterior and oblique projections. The examination is concluded with a spot radiograph of the conus medullaris in the supine position with the patient's head flexed to avoid rapid ascent of the metrizamide (Fig 4–30,B). This may require a brief 5–10-degree craniad tilt of the table, after which the table is again returned to the horizontal position. For the oblique views, the

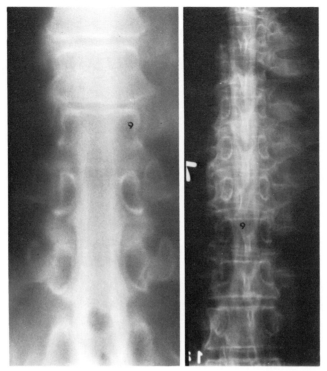

Fig 4–29.—AP tomogram *(left)* of a patient who underwent thoracic metrizamide mye-lography because of left-sided thoracic root pain at the T9-10 level. The conventional film *(right)* visualized this region poorly because of dilution. The tomogram saved the day and ruled out a lesion at this level.

patient is asked not to move spontaneously but to permit the examiner to move him gently, thereby minimizing turbulence of the metrizamide in the CSF.

Some examiners prefer to use the overhead tube for radiography instead of spot films. If available, a C arm is helpful. The tube is angled 45 degrees to the center of the film for the oblique projections (Fig 4–31). This entirely eliminates patient motion. Other examiners prefer to conduct the examination with the patient in the lateral decubitus position with a horizontal beam. I have found all of these methods to be equally satisfactory.

Rarely (e.g., in cases of severe spinal stenosis or local infection), lumbar myelog-raphy is best performed via a C1-2 puncture. In such cases, the table is tilted 45 degrees or more caudad after injection of the metrizamide (10 ml of 250 mg I/ml). In spinal dysraphism, I use the posterolateral lumbar approach routinely in children to avoid possible entry of the contrast medium into the intracranial subarachnoid space. In adults with this lesion, either the lumbar or the cervical route can be employed.

I have satisfactorily performed several thousand Pantopaque cervical and lumbar myelograms on outpatients through the years. During the past 3 years, I have also been involved in approximately 500 metrizamide lumbar myelograms on outpa-tients without serious incident. I limit the latter procedure to patients 50 years or younger in good health who speak and understand English. I thoroughly brief the

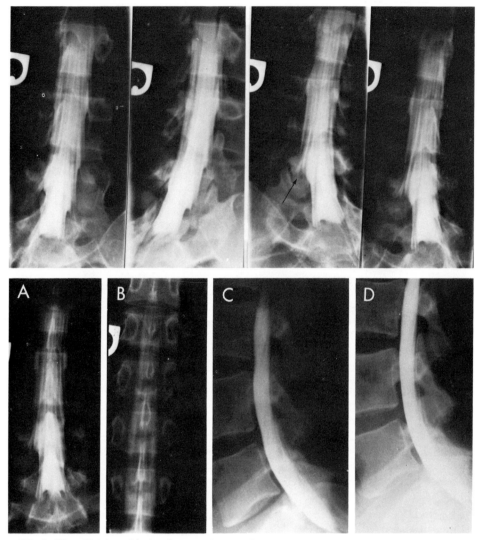

Fig 4–30.—Metrizamide lumbar myelogram in a patient with a herniated disk at L5-S1 on the right *(arrows)*. **Upper,** oblique (20 and 40 degrees) spot films. **Lower,** anteroposterior views of distal cauda equina *(a)*, the conus medullaris *(b)*, and lateral shoot-through radiographs (with horizontal beam) of the distal cauda equina in the erect *(c)* and prone *(d)* positions.

patients on the possible complications and insist that they be accompanied by a relative or friend. I give the patients my telephone number and tell them to call me if they have any problems. I do not perform metrizamide cervical myelography on an outpatient basis because of the greater risk of seizures.

Thoracic Myelography

Metrizamide (12 ml of 220 mg I/ml; total dose, 2,440 mg I) is injected into the lumbar subarachnoid space with the table in the horizontal position. If the patient

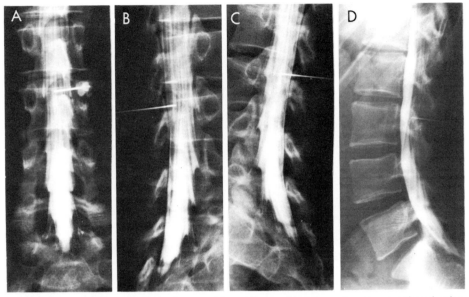

Fig 4–31.—A–C, normal lumbar metrizamide myelogram, using the overhead tube. The patient remains straight in the prone position and the tube is angled. **D,** lateral shoot-through film of the same patient.

does not have a significant dorsolumbar kyphos, the contrast medium is directed into the thoracic region by slowly tilting the table 15 degrees or more craniad with the patient prone and the head hyperextended to avoid passage of the contrast material into the high cervical region. Anteroposterior spot films are made of various segments of the thoracic cord until the entire thoracic region is covered. The patient is then placed in the lateral position, and one or more radiographs are made with the overhead tube. Finally, the patient is gently turned into the supine position. An overhead radiograph is taken with the vertical beam, followed by a lateral radiograph with the horizontal beam (Fig 4–32). The table is then tilted 45 degrees caudad to displace the metrizamide into the lumbar sac.

In patients with a pronounced thoracolumbar kyphosis, the metrizamide is injected with the patient in the lateral decubitus position. The hyperbaric metrizamide gravitates to the dependent gutter. In this position, with the head and neck hyperextended and a pillow under the head, there is no difficulty in getting the contrast to flow up into the thoracic subarachnoid space. When all the contrast is in the thoracic and lower cervical region, the table is returned to a horizontal position. The patient is then gently turned into the supine position for vertical beam anteroposterior radiography and lateral filming with the horizontal beam. Finally, the table is tilted 45 degrees caudad to facilitate flow of the contrast medium into the caudal sac.

Thoracic myelography can also be carried out by a lateral C1-2 puncture with the patient supine, thus eliminating the need to turn the patient over. Indeed, the conus medullaris is best visualized with the patient supine. Also, the supine position facilitates the collection of contrast medium in the concavity of the thoracic spine, thereby giving the examiner greater control.

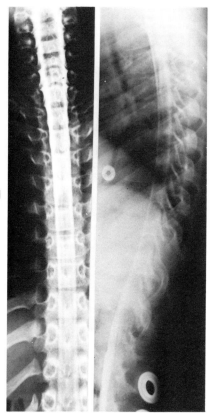

Fig 4–32.—Anteroposterior and lateral radiographs of a normal thoracic metrizamide myelogram.

Cervical Myelography

This procedure can usually be performed satisfactorily either by lumbar puncture or by a lateral C1-2 puncture. The C1-2 puncture is preferable in patients with an exaggerated dorsal kyphosis or a straight cervical spine. With the lumbar approach, the puncture is made at L2-3, and 10 ml of a metrizamide solution containing 250 mg I/ml are injected (total dose, 2,500 mg I) with the patient's head in hyperextension and the table tilted 5 degrees craniad. The needle is then removed. The table is then slowly tilted 25–20 degrees craniad to facilitate ascent of the metrizamide into the cervical subarachnoid space. One should not try to visualize the ascent of the contrast medium through the thoracic region by fluoroscopy. When the metrizamide reaches the cervical area, the table is returned to the horizontal. It is important to keep the head and neck hyperextended until the metrizamide is trapped in the cervical lordotic curve. The degree of hyperextension of the head and neck may be varied by the examiner, depending upon the level of the suspected cervical lesion. At this point, I take anteroposterior and oblique spot films as in lumbar myelography (Fig 4–33). I follow the spot films with radiographs in the lateral and swimmer's positions, using a horizontal beam. Whenever necessary, I gently turn the patient into the supine position and take an anteroposterior radiograph with the horizontal beam.

As in lumbar myelography, the examiner can, if he wishes, omit the spot films

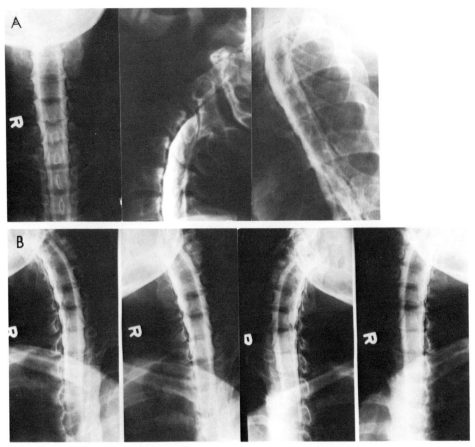

Fig 4–33.—Normal cervical metrizamide myelogram performed via a lumbar injection. **A,** anteroposterior spot film *(left),* lateral shoot-through *(middle),* and swimmer's view *(right).* **B,** right and left oblique spot films (20 and 45 degrees).

and use the overhead tube for anteroposterior and oblique radiography without moving the patient (Fig 4–34). Cross-table oblique radiography with a horizontal beam can also be employed by those who prefer this method. After obtaining the necessary films, the table is steeply tilted toward the feet (45–60 degrees) to promote flow of the metrizamide into the lumbar area. The patient is kept in this position for 5 minutes and then managed as in lumbar myelography.

I prefer to carry out cervical and high thoracic (T1-4) myelography via a lateral C1-2 puncture (Fig 4–35). If a C arm is available, I like to do the puncture with the patient prone to avoid possible movement of the needle tip. If a C arm is not available, I do the puncture with the patient in the lateral decubitus position. In either case, when CSF appears in the hub of the spinal needle, I rotate the tip of the needle downward. The table is tilted approximately 5–10 degrees toward the feet, and 1 ml of metrizamide is injected under fluoroscopic control. Metrizamide in the subarachnoid space flows caudad without delay. If the puncture is done with the patient prone, the rest of the contrast medium is slowly injected under fluoroscopic control. If the puncture is performed in the lateral decubitus position, the

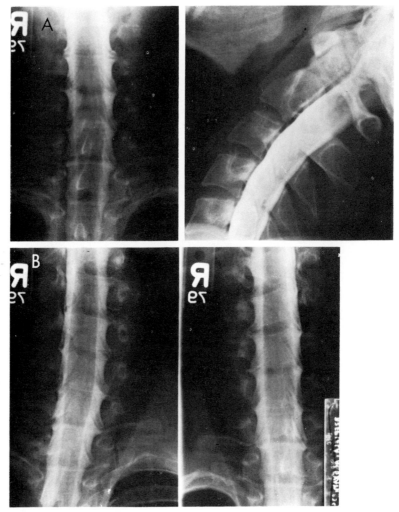

Fig 4–34.—Anteroposterior, lateral shoot-through **(A)** and bilateral oblique radiographs **(B)** made with the patient prone and the overhead x-ray tube appropriately positioned.

patient is carefully turned into the prone position. The needle is checked to confirm good flow of CSF, and the remainder of the contrast bolus is slowly injected under fluoroscopic guidance. The injection is made with the patient's head hyperextended. I use a total volume of 7 ml of metrizamide (250 mg I/ml; total dose, 1,750 mg I).

This technique affords the operator complete control over the contrast column and avoids the rapid entrance of a significant amount of concentrated contrast medium into the intracranial subarachnoid space. This, in turn, decreases the likelihood of severe cerebral neurotoxic complications, i.e., seizure, aphasia, marked diminution of the level of cerebral consciousness, etc. After the study is completed, I slowly tilt the table to the upright position and transfer the patient to a wheelchair, if feasible. Otherwise, the patient is transferred to a stretcher with the head and neck propped up to approximately 40–50 degrees.

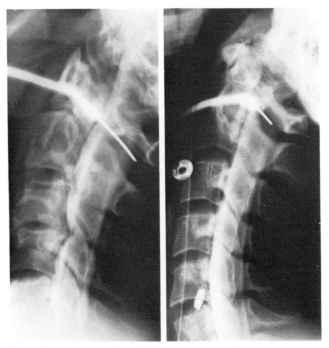

Fig 4–35.—Lateral shoot-through radiographs of two different patients who underwent cervical myelography via a C1-2 puncture.

Total Myelography

At times, it may be necessary to opacify the entire cervical, thoracic, and lumbar subarachnoid space. Adequate to good opacification can be achieved in most instances in a cooperative patient. However, this technique requires rapid execution by the examiner and a relatively high iodine concentration (10–12 ml of 250 mg I/ml; total dose, 2,500–3,000 mg I). In addition, the other conditions that promote good metrizamide myelography—i.e., slow injection and minimal patient motion—must be observed. The study can be accomplished either via lumbar puncture or by a lateral C1-2 injection. If lumbar puncture is the choice, the lumbar region is examined first. After the upright films are obtained, the table is returned to the horizontal position; and anteroposterior, oblique, and cross-table lateral views of the upper lumbar area are taken.

With the patient prone and the head and neck hyperextended, the contrast medium is transferred first to the thoracic and then to the cervical region by progressive, smooth craniad tilting of the table. Anteroposterior spot films of the low and midthoracic areas are obtained as the metrizamide flows up to the cervical area. When the metrizamide reaches the cervical region, films are taken as described for cervical myelography. Extreme kyphosis may interrupt smooth craniad flow of the contrast material with resulting dilution and poor opacification. According to Fox and his co-workers, smooth ascent of the metrizamide can be enhanced with the patient prone if the head is straight and hyperextended and the body is turned obliquely into a semilateral decubitus position.

COMPLETE OR HIGH-GRADE OBSTRUCTION

Many obstructions which appear to be total, particularly with Pantopaque, are not absolute. Thus, Pantopaque introduced via a lateral C1-2 puncture can frequently be demonstrated below the site of a "complete obstruction" on a 24-hour delayed film. Levine and Olmstead suggested the injection of an additional small aliquot of Pantopaque or saline in the Trendelenburg position in nontraumatized patients with an apparent complete block at Pantopaque myelography. In their experience, this obviated the need to introduce additional Pantopaque from above. Kendall and Valentine have also found this technique to be safe and effective with metrizamide myelography. With the patient in the lateral decubitus position and the site of obstruction dependent, the spine is bowed to place the area that is proximal to the obstruction above the horizontal plane. Additional metrizamide is injected slowly under fluoroscopic control, and the table is tilted to pool the contrast medium around the site of obstruction. Anteroposterior and lateral radiographs are then made without changing the position of the patient. Thereafter, supine or prone films can be taken if desired. In the uncommon instance where this technique is unsuccessful, additional metrizamide or air can be introduced by lateral C1-2 injection in order to outline the superior extent of the lesion.

In a few patients with a complete block in the lumbar region at metrizamide myelography, I have removed the contrast medium in an effort to prevent irritation of the cauda equina. Under these circumstances, the patient should be carefully watched for possible exacerbation of the neurologic findings due to the altered CSF dynamics.

MYELOCYSTOGRAPHY (ENDOMYELOGRAPHY)

When enlargement of the spinal cord is demonstrated by Pantopaque, metrizamide, or air myelography, percutaneous puncture of the spinal cord can be carried out. Dilated or abnormal blood vessels can be visualized by positive contrast myelography but cannot be recognized by pneumomyelography. If a vascular lesion is strongly suspected, myelocystography should probably be eschewed because of the risk of hemorrhage.

The cord is punctured in the midline with a 20-gauge spinal needle under fluoroscopic control. The needle is inserted in the midline between the spinous processes and slowly advanced into the subarachnoid space. A sample of CSF is taken for cytologic and chemical examination. The stylet is removed, and the needle is cautiously advanced into the cystic lesion. Fluid is aspirated from the cyst itself for cytologic and chemical study, but the cyst should not be collapsed. At this point, 1–2 ml of positive contrast medium are injected and the needle is removed. The superior and inferior margins of the cystic lesion are then visualized by films in the prone and supine positions.

ASSESSMENT OF THECOPERITONEAL SHUNT PATENCY

West and Grebbell reported the use of metrizamide to determine the patency of a lumboperitoneal shunt. They recommend lumbar puncture with the patient in the sitting position, followed by slow intrathecal injection of 10 ml of metrizamide (170 mg I/ml). PA and lateral films are made immediately, and 5 minutes, after injection. A functioning shunt should show contrast outlining the tube and coating the outer surface of bowel loops. Failure to opacify the tubing indicates shunt obstruction or migration.

BIBLIOGRAPHY

Ahlgren P.: Myelography with metrizamide in the cervical region. *Acta Radiol.* (Suppl.) 355:98, 1977.

Ahmadi J., Potts D.G.: A new device for myelography. *Radiology* 129:821, 1978.

Albrecht K., Dressler W.: Contrast roentgenography of peridural space. Diagnosis of pathologic changes of vertebral bodies and intervertebral disks. *Fortschr. Geb. Röntgenstrahlen* 72:703, 1950.

Amundsen P.: Metrizamide in cervical myelography. *Acta Radiol.* (Suppl.) 355:85, 1977.

Amundsen P., Helsingen P., Kristiansen K.: Evaluation of lumbar radiculography ("Myelography") with water-soluble contrast media. *Acta Radiol. (Diagn.)* 1:659, 1963.

Anderson T., Chrom S.A.: Gas myelography in sciatica patients. *Nord. Med.* 14:1619, 1942.

Ayer J.B., Mixter W.J.: Radiography following the injection of Iodipin into the spinal subarachnoid space. *Arch. Neurol. Psychiatr.* 11:499, 1924.

Baker H.L., Jr.: Myelographic examination of posterior fossa with positive contrast medium. *Radiology* 81:791, 1963.

Bartelink D.L.: Myelography in disc protrusion. Horizontal beam examination with patient prone. *Radiology* 50:202, 1948.

Bauer F.K., Yuhl E.T.: Myelography by means of I^{131}. *Neurology* 3:341, 1953.

Bell A.L.L., et al.: Erect method of myelography. *Am. J. Surg.* 79:259, 1950.

Bell J.C.: Apparatus for the study of opaque media in the spinal canal. *Am. J. Roentgenol.* 37:416, 1937.

Bell J.C., Spurling R.G.: Concerning the diagnosis of lesions in the lower spinal canal. *Radiology* 31:473, 1938.

Bergstrom K., Mostrom U.: Technique of cervical myelography with metrizamide. *Acta Radiol.* (Suppl.) 355:105, 1977.

Bleasel K.: Nerve root radiography. *Br. J. Radiol.* 34:596, 1961.

Bonte G., Delfosse C.: Diagnostic des myélopathies cervicales d'origine discale par la myélotomographie gazeuse par voie lombaire. *Acta Radiol. (Diagn.)* 1:665, 1963.

Bradac G.B., Simon R.S.: Cervical air myelography—an improved technique. *Fortschr. Geb. Röntgenstrahlen* 115:73, 1971.

Breig A.: *Biomechanics of the Central Nervous System.* Stockholm, Almqvist & Wiksell, 1970, p. 183.

Breit A., Wiedenmann O.: Experiences with gas myelography. *Fortschr. Geb. Röntgenstrahlen* 81:761, 1954.

Brierre J.T., Colclough J.R.: Total myelography. *Radiology* 64:81, 1955.

Bücker J.: Air myelography in prolapse of intervertebral disks. *Fortschr. Geb. Röntgenstrahlen* 72:493, 1950.

Burgers E., Anderson R.: Nonoperative removal of intraspinal Lipiodol and Thorotrast. *Northwest Med.* 41:158, 1942.

Burrows E.H.: Positive contrast examination (cerebellopontine cisternography) in extrameatal acoustic neurofibromas. *Br. J. Radiol.* 42:902, 1969.

Camp J.D., Addington E.A.: Intraspinal lesions associated with low back pain and sciatic pain and their localization by means of Lipiodol within the subarachnoid space. *Radiology* 33:701, 1939.

Chakers D., Howieson D.C.: Lateral C2-C3 subarachnoid puncture for metrizamide myelography or cisternography. *A.J.N.R.* 2:280, 1981.

Chamberlain W.E., Young B.R.: The diagnosis of intervertebral disk protrusion by intraspinal injection of air. *J.A.M.A.* 113:2022, 1939.

Coin C.G., Scanlan R.L.: Technique for internal auditory cisternography. *Acta Radiol.* (Suppl.) 347:53, 1976.

Copleman B.: Pantopaque myelography. Indications and technic. *J. Med. Soc. New Jersey* 43:460, 1946.

Cronqvist S.: Thoracic myelography with metrizamide. *Acta Radiol.* (Suppl.) 355:64, 1977.

Cronqvist S., Brismar J.: Cervical myelography with metrizamide. *Acta Radiol.* (Suppl.) 355:110, 1977.

Cuatico W., Gannon W., Samouhos E.: A needle designed for myelography. Technical note. *J. Neurosurg.* 28:87, 1968.

Dalith F.: Cervical oil myelography with full hyperextension of the neck. A modified technique. *Radiol. Clin.* 25:212, 1956.

Davies H.W.: Positive contrast myelography. *Proc. Roy. Soc. Med.* 44:881, 1951.

Del Prado E.A., Enditz L.J.: La myélographie gazeuse cervicale; méthode et essai d'interprétation: à propos de 40 observations. *J. Belge de Radiol.* 42:523, 1959.

de van Niekerk J.P.: Myelography using water-soluble contrast media as an outpatient procedure. *S. Afr. Med. J.* 55:550, 1979.

deVilliers P.D.: The use of metrizamide for myelography. *S. Afr. Med. J.* 56:631, 1979.

Edholm P., Fernstrom I., Lindblom K.: Extradural lumbar disk puncture. *Acta Radiol. (Diagn.)* 6:322, 1967.

Edling L., Ingvar S.: Über Myelographie mit kleinen Kontrastmengen. *Acta Radiol.* 13:239, 1932.

Eldevik O.P., Haughton V.M., Ho K.-C., Williams A.L., et al.: Ineffectiveness of prophylactic intrathecal methylprednisolone in myelography with aqueous media. *Radiology* 129:99, 1978.

Eldevik O.P., Nakken K.O., Haughton V.M.: The effect of dehydration on the side effects of metrizamide myelography. *Radiology* 129:715, 1978.

Eldevik O.P., Nakken K.O., Haughton V.M.: The effect of hydration on the acute and chronic complications of aqueous myelography. An experimental study. *Radiology* 129:713, 1978.

El Gammal T.: Cervical myelography and posterior fossa examinations with Amipaque: Use of magnification and subtraction. *Radiology* 136:219, 1980.

Epstein B.S.: Effect of increased intraspinal pressure on movement of iodized oil within spinal canal. *Am. J. Roentgenol.* 52:196, 1944.

Epstein B.S.: Evacuation of Pantopaque from lumbar spinal canal by siphon action. *Radiology* 83:472, 1964.

Epstein B.S., Epstein J.A.: The siphonage technique for the removal of Pantopaque following myelography. *Radiology* 103:353, 1972.

Finney L.M.: The McCallum liquid goniometer for gas encephalography and myelography. *Radiography* 42:197, 1976.

Finney L.M.: The McCallum radio-opaque liquid goniometer for encephalography and myelography. 43:107, 1977.

Fitz C.R., Harwood-Nash D.C., Barry J.F., Byrd S.E.: Pediatric myelography with metrizamide. *Acta Radiol.* (Suppl.) 355:182, 1977.

Forestier J., Sicard A., Oeconomo D.: Roentgenologic examination by means of Lipiodol (iodized oil) introduced epidurally through sound. *Rev. Neurol.* 8:119, 1949.

Fox A.J., Vinuela F., Debrun, G.: Complete myelography with metrizamide. *A.J.N.R.* 2:79, 1981.

Fullenlove T.M.: Factors in globule formation with Pantopaque myelography. *Am. J. Roentgenol.* 63:378, 1950.

Gabrielson T.O., Seeger J.F., Knake J.E., et al.: C1-C2 puncture with the patient supine for thoracic metrizamide myelography. *Radiology* 136:229, 1980.

Gass H.: Pantopaque anterior basal cisternography of the posterior fossa. *Am. J. Roentgenol.* 90:1197, 1963.

Gates G.F.: 45-degree central ray angulation for improved lumbosacral myelography. *Radiol. Technol.* 47:301, 1976.

Globus J.H.: Contribution made by roentgenographic evidence after the injection of iodized oil. *Arch. Neurol. Psychiatr.* 37:1077, 1937.

Globus J.H., Strauss I.: Intraspinal iodolography: Subarachnoid injection of iodized oil as an aid in the detection and localization of lesions compressing the spinal cord. *Arch. Neurol. Psychiatr.* 21:1331, 1929.

Gold L.H.A., Leach C.G., Kieffer S.A., et al.: Large volume myelography. An aid in the evaluation of curvatures of the spine. *Radiology* 97:531, 1970.

Gonsette R.E.: Cervical myelography with metrizamide by suboccipital puncture. *Acta Radiol.* (Suppl.) 355:121, 1977.

Goodman J.M.: Myelography in acute cervical injuries: Technical note. *Am. J. Roentgenol.* 107:491, 1969.

Grainger R.G.: Lumbar myelography with metrizamide—a new non-ionic contrast medium. *Br. J. Radiol.* 49:996, 1976.

Grainger R.G.: Technique of lumbar myelography with metrizamide. *Acta Radiol.* (Suppl.) 355:31, 1977.

Grayson C.E., Black H.A.: Myelography, diagnostic value in lesions of lumbar discs with variation in technic. *California Med.* 70:464, 1949.

Gutterman P., Bezier H.S.: Prophylaxis of postmyelogram headaches. *J. Neurosurg.* 49:869, 1978.

Haft H., Weinstein C.E., Krueger E.G.: Large volume Pantopaque lumbar myelography. *Radiology* 74:605, 1960.

Haggart G.E., Albers J.H., Zintl W.J.: Introduction and removal of Lipiodol for spinal studies. *Surg. Clin. North Am.* 22:857, 1942.

Haggart G.E., Grannis W.R.: Pantopaque myelography in low back and sciatic pain: Indications and technic. *Surg. Clin. North Am.* 32:695, 1952.

Hammer B.: Experiences with intrathecally enhanced computed tomography. *Neuroradiology* 19:221, 1980.

Hansen E.B., Praestholm J., Fahrenkrug A., Bjerrum J.: A clinical trial of Amipaque in lumbar myelography. *Br. J. Radiol.* 49:34, 1976.

Harwood-Nash D.C., Fitz C.R.: Myelography and syringomyelia in infancy and childhood. *Radiology* 113:661, 1974.

Harwood-Nash D.C., Fitz C.R., Resjo I.M., Chuang S.: Spinal and cord lesions in children and computed tomographic metrizamide myelography. *Neuroradiology* 16:69, 1978.

Haughton V.M., Correa-Paz F.: Double contrast myelography. *Invest. Radiol.* 12:552, 1977.

Haughton V.M., Williams C., Jr., Meyer G.A.: A myelographic technique for cysts in the spinal canal and spinal cord. *Radiology* 129:717, 1978.

Haverling M.: Trans-sacral puncture of the arachnoidal sac–an alternative procedure to lumbar puncture. *Acta Radiol. (Diagn.)* 12:1, 1972.

Heckster R.E.M., Prins H.J., Pennings-Braun A.G.M.: Lumbar myelography with metrizamide. *Acta Radiol.* (Suppl.) 355:38, 1977.

Heinz E.R., Goldman R.L.: The role of gas myelography in neuroradiologic diagnosis. *Radiology* 102:629, 1972.

Herskowitz A., Graebner R., Naidech H.: A technique for supine myelography. Technical note. *J. Neurosurg.* 40:549, 1974.

Hinck V.C.: The myelography needle. A new cannula for aspiration. *Radiology* 120:731, 1976.

Hinck V.C.: Simplified supine thoracic myelography. *A.J.R.* 133:1197, 1979.

Hindmarsh T.: Myelography with the non-ionic water-soluble contrast medium metrizamide. *Acta Radiol. (Diagn.)* 16:417, 1975.

Hindmarsh T.: Metrizamide in selective cervical myelography. *Acta Radiol.* (Suppl.) 355:127, 1977.

Hitselberger W.E., House W.F.: Polytome-Pantopaque: A technique for the diagnosis of small acoustic tumors. Technical note. *J. Neurosurg.* 29:214, 1968.

Horton J.A., et al.: Guiding the thin spinal needle. *A.J.R.* 134:845, 1980.

Hugosson C., Hindmarsh T., Bergstrom K.: Myelography with metrizamide in infants and children. *Acta Radiol.* (Suppl.) 355: 193, 1977.

Hungerford G.D., Powers J.M.: Avulsion of nerve rootlets with the Cuatico needle during Pantopaque removal after myelography. *A.J.R.* 129:485, 1977.

Hurwitz S.R., Suydam M., Steinberg A.: Aspiration of metrizamide following lumbar myelography. *Radiology* 136:789, 1980.

Irstam L.: Lumbar myelography with Amipaque. *Spine* 3:70, 1978.

Jirout J.: Pneumographic examination of lumbar disc lesions. A new method. *Acta Radiol. (Diagn.)* 9:727, 1969.

Juers E.H., Petersen H.O.: Simple method for removal of iodized oil from subarachnoid space. *Minnesota Med.* 25:270, 1942.

Kaplan J.O., Quencer R.M., Stokes N.A., Post M.J.D.: Improved technique for cervical metrizamide myelography. *Radiology* 135:519, 1980.

Kauman G.R., Medelman J.P.: Removal of iodized oil after roentgen diagnosis. *Minnesota Med.* 25:273, 1942.

Kehrer H.E.: Myelography with oxygen in diagnosis of disk prolapse. *Deutsche Med. Wehnschr.* 74:700, 1949.

Kelly D.L., Alexander E., Jr.: Lateral cervical puncture for myelography. Technical note. *J. Neurosurg.* 29:106, 1968.

Kendall B.E., Valentine A.R.: Myelographic study of the obstructed spinal theca with water-soluble contrast medium. *Br. J. Radiol.* 54:408, 1981.

Kennedy T.F., Steinfeld J.R.: Nerve rootlet avulsion as a complication of myelography with the Cuatico needle. *Radiology* 119:389, 1976.

Kesala B.A., Baker D., Morin M., Sue H.: A new device to support handicapped patients during venography or myelography. *Radiology* 128:507, 1978.

Kieffer S.A., Binet E.F., Esquerra J.V., et al.: Contrast agents for myelography: Clinical and radiological evaluation of Amipaque and Pantopaque. *Radiology* 129:695, 1978.

Kieffer S.A., Peterson H.O., Gold L.H.A., Binet E.F.: Evaluation of dilute Pantopaque for large-volume myelography. *Radiology* 96:69, 1970.

Knutsson F.: Experiences with epidural contrast investigation of the lumbosacral canal in disc prolapse (Perabrodil). *Acta Radiol.* 22:694, 1941.

Knutsson F.: Lumbar myelography with water-soluble contrast in cases of disc prolapse. *Acta Orthop. Scandinav.* 20:294, 1951.

Kohout J.: Epidural pneumomyelography. *Acta Radiol.* 50:217, 1958.

Kricheff I.I., Pinto R.S., Bergeron R.T., Cohen N.: Air CT cisternography and canalography for small acoustic neuromas. *A.J.N.R.* 1:57, 1980.

Krupka J.J., D'Angelo C.M.: Artifactual midline cervical defect seen during myelography. *Spine* 3:210, 1978.

Kubik C.S., Hampton A.O.: Removal of iodized oil by lumbar puncture. *N. Engl. J. Med.* 224:455, 1941.

Kvernland B.N., Grewe R.V., Wooley L.M.: Upright large-volume dynamic myelography. *Radiology* 72:562, 1959.

Legge D., Staunton H.: Minimizing side effects in lumbar radiculography. *Clin. Radiol.* 30:559, 1979.

Levine H.L., Olmstead E.J.: Myelographic evaluation of non-traumatic spinal canal obstruction: A new approach. *A.J.R.* 133:715, 1979.

Lindblom K.: Technic and results in myelography and disk puncture. *Acta Radiol.* 34:321, 1950.

Lindblom K.: Technic and results of diagnostic disk puncture and injection (discography) in lumbar region. *Acta Orthop. Scandinav.* 20:315, 1951.

Lindgren E.: Radiologic examination of the brain and spinal cord. *Acta Radiol.* (Suppl.) 151, 1957.

Long J.M., Kier E.L., Hilding D.A.: Pitfalls of posterior fossa cisternography using 2 ml of iophendylate (Pantopaque). *Radiology* 102:71, 1972.

Lowman R.M., Finkelstein A.: Air myelography for demonstration of the cervical spinal cord. *Radiology* 39:700, 1942.

Luyendijk W.: Canalography. Röntgenological examination of the peridural space in the lumbosacral part of the vertebral canal. *J. Belge de Radiol.* 46:236, 1963.

Malis L.I.: Myelographic examination of the foramen magnum. *Radiology* 70:196, 1958.

Malis L.I., Newman C.M., Wolf B.S.: Full-column technique in lumbar disk myelography. *Radiology* 60:18, 1953.

Margolis M.T.: A simple myelographic maneuver for the detection of mass lesions at the foramen magnum. *Radiology* 119:482, 1976.

Martinez G.T., Olivera V.C.: Epidurograma. *Radiologia* (Panama) 3:21, 1952.

McClendon L.K.: Flying lateral technique for thoracic myelography. *Radiol. Technol.* 50:9, 1978.

McGrath T.W.: The oblique approach to the spinal canal for myelography. *Neuroradiology* 19:149, 1980.

Mones R., Werman R.: Pantopaque myeloencephalography. *Radiology* 72:803, 1959.

Morris J.L., Cail Wayne S.: A head rest for cervical myelography. *Radiology* 135:228, 1980.

Mullan S., Hekmatpanah J., Dobben G., Beckman F.: Percutaneous, intramedullary cordotomy utilizing the unipolar anodal electrolytic lesion. *J. Neurosurg.* 22:548, 1965.

Murtagh F., et al.: Cervical air myelography. A review of 130 cases. *Am. J. Roentgenol.* 74:1, 1955.

Negrin J.: A catheter device for myelography. Presented before the New York Society of Neurosurgeons, Jan. 20, 1959.

Nordentoft J.: Myelography with Skiodan. *Nord. Med.* 21:255, 1944.

Oden S.: Diagnosis of spinal tumours by means of gas myelography. *Acta Radiol.* 40:301, 1953.

Olsson O.: Technic of lumbar pneumomyelography. *Acta Radiol.* 29:107, 1948.

O'Reilly I.: The McCallum "breathing" head support for myelography. *Radiography* 45:150, 1979.

Padberg F.T.: Myelography with Pantopaque. *Quart. Bull. Northwestern Univ. M. School* 25:320, 1951.

Perryman C.R., Noble P.R., Bragdon F.H.: Myeloscintigraphy: A useful procedure for localization of spinal block lesions. *Am. J. Roentgenol.* 80:104, 1958.

Poppen J.L.: Use of oxygen in demonstrating posterior herniation of intervertebral disks. *N. Engl. J. Med.* 223:978, 1940.

Pribram H.F.W.: A simple biplane myelographic table. *Am. J. Roentgenol.* 105:411, 1969.

Reichert T.L.: Injection of air for localization of lesions in spinal canal–pneumomyelography. *West J. Surg.* 47:297, 1939.

Rice J.F., Bathia A.L.: Lateral C1-2 puncture for myelography: Posterior approach. *Radiology* 132:760, 1979.

Robertson W.D., LaPointe J.S., Nugent R.A., et al.: Positioning of patients after metrizamide lumbar myelography. *A.J.R.* 134:947, 1980.

Rosomoff H.L., Brown C.J., Sheptak P.: Percutaneous radiofrequency cervical cordotomy: Technique. *J. Neurosurg.* 23:639, 1965.

Roth M.: Gas myelography by the lumbar route. *Acta Radiol.* (Suppl.) 1:53, 1963.

Russell E.J., Pinto R., Kricheff I.I.: Supine metrizamide myelography: A technique for achieving excellent visualization of the thoracic cord and conus medullaris. *Radiology* 135:227, 1980.

Sackett J.F.: Cervical and lumbar routes for metrizamide cervical examination. *Neuroradiology* 16:273, 1978.

Sackett J.F., Hausserman S.A., Okagaki H.I., Breed A.L.: Myelography with metrizamide in intraspinal and spinal abnormalities. *Acta Radiol.* (Suppl.) 355:135, 1977.

Sackett J.F., Quaglieri C.E., et al.: Metrizamide—CSF contrast medium. Analysis of clinical application in 215 patients. *Radiology* 123:779, 1977.

Salmon J.H.: Transventricular spinal myelography in the infant. *Radiology* 91:1041, 1968.

Sanford H., Doub H.P.: Epidurography: A method of roentgenologic visualization of protruded intervertebral disks. *Radiology* 36:172, 1941.

Scanlan R.L.: Positive contrast medium (Iophendylate) in diagnosis of acoustic neuroma. *Arch. Otolaryng.* 80:698, 1964.

Schmidt R.C.: Cervical double contrast myelocisternography by the lateral approach: Technical note. *Neuroradiology* 174:183, 1979.

Scholten E.T., Hekster R.E.M.: Visualization of the craniocervical subarachnoid spaces. *Neuroradiology* 14:139, 1977.

Schultz E.H., Jr., Bragdon B.G.: Problem of subdural placement in myelography. *Radiology* 79:91, 1962.

Scott W.C., Furlow L.T.: Myelography with Pantopaque and new technic for its removal. *Radiology* 43:241, 1944.

Seyfert S., et al.: Abducens palsy after lumbar myelography with water-soluble contrast media. *J. Neurol.* 219:213, 1978.

Sgalitzer M.: Myelography with descending and ascending Lipiodol. *Acta Radiol.* 9:136, 1928.

Shipp F.L.: Technique and value of myelography. *J.A.M.A.* 151:185, 1953.

Sisson W.R., Jr.: Lateral cervical myelography. *N. Engl. J. Med.* 250:651, 1954.

Skalpe I.O., et al.: Lumbar myelography with metrizamide. *Acta Radiol.* (Suppl.) 335:367, 1973.

Skalpe I.O., et al.: Cervical myelography with metrizamide (Amipaque): A comparison between conventional and computer-assisted myelography with special reference to the upper cervical and foramen magnum region. *Neuroradiology* 16:275, 1978.

Skalpe I.O., Sortland O.: Thoracic myelography with metrizamide. *Acta Radiol.* (Suppl.) 355:57, 1977.

Smith F.P., Pitts F.R., Jr., Rogoff S.M.: Cinemyelography. *J. Neurosurg.* 17:1112, 1960.

Sortland O.: Cervical myelography with metrizamide using lumbar injection. *Acta Radiol.* (Suppl.) 355:141, 1977.

Sortland O.: Computed tomography combined with gas cisternography for the diagnosis of expanding lesions in the cerebellopontine angle. *Neuroradiology* 18:19, 1979.

Sortland O., Hovind, K.: Myelography with metrizamide in children. *Acta Radiol.* (Suppl.) 355:211, 1977.

Sortland O., Skalpe I.O.: Cervical myelography by lateral cervical and lumbar injection of metrizamide. *Acta Radiol.* (Suppl.) 355:154, 1977.

Southworth L.E., Jiminez J.P., Goree J.A.: A practical approach to cervical air myelography. *Am. J. Roentgenol.* 107:486, 1969.

Stitt H.L., Dunbar H.S., Schick R.W., Dunn A.A.: Pontocerebellar cisternography. *Radiology* 90:942, 1968.

Stovring J., Saksanen S.J., Fernando L.T., Roberson G.H.: Successful myelography after dry spinal puncture. *Radiology* 143:265, 1982.

Strand R.D., Baker R.A., Rosenbaum A.E., Drayer B.P.: Myelography with metrizamide in infants and children. *Acta Radiol.* (Suppl.) 335:171, 1977.

Sty J.R., et al.: Cervical metrizamide myelography by lumbar puncture. *Pediatr. Radiol.* 7:133, 1978.

Swann G.F.: Technique of positive contrast myelography. *Proc. Roy. Soc. Med.* 53:448, 1960.

Sypert G.W., Mozingo J.R.: A technique for early Pantopaque myelography in cervical spinal cord injuries. *Surg. Neurol.* 6:221, 1976.

Thomas H.A., Sievers R.E.: The Cuatico aspiration cannula as a depth guide during myelography. *Radiology* 133:796, 1979.

Toth J.: Diagnostic value of myelography. *Röntgenpraxis* 13:285, 1941.

Tourtellotte W.W., Henderson W.G., Tucker R.P., et al.: A randomized, double-blind clinical trial comparing the 22- versus 26-gauge needle in the production of the postlumbar puncture syndrome in normal individuals. *Headache* 12:73, 1972.

Valk J.: Thoracic myelography with metrizamide. *Acta Radiol.* (Suppl.) 355:77, 1977.

Vogelsang H., Schmidt R.: Cervical myelography and lateral C1-C2 approach. *Acta Radiol.* (Suppl.) 355:164, 1977.

von Briesen H.: Removal of Lipiodol after myelography. *Am. J. Roentgenol.* 42:525, 1939.

Weber H.M.: Epidural air injection in diagnosis of spinal canal masses. *Calif. & West. Med.* 54:27, 1941.

Weidenman O.: Method for demonstration of upper thoracic spinal cord in positive myelography. *Fortschr. Geb. Röntgenstrahlen* 92:170, 1960.

Wendth A.J., Jr., Moriarty D.J.: A simplified method for the rapid removal of myelographic contrast medium. *Radiology* 93:1092, 1969.

West C.G.H., Grebbell F.S.: A means of assessing theco-peritoneal shunt patency. *Br. J. Radiol.* 53:647, 1980.

Whitcomb B.B., Wyatt G.M.: Technic of Pantopaque myelography. *J. Neurosurg.* 3:95, 1946.

Wood E.H.: Myelography with Pantopaque. *Med. Radiogr. Photogr.* 28:47, 1952.

Woodhall B.: Aspiration of Lipiodol injected for diagnosis and localization of ruptured intervertebral discs. *North Carolina Med. J.* 2:655, 1941.

Young B.R., Scott M.: Air myelography: Substitution of air for Lipiodol in roentgen visualization of tumors and their structures in spinal canal. *Am. J. Roentgenol.* 39:187, 1938.

5

Radiation Dosage in Myelography

ROHRER AND HIS CO-WORKERS at Emory University have studied the radiation dosage to various organs of the patient during Pantopaque myelography. The data were obtained by a system that recorded the fluoroscopic procedure in 58 patients undergoing myelography and in a phantom with multiple ion dosimeters. An image intensifier was always used during fluoroscopy with settings of 90 kvp at 1.5 ma and 2.0 ma. Several examiners with varying experience performed the myelograms.

Ovarian exposures varied from less than 400 mR per examination to a high of 4 R. Eighty per cent of the procedures resulted in an ovarian dose less than 2 rad, 50% in doses less than 800 mrad, and 35% in doses less than 400 mrad. In the lowest dose range, there was a somewhat greater contribution from cervical, as compared with lumbar, myelograms.

A wider range of dosage to the spleen was found. In general, the average splenic dose was greater than the average ovarian dose, and there was more uniform distribution between the cervical and lumbar examinations. Eighty-five per cent of the procedures resulted in a splenic dose less than 2 rad and 42% in doses less than 800 mrad.

The dosimeter placed in the third lumbar vertebral body recorded several doses in the 5-rad range, but the distribution appeared to reach a maximum in the neighborhood of 1 rad. Seventy-two per cent of the examinations resulted in doses less than 2 rad, and 19% in doses less than 800 mrad. Contributions from the cervical and lumbar examinations were fairly equal.

In general, there was a greater average radiation dose to the spleen and lumbar vertebrae from cervical myelography and a higher ovarian exposure during lumbar myelography. The average exposure time for the cervical examinations was longer than for lumbar myelography because of a small number of cases that required a prolonged period of study. The relatively high radiation dose to the ovaries and lumbar spine during cervical myelography is explained by the fact that these examinations were really combined cervicolumbar myelograms rather than pure cervical examinations.

On the average, large doses seem to be caused by the use of large field areas and prolonged use of the fluoroscope by inexperienced examiners.

The radiation dosage is significantly reduced in metrizamide myelography because of the shorter fluoroscopic time. I have performed complete lumbar metrizamide myelography with four oblique and two anteroposterior spot films and two lateral shoot-through radiographs with a total radiation dose of 180 mrad (1.8 mGy) to the gonads, 13 mrad (0.13 mGy) to the thyroid gland, and 566 mrad (5.7 mGy) to the active bone marrow. I have carried out metrizamide cervical myelography via the lumbar approach with a dose of 62 mrad (0.6 mGy) to the gonads, 5 mrad (0.05 mGy) to the thyroid gland, and 183 mrad (0.2 mGy) to the active bone marrow.*

BIBLIOGRAPHY

Rohrer R.H., Sprawls P., Jr., Miller W.B., Jr., Weens H.S.: Radiation doses received in myelographic examinations. *Radiology* 82:106, 1964.

---

*Measurements made by Edward V. Kennelly, M.S.

6

Roentgen Examination of the Spine

PLAIN ROENTGENOGRAMS OF THE SPINE should always be taken and carefully studied prior to myelography (Figs 6–1 to 6–4). It is important to be familiar with the many normal variants and minor anomalies affecting the spine. Thus, in the lateral roentgenograms of the cervical spine in adults with the neck flexed, the body of each vertebra is displaced slightly anteriorly with respect to the subjacent vertebra. In infants and children, this displacement may be exaggerated, particularly at the level of C2-3, so that a "step-off" of 2–3 mm at this interspace should not be mistaken for a dislocation (Fig 6–5). In children also, all of the cervical intervertebral foramina are ovoid in shape, whereas in adults the lower intervertebral foramina are shaped like the sole of a shoe. The adult intervertebral foramen at C2-3 is commonly larger than at any other level. This should not be considered abnormal unless there is evidence of bone erosion. Simple failure of segmentation is not uncommon in the cervical spine.

Minor anomalies of the thoracic spine are less frequent, except for the variant of eleven rib-bearing thoracic vertebrae associated with six non-rib-bearing vertebrae of the lumbar type. The fifth lumbar vertebra is a common site for variations. Thus, instead of being vertically oriented, the facets of L-5 may lie in a coronal or oblique plane. Furthermore, the disposition of these facets may not be symmetric bilaterally. One or both transverse processes of L-5 may be sacralized, or the first sacral segment may be lumbarized. Incomplete bony fusion of the neural arch of L-5 and S-1 or S-2 is quite common. Although spina bifida usually exists alone as a bony defect without accompanying anomalies of the spinal cord or its membranes, varying forms of myelodysplasia (e.g., meningocele, meningomyelocele, etc.) may accompany it. In some instances, a congenital dermoid tumor of the spinal cord or cauda equina may be associated with spina bifida occulta. Defects in the pars interarticularis most commonly involve L-5 and may be unilateral or bilateral (spondylolysis). Anterior displacement of one vertebral body relative to another (spondylolisthesis) may occur with or without spondylolysis (Fig 6–6). In the latter circumstance, the displacement is due to degenerative changes in the zygapophyseal joints with loss of articular cartilage and subchondral sclerosis. Consequently, there is excessive forward motion of the vertebra. As a result of the forward slipping

73

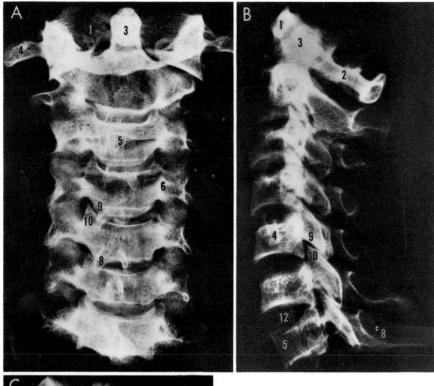

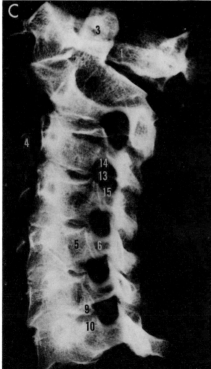

Fig 6–1,—Radiographs of dried specimen of the cervical spine. **A,** anteroposterior; **B,** lateral; **C,** oblique.

Key for Figs 6–1 through 6–4.—*1,* Anterior arch of atlas; *2,* posterior arch of atlas; *3,* dens; *4,* transverse process; *5,* body; *6,* pedicle; *7,* lamina; *8,* spinous process; *9,* inferior articular process; *10,* superior articular process; *11,* pars interarticularis; *12,* intervertebral disk; *13,* intervertebral foramen; *14,* superior vertebral notch; *15,* inferior vertebral notch; *16,* anterior tubercle; *17,* cross-section of opposite lamina, *18,* foramen transversarium; *19,* superior articular facet; and *20,* vertebral foramen.

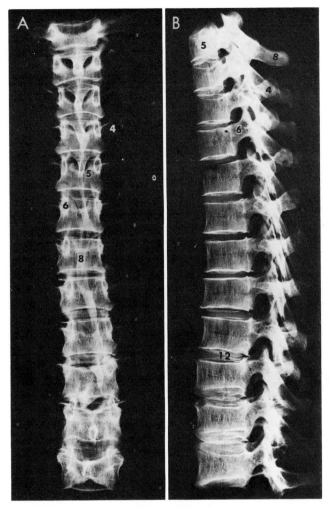

Fig 6–2.—Radiographs of dried specimen of the thoracic spine. **A,** anteroposterior; **B,** lateral.

of the pedicles, superior articular processes, and the vertebral body, there is narrowing of the involved invertebral foramen, which may produce nerve root compression. There may or may not be associated herniation of the intervertebral disk. Hypoplasia of a lumbar vertebral body resulting in a short sagittal diameter should not be mistaken for true spondylolisthesis.

In 1934, Elsberg and Dyke published data on normal adult measurements of the interpediculate distances of the spine in the anteroposterior projection (Fig 6–7). These measurements, which are applicable with a target-film distance of 36–40 inches, should be made from the most medial border of the pedicles. Schwarz introduced a graph with a family of curves for the maximal predicted width of the spinal canal related to age (Fig 6–8). Schwarz's data indicate that the various segments of the spine grow at different rates, with minimal growth at T-4 and maximal growth at S-1. Growth of the spinal canal stops at approximately 18–25 years of age. These graphs are best utilized if the interpediculate measurements are charted

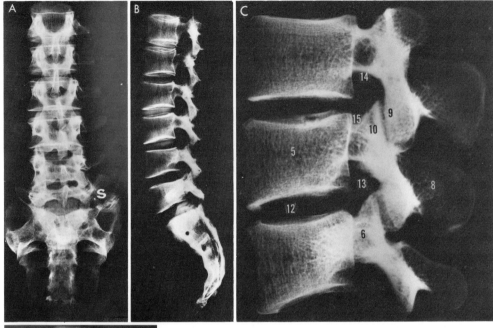

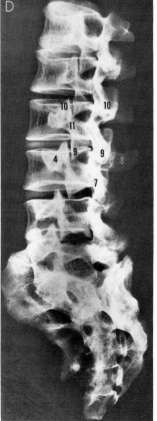

Fig 6–3.—Radiographs of dried specimen of the lumbosacral spine. **A,** anteroposterior; **B** and **C,** lateral; **D,** oblique. Note the six presacral, non-rib-bearing vertebrae with unilateral sacralization of the transverse process of the last vertebra *(S)*.

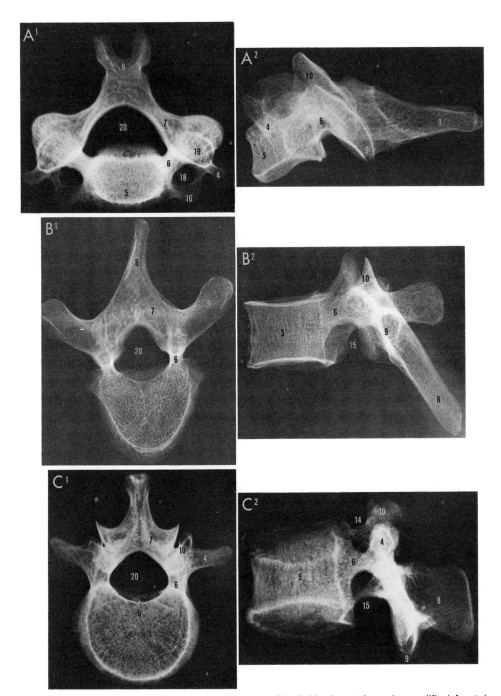

Fig 6–4.—Radiographs of dried specimens of individual vertebrae in modified frontal and lateral projections demonstrating detailed anatomical features. **A,** cervical; **B,** thoracic; **C,** lumbar.

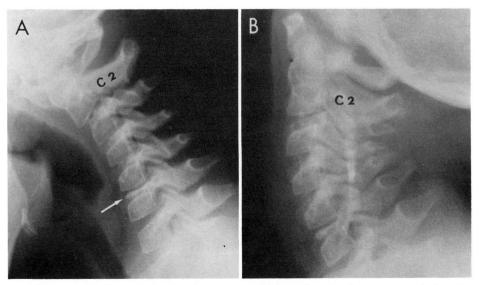

Fig 6–5.—Lateral cervical spine in a 4-year-old boy. **A,** note the normal anterior displacement of C-2 on C-3 in flexion and, **B,** the straight alignment of the vertebrae in extension. There is a calcified intervertebral disk at C5-6 *(arrow)*.

on paper, the points connected by straight lines, and a curve derived for the particular spine under study. Some lack of parallelism between the patient's curve and the predicted curve is not abnormal per se. A more important indication of an intraspinal lesion is an abnormal trend of the patient's curve in a direction opposite to that of the predicted curve. An abrupt change in measurement at successive vertebral levels is also significant.

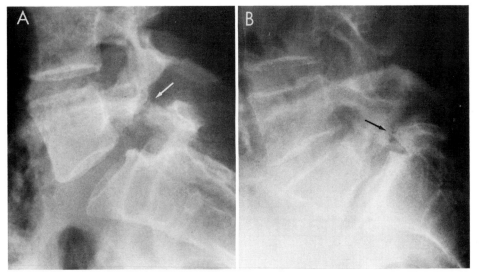

Fig 6–6.—Lateral radiographs demonstrating varying degrees of spondylolisthesis at L5-S1 in two patients. **A,** slight; **B,** marked. The bony defects in the pars interarticularis are identified by arrows.

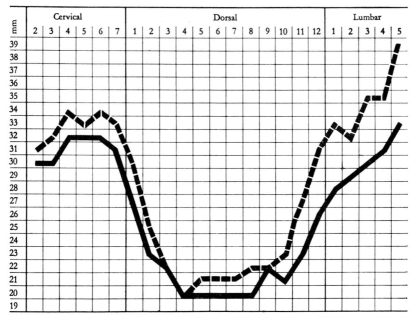

Fig 6–7.—Diagram of the spinal interpediculate distances (after Elsberg and Dyke); the broken line indicates the extreme upper limits, and the continuous line the usual upper limits of normalcy.

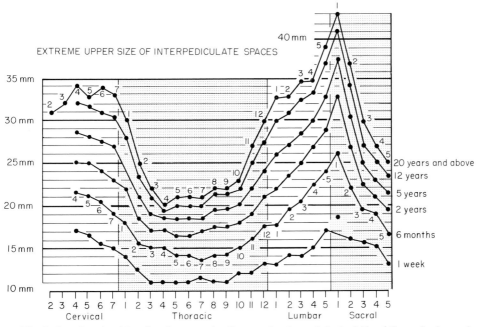

Fig 6–8.—Graph of family of curves for the maximal predicted width of the spinal canal. (Reprinted by permission of Charles C Thomas, Publisher, and G. S. Schwarz, *Am. J. Roentgenol.* 76:479, 1956.)

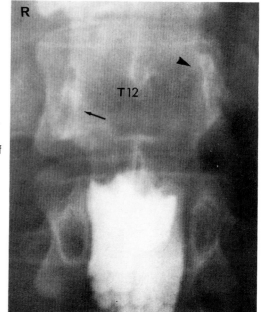

Fig 6–9.—Myelogram of a 50-year-old male with an intradural neurilemoma. Note loss of definition of the right pedicle *(arrow)* and erosion of the left pedicle of T-12 *(arrowhead).*

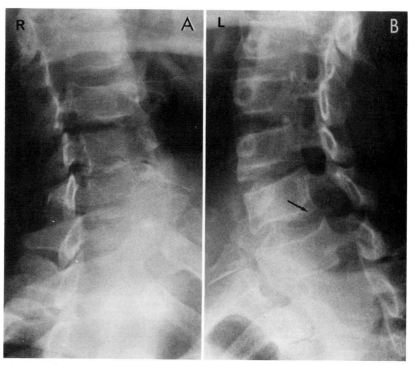

Fig 6–10.—Oblique views of the cervical spine in a patient with a dumbbell neurilemoma: **A,** normal right side; **B,** abnormal left side with enlargement of the intervertebral foramen at C7-T1 *(arrow).*

Although the Elsberg-Dyke chart and its modifications are helpful, there are a number of inherent imprecisions. The gamut of normalcy is great, the measurements involve only one diameter of the spinal canal, and the pedicles may be difficult to visualize (particularly in the cervical region). In my experience, changes in the bony structure of the pedicles and the vertebral canal frequently are more valuable in the early recognition of an intraspinal lesion. The first bone change that can be appreciated is erosion of the medial margin of one or more pedicles (Fig 6–9). As an intraspinal mass grows, particularly if growth is slow over a long period of time, pressure erosion and widening of the vertebral canal may occur, with scalloping of the posterior margins of one or more vertebrae and thinning of the pedicles and laminae (Figs 6–10 and 6–11). According to Camp et al., approximately 30% of intraspinal lesions produce bony changes that are roentgenologically demonstrable. Calcification in intraspinal lesions is uncommon and likely to be associated with meningioma or a herniated disk fragment (Fig 6–12). It is extremely rare in neurilemomas (Fig 6–13).

Haun, and Newmark et al. have called attention to calcification in the tendon of the longus colli muscle secondary to inflammation, i.e., peritendinitis. Characteristically, the calcification lies anterior to the spine, below the anterior arch of C-1.

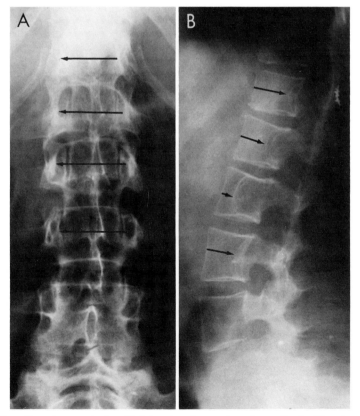

Fig 6–11.—A, anteroposterior, **B,** lateral radiographs of a patient with a long-standing ependymoma of the conus medullaris and cauda equina, demonstrating marked scalloping of the posterior margins of the vertebrae and widening of the spinal canal *(arrows).*

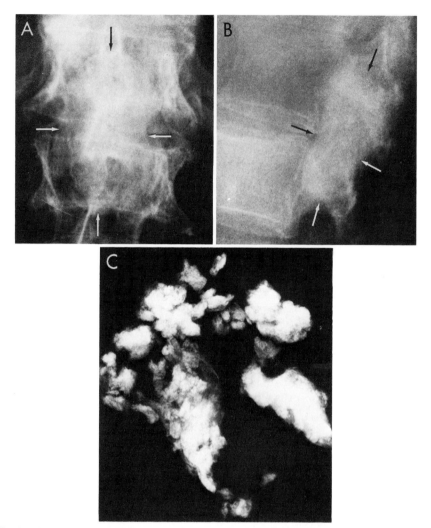

Fig 6–12.—A, anteroposterior, **B,** lateral radiographs of the thoracolumbar region of the spine in a middle-aged female with a large intraspinal meningioma. Note the massive calcification in the films of the spine *(arrows)* (**A** and **B**) and in the postoperative specimen **(C).**   *(Continued.)*.

During the inflammatory process, there may be associated swelling of the prevertebral soft tissues from C-1 through C-4 (Fig 6–14). This should not be confused with the congenital small ossicle that lies below the anterior arch of C-1 and has a well-defined cortical rim. It should also not be confused with an old hyperextension fracture of the anterior arch of the atlas.

Benzian et al. have pointed out that localized unilateral or bilateral flattening of the pedicles may occur as a normal variant (7%) at the thoracolumbar junction, i.e., T-12, L-1. The involved pedicle is thinner than normal, with a flat or concave lateral border; the medial border may be convex, straight, or, less commonly, concave. Differentiation from an expanding intraspinal mass is facilitated by (1) the presence of intact cortical margins, (2) a normal interpediculate distance, (3) a con-

D

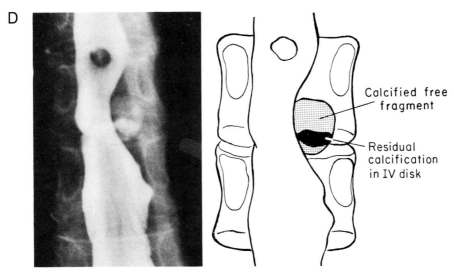

Calcified free
fragment

Residual
calcification
in IV disk

Fig 6–12 (cont.).—D, anteroposterior spot film of a different patient made during myelography, demonstrating a defect of the Pantopaque column on the left side in the midthoracic region. Note the calcification in the disk space and the large, round, calcified
density representing a free disk fragment in the spinal canal (retouched).

vex medial border with a concave lateral border, (4) the absence of erosion of the
posterior aspect of the vertebral body (Fig 6–15).

Erosion of one or more cervical pedicles with enlargement of the corresponding
intervertebral foramina can be produced by tortuosity of the vertebral artery. The
bone defect may range from subtle erosion of the posterolateral aspect of the vertebral body to complete erosion of the pedicle (Fig 6–16). The cases reported in
the literature have been predominantly on the left side at the level of C-4 in middle-aged or elderly patients. Because the tortuous artery loops anteromedially and
superiorly, the foraminal enlargement tends to be in the same direction and less
symmetric than in neurogenic tumors. This is helpful in differential diagnosis. Enlargement of the cervical intervertebral foramina has also been reported in hypertrophic interstitial polyneuritis (Dejerine-Sottas disease).

Pedicular erosion should not be confused with congenital hypoplasia of a pedicle
associated with underdevelopment of the corresponding lamina (Fig 6–17). The
presence of the sharp, white cortical line around the pedicle, along with the well-
defined absence of part or all of the ipsilateral lamina, will establish the correct
diagnosis. The findings can be confirmed by body section radiography. Unilateral
aplasia or hypoplasia of a pedicle may be associated with sclerotic hypertrophy of
the contralateral arch. This combination frequently produces rotational instability.
The clue to the correct diagnosis is the tilt of the spinous process toward the side
of the defect, along with asymmetry of the pedicles and arches. These changes
should readily differentiate this condition from old fracture (Fig 6–18). One may
also find sclerosis of a pedicle on the side opposite a unilateral defect of the pars
interarticularis, at times associated with some scoliosis. Presumably, the sclerosis is
the result of an effort to compensate for the shift in weight bearing. This can be
differentiated from osteoid osteoma of the pedicle by demonstrating the contralateral spondylolysis and by the absence of a "nidus" on body section radiography.
Both conditions may be associated with a positive bone scan.

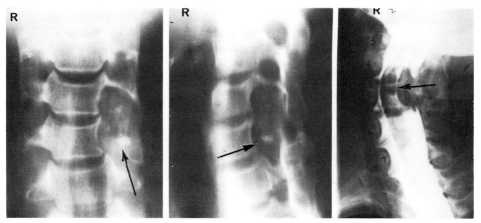

Fig 6–13.—Gross calcification in a large neurilemoma at C-4 and C-5 in a 49-year-old woman. This is the only case of gross calcification in a neurilemoma that I have seen. The anteroposterior and oblique tomograms show the calcification *(arrow)* and the markedly enlarged left C-4 and C-5 intervertebral foramina. The myelogram demonstrates cord displacement to the right *(arrow)* by the intradural extramedullary tumor lying on the left posterolateral surface of the cord.

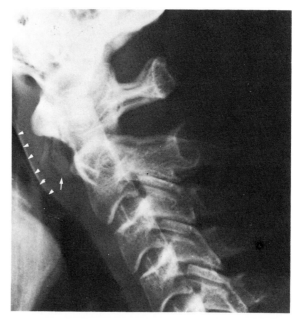

Fig 6–14.—The patient, a 42-year-old male, complained of increasing neck pain over several days. The pain was increased by cervical motion and not relieved by over-the-counter analgesics. Physical examination revealed some spasm and tenderness in the region of the anterior neck muscles. Note the prevertebral soft tissue swelling *(arrowheads)* and the characteristic amorphous calcification *(arrow)* just below the anterior arch of C-1 in the tendon of the longus colli muscle.

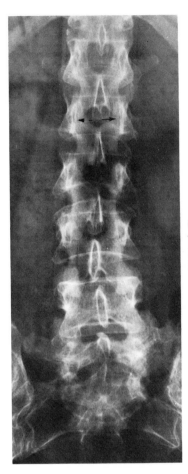

Fig 6–15.—Normal thinning of the pedicles of L-1 in a patient with six presacral non-rib-bearing vertebrae. Note the straight, flat medial and lateral borders of the pedicles as well as their intact cortical margins (arrows).

I have seen a number of patients with advanced disk degeneration or Schmorl's node accompanied by marked sclerosis of the adjacent vertebral bodies. This should not be confused with osteoblastic metastases. The salient differential features are (1) a tendency for the bony sclerosis to fade off with increasing distance from the abnormal disk space and (2) marked narrowing of the intervertebral disk space, frequently with intradiskal gas, between two sclerotic vertebrae (Fig 6–19).

Developmental enlargement of the spinal canal may occur in the absence of an intraspinal lesion. This was pointed out as early as 1944 by Walker, and re-emphasized by Jefferson in 1955 (Fig 6–20). At times, enlargement of the spinal canal may be associated with a congenital abnormality of the spinal cord, in the absence of an intraspinal neoplasm. Presumably, the spinal canal enlargement occurs during development of the vertebrae. It is important, therefore, not to make an unequivocal diagnosis of an expanding intraspinal mass solely on the presence of a wide canal, if the bony margins of the canal, the pedicles, and the posterior aspects of the vertebral bodies are intact. Rarely, long-standing chronic, increased intracranial pressure can produce enlargement of the spinal canal and scalloping of the posterior aspects of the vertebral bodies. Hence, the finding of an enlarged bony canal should prompt radiographic examination of the skull (Fig 6–21). In this regard, it is inter-

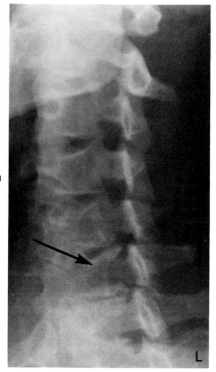

Fig 6–16.—Asymmetric erosion of the anteromedial aspect of the left C-6 foramen by a tortuous vertebral artery in a 67-year-old male.

esting that patients with Ehlers-Danlos and Marfan's syndromes may have enlargement of the spinal canal in one or both diameters as an expression of the diffuse connective tissue defect, along with narrowing of the pedicles and a concave appearance of the posterior aspect of the vertebral bodies (Fig 6–22). However, the well-defined cortical outlines of the pedicles and the vertebral bodies are pre-

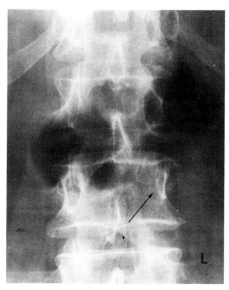

Fig 6–17.—Anteroposterior roentgenogram demonstrating hypoplasia of left pedicle of L-2 with failure of development of the lateral portion of the lamina *(arrow)*. Note the intact cortex. The findings were confirmed by oblique films and body section radiography.

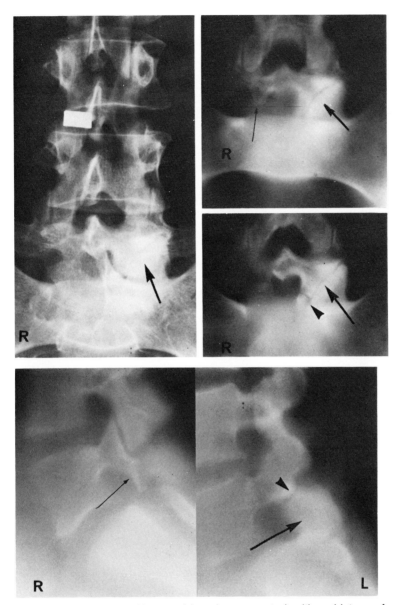

Fig 6–18.—The patient, a 40-year-old male, presented with a history of previous trauma and low back pain upon arising in the morning. He was sent to the emergency department with a diagnosis of a fracture of L-5, based upon radiographs made elsewhere. The anteroposterior plain radiographs and tomographic sections *(top)* clearly show hypoplasia of the right inferior articular process of L-5 *(thin arrow),* and marked sclerotic hypertrophy of the contralateral inferior articular process of L-5 and superior articular process of S-1 *(thick arrow).* Note the slight rotation of the spinous processes to the right. There is also an associated bifid left inferior articular process or stress fracture *(arrowhead).* The lateral tomograms *(bottom)* clearly show the hypoplastic right inferior articular process of L-5 *(thin arrow)* and marked hypertrophy of the left inferior articular process *(thick arrow)* with an associated defect of the isthmus *(arrowhead).*

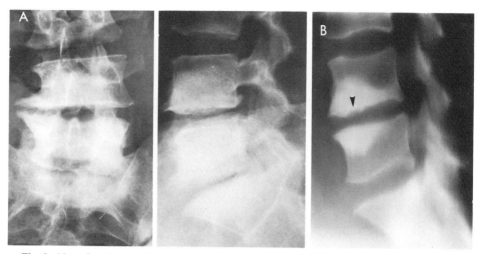

Fig 6–19.—**A,** advanced degenerative disk disease at L4-5 and to a greater extent at L5-S1. Note the pronounced sclerosis of the body of L-5, the inferior margin of the body of L-4, and the superior aspect of S-1. Note also the gas in the narrowed lumbosacral disk space. **B,** striking sclerosis of the vertebral bodies at L4-5 associated with disk degeneration and Schmorl's nodes *(arrowhead).* Note that the sclerosis tails off at the upper half of L-4 and the lower half of L-5, i.e., with increasing distance from the involved disk space.

served. Scalloping of the posterior surfaces of the vertebral bodies may also occur as a developmental anomaly in neurofibromatosis (Fig 6–23). In these patients, diffuse scalloping is due to dural ectasia and not to erosion by an intraspinal tumor.

Scalloping of the vertebral bodies also occurs as a normal variant (Fig 6–24), in mucopolysaccharide disorders (Morquio, Hurler syndromes), and in achondroplasia (Fig 6–25).

Generalized narrowing of the spinal canal is also present in achondroplastic dwarfs (Fig 6–25). These patients have an inherent defect in enchondral ossification. The vertebral bodies are diminished in height because of interference with normal longitudinal growth at the epiphyseal plates and exhibit enlargement and mushrooming of their cranial and caudal surfaces. In addition, premature fusion of the cartilaginous neurocentral synchondroses interferes with growth of the neural arch. The associated increased periosteal bone formation produces thickening of the pedicles and laminae. Often the intervertebral disks demonstrate generalized bulging. Approximately one third of these patients have a thoracolumbar kyphosis with localizing vertebral wedging (one or more vertebrae from T-11 to L-2) at the apex of the kyphotic curve. The effect of these abnormalities is to decrease the size of the spinal canal. Since growth of the spinal cord and the cauda equina is not impaired, these structures become crowded in their greatly reduced bony casing. It is interesting that many of these patients have no neurologic difficulty until a herniated disk or spondylosis intervenes. Acute herniation of a lumbar disk may lead to an acute cauda equina syndrome. Chronic disk herniation and spondylosis tend to produce a chronic cauda equina syndrome. Progressive paraparesis may also be associated with the thoracolumbar kyphosis.

Reduction in size of the spinal canal, usually in the sagittal diameter, may occur

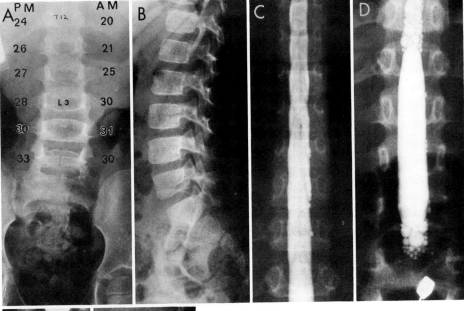

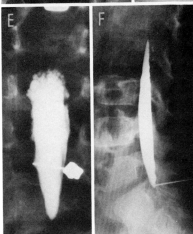

Fig 6–20.—The patient, a 5-year-old girl, had had a spastic paraplegia since birth due to cerebral palsy. Radiography of the spine at another institution (**A** and **B**) showed widening of the interpediculate measurements at L-3. *AM* refers to actual measurements. *PM* to predicted measurements. Myelography was suggested because of the suspicion of an intraspinal tumor. **C-F,** examination of the entire subarachnoid space was negative. This is an example of a normal variation in the size of the spinal canal.

particularly in the thoracic and lumbar regions in the absence of any other congenital lesion. In addition, localized narrowing of the canal may result from enlargement of an articular process or pedicle in the lumbar region. This will be considered more fully in the section dealing with spondylosis.

Burrows, Boijsen, Payne and Spillane, and Wolf and his associates studied the sagittal diameter of the normal spinal canal in the cervical region (Table 6–1). Burrows used a standard lateral radiograph of the cervical spine with the patient sitting upright and a focus-grid distance of 72 inches (magnification with a 40-inch distance is approximately 2 mm). The bony landmarks used for measurement were (1) the middle of the posterior surface of the vertebral body and (2) the closest point on the cortical line marking the fusion of the corresponding laminae and spinous process (Fig 6–26). The measurements were not influenced by position of the head or

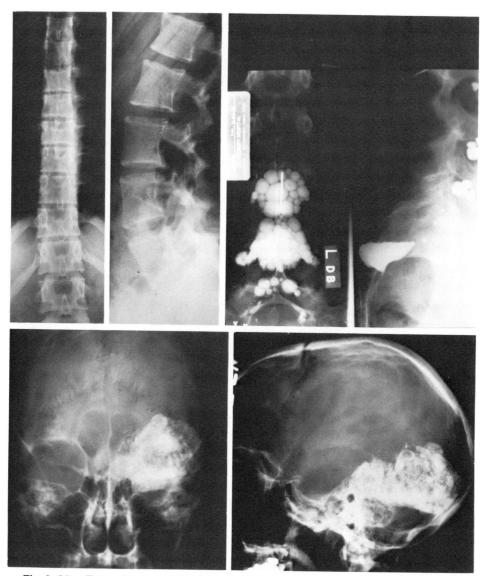

Fig 6–21.—Top, widening of the interpediculate distances, scalloping of the vertebral bodies, and dural ectasia in an 18-year-old girl with chronic increased intracranial pressure due to a large calcified left occipital tumor (? angiolipoma). **Bottom,** note the spreading of the coronal sutures, as well as the secondary sella. (Courtesy of A. Youngberg.)

neck and there was no significant sex difference. As might be expected, there was a significant individual variation. Nonetheless, a sagittal diameter of the cervical spinal canal less than 12 mm should be viewed with suspicion in a patient with appropriate neurologic findings. The truly narrow canal can be recognized by inspection because the articular pillars overlap the vertebral bodies to a greater degree than normally, i.e., normally, the articular pillars lie considerably anterior to the posterior wall of the bony canal.

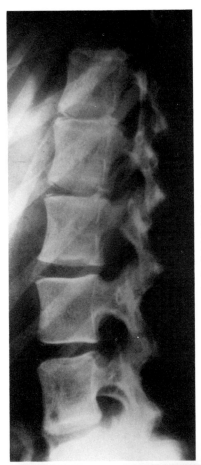

Fig 6–22.—Lateral radiograph of the lumbar spine in a patient with Marfan's syndrome demonstrating enlargement of the spinal canal. Note the normal cortical margins of the canal and of the vertebral bodies. **B,** young woman with Marfan's syndrome. Note the tall thoracic vertebrae with enlargement of the spinal canal *(1)*, and excavation of the posterior surface of L-5 *(arrowhead) (2)*, due to diffuse dural ectasia *(3)*.

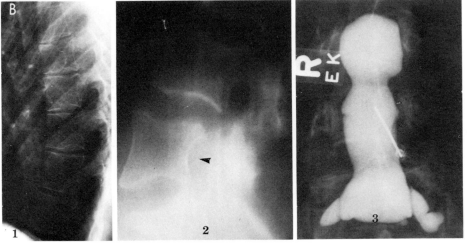

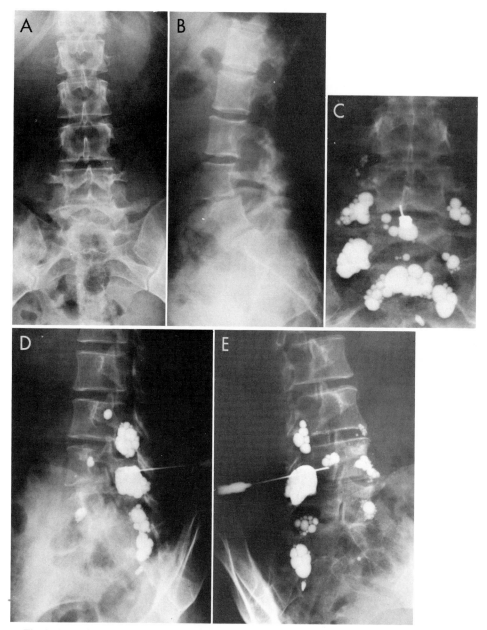

Fig 6–23.—Scalloping of the vertebrae and thinning of the pedicles due to dural ectasia in a 31-year-old woman with generalized neurofibromatosis. (Courtesy of A. Grugan.)

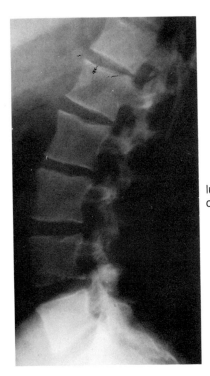

Fig 6–24.—Physiologic scalloping of the lumbar vertebral bodies in a normal 30-year-old male.

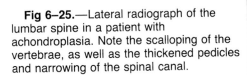

Fig 6–25.—Lateral radiograph of the lumbar spine in a patient with achondroplasia. Note the scalloping of the vertebrae, as well as the thickened pedicles and narrowing of the spinal canal.

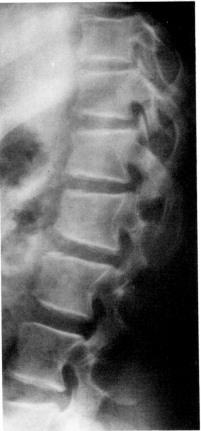

TABLE 6–1.—NORMAL RANGE OF VARIATIONS*

AUTHOR	FOCUS FILM DISTANCE (IN.)	MEASUREMENTS (MM)						
		C-1	C-2	C-3	C-4	C-5	C-6	C-7
Boijsen	59.9	19–32	16–27	15–25	14–24	14–23	14–23	14–23
Wolf et al.	72	16–30	15–27	13–22	13–22	12–21	13–22	12–22
Payne and Spillane	72	16–26	15–23	12.5–22	12–20	12–22	11–20	11–20
Burrows	72	16–27	15–25	12–23	12–22	12–22	12–21	12–21
		(av. 22.9)	(av. 20.3)	(av. 18.5)	(av. 17.7)	(av. 17.7)	(av. 17.5)	(av. 17.3)

*After Burrows.

Hinck, Hopkins, and Savara made similar measurements in 48 children with a target-midsagittal distance of 5 feet but were unable to measure C-6 and C-7 adequately (Table 6–2).

In general, the cervical bony canal is disproportionately wide in children. Hence, Yousefzadeh et al. suggest that relative widening of the lower cervical canal per se in asymptomatic children without clinical findings does not warrant further investigation.

The posterior paraspinal line is a linear density paralleling the left side of the thoracic spine in patients with a left descending aorta. It extends from T-4 to T-11 or T-12. It is produced by the interface of the water-density paravertebral soft tissues and the contiguous air-containing lung (Fig 6–27). The paraspinal line is medial to the descending thoracic aorta. Normally, there is no posterior paraspinal line on the right because of obliquity of the posteromedial border of the right lung. Many pathologic processes can produce lateral deviation of the posterior paraspinal line, including granulomas, abscess, and tumor.

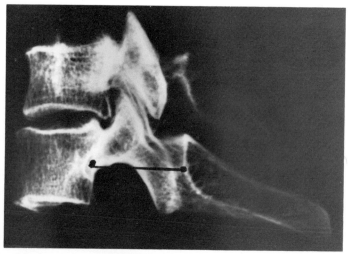

Fig 6–26.—Lateral view of dried specimen of the sixth and seventh cervical vertebrae, demonstrating the bony landmarks for measurement of the sagittal diameter of the spinal canal.

TABLE 6–2.—Sagittal Diameter Measurements
of Cervical Spinal Canal in Normal Children*

| LEVEL | AGE (YRS) | MEAN (MM) | 90% TOLERANCE RANGE | |
			Lower Limit	Upper Limit
C-2	3	17.2	14.0	20.4
	8	17.8	14.6	21.0
	13	18.6	15.4	21.8
	18	19.4	16.2	22.6
C-3	3	15.0	12.0	18.0
	8	15.8	12.8	18.8
	13	16.6	13.6	19.6
	18	17.3	14.3	20.3
C-4	3	14.8	11.9	17.7
	8	15.6	12.7	18.5
	13	16.3	13.4	19.2
	18	17.1	14.2	20.0
C-5	3	15.0	12.3	17.7
	8	15.6	12.8	18.3
	13	16.1	13.3	18.8
	18	16.7	13.9	19.4

*After Hinck et al., 1962.

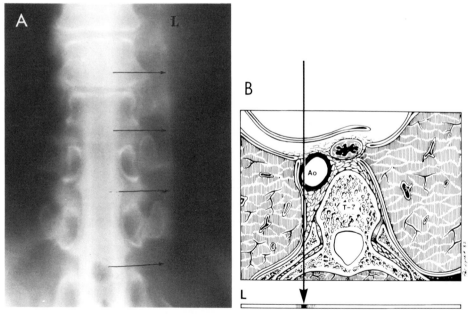

Fig 6–27.—A, AP tomogram of thoracic spine demonstrating a normal left paraspinal line *(arrows)* in a patient who had a metrizamide myelogram. **B,** diagram of axial section at level of T-7, demonstrating the posteromedial margin of the left lung forming the paraspinal line.

BIBLIOGRAPHY

Anderson R.E., Shealy C.: Cervical pedicle erosion and rootlet compression caused by tortuous vertebral artery. *Radiology* 96:537, 1970.

Benzian S.R., Mainzer F., Gooding C.A.: Pediculate thinning: A normal variant at the thoracolumbar junction. *Br. J. Radiol.* 44:936, 1971.

Boijsen E.: The cervical spinal canal in intraspinal erosive processes. *Acta Radiol.* 42:101, 1954.

Burrows E.H.: The sagittal diameter of the spinal canal in cervical spondylosis. *Clin. Radiol.* 14:77, 1963.

Camp J.D., Adson A.W., Shugrue J.J.: Roentgenographic findings associated with tumors of spinal column, spinal cord and associated tissues. *Am. J. Cancer* 17:348, 1933.

Duvoisin R.C., Yahr M.D.: Compressive spinal cord and root syndromes in achondroplastic dwarfs. *Neurology* 12:202, 1962.

Elsberg C.A., Dyke C.G.: Diagnosis and localization of tumors of the spinal cord by means of measurements made on x-ray films of vertebrae, and the correlation of clinical and x-ray findings. *Bull. Neurol. Inst., New York* 3:359, 1934.

Haun C.L.: Retropharyngeal tendinitis. *A.J.R.* 130:1137, 1978.

Haworth J.B., Keillor G.W.: Use of transparencies in evaluating the width of the spinal canal in infants, children and adults. *Radiology* 79:109, 1962.

Hinck V.C., Hopkins C.E., Savara B.S.: Diagnostic criteria of basilar impression. *Radiology* 76:572, 1961.

Hinck V.C., Hopkins C.E., Savara B.S.: Sagittal diameter of the cervical spinal canal in children. *Radiology* 79:97, 1962.

Jefferson A.: Localized enlargement of the spinal canal in the absence of tumour: A congenital abnormality. *J. Neurol., Neurosurg. Psychiatr.* 18:305, 1955.

Leeds N.E., Jacobson H.G.: Plain film examination of the spinal canal. *Sem. Radiol.* 7:179, 1972.

Lombardi G., Morello G.: Rare causes of enlargement of the spinal canal. *Acta Radiol.* 50:230, 1958.

McRae D.L.: The significance of abnormalities of the cervical spine. *Am. J. Roentgenol.* 84:3, 1960.

Maldague B.E., Malghen J.J.: Unilateral arch hypertrophy with spinous process tilt: A sign of arch deficiency. *Radiology* 121:567, 1976.

Mitchell G.E., Louie H., Berne A.G.: The various causes of scalloped vertebrae with notes on their pathogenesis. *Radiology* 89:67, 1967.

Morin M.E., Palacios E.: The aplastic hypoplastic lumbar pedicle. *A.J.R.* 122:639, 1974.

Newmark H., III, Forrester D.M., Brown J.C., et al.: Calcific tendinitis of the neck. *Radiology* 128:355, 1978.

Pallis C., Jones A.M., Spillane J.D.: Cervical spondylosis: Incidence and implications. *Brain* 77:274, 1954.

Payne E.E., Spillane J.D.: Cervical spine: Anatomic-pathological study of 70 specimens (using a special technique) with reference to problem of cervical spondylosis. *Brain* 80:571, 1957.

Schechter L.S., Smith A., Pearl M.: Intervertebral disk calcification in childhood. *Am. J. Dis. Child.* 123:608, 1972.

Schreiber F., Rosenthal H.: Paraplegia from ruptured lumbar discs in achondroplastic dwarfs. *J. Neurosurg.* 9:648, 1952.

Schwarz G.S.: The width of the spinal canal in the growing vertebra with special reference to the sacrum. Maximal interpediculate distances in adults and children. *Am. J. Roentgenol.* 76:476, 1956.

Shealy C.N., LeMay M., Hadded F.S.: Posterior scalloping of vertebral bodies in uncontrolled hydrocephalus. *J. Neurol., Neurosurg. Psychiatr.* 27:567, 1964.

Simril W.A., Thurston D.: The normal interpediculate space in the spines of infants and children. *Radiology* 64:340, 1955.

Slover W.P., Kiley R.F.: Cervical vertebral erosion caused by tortuous vertebral artery. *Radiology* 84:112, 1965.

Vogl A., Osborne R.L.: Lesions of the spinal cord (transverse myelopathy) in achondroplasia. *Arch. Neurol. Psychiatr.* 61:644, 1949.

Walker A.E.: Dilatation of the vertebral canal with congenital anomalies of spinal cord. *Am. J. Roentgenol.* 52:571, 1944.

Whelan M.A., Feldman F.: The variant lumbar pedicle. *Neuroradiology* 22:235, 1982.

Wolf B.S., Khilnani M., Malis L.J.: The sagittal diameter of the bony cervical spinal canal and its significance in cervical spondylosis. *J. Mt. Sinai Hosp.* 23:283, 1956.

Yousefzadeh D.K., El-Khoury G.Y., Smith W.L.: Normal sagittal diameter and variation in the pediatric cervical spine. *Radiology* 144:319, 1982.

Zimmerman A.B., Farrell W.J.: Cervical vertebral erosion caused by vertebral artery tortuosity. *Am. J. Roentgenol.* 108:767, 1970.

7

Anatomy

EACH VERTEBRAL BODY is joined to the vertebra above and below by a fibrocartilaginous intervertebral disk. The bodies are also united by the anterior and posterior longitudinal ligaments. The former are firmly attached to the intervertebral disks and the margins of the vertebral bodies but loosely attached at the level of the bodies (Fig 7–1). The posterior longitudinal ligament is attached to the posterior surface of the vertebral bodies within the spinal canal; it is separated from the bodies at the sites of emergence of the basivertebral veins.

Each vertebra also articulates with the vertebra above and below by fairly flat articular processes. The joints formed by these articulations are covered with hyaline cartilage lined with a secretory synovial membrane. The articular cartilage itself lacks blood vessels, lymphatics, and nerves. However, the synovial membrane is supplied with a periarticular arterial plexus and accompanying lymphatics that pierce the capsule. Each vertebral arch joint is covered by a thin, loose articular capsule attached to the edges of the adjacent articular processes. The capsule is also lined by a thin synovial membrane and innervated by the posterior ramus of the spinal nerves. The branch also supplies the ligamentum flavum and the interspinous ligaments. The nerve fibers supplying the joint capsule and associated ligaments transmit pain and stretch sensation, for the most part.

The laminae and the spinous and transverse processes are connected by the ligamenta flava, supraspinous, interspinous, and intertransverse ligaments. The ligamenta flava connect the laminae of adjacent vertebrae and are thickest in the lumbar region. The supraspinous ligament, which connects the tips of the vertebral spines, is also thickest and broadest in the lumbar region. The thin interspinous ligaments connect adjacent vertebral spines, and the thin intertransverse ligaments are attached to the transverse processes of adjoining vertebrae.

The sinuvertebral nerve, a recurrent branch of each spinal nerve, traverses the intervertebral foramen to supply fibers to the articular connective tissue, periosteum, dura, and epidural vessels. The sinuvertebral nerve arises just beyond the dorsal root ganglion, passes through the superior half of the intervertebral foramen, and curves up around the base of the pedicle. It divides into superior and inferior branches near the posterior longitudinal ligament (Fig 7–2). There is probably overlap in the levels of the sinuvertebral nerve endings. Hence, accurate localization of diskogenic pain may not always be possible.

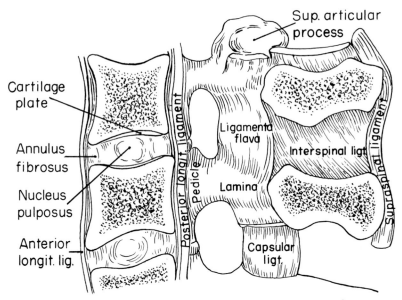

Cartilage
plate

Annulus
fibrosus

Nucleus
pulposus

Anterior
longit. lig.

Sup. articular
process

Posterior longit. ligament

Pedicle

Ligamenta
flava

Lamina

Interspinal ligt.

Supraspinal ligament

Capsular
ligt.

Fig 7–1.—Median sagittal section through midlumbar spine.

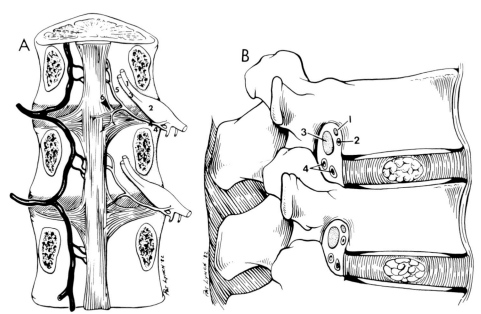

A

B

Fig 7–2.—**A,** schematic diagram of the sinuvertebral nerve and its branches (after Rothman and Simeone). *1,* dorsal root. *2,* dorsal root ganglion. *3,* ventral root. *4,* sinuvertebral nerve. *5,* superior branch. *6,* inferior branch. **B,** lateral schematic diagram demonstrating the position of the sinuvertebral nerve ventral to the spinal nerve. *1,* sinuvertebral nerve. *2,* sinuvertebral artery. *3,* spinal nerve. *4,* radicular veins.

THE SPINAL CORD AND MENINGES

THE SPINAL CORD AND MENINGES are encased in the bony vertebral canal, which begins as a large triangular structure in the cervical region. Widest at C3-5, it rapidly decreases in size to a small circular lumen throughout the thoracic area (smallest at T5-9) and enlarges again in the lumbar region (L3-S1). Throughout the cervical region, the transverse diameter of the spinal canal is almost twice the anteroposterior (sagittal) diameter. Thus, the spinal cord has ample room to expand laterally but considerably less room in the anteroposterior direction. Although the lumbar canal is usually triangular in shape, at times it may be somewhat cloverleaf-shaped or even rounded (Fig 7–3). The latter types tend to have a diminished dorsoventral diameter and narrow lateral recesses. This may be important later in life when degenerative disk disease or spondylosis further restricts the available space in the spinal canal. Anteriorly, the spinal canal is formed by the posterior surface of the vertebral bodies and the posterior longitudinal ligament. Posteriorly, the canal is capped by the ligamenta flava and the upper third of the anterior surfaces of the laminae. The lateral walls of the canal are formed by the ligamenta flava, the posterior intervertebral joints and the pedicles. The intervertebral fora-

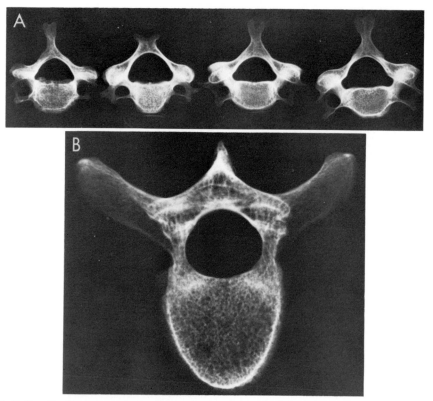

Fig 7–3.—Radiographs of dried specimens of vertebrae demonstrating variations in the shape of the spinal canal. **A,** cervical; **B,** thoracic—the round thoracic canal varies the least. *(Continued.)*

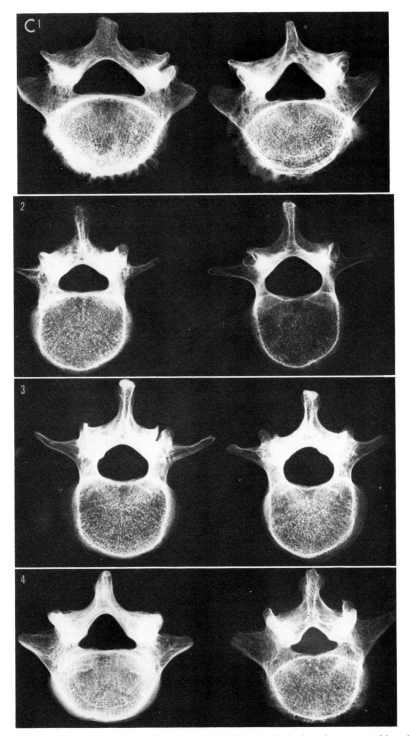

Fig 7–3 (cont.).—C, lumbar—(1) triangular; (2) rounded triangle, a transitional form between the triangular and the rounded; (3) rounded; (4) cloverleaf.

mina lie anterior to the posterior intervertebral joints below each pedicle (see Fig 7–1). The roof of the intervertebral foramen is formed by the inferior aspect of the posterior articular facet and the adjacent tip of the anterior articular facet.

The regional variations in size and shape of the vertebral canal parallel the size and shape of the spinal cord. The latter ranges from the small circular thoracic cord to the expanded cervical and lumbar segments, which give rise to the limb innervations. The cervical enlargement of the cord begins at the third cervical vertebra, is maximal at C5-6, and extends down to T1-2. From T-2 to T-10, there is a fairly uniform decrease in the caliber of the cord. The slightly smaller caudal expansion starts at the tenth thoracic vertebra and extends down to the level of L-1. The tapered conus medullaris below the end of the caudal expansion is surrounded by the nerve roots of the cauda equina. The cervical and lumbar enlargements of the spinal cord are due to an increase in the transverse diameter. The anteroposterior diameter, approximately 9–10 mm, is relatively constant throughout the entire length of the cord. Because the spinal cord follows the normal bony curvatures, it has a slight lordosis in the cervical region and a slight kyphotic curve in the midthoracic region.

Proximally, the spinal cord begins at the inferior margin of the foramen magnum, where it merges with the medulla oblongata. Distally, the termination of the cord is somewhat variable. Until the third fetal month, the spinal cord and vertebral column are equal in length. Thereafter, because the spine grows more rapidly than the cord, the lower end of the cord comes to lie opposite the third lumbar vertebra at birth (Figs 7–4, 7–5). By 4 months of age, the conus reaches the L-1 level. At 5–10 years of age, the tip of the normal conus lies above the inferior margin of L-2. By 12 years of age, the normal conus should not lie below the midbody of L-2, and the normal filum should not exceed 2 mm in diameter. Normal variations in the location of the tip of the adult conus range from T12-L1 to the inferior aspect of L-2.

The average length of the adult spinal cord from the inferior rim of the foramen magnum to the lower margin of L-1 is approximately 45 cm (normal range 40–45 cm). The conus medullaris ends in the thread-like filum terminale, which passes through the distal sacral canal to attach to the back of the coccyx. The filum terminale, surrounded by the roots of the cauda equina in its intradural portion, is approximately 15 cm long. The filum blends into the dura at the level of S-2 and continues caudally as an extradural structure to insert into the first coccygeal segment, where it fuses with the periosteum. According to Streeter, the filum terminale represents the portion of the spinal cord distal to the second coccygeal segment that has dedifferentiated into a fibrous strand.

The spinal cord is incompletely divided into symmetric halves throughout its entire length by anterior and posterior fissures. The deep anterior median fissure contains a pial fold that encloses the anterior spinal artery. The posterior median fissure is a shallower groove that also contains some blood vessels. On either side of the posterior median fissure are the posterolateral sulci marking the sites of attachment of the posterior spinal roots. The sites of attachment of the anterior spinal roots are less readily identifiable as anterolateral sulci (Figs 7–6, 7–7).

The blood supply of the spinal cord is considered in Chapter 15.

The cord is divided into segments corresponding to the attachments of the 31 pairs of spinal nerve roots (8 cervical, 12 thoracic, 5 lumbar, 5 sacral, and 1 coccy-

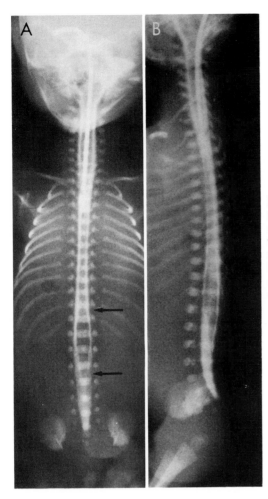

Fig 7–4.—A, anteroposterior and **B,** lateral radiographs made during myelography in newborn infant at term (stillbirth). A catheter was inserted into the cisterna magna and then into the upper cervical subarachnoid space. Note the lumbar intumescence *(arrows)* of the cord, with termination of the conus medullaris at the upper border of the fourth lumbar vertebra.

geal). The first cervical nerve emerges from the vertebral canal at the atlanto-occipital junction, and the eighth cervical nerve between the seventh cervical and the first thoracic vertebrae. Throughout the rest of the spine, each nerve emerges below the corresponding vertebra and is so designated. For instance, the eighth thoracic nerve exits below the eighth thoracic vertebra (Fig 7–8).

THE SPINAL NERVES

Each spinal nerve is formed by the union of an anterior (ventral) motor root and a posterior (dorsal) sensory root. The anterior roots contain axons of neurons in the ventral and lateral gray matter of the spinal cord. The posterior roots contain fibers that originate in the dorsal root ganglia. The anterior and posterior roots course laterally through the subarachnoid space and pierce the dura separately. Usually they fuse at, or somewhat beyond, the point where they pierce the dura in the intervertebral foramen. The individual nerve bundles fan out from the cord to converge as they pierce the dura. In the cervical region, the nerve root filaments unite

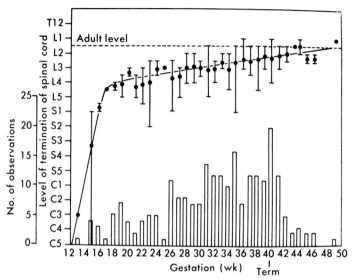

Fig 7–5.—Level of termination of the spinal cord, demonstrating migration of the conus in the pre- and postnatal periods. (From Bárson A.J.: *J. Anat.* 106:492, 1970.)

into two or more bundles before they penetrate the dura (Fig 7–9). In the thoracolumbar region, the nerve bundles join in a single trunk before piercing the dura.

The first four cervical nerves give rise to the cervical plexus, which supplies sensory and motor fibers to the back of the scalp, neck, and upper chest. The lower four cervical nerves and the first thoracic nerve unite in the axilla to form the trunks of the brachial plexus. The latter provides the sensory and motor supply to the upper extremities. The phrenic nerve, principally derived from the fourth cervical nerve, also receives some fibers from the third and fifth cranial nerves.

The thoracic roots T2-12 give rise to the intercostal nerves, which carry sympathetic and autonomic fibers as well as sensory and motor innervation to the thorax and abdomen. The first four lumbar nerves and, often, a branch from the 12th thoracic nerve unite within the psoas muscle to form the lumbar plexus. The fifth lumbar nerve fuses with a branch of the anterior ramus of the fourth lumbar nerve to form the lumbosacral trunk. The latter joins the anterior rami of the first three sacral nerves and a branch of the anterior ramus of the fourth sacral nerve to form the sacral plexus. The coccygeal plexus is formed by the fusion of the coccygeal nerve with a branch of the fourth sacral nerve and the anterior ramus of the fifth sacral nerve. The lumbar, sacral, and coccygeal plexi provide sensory and motor innervation to the lower extremities, buttocks, and genitalia.

The course of the spinal roots varies considerably at different levels because of the discrepancy between the length of the spinal cord and the bony canal (Fig 7–10). The first cervical nerve root runs a horizontal course through the subarachnoid space to exit above the lateral aspect of the atlas. The first and second cervical nerves, which have no intervertebral foramina, pass over the arches of C-1 and C-2, respectively. The posterior root of the second cervical nerve and its prominent ovoid ganglion are the largest of the cervical nerves. The points of exit of the first two cervical nerves are somewhat posterior to the sites of exit of the other cervical

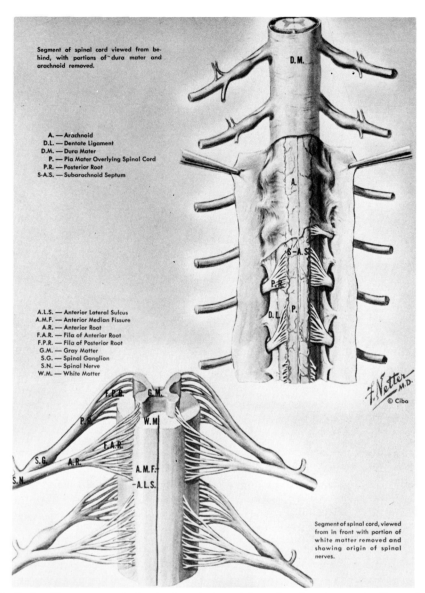

Segment of spinal cord viewed from behind, with portions of dura mater and
arachnoid removed.

A. — Arachnoid
D.L. — Dentate Ligament
D.M. — Dura Mater
P. — Pia Mater Overlying Spinal Cord
P.R. — Posterior Root
S-A.S. — Subarachnoid Septum

A.L.S. — Anterior Lateral Sulcus
A.M.F. — Anterior Median Fissure
A.R. — Anterior Root
F.A.R. — Fila of Anterior Root
F.P.R. — Fila of Posterior Root
G.M. — Gray Matter
S.G. — Spinal Ganglion
S.N. — Spinal Nerve
W.M. — White Matter

Segment of spinal cord, viewed
from in front with portion of
white matter removed and
showing origin of spinal
nerves.

Fig 7–6.—Top, segment of spinal cord viewed from the dorsal aspect with portion of the dura mater and arachnoid removed; **bottom,** segment of spinal cord viewed from the ventral aspect with portion of white matter removed, showing the origin of the spinal nerves. (Reprinted, with permission, from the Ciba Collection of Medical Illustrations by Frank H. Netter, M.D., Copyright, Ciba.)

nerves. All of the other cervical roots exit from the dura with a slight upward inclination as they course toward the intervertebral foramina. They tend to leave the intervertebral foramina fairly perpendicular to the long axis of the cord. From the eighth cervical to the midthoracic area, each root tilts downward from the cord until it approaches the dura, where it angles up quite sharply at approximately 45 degrees. In the lower thoracic and lumbar areas, the roots course inferiorly and

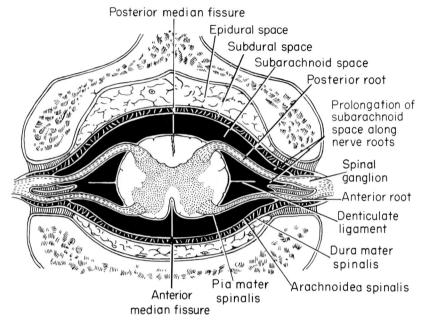

Posterior median fissure
Epidural space
Subdural space
Subarachnoid space
Posterior root

Prolongation of subarachnoid space along nerve roots

Spinal ganglion

Anterior root

Denticulate ligament

Dura mater spinalis

Pia mater spinalis

Arachnoidea spinalis

Anterior median fissure

Fig 7–7.—Diagrammatic cross section of the spinal cord.

laterally. In general, the farther one passes down the spine, the greater the slope of the nerve roots and their emerging nerves. The lowermost nerves (lumbar and sacral) pass directly downward in an almost parallel fashion to form the cauda equina around the filum terminale (Fig 7–11).

The relationship of the various segments of the cord and the nerve roots to the vertebral spinous processes is important clinically. This relationship can be best understood by referring to Figure 7–8, which shows the origin of the upper cervical nerve roots at the same level as their site of emergence from the vertebral canal. The lower the nerve root, the greater the distance between its origin from the cord and its site of exit from the vertebral canal. Thus, the relationship between the segmental level of the spinal cord and the vertebral level varies; i.e., the segmental cord level is approximately one vertebral segment cephalad in the cervical region and two to three segments cephalad in the thoracic and upper lumbar regions.

Sunderland has shown that the nerves, their meningeal sleeves, and their fibrous sheaths are freely mobile in the intervertebral foramen and can readily adjust to normal movements of the spinal column. However, the nerve complex does not have unlimited freedom of movement throughout the vertebral foramen because of continuity of the nerve sheath with the dural sac and the plugging action of the dural funnel at the foramen. In the lower cervical region, where the wide range of motion puts additional strain on cervical nerves 4, 5, 6, the latter are firmly attached to the gutters of the corresponding transverse processes. This unique arrangement is not present anywhere else in the spine, including the lumbosacral region, where stresses are dissipated over the long lengths of the lumbosacral nerves and their roots.

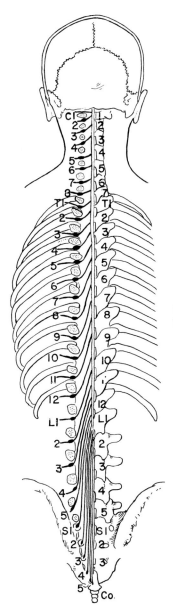

Fig 7–8.—Diagram showing the relationship of the spinal nerves to the vertebral spinous processes.

THE SUBARACHNOID SPACE

The spinal subarachnoid space filled with cerebrospinal fluid is bounded internally by the pia mater, which invests the spinal cord. Externally, it is limited by the delicate arachnoid, which, in turn, is separated from the smooth inner surface of the dura by the slit-like subdural space. Since the spinal membranes are intimately related to the cord, the shape of the subarachnoid space is determined by the configuration of the cord. Thus, the subarachnoid space is narrow and circular in the thoracic region, becoming wider and more triangular in the cervical and

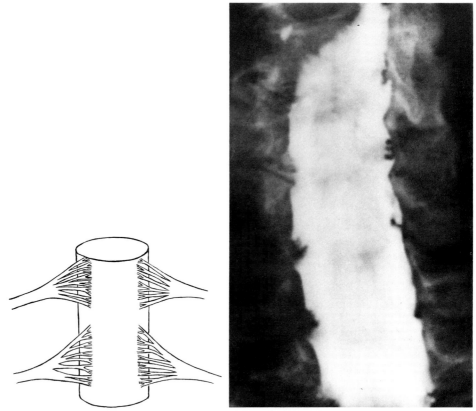

Fig 7–9.—Left, diagram illustrating coalition of multiple nerve filaments arising from the cervical cord into several individual bundles which finally unite to form a single nerve root. **Right,** radiograph demonstrating three individual nerve bundles at C-5 on the left, prior to fusing into a single root.

lumbar areas (Figs 7–12, 7–13). At the levels of the intervertebral foramina, the subarachnoid space accompanies the nerve roots laterally for a varying distance. Below the level of the cord, the subarachnoid space surrounds the cauda equina, terminating in a tip of varying length and shape. The terminal subdural space likewise varies considerably. It may be slit-like or wide, funnel-shaped, blunted, or diverticular (Fig 7–14); it may be as high as the lumbosacral interspace or as low as the fourth sacral vertebra.

The subarachnoid space is divided incompletely into anterior and posterior compartments by the thin, serrated denticulate (dentate) ligaments. These ligaments arise from the pia on either side of the cord at the level of the foramen magnum and fan out to attach to the inner surface of the dura down to the level of L-1. The ligaments are thickest in the cervical region.

The anterior subarachnoid space is a simple compartment through which nerve root bundles pass on either side of the cord as they converge to form the anterior motor roots. The latter pursue a horizontal course in the upper cervical region, passing more obliquely downward as one proceeds down the cord. The anterior subarachnoid space is widest at C-1, begins to diminish in depth at C-2, and then

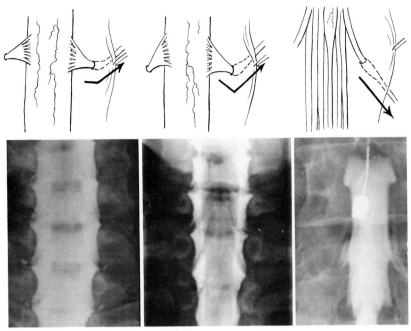

Fig 7–10.—Top, diagrams demonstrating the regional variation in the course of the spinal roots. **Bottom,** radiographs showing the varying course of the nerve roots in the cervical, thoracic, and lumbar regions.

maintains a fairly uniform caliber caudally except for gradual narrowing at the level of the lumbar enlargement of the cord. Nordqvist's data indicate no sex difference in the sagittal diameter of the subarachnoid space, except for a slight increase in the thoracic region in females in the 70–88-year age group. Nordqvist suggests that the latter difference may be due to increased osteoporosis and atrophy of the extradural tissues in these women. In patients with pronounced kyphosis, the anterior subarachnoid space in the thoracic region may be diminished because of a tendency for the spinal cord to approximate the anterior wall of the sac at the level of the maximal vertebral convexity.

The posterior subarachnoid space is divided into two compartments by the midline membranous septum posticum (Fig 7–15, A). DiChiro and Timins have pointed out that this structure consists of irregular, discontinuous bands in the upper cervical region that become thicker and fuse into a distinct membrane at the lower cervical cord level. In the thoracic and lumbar areas, the septum usually is a discrete membrane, often with irregular perforations, terminating at the conus. There is a network of arachnoid trabeculae between the septum posticum and the dentate ligaments. According to DiChiro and Timins, the septum thickens with increasing age, whereas the converse is true of the trabeculae. The arachnoidal trabecular rete should not be misinterpreted as abnormal vessels of a vascular malformation. Because of its posterior position, the septum posticum can be visualized only during myelography in the supine position. The latter is particularly useful in demonstrating (1) arteriovenous malformations, which commonly lie on the dorsal aspect of the cord, (2) dorsal arachnoidal diverticulae, (3) tumors on the dorsal

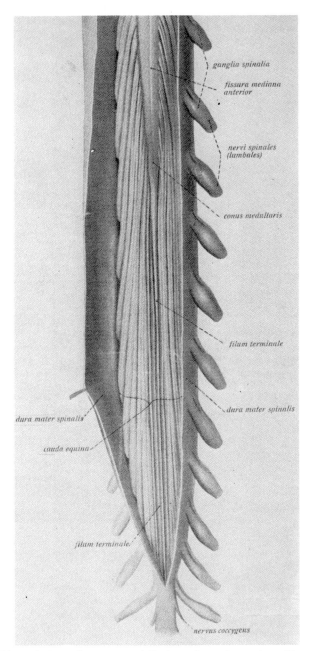

ganglia spinalia

fissura mediana anterior

nervi spinales (lumbales)

conus medullaris

filum terminale

dura mater spinalis

dura mater spinalis

cauda equina

filum terminale

nervus coccygeus

Fig 7–11.—Ventral view of conus medullaris and cauda equina. (Reprinted from Sobotta, *Atlas of Human Anatomy,* ed. 8, with permission of Hafner Publishing Company, N.Y., and Urban and Schwarzenburg, Munich.)

surface of the cord and cauda, and (4) the low position of the cerebellar tonsils in the Arnold-Chiari malformation.

The posterior subarachnoid space is not defined as clearly as its anterior counterpart because the cord tends to hug the posterior wall of the meninges, particularly in the lower thoracic region. As in the anterior subarachnoid space, the nerve root

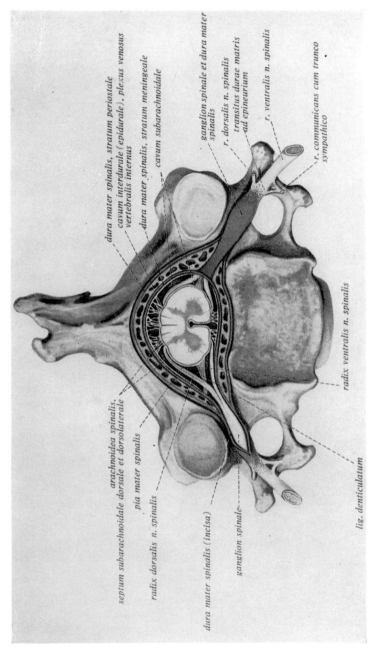

Fig 7–12.—Transverse section through the cervical spine, showing the spinal cord and its investing membranes in cross section. (Reprinted from Sobotta, *Atlas of Human Anatomy*, ed. 8, with permission of Hafner Publishing Company, N.Y., and Urban and Schwarzenburg, Munich.)

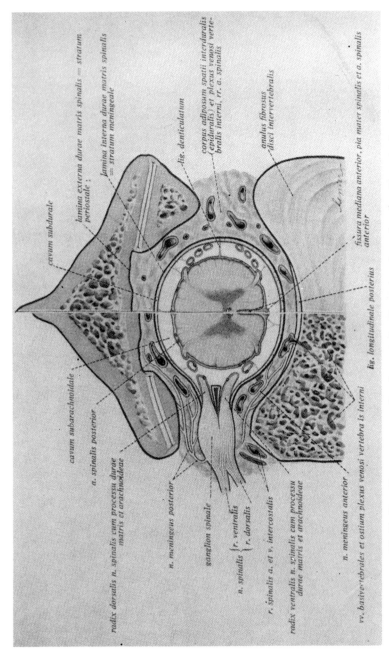

Fig 7–13.—Transverse section through the thoracic spine, showing the spinal cord and the investing membranes in cross-section. The cut is at the level of the vertebral body on the right side and at the level of the intervertebral disk on the left side. (Reprinted from Sobotta [after Fernkopf], *Atlas of Human Anatomy*, ed. 8, with permission of Hafner Publishing Company, N.Y., and Urban and Schwarzenburg, Munich.)

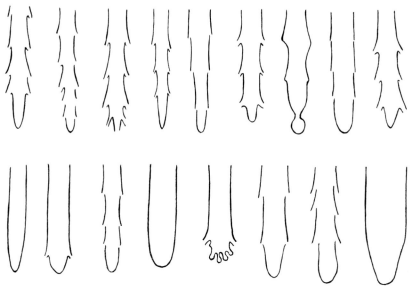

Fig 7–14.—Tracings from myelograms, illustrating the variability in termination of the caudal sac.

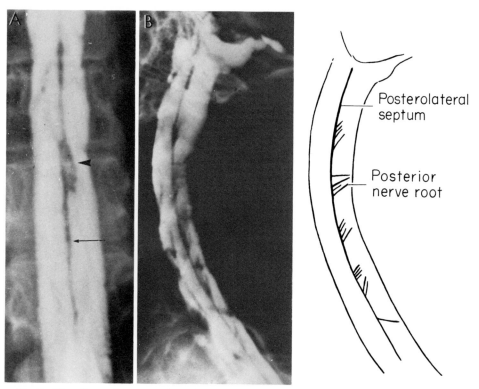

Fig 7–15.—**A,** supine normal myelogram in a 28-year-old woman showing the septum posticum *(arrow)* and trabecula *(arrowhead)* in the lower thoracic region. **B,** oblique radiograph and line drawing of a cervical myelogram demonstrating the posterior nerve roots and their origin from the posterolateral septum.

fibers also traverse the posterior space to form the posterior sensory roots on either side of the cord (Fig 7–15, *B*). The course of the posterior roots corresponds to that of the anterior roots.

THE EXTRADURAL SPACE

The dura is separated from the bony wall of the spine by the extradural (epidural) space containing fatty areolar tissue and a rich plexus of veins. Anteriorly, it is only a potential space (Fig 7–16); posteriorly, however, the extradural space is fairly deep. This relationship commonly is reversed in the lower lumbar and sacral regions. Malinowsky measured the distance between the dura and the vertebral bodies and neural arches in several sections of frozen vertebral columns. In the cervical region, he found this distance to be 1–3 mm anteriorly and 2–6 mm posteriorly, with the largest space in the midcervical region. In the thoracic region, the distances were 1–3 mm anteriorly and 2–6 mm posteriorly; in the lumbar region, 1–3 mm anteriorly and 2–7 mm posteriorly; in the sacral region, 3–5 mm both anteriorly and posteriorly. The dura itself is attached by connective tissue strands to the anterior and posterior walls of the vertebral canal, particularly at its cranial and caudal extremities. The extradural soft tissue space tends to increase in prominence as one proceeds caudad from L-1 to S-1. Indeed, at the lumbosacral level, the ventral extradural space may, at times, occupy considerably more than half of the cross-sectional area of the spinal canal.

The extradural venous plexus manifests itself indirectly at myelography under various physiologic circumstances that alter its filling. Thus, increased venous filling

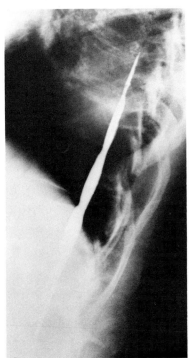

Fig 7–16.—Lateral prone radiograph of the thoracic region made with the horizontal beam during myelography. Note the close approximation of the ventral aspect of the Pantopaque column to the posterior surface of the vertebral bodies, indicating the existence of only a potential ventral extradural space.

(during deep inspiration, abdominal compression, or a modified Valsalva maneuver, i.e., coughing, straining, or retching) diminishes the available subarachnoid space, thereby narrowing and displacing the Pantopaque column craniad (Fig 7–17). Conversely, jugular compression, which diminishes the degree of filling of the extradural venous plexus, increases filling of the subarachnoid space. As a result, the Pantopaque column widens during bilateral jugular compression. Likewise, because the extradural veins are valveless and empty out in the erect position, the anterior soft tissue shadow of the extradural space is narrower in the erect, compared with the horizontal, position (Fig 7–18).

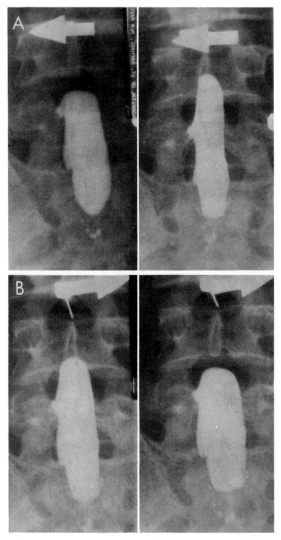

Fig 7–17.—A, lumbar myelogram with the patient in the prone position (6 ml Pantopaque). **Left,** control. **Right,** narrowing and cranial displacement of the subarachnoid space during deep inspiration. **B,** same patient. **Left,** control. **Right,** widening of the oil-filled subarachnoid space during jugular compression.

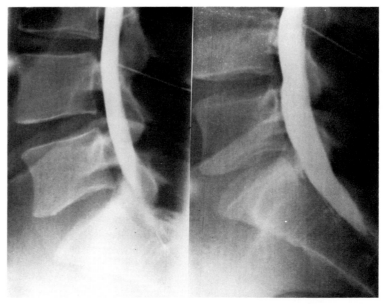

Fig 7–18.—Lateral shoot-through radiographs of lumbar myelogram. Note the closer approximation of the ventral aspect of the Pantopaque column to the posterior surface of the vertebral bodies **(right)** in the erect position compared with the prone position **(left).** This is due to the fact that the valveless extradural venous plexus empties out in the erect position and is filled when the patient is prone.

Fig 7–19.—Lateral shoot-through radiograph with the horizontal beam, showing Pantopaque in the slit-like anterior subdural space (thin white streak) and in the more ample posterior subdural space (wider collection of oil at the L4-5 level).

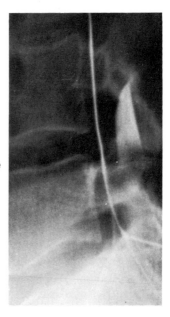

THE SUBDURAL SPACE

The spinal subdural space is only a potential space between the dura mater and the arachnoid (Fig 7–19). In essence, the dura and arachnoid are in close contact with one another. The spinal and cranial subdural spaces are continuous. The spinal dura is attached to the margins of the foramen magnum, the arches of C-1 and C-2, and the walls of the intervertebral foramina.

BIBLIOGRAPHY

Adamkiewicz A.: Die Blutgefässe der menschlichen Rückenmarksoberfläche. Sitz. Akad. Wiss. Wien, Math. Natur. Klasse 85:101, 1882.

Atkinson W.J.: Anterior-inferior cerebellar artery. *J. Neurol., Neurosurg. Psychiatr.* 12:137, 1949.

Böhmig R.: Die Blutgefässversorgung der Wirbelbandscheiben, das Verhalten des intervertebralen Chordasegments und die Bedeutung beider für die Bandscheiben Degeneration; zugleich ein Beitrag zur enchondralen Ossifikation der Wirbelkörper. *Arch. Klin. Chir.* 185:374, 1930.

Brown F.M., Aye R.C.: Myelographic demonstration of the basilar artery. *Am. J. Roentgenol.* 73:32, 1955.

Danforth M.S., Wilson P.D.: The anatomy of the lumbosacral region in relation to sciatic pain. *J. Bone Joint Surg.* 7:109, 1924.

DiChiro G., Timins E.L.: Supine myelography and the septum posticum. *Radiology* 111:319, 1974.

Dyke C.G., Deery E.M.: An observation on relationship of subarachnoidal and perineural spaces. *Bull. Neurol. Inst., New York* 1:593, 1931.

Elliott H.C.: Cross sectional diameters and areas of human spinal cord. *Anat. Rec.* 93:287, 1945.

Epstein B.S.: The effect of increased intraspinal pressure on the movement of iodized oil within the spinal canal. *Am. J. Roentgenol.* 52:196, 1944.

Frykholm R.: Deformities of dural pouches and strictures of dural sheaths in the cervical region producing nerve root compression. A contribution to the etiology and operative treatment of brachial neuralgia. *J. Neurosurg.* 4:403, 1947.

Howieson J., Norrell H.A., Wilson C.B.: Expansion of subarachnoid space in lumbosacral region. *Radiology* 90:488, 1968.

Jirout J.: Position of the lumbar intumescence of the spinal cord. *Acta Radiol. (Diagn.)* 7:509, 1968.

Joplin R.J.: Intervertebral disc. Embryology, anatomy, physiology and pathology. *Surg., Gynecol. Obstet.* 61:591, 1935.

Keegan J.J.: Relations of nerve roots to abnormalities of lumbar and cervical portions of the spine. *Arch. Surg.* 55:246, 1947.

Keyes D.C., Compere E.J.: Normal and pathological physiology of the nucleus pulposus of the intervertebral disc. *J. Bone Joint Surg.* 14:897, 1932.

Liliequist B.: Gas myelography in the cervical region. *Acta Radiol. (Diagn.)* 4:79, 1966.

Lindblom K.: The subarachnoid spaces of the root sheaths in the lumbar region. *Acta Radiol.* 30:419, 1948.

Malinowsky K.: Quoted by Nordqvist, L., *Acta Radiol.* (Suppl.) 227:85, 1964.

Nordqvist L..: The sagittal diameter of the spinal cord and subarachnoid space in different age groups. *Acta Radiol.* (Suppl.) 227, 1964.

Onofrio B.M.: Cervical spinal cord and dentate ligament delineation in percutaneous radiofrequency cordotomy at the level of the first to second cervical vertebrae. *Surg., Gynecol. Obstet.* 133:30, 1971.

Porter E.C.: Measurement of the cervical spinal cord in Pantopaque myelography. *Am. J. Roentgenol.* 76:270, 1956.

Reid J.D.: Ascending nerve roots. *J. Neurol., Neurosurg. Psychiatr.* 23:148, 1960.

Reitan H.: On movements of fluid inside the cerebrospinal space. *Acta Radiol.* 22:762, 1941.

Rothman R.H., Simeone F.A.: *The Spine.* Philadelphia, W.B. Saunders Co., 1975.

Streeter G.L.: Factors involved in the formation of the filum terminale. *Am J. Anat.* 25:1, 1919.

Sunderland S.: Meningeal-neural relations in the intervertebral foramen. *J. Neurosurg.* 40:756, 1974.

Teng, P.: Myelographic identification of the dentate ligament. *Radiology* 74:944, 1960.

Wolf B.S., Khilnani M., Malis L.I.: The sagittal diameter of the bony cervical spinal canal and its significance in cervical spondylosis. *J. Mt. Sinai Hosp.* 23:283, 1956.

8

Normal Neurovertebral Relations

Milan Roth, M.D., C.S.C.

NEURAL SUBSTANCE—THE MORPHOGENIC FACTOR IN NEUROSPINAL AND NEUROCRANIAL DEVELOPMENT

The bony and neural tissues are intimately related at the gross morphologic level from earliest development. Although this relationship is universally accepted in the head, the spinal neural contents and their bony envelope have been regarded as two completely separate structures (Fig 8–1). This may be due to the fact that the spinal column is more complex than the calvaria because of the intricate arrangement of its neural elements compared with the simple ovoid shape of the brain. The cranial and the axial skeleton both represent protective coverings for the delicate neural contents. The shape of the bony envelope in both instances is adapted to the enclosed neural structures laid down earlier. The neurospinal relationship during embryogenesis, when the primordia of the axial skeleton clearly mirror the anatomical features of the relatively huge spinal cord and ganglia (Fig 8–2,C), is vaguely mentioned by several authors (Blechschmidt, Detwiler and Holtzer, Holtzer, Töndury).

In later fetal and postnatal stages, however, the morphogenic influence of the neural contents upon the growing vertebral column has been largely ignored because spinal cord ascent has been regarded as a growth dissociation of the spinal cord and spine. After ascent, the two structures have been thought to develop independently of one another. Dissociation of spinal cord–spine growth fails to explain the intimate relationship of the "ascending cord" to the growing spine reflected by the paired spinal nerve roots angulated around the pedicles like reins (Fig 8–3).

THE PHYSIOLOGIC NEUROVERTEBRAL GROWTH DIFFERENTIAL

Neurovertebral growth dependence is significantly modified by neurovertebral growth differential. Traditionally, onset of spinal cord ascent by the end of the third

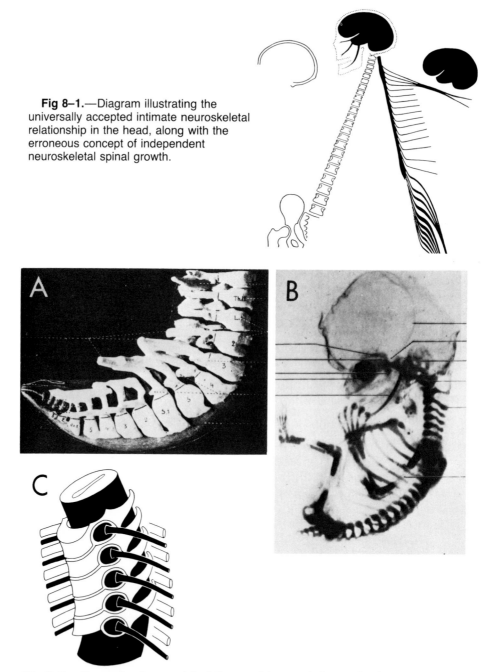

Fig 8–1.—Diagram illustrating the universally accepted intimate neuroskeletal relationship in the head, along with the erroneous concept of independent neuroskeletal spinal growth.

Fig 8–2.—Reconstruction model of the caudal part of the trunk of a 15-mm human embryo (from Holmdahl). **A,** the white structures resembling vertebrae are in fact the spinal ganglia and spinal nerves, both relatively enormous at this early period. The beginnings of the axial skeleton appear between them. The early skeleton consists essentially of neural tissue. **B,** cartilaginous skeleton of a 52-mm human fetus (from Theiler). **C,** the shape of the spinal skeletogenic envelope mirrors the gross anatomical features of the enclosed neural contents in the fetus and adult.

fetal month has been considered to be the first manifestation of a neurovertebral growth differential associated with an increasingly oblique course of the spinal nerve roots. However, obliquity of the lumbosacral nerve roots is evident as early as 7 weeks of gestation (Fig 8–3,A), i.e., prior to onset of ascent (Bardeen and Lewis, Lebedkin). This means that ascent of the cord is a phenomenon "grafted" on an already preexisting growth differential between the axial neural and bony tissues. Actually, ascent of the cord is the most conspicuous manifestation of craniocaudal developmental direction, i.e., growth in length of the vertebrate body proceeds from the head to the tail. This biologic law has for the most part been ignored in medicine. An appreciation of this law is indispensable for correct understanding of neurovertebral developmental events. Hence, diagrams illustrating

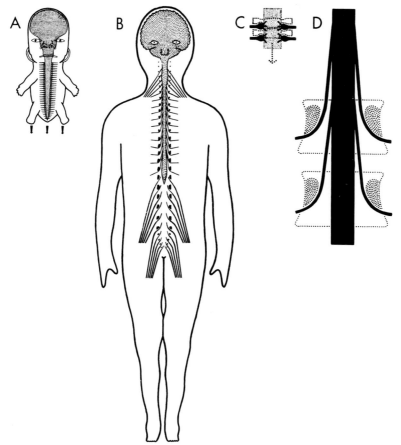

Fig 8–3.—Diagram illustrating the law of craniocaudal direction of body growth. **A,** human embryo at the end of the second month of gestation. Note the relatively enormous head and spinal cord filling the entire length of the spinal canal. The spinal nerves leave the cord at right angles (compare with **B**). The ensuing rapid growth distally is indicated by arrows. **B,** 8-year-old child showing continuing distad-directed growth of the skeleton and extensive growth of the neural structure. **C,** upper left detail from **A** demonstrates the embryonic arrangement of the relatively massive spinal cord, spinal nerves, and primitive vertebrae. The direction of growth is indicated by an arrow. **D,** the longitudinal growth of the individual vertebrae is governed by the slower growth of the rein-like arrangement of the spinal nerve roots.

these events must be placed with their upper, not lower, ends at the same level.

The neurovertebral growth disproportion is related to the following sequence: In the early embryonic period, the anlages of the intraspinal neural structures and of the axial skeleton grow by division and multiplication of neuroblasts and skeletogenic cells, i.e., by mitosis. Thus, their growth in length proceeds at the same rate, with the spinal cord occupying the entire length of the spinal canal and the spinal nerves attached to the cord at right angles (Fig 8–4). During the early weeks of development, a second type of neural growth manifests itself, i.e., growth by neural extension. At the same time, there is a decline in the rate of mitotic activity of the neuroblasts. Growth by neural extension is characterized by the formation of processes several decimeters long from a single cell body. This produces the neuron and its processes with a shape totally different from the globular shape of the original neuroblast. Growth by neural extension involves a much greater metabolic and energy requirement than mitosis (Fig 8–5). Thus, the original single mitotic type of growth of the vertebrate body changes to two types, proceeding distally side by side at different energy levels. This is the factor which appears to be responsible for neurovertebral growth differential. The obliquity of the nerve roots evident as early as the 20-mm (7-week) embryo reflects a shift of the neural primordia from the mitotic to the extension type of growth.

Ascent of the cord and formation of the cauda equina have been linked with the concept of growth passivity of the spinal neural elements. According to this erro-

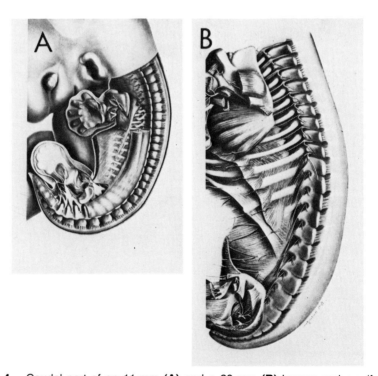

Fig 8–4.—Caudal part of an 11-mm **(A)** and a 20-mm **(B)** human embryo (from Bardeen and Lewis). The obliquity of the lumbosacral nerve roots, indicating the onset of a neurovertebral growth differential, is clearly visible in **B.** However, the spinal cord still occupies the entire length of the spinal canal.

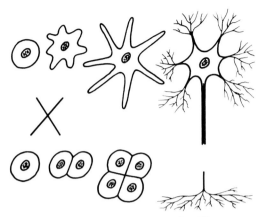

Fig 8–5.—Diagram illustrating the two fundamentally different types of growth proceeding side by side in the developing axial organ, i.e., mitotic growth of bones, and growth of the spinal cord and nerve roots by forming long processes from a single neuroblast. Because the latter type of growth requires a greater energy supply, it is more susceptible to inhibitory conditions than the mitotic type of cellular bone growth.

neous concept, the degree of longitudinal outgrowth of the nerve roots is determined by the extent of growth in length of the vertebral column. The reverse, however, is more likely to be correct in the light of what we know about similar events in the head. Growth in length of the vertebral column depends upon the growth in length potential of the cord–nerve root complex (Fig 8–6).

THE SPINE AS A WHOLE—NEUROVERTEBRAL GROWTH MECHANISM OF PHYSIOLOGIC CURVATURES

The hyperkyphotic curvature of the early embryo is attributed to the intense mitotic proliferation of neuroblasts in the relatively huge primordia of the central nervous system which are dorsal in location (see Fig 8–2,A). The latter are laid down in the hyperkyphotic curvature of the slower growing, scanty supporting tissue. With the onset of the neurovertebral growth differential, the roles become reversed. The extensively growing spinal neural structures become a retarding factor relative to the now more rapidly growing vertebral column. In so doing, they exert a "braking" effect on the spine. During the entire developmental period, the growing spine constantly encounters the resistance of the slower growing neural elements. The neural "braking" effect results in gradual straightening of the axial organ, culminating in the appearance of a lumbar lordosis in man (Fig 8–7,F). In the quadruped with its comparatively longer spinal cord–nerve root complex, the neural braking effect is less pronounced and a lumbar lordosis does not evolve (Fig 8–7,D). The physiologic thoracic kyphosis in man should be looked upon as a remnant of the primordial embryonic hyperkyphosis. The normal cervical lordosis which appears at approximately 9 weeks of gestation (Bagnall et al.) has the same relationship to neurovertebral growth disproportion as the lumbar curve.

Differences in rates of growth of body parts are an important morphogenic factor in embryology. Neurovertebral growth disproportion is a striking example of growth differential in embryonic and postnatal life which decisively influences the

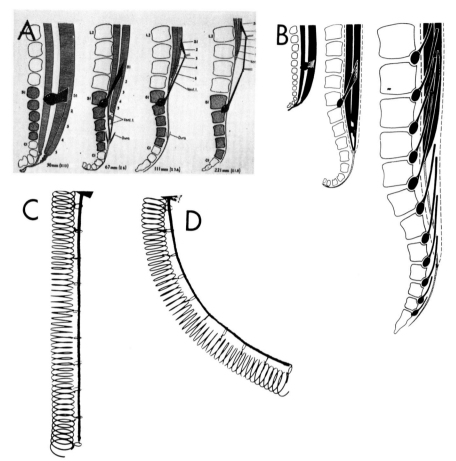

Fig 8–6.—A, the classic diagram by Streeter illustrating ascent of the spinal cord. **B,** same diagram redrawn with regard to the actual length of the individual developmental stages and to the craniocaudal neurovertebral longitudinal growth. The slower growing spinal neural structures impart a lordotic tendency to the more rapidly growing spine. **C** and **D,** a model of the neurovertebral mechanism of lumbar lordosis and hyperlordosis in man. The spring **(C)** represents the axial skeleton; and the string **(D),** the spinal neural structures, which are much larger in the embryo. With the shortening, i.e., "growth retardation" of the string relative to the spring, the latter acquires a lordotic curvature. The gross mechanistic features of the model imitate the gradual plastic adaptation of the growing axial skeleton on the normal, or the pathologically enhanced growth retardation of the spinal neural structures.

general shape of the vertebrate body. The spinal cord is the "Hauptmotor" in the development of the spine (Blechschmidt).

NEUROVERTEBRAL FEATURES OF THE INDIVIDUAL VERTEBRAE

Length and Width of the Vertebral Body

The developing axial skeleton mirrors not only the width but also the length of the enclosed neural contents. The comparatively short cord–nerve root complex in man is encased by shorter, broader vertebrae, whereas the relatively long spinal cord in the quadruped is associated with longer, more slender vertebrae (Figs 8–7,*D, E*; 8–8; 8–9). The spatial distribution of skeletogenic material, which is quantitatively fairly stable during phylogenetic development of higher vertebrates, depends upon the space available along the spinal neural structures.

Girth of the Vertebral Body

The more rapid growth in length of the vertebral column relative to its neural contents implies that each vertebra has a surplus of growth potential that cannot be realized in the longitudinal direction because of the "curbing" effect of the slower-growing neural contents. The skeletogenic surplus, therefore, manifests itself in the transverse direction by forming circumferential excrescences at the cranial and caudal ends of the vertebral bodies, where new enchondral growth occurs. The beginning of this process coincides with the onset of neurovertebral growth disproportion (see Fig 8–8) and is reflected in the girth of the vertebral body, i.e., in the concavity most pronounced on its ventral and lateral surfaces.

Shape of the Intervertebral Foramina

The shape of the intervertebral foramina reflects the cross-sectional shape of the spinal cord, i.e., transverse oval in the cervical, circular in the thoracic region (Figs 8–9 and 8–10). The shape of the lumbar vertebral foramina is related to the specific cross-sectional arrangement of the cauda equina, which comprises approximately 40 circular or slightly oval paired dorsal and ventral lumbosacral nerve roots. The cross-section of the cauda equina at the level of the thoracolumbar junction decreases gradually and becomes triangular in the lower lumbar area because of the more ventrolateral exit of the spinal nerves (Figs 8–11; 8–12; 8–13,*C*). Despite the lack of a rigid, fixed position of the nerve roots within the spinal canal, the sum of all "morphogenic fields" (Holtzer) surrounding the individual nerve roots comprises a complex oval or triangular cross-sectional area responsible for the adaptive shape of the lumbar vertebral foramina (Fig 8–13,*A, B*). The ventrolateral recesses of the L-4 and L-5 foramina represent an "imprint" of the respective spinal nerves running ventrolaterally through the foramina, in contrast to the direct lateral course of the L1-2 nerves. The analogous recesses of the cervical vertebral foramina reflect the ventrolateral course of the cervical spinal nerves.

Neurovertebral Features of the Intervertebral Foramina

The primordial intervertebral foramina have a transversely oriented oval shape in accordance with the shape of the embryonic spinal ganglia and their short nerve roots (see Fig 8–2). With cord ascent, each ganglion assumes a craniad eccentric position within its foramen. At the same time, the vertebral groove in man forms on either side of the midline (Figs 8–12 and 8–15). The appearance of the groove coincides with straightening of the hyperkyphotic embryonic body (Bardeen). The embryonic spinal nerves running within the thoracic wall are intimately involved in the process of vertebral groove formation (Becker). They are exposed to two "microtension" components—one cranially directed, derived from ascent of the cord, and the other dorsally directed, derived from formation of the vertebral

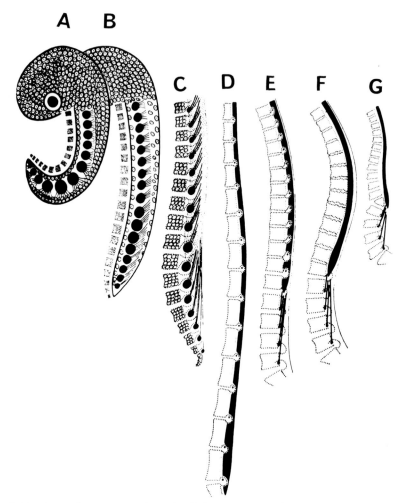

Fig 8–7.—Lateral representation of relative neurovertebral growth dynamics in the course of development. In the early embryo *(A),* composed almost exclusively of neural tissue, the primordia of the brain and spinal cord, growing rapidly by mitotic proliferation of neuroblasts, are thrown into a hyperkyphotic curvature in the still meager, slower growing surroundings. With the shift of the neural primordia to the extensive growth type *(B,* 7-wk. embryo; *C,* full-term fetus), the neural structures become the retarding factor with respect to the more rapidly growing vertebral column. This "neural braking effect," more pronounced in man than in quadrupeds *(D),* results in lumbar lordosis in man *(E).* Exaggerated neurovertebral growth differential, brought about by insufficient neural growth, results in pathologic curvatures of the spine with adaptive transformation of vertebral shape (Scheuermann's disease *(F),* and platyspondyly with a wedged vertebra in bone dysplasias *(G).*

groove. The definitive shape of the intervertebral foramina depends upon the predominance of one of these two components, i.e., on the direction of their resultant. Thus, the thoracic foramina gradually become pear-shaped (Figs 8–14 and 8–16) and the lumbar foramina kidney-shaped with their most cranial point situated ventrally. The kidney shape of the lumbar foramina is due to the fact that the lumbar nerves lack the dorsal traction component and run distally in a ventral direction through the cranioventral portion of the intervertebral foramina. The course of the

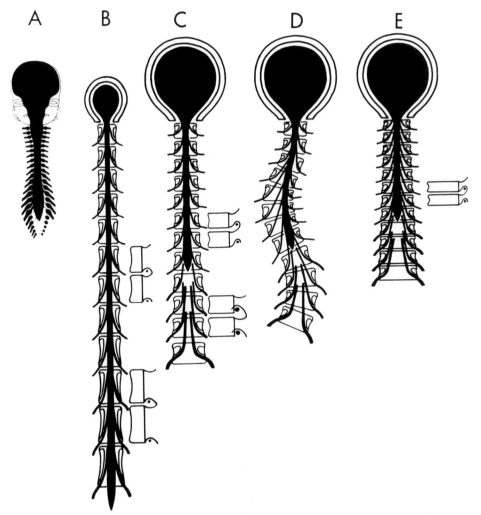

Fig 8–7.—Anteroposterior representation of the same process. The growth of the axial skeleton is adapted to the growth and shape of the neural structures, and not the reverse. This is similar to the growth interrelations between the brain and its bony case. According to the phylogenetically evolved extensive growth capacity of the neural structures, the vertebrae grow either long and slender (B, quadruped) or short and broad (C, man). The phylogenetic process of neural-dependent shortening of the axial skeleton can reach pathologic levels, i.e., kyphoscoliosis (D), platyspondyly (E), broad, short vertebrae that do not have enough space along growth-insufficient neural structures. The shape of the incisura vertebrae caudalis is determined by the more (C) or less (B) deep "cutting in" of the spinal nerves. Thus, the craniocaudal length of the vertebral arch depends on the neural structures. The length of the schematic drawings in these figures does not correspond exactly to the natural state. For the purpose of simplicity, only 12 vertebrae are shown.

lumbar spinal nerves after leaving the spinal canal accounts for the more ventral position of the lower lumbar intervertebral foramina and their pedicles, compared with the upper lumbar foramina (Figs 8–14 and 8–17). While the upper lumbar foramina look directly laterally, the lower foramina are directed ventrolaterally. In the lateral roentgenogram, this gives the impression that the L4-5 foramina are

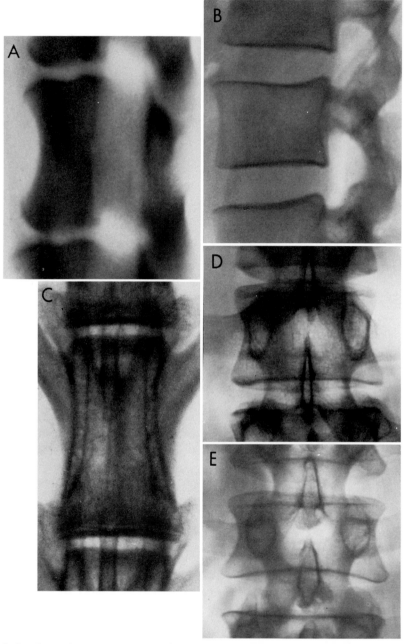

Fig 8–8.—Lateral roentgenograms (**A,** dog; **B,** man) and AP roentgenograms of lumbar vertebrae reproduced in the same relative size (**C,** rabbit; **D** and **E,** man). The different spatial distribution of the same relative quantity of bony material depends on the growth-in-length capacity of the intraspinal neural structures. Note especially the shape of the pedicles in **C, D,** and **E,** as well as the different lengths of the vertebral arch in quadrupeds and in man.

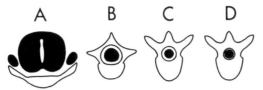

Fig 8–9.—Quantitative osteoneural shift during development demonstrated in schematic cross-sectional diagrams of the spine in the embryo **(A)**, newborn **(B)**, and adult **(C)**. The size of the vertebral foramen is a function of the enclosed neural structures from the surface of which the skeletogenic masses maintain a certain distance. Abnormal reduction of this distance results in a tight spinal canal **(D)**.

smaller than the others. In fact, however, their sagittal diameter is not significantly reduced, although their craniocaudal diameter is somewhat reduced because of the lumbosacral lordosis (Figs 8–13,C and 8–17).

The dorsocranial position of the nerves within the thoracic foramina is well demonstrated by pneumoperidurography (Fig 8–18). The ventrocranial position of the nerves within the lumbar foramina is a well-established anatomical fact. In quadrupeds, the dorsal microtraction component of the thoracic nerves is absent, in keeping with the lack of a vertebral groove (see Fig 8–15,B). Thus, the thoracic

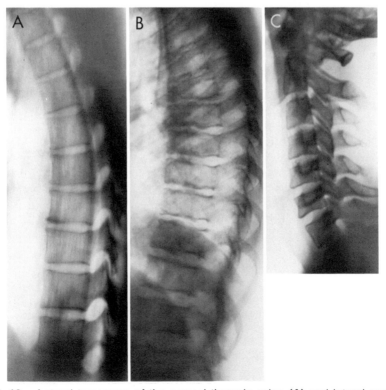

Fig 8–10.—Lateral tomogram of the normal thoracic spine **(A)** and lateral roentgenogram of the thoracic spine **(B)** in a patient with platyspondyly. Combination of cervical dolicho- and brachyspondyly **(C)** related to the amount of space available for the vertebrae along the intraspinal neural structures.

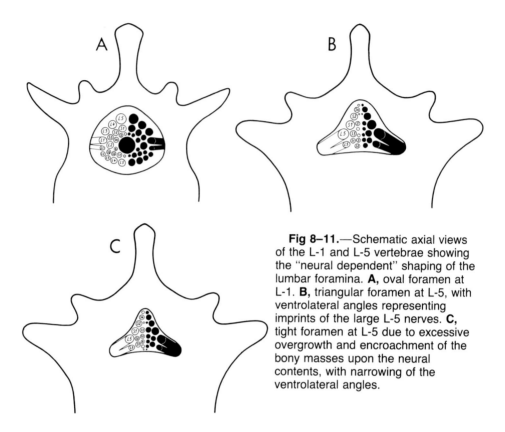

Fig 8–11.—Schematic axial views of the L-1 and L-5 vertebrae showing the "neural dependent" shaping of the lumbar foramina. **A,** oval foramen at L-1. **B,** triangular foramen at L-5, with ventrolateral angles representing imprints of the large L-5 nerves. **C,** tight foramen at L-5 due to excessive overgrowth and encroachment of the bony masses upon the neural contents, with narrowing of the ventrolateral angles.

intervertebral foramina in the dog do not extend as far dorsally as they do in man (see Fig 8–16,C).

It is helpful to think of the nerve trunk traversing the intervertebral foramen as a glowing wire plunged into a plate of fusible metal. A halo is formed around the wire that follows it with every displacement. The plastic modeling of the intervertebral foramina is best understood as an endless sequence of successive cranial eccentricities of the spinal ganglion and nerve with respect to the foramen, followed by a "melting reaction" of the nearby skeletogenic tissue (Fig 8–18,B). Either "Microtension" or "microtraction" on the nerve roots, although irreconcilable with known neurophysiologic data, is a useful term to indicate the intimate attachment

Fig 8–12.—Paramedian section through two thoracic vertebrae in a 75-mm fetus (from Töndury). Note the dorsocranial eccentricity of the spinal ganglia within the intervertebral foramina *(lines)* and the already established girth of the vertebral body. The girth strongly evokes the impression of some axial force already acting upon the spine at that early stage to "compress" the vertebral bodies. In fact, however, the girth is the result of "crowding" of the rapidly growing vertebrae along the cord–nerve complex, which lags behind.

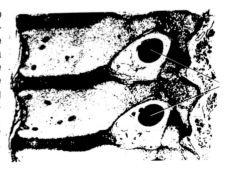

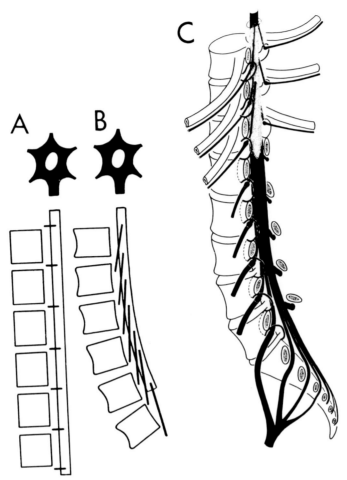

Fig 8–13.—**A,** if the neural and vertebral growth rates were identical, lumbar lordosis would not occur. **B,** the girth of the vertebral bodies and the lumbar lordosis are produced by "crowding" of the vertebrae along the slower growing cord–nerve complex (compare Fig 8–6, **C**). **C,** perspective diagram of the neurovertebral structures of the lower thoracic and lumbar spine. The "braking" neural structures retain a distinct "length reserve" relative to the spine.

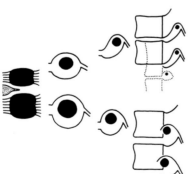

Fig 8–14.—Molding of the primitive intervertebral foramina (left) by the dorsocranial thoracic (upper row) and the ventrocranial lumbar *(lower row)* eccentricity of the spinal ganglia. The arrangement in the quadruped is indicated in dots *(upper right).*

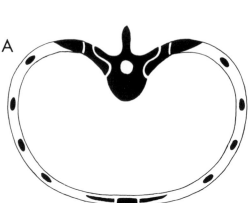

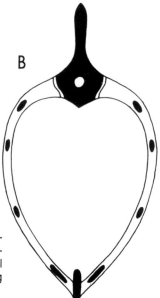

Fig 8–15.—The vertebral groove is a characteristic feature in man **(A)** but does not exist in quadrupeds **(B).** Accordingly, the intercostal nerves in man take a dorsolateral course after leaving the spinal canal, with corresponding dorsocranial eccentricity of the thoracic spinal ganglia.

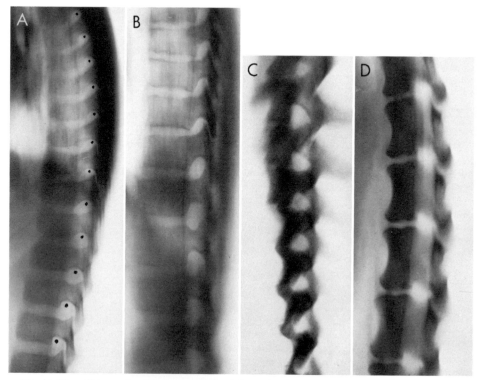

Fig 8–16.—Thoracolumbar intervertebral foramina in an 8-year-old child **(A)** and in an adult **(B).** Tomograms of thoracic **(C)** and lumbar **(D)** foramina in a dog. In **A,** the position of the spinal nerves within the intervertebral foramina is indicated by black dots.

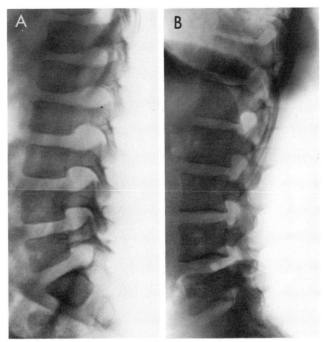

Fig 8–17.—Lateral roentgenograms of the lumbar spine in an 8-year-old child **(A)** and in an adult **(B)**. Note the size relationship between the bony parts and the intervertebral foramina that still retain the embryonal transverse-oval shape in the child (cf. Fig 8–2,*B*). The two pictures reflect the quantitative osteoneural shift that occurs during development, i.e., the steady relative decrease in size of the neural structures compared with the increase in size of the bony parts.

of the nerve at the cranial end of the intervertebral foramen followed by the "melting reaction" of the skeletogenic tissue. In this way, the nerve more or less cuts into the vertebral arch from below. This notching effect of the nerve is responsible for the shape and size of the incisura vertebrae caudalis.

The underlying mechanism of the "melting reaction" of the skeletogenic tissue has been studied experimentally by Holtzer in amphibian embryos. By maintaining a suitable distance from the neural tissue, the prechondral mesenchymal cells line up to form a lumen in the developing cartilage. The size of the lumen is a function of the enclosed nerve bundle. Holtzer suggests that a metabolic product may possibly be released from the surface of the nerve fibers to which chondroblasts react in a negative chemotactic fashion. Similar findings have been reported by Baumann, who metaphorically refers to the "victory" of the neural over the skeletogenic tissue. This mechanism is involved in the morphogenesis of the intervertebral, as well as the vertebral, foramina in man. The active effect of the nervous tissue upon the surrounding skeletogenic mass safeguards the integrity of the former, i.e., the developing neural structures never come into direct contact with their cartilaginous or bony surroundings.

The early appearance of the girth of the vertebral bodies and the formation of the intervertebral foramina can be followed in histologic sections (see Fig 8–12). However, such single sections demonstrate merely a fragment of the macroscopic

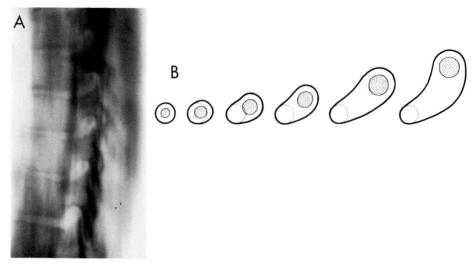

Fig 8–18.—A, accidental pneumoperidurography. The spinal nerves in the intervertebral foramina appear as rounded densities. **B,** schema of the plastic modeling of a thoracic intervertebral foramen. Eccentricity of the spinal nerve, brought about by the ascent and by the formation of the vertebral groove, is accompanied by the corresponding shaping of the foramen. The underlying biologic mechanism may be compared to a glowing wire put into a plate of easily fusible metal. Displacement of the wire is accompanied by a halo.

whole, which can only be grasped by a global approach to the neurovertebral growth dynamics of the entire organ system. With cessation of growth, the vertebral column and its neural contents lie alongside each other without any further dramatic morphogenic changes, not unlike the adult brain and its bony case.

QUANTITATIVE NEUROVERTEBRAL DEVELOPMENT SHIFT

An understanding of the dynamics of the neurovertebral growth relationship must account for the profound quantitative shift between the neural and bony tissues that occurs during development. This is reflected in the evolving shape and size of the intervertebral and vertebral foramina. The embryonic spinal ganglia and the spinal cord are relatively enormous, as are the corresponding primitive intervertebral foramina. In the lumbar region, for example, the size of the foramina exceeds the size of the primitive vertebral bodies, a ratio which persists in the newborn. The relative size of the spinal ganglia decreases steadily in keeping with the relative reduction in volume of the entire central nervous system. The bulk of the surrounding skeletogenic structures, on the other hand, steadily increases. The neural decrease and the bony increase, precisely balanced, are reflected in the lateral roentgenogram of the lumbar spine (see Fig 8–17,A,B). The infantile spine is characterized by large, transversely oriented oval foramina. Its vertebral arch is thin, especially in the interarticular portion. With increasing bone growth, the vertebral arches get thicker, the vertebral bodies larger, and the intervertebral foramina smaller, reflecting the relative reduction in size of the neural components.

The same quantitative osteoneural shift can be observed in the vertebral foramen (see Figs 8–2,C and 8–9,A–C). The relatively enormous embyonic spinal cord is only partly covered by the vertebral body anlage as the neuroapophyses diverge widely to partially embrace the cord. In the course of further development, however, the neuroapophyses gradually close to form a complete arch. The almost frontal orientation of the pedicles in early embryonic life changes to a sagittal orientation, with the pedicles attached at right angles to the dorsal surface of the vertebral body. Hence, the pedicles in the adult do not overlap the lateral outlines of the vertebral body in the frontal roentgenogram. In the newborn, the pedicles project somewhat lateral to the vertebral body because of a relatively wide spinal canal.

THE ROLE OF MUSCLES IN VERTEBRAL MORPHOGENESIS

The muscles are credited with an important role in morphogenesis of the axial skeleton, particularly with respect to the development of spinal curvatures. However, the neurovertebrally shaped skeletal parts are set in motion by the muscles according to the immediate needs of the organism with respect to antigravity, locomotion, and function. At the sites of muscle insertions, local modifications of the bony surface develop, i.e., tuberosities, protuberances, and processes, according to the bulk of the inserting muscle mass. These myogenically dependent external prominences include the external occipital protuberance in man and the more massive bony calvarial crests in some mammals.

DISPENSABILITY OF THE NOTOCHORD

The notochord is generally credited with an important role in the normal and pathologic development of the axial skeleton. Although a prominent structure in fishes, amphibians, and reptiles, the notochord is vestigial in higher mammals; its morphogenic role in the developmental events of the spine is grossly overestimated (Holtzer). In human embryos, the notochord in the early neural tube stage is approximately ¹⁄₂₀ the diameter of the spinal cord (Holtzer). It is soon replaced by the definitive axial skeleton, which remains in intimate relationship with the spinal cord and nerve roots during the entire developmental period of life. The significance of the notochord during early development cannot be denied. However, its role is transient compared with the lasting importance of the neurovertebral relationship in morphogenesis of the axial skeleton.

PATHOLOGIC NEUROVERTEBRAL RELATIONSHIPS

Analysis of gross morphologic neurovertebral developmental events offers a clue to the understanding of several hitherto obscure pathologic spinal conditions that begin and progress during growth. An explanation for these abnormalities has been unsuccessfully sought for in the growing axial skeleton. Perhaps the explanation is rooted in a disturbance of the normal growth relationship between the growing spine and its neural contents. Possibly, the normal neurovertebral growth relationship overshoots the mark in both the transverse and the longitudinal directions.

Tight Spinal Canal (Spinal Stenosis)

Maintenance of the indispensable neurovertebral balance during the developmental quantitative shift, i.e., keeping a safe "living space" for the neural structures, is an inherent function of the "instinct of neural self-preservation." Failure of this protective mechanism, possibly related to a metabolic abnormality of the neural tissue, results in a closer than normal encroachment of the bony masses upon the intraspinal neural structures, i.e., a tight spinal canal and tight intervertebral foramina (see Fig 8–9,*D*). The tightness of the canal and the foramina may be thought of as an exaggeration of the normal neurovertebral quantitative shift, with the bony tissue gaining the upper hand. Disproportionately massive vertebral bodies and arches are a characteristic radiographic and operative finding in developmental spinal stenosis. In the tight lumbar spinal canal, bony overgrowth results in an accentuation of the ventrolateral recess of the vertebral foramen of the L-4 and L-5 vertebrae (see Fig 8–11,*C*).

Developmental Platyspondyly

Platyspondyly (more appropriately, "brachyspondyly") is characteristic of a number of bone dysplasias. Phylogenetically, it can be thought of as an abnormal "overshooting of the mark" of the growing vertebrae in response to deficient growth (but normal function) of the cord–nerve root complex. This type of neurovertebral growth adaptation occurs during the prenatal or early postnatal period, when the growing vertebrae still have a high degree of adaptive plasticity. The early unossified vertebral primordia have no difficulty in spreading more in the transverse than in the longitudinal direction (see Fig 8–7).

Idiopathic Scoliosis and Scheuermann's Disease

During childhood and adolescence, the fairly advanced ossification process permits only a limited degree of adaptive change in vertebral shape in patients who develop neurovertebral growth disproportion at that time. Adaptive changes of the growing spine in the form of pathologic curvatures are necessary to compensate for increased neurovertebral growth disproportion. In this regard, normal growth spurts, i.e., the periods of accelerated growth in body length, are critical since the vertebral growth spurt may be too rapid to keep pace with the slower cord–nerve root growth rate. The resulting pathologic growth disproportion between the normal vertebral column and normal cord–nerve root complex is compensated for by adaptive scoliotic or hyperkyphotic curvatures (Fig 8–19). Scoliosis and juvenile hyperkyphosis may thus represent highly purposeful adaptations of a too rapidly growing spine to a cord–nerve complex that lags too much behind (see Fig 8–7). If the spine grew in length rapidly in the face of the slower growth rate of the spinal cord and nerve roots, traction on the latter would result in catastrophic clinical sequelae unless some accommodation were made.

The appearance of scoliosis or of Scheuermann's hyperkyphosis probably depends upon the acuteness and severity of the underlying neurovertebral growth disproportion. With a milder disproportion occurring slowly, a simple hyperkyphosis of the Scheuermann's type, with sagittal adaptive wedging of the vertebrae, is pro-

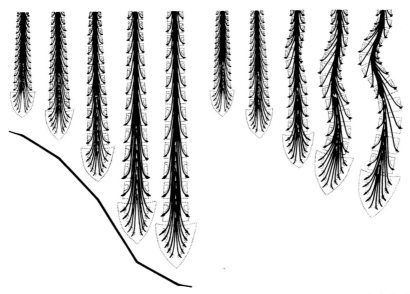

Fig 8–19.—Diagram of craniocaudal growth in length of the axial organ. *Left,* indication of a growth spurt. *Right,* inability of the spinal cord and nerve roots to keep pace with the accelerated growth of the spine results in an adaptive scoliotic (kyphoscoliotic, lordoscoliotic) deformity.

duced. With a more severe acute disproportion, adaptive curvatures of the spine in the frontal plane with lateral wedging are necessary to compensate for the critical neurovertebral growth abnormality.

Congenital scoliosis and kypholordosis with hemivertebrae may be related to the same neurovertebral growth mechanism at a very early developmental stage (Fig 8–20). Because of rapid growth of the axial organ and the high plasticity of its skeletogenic elements, congenital deformities, although exhibiting similar basic traits, are more bizarre than those which appear after birth. The wedged hemivertebra (lateral or dorsal), the most common deformity in congenital scoliosis or kypholordosis, seems to represent an exaggeration of the milder wedged vertebra in idiopathic scoliosis and Scheuermann's hyperkyphosis. The neurovertebral growth disproportion in congenital malformations of this type is so severe that there is no room for some vertebrae to develop normally along the cord–nerve root complex. "Aplasia" of one-half (lateral or ventral) of a hemivertebra is related to a lack of space along the cord. The wedged hemivertebra is not the cause, but the consequence, of the neurovertebral deformity.

Dysplasia of the Vertebral Isthmus

Dysplasia of the isthmic portion of the vertebral arch, most frequent at L-5, is a common finding predisposing to spondylolysis. While the spinal nerve leaving the spinal canal in the adult lies in the ventrocranial portion of the intervertebral foramen, i.e., rather far from the isthmus, the oblique dorsal roots in the embryo cross the isthmic portion of the future vertebral arch (see Fig 8–4,*B*). The craniocaudal length or "thickness" of the isthmus depends upon the length of the distance be-

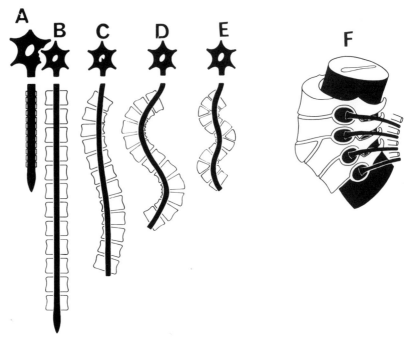

Fig 8–20.—Congenital scoliosis with wedged hemivertebra **(E,F)**, a manifestation of exaggerated neurovertebral growth disproportion appearing at a very early stage of development. There was not enough room left along the cord-nerve complex for the wedged vertebrae to develop normally. The wedged vertebrae represent an exaggerated degree of the milder wedged vertebrae in idiopathic scoliosis **(C,D).** An analogous mechanism appears responsible for the dorsal hemivertebra. Normal neurovertebral growth in **A** and **B.** The cord-nerve complex curves together with the spine **(C,E)** and becomes victimized by the deformity originally evoked by the cord itself. Reduced craniocaudal distances of pedicles frequently found in congenital malformation with or without scoliosis seem to reflect the reduced distances between the spinal ganglia, i.e., insufficient medulloradicular growth in length.

Fig 8–21.—The craniocaudal length, i.e., thickness of the vertebral arch, depends on the distances between the spinal ganglia in the fetus and adult. The dysplastic thinning on the isthmus may be related to an embryonic neuroforaminal (or ganglioforaminal) disturbance *(upper right).* Cross-hatching indicates a growth insufficiency of the nerve root.

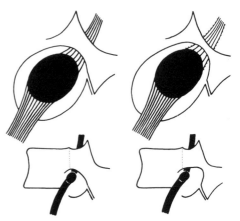

tween the individual spinal ganglia (see Figs 8–7 and 8–8). It is not difficult to imagine a local growth retardation of the L-5 nerve roots and accentuated craniad eccentricity of the spinal ganglion as the cause of "dysplastic" thinning of the L-5 isthmus (Fig 8–21). The dysplastic, thin isthmus in the adult possibly represents the residuum of this local embryonic neurovertebral disturbance.

The proposed explanation of curvatures and other neurovertebral spinal relationships may initially conjure up a mechanical pull of the nerve roots upon the growing spine. Nothing like that takes place. The growing axial skeleton gradually adapts to the shape of the spinal neural structures, which lag somewhat behind and maintain the surrounding skeletogenic masses at a "respectful" distance in both the transverse and longitudinal directions. In this way, the neural structures protect themselves against transverse compression and longitudinal overstretching. Because of this, the cord and nerve roots retain a slightly wavy course, which acts as an indispensable "length reserve" for the excursions of the spine. The nerve roots are not stretched, except in maximal lateral flexion or hyperflexion of the spine (Breig, 1978).

BIBLIOGRAPHY

Bagnall K.M., Harris P.F., Jones P.R.M.: A radiographic study of the human fetal spine. *J. Anat.* (Lond.) 123:777, 1977.

Bardeen C.R.: The development of the thoracic vertebrae in man. *Am. J. Anat.* 4:163, 1905.

Bardeen C.R., Lewis W.H.: Development of the limbs, body-wall and back in man. *Am. J. Anat.* 1:1, 1901–02.

Baumann J.A.: Fibre nerveuse et cartilage: Un exemple d'incompatibilité intertissulaire. *Arch. Anat. Hist. Embr.* 34:55, 1951–52.

Becker A.: Über Lageveränderungen der Spinalnervenwurzeln und der Spinalnerven während der ontogenetischen Entwicklung. *Gegenbaurs Morphol. Jahrb.* 84:17, 1940.

Blechschmidt E.: Entwicklungsfunktionelle Untersuchungen am Nervensystem. Entstehung von Wachstumskoordinationen. *Zschr. Anat.* 119:112, 1956.

Breig A.: *Biomechanics of the Central Nervous System.* Stockholm, Almqvist & Wiksell, 1970, p. 183.

Breig A.: *Adverse Mechanical Tension in the Central Nervous System.* Stockholm, Almqvist & Wiksell, 1978.

Detwiler S.R., Holtzer H.: The inductive and formative influence of the spinal cord upon the vertebral column. *Bull. Hosp. Joint Dis.* 15:114, 1954.

Evison G., Windsor P., Duck F.: Myelographic features of the normal sacral sac. *Br. J. Radiol.* 52:777, 1979.

Holmdahl D.E.: Utvecklingen av den kaudala delen av ryggmargen hos manniskan. Lund, 1918.

Holtzer H.: Experimental analysis of development of spinal column. I. Response of precartilage cells to size variations of spinal cord. *J. Exper. Zool.* 121:121, 1952.

Holtzer H.: An experimental analysis of the development of the spinal column. II. The dispensability of the notochord. *J. Exper. Zool.* 121:573, 1952a.

Krupka J.J., D'Angelo C.M.: Artifactual midline cervical defect seen during myelography. *Spine* 3:210, 1978.

Lamont A.C., Zachary J., Sheldon P.W.E.: Cervical cord size in metrizamide myelography. *Clin. Radiol.* 32:409, 1981.

Lebedkin S.I.: Length variations of the spinal cord segments and of the vertebrae during the development in man and in swine. (Russian text, Izvest. nautsh. instit. im. P.F. Lesgafta, Vol. 20, vyp. I.) Moscow, 1936, pp. 13–102.

Roth M.: Idiopathic scoliosis from the point of view of the neuroradiologist. *Neuroradiology* 21:133, 1981.

Roth M.: Idiopathische Skoliose und Scheuermannsche Erkrankung: Wesensgleiche Erscheinungsformen der neurovertebralen Wachstumsdisproportion. *Radiol. Diagn.* 22:380, 1981.

Roth M., Krkoska J., Toman I.: Morphogenesis of the spinal canal, normal and stenotic. *Neuroradiology* 10:277, 1976.

Streeter G.L.: Factors involved in the formation of the filum terminale. *Am. J. Anat.* 25:1, 1919.

Theiler K.: Embryonale und postnatale Entwicklung des Schädels, in *Handbuch der Medizinischen Radiologie*, Bd. VII/1. Berlin, Springer, 1963, pp. 22–60.

Töndury G.: Entwicklungsgeschichte und Fehlbildungen der Wirbelsäule. Stuttgart, Hippokrates, Verlag, 1958.

9

The Normal Myelogram

In MYELOGRAPHY with oily media, the oil settles to the most dependent portion of the subarachnoid space because of its greater specific gravity. This is less pronounced with metrizamide, although the latter is also hyperbaric (sp. gr. 1.184; sp. gr. of CSF, 1.006–1.008). Thus, in the prone position the oil fills the ventral aspect of the subarachnoid space, whereas in the supine position it accumulates in the dorsal portion of this space. In the frontal projection, the cervicodorsal subarachnoid space appears as a peripheral opaque band on either side of the wider, less dense central zone which corresponds to the spinal cord (Fig 9–1). The opaque bands representing the lateral margins of the subarachnoid space are relatively wide in the lower cervical and upper thoracic regions; they taper sharply to their narrowest width in the midthoracic area and again become wider in the lower thoracic region. Below the termination of the spinal cord the differential density between the lateral and central portions of the opaque column disappears, leaving a single uniform lumbar opacity. Because metrizamide is less opaque than Pantopaque, the individual nerve roots can be better distinguished with the former.

Perhaps the most striking single characteristic of the normal myelogram throughout the spinal subarachnoid space is the symmetry of the column of contrast material in the frontal projection.

CERVICAL

The enlargement of the cervical cord for the brachial plexus commences at the level of the third cervical vertebra, is maximal opposite C5-6, and diminishes down to T-2. The cervical intumescence essentially involves the transverse diameter and, therefore, can be appreciated only in the frontal projection. Myelography with air or metrizamide in the lateral projection reveals a fairly uniform sagittal diameter of the cervical cord from C-2 to C-6. A gross alteration in the transverse diameter of the spinal cord can readily be recognized by myelography in the frontal projection. However, a subtle change is more difficult to detect and may go unrecognized. It is important, therefore, to establish a range of normalcy for the diameters of the spinal cord. Routine Pantopaque myelography in the prone position visualizes only the ventral aspect of the subarachnoid space. Hence, the sagittal diameter of the

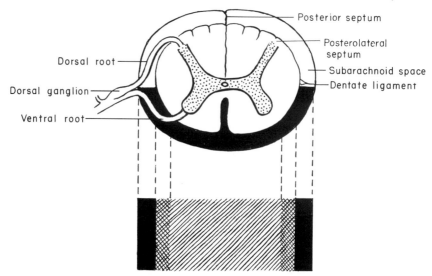

Fig 9–1.—Diagrammatic cross-section of the thoracic spinal cord with Pantopaque filling the ventral half of the subarachnoid space (patient prone). The contrast-filled subarachnoid space is projected as an opaque band on either side of the dense central zone representing the spinal cord.

cord cannot be determined with this technique unless the entire subarachnoid space is filled with oil or the patient is also examined in the supine position. Measurement of the sagittal diameter is readily accomplished by air or metrizamide, which clearly delineates the cord between the contrast-filled anterior and posterior subarachnoid spaces. The dorsal margin of the posterior subarachnoid space has a straight or slightly concave margin. At its cranial end, it extends from the anterior surface of the posterior arch of the atlas to the middle of the posterior rim of the foramen magnum, where it merges imperceptibly with the cisterna magna.

The introduction of metrizamide has facilitated more accurate measurement of the size of the cervical cord. Lamont, Zachary, and Sheldon measured the transverse and sagittal diameters of the cervical cord in 282 patients between the ages of 18 and 68 years. All of the patients had metrizamide cervical myelography performed with a focus-film distance of 100 cm and an object-film distance averaging 25 cm. The sagittal and coronal measurements (made at the midvertebral body level from C-1 to T-1 on the lateral view and from C-2 to T-5 on the posteroanterior view) are given in Tables 9–1 and 9–2.

In 1959, Paul and Chandler suggested the ratio of spinal cord width to the width of the subarachnoid space (C/SAS) as an index of spinal cord size. The normal range for this measurement was reported by Paul and Chandler as 0.52–0.73, with a mean value of 0.63 (35 cases), and by Khilnani and Wolf as 0.53–0.78, with a mean value of 0.67 (80 cases). A difference of more than 3 mm in the transverse diameter of adjacent cervical cord segments and a cord-subarachnoid ratio greater than 80% or less than 50% should be viewed with suspicion.

Nordqvist made a detailed postmortem study of the spinal cord and subarachnoid space in different age groups. According to him, the greatest frontal diameter of the cervical cord lies at the level of C-5. The spinal cord has an elliptic cross-section

TABLE 9–1.—SAGITTAL MEASUREMENTS (CORD DEPTH),
IN MILLIMETERS*

VERTEBRAL LEVEL	NO. CASES	AVERAGE MEASUREMENT	STANDARD DEVIATION × 2	MEASUREMENT AFTER MAGNIFICATION CORRECTION
C-1	58	11.3	1.9	8.5
C-2	64	11.5	3.0	8.6
C-3	63	10.6	3.2	8.0
C-4	65	10.3	1.8	7.7
C-5	64	9.9	1.6	7.4
C-6	57	9.5	1.8	7.1
C-7	33	9.9	1.4	7.5
T-1	9	9.3	1.8	7.0

*From Lamont et al.

in the lower cervical region. The thoracic cord, which extends from the third to the tenth thoracic vertebral body, has its smallest sagittal diameter at T5-8 and its smallest frontal diameter at T8-9. The lumbar enlargement begins at the level of T-10 (judged by its sagittal diameter) and, together with the cauda equina, forms a single structure which broadens toward L-1 in both the frontal and sagittal diameters. Nordqvist established curves for the normal sagittal and transverse diameters of the cord for various age groups (Figs 9–2 and 9–3). For practical purposes, there was no significant distortion when the myelographic measurements were compared with those taken directly from the cord. The sagittal diameters of the cord and subarachnoid space in children are relatively large at birth and increase rapidly during the first 10 years. At age 9, the average sagittal diameter of the cord is 0.65 mm less and the average sagittal diameter of the subarachnoid space 0.56 mm less than the adult mean values. There apparently is no significant sex difference in the sagittal diameter of the cord. The sagittal diameter of the cord decreases in old age. The sagittal diameter of the subarachnoid space also diminishes with age in the cervical region, perhaps secondary to degenerative changes in the spinal column. On the other hand, the sagittal diameter of the thoracic subarachnoid space increases with advancing age. At the level of T-10, i.e., the upper limit of lumbar enlargement, the subarachnoid space suddenly increases in size in all age groups.

In the lateral projection, the anterior surface of the cervical subarachnoid space hugs the posterior aspect of the vertebrae rather closely, forming a fairly straight

TABLE 9–2.—CORONAL MEASUREMENTS (CORD WIDTH),
IN MILLIMETERS*

VERTEBRAL LEVEL	NO. CASES	AVERAGE MEASUREMENT	STANDARD DEVIATION × 2	MEASUREMENT AFTER MAGNIFICATION CORRECTION
C-1	2	15	—	11.3
C-2	23	14.9	6.8	11.2
C-3	48	15.9	8.3	11.9
C-4	60	16.9	4.8	12.7
C-5	61	17.4	2.8	13.0
C-6	62	17.0	2.8	12.8
C-7	64	15.9	3.6	11.9
T-1	61	13.4	3.6	10.1

*From Lamont et al.

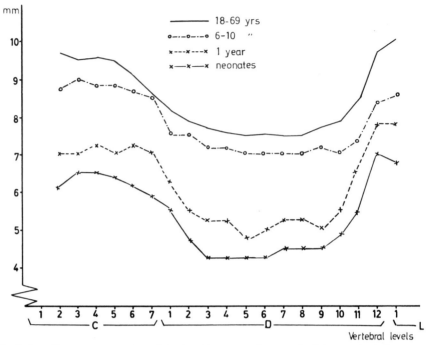

Fig 9–2.—Group mean values (obtained from myelograms) of the sagittal diameters of the spinal cord at various vertebral levels in children aged 0–10 years; values from the age group 18–69 years are included for comparison. (Reprinted, with permission, from L. Nordqvist, *Acta Radiol.,* Suppl. 227, 1964.)

line (Fig 9–4). The latter may be indented by the posterior margin of the intervertebral disks at the interspaces. The spinal canal of cervical vertebrae 2–6 is not perfectly triangular in cross-section because of the posterior bulge of the centrum, which creates a shallow gutter on either side. Some of the contrast medium that projects anteriorly in the lateral view lies in the lateral gutters. Hence, the anterior margin of the contrast column in the lateral prone projection may not necessarily represent the anterior aspect of the subarachnoid space (Fig 9–5). This is important in dealing with midline cervical disk herniations. The anterior surface of the opacified subarachnoid space usually presents a shallow concavity, beginning at the caudal margin of the dens and extending up to the anterior rim of the foramen magnum (Fig 9–6). This is due to the transverse ligament. Craniad to this point, the anterior aspect of the column resumes its flat configuration. The radiopacity of the Pantopaque column frequently makes it difficult to distinguish the anterior surface of the spinal cord. When this structure is visible, particularly in slightly overexposed films, it usually lies approximately 3 mm posterior to the anterior aspect of the Pantopaque column. Not infrequently, the posterior margin of the opaque contrast column (with the patient prone) is indented to a varying degree by the posterior nerve roots. The dentate ligament is visualized through the opaque column as a thin vertical radiolucency between the radiolucent streaks of the posterior nerve roots dorsally and the opaque contrast under the ventral surface of the ligament. This appearance is more striking in the cervical region, where the ligament is thickest. In patients with a narrow sagittal diameter of the cervical bony canal

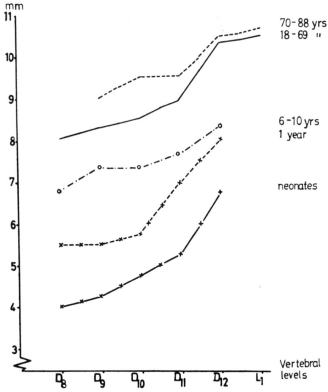

Fig 9–3.—Group mean values (obtained from myelograms) for frontal diameters of the spinal cord between vertebral levels T8-L1 for age groups 0–88 years. (Reprinted, with permission, from L. Nordqvist, *Acta Radiol.,* Suppl. 227, 1964.)

and spondylosis, the indentations on the posterior aspect of the contrast column are particularly prominent and deep, especially in hyperextension. This accentuation of the normal posterior indentations is due to forward bulging of the ligamentum flavum (Fig 9–7).

The course of the nerve roots varies at different levels in the cord. The roots are almost horizontal in the upper cervical region and traverse an obliquely inferior course in the thoracic region, with increasing obliqueness in the lumbar area. The lower cervical roots that form the brachial plexus are much larger than the more proximal cervical roots. In addition, the lower cervical roots come off the spinal cord at a considerably higher level than the intervertebral foramina through which they exit. The posterior roots in the cervical region are disproportionately larger than their anterior counterparts, much more so than in the thoracolumbar area.

As the individual nerve filaments leave the thoracolumbar cord, they promptly merge to form a single nerve root. In the cervical region, however, the filaments may fuse to form two or more bundles that maintain their identity as far out as the axillary pouch before uniting to form a single root. The subarachnoid space is continuous over each root for a varying distance lateral to the ganglion in the intervertebral foramen.

In the frontal projection, the cervical myelogram appears as a vertical column

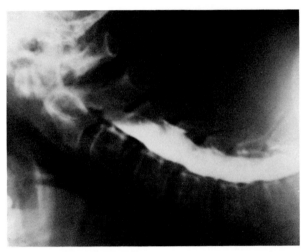

Fig 9–4.—Lateral shoot-through film with the horizontal beam, demonstrating the normal close relationship between the anterior aspect of the subarachnoid space and the posterior vertebral surfaces (prone position).

with a thin, dense band on either side of a much wider, less dense, central opacity (Figs 9–8 and 9–9). The opaque column presents a symmetric concave indentation on either side of the vertebral bodies. Above and below these indentations, the dura and arachnoid pouch out at right angles to the main column at the points of exit of the nerve roots from the thecal sac (axillary pouch of Hampton and Robinson). Within the contrast-filled axillary pouch, it is possible to see the nerve root (anterior root in the prone position) or two or more bundles of nerve fibers before they fuse more laterally to form the root. The axillary pouches usually are symmetrically filled. The pathologic pouch is characterized by deformity or displacement (Fig 9–10). Filling and visualization of the nerve root pouches is vastly improved with metrizamide.

The anterior spinal artery is usually demonstrable as a thin, linear, midline radiolucency in the oil column in the prone position. In well-penetrated prone films, the arteria radicularis magna can also frequently be seen in the thoracolumbar area (Fig 9–11). In addition, one often sees anterior radicular arterial branches accompanying the anterior roots at various segmental levels (Fig 9–12). The roots can be distinguished from the radicular arteries because the former do not extend to the midline, whereas the latter join the anterior spinal artery in the midline.

With the patient in the supine position, a somewhat irregular, thin, midline, vertical, radiolucent streak can often be visualized in the thoracic region that probably represents the septum posticum.

The dens, when prominent, is visualized as a central, oval-shaped defect in the oil column. When the dens does not protrude prominently into the oil column, the subarachnoid space dorsal to it may be quite deep. As a result, the column of oil tends to fill the central portion of the subarachnoid space first, leaving the lateral portions relatively unfilled. This type of central constriction should not be misinterpreted as pathologic (Fig 9–13). It is important to be familiar with the effect of rotation of the head and neck on the appearance of the contrast column in the atlanto-axial and atlanto-occipital regions. With the neck in the straight anteropos-

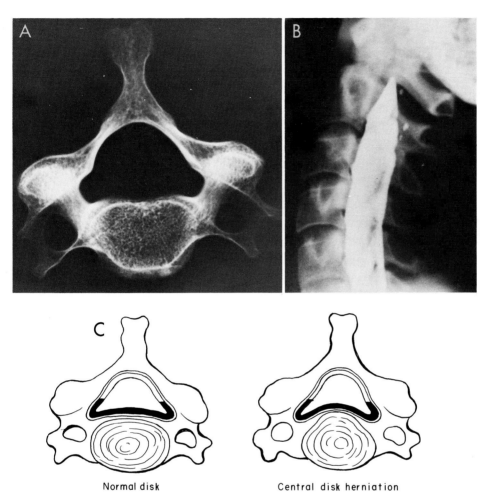

Fig 9–5.—A, radiograph of a dried cervical vertebra demonstrating the lateral gutters of the spinal canal. **B,** lateral cervical myelogram taken with the horizontal beam and the patient in the prone position. **C,** cross-sectional diagrams of the cervical spinal canal in the presence of a normal disk and a central disk herniation; the ventral half of the sub-arachnoid space is filled with Pantopaque. Note that the Pantopaque-filled lateral gutters project anteriorly in the lateral view, thereby obscuring the midline defect produced by a central disk herniation.

terior position, rotation of the head causes the cranial end of the oil column to flow around the dens toward the occiput (Fig 9–14). Thereafter, the oil passes either forward up the clivus if the head is flexed or into the cisterna magna if the head is extended. With the neck and the head turned obliquely or laterally, the Panto-paque gravitates posteriorly into the dependent cisterna magna. In either instance, spurious defects may be produced, particularly when a small amount of oil flows craniad. This is not a problem with metrizamide. In examining for a suspected lesion in the area of the foramen magnum, it is necessary to use an ample amount of contrast and to study the column in the conventional anteroposterior and lateral projections (using the horizontal beam) with the head and neck in the midline (Fig 9–15).

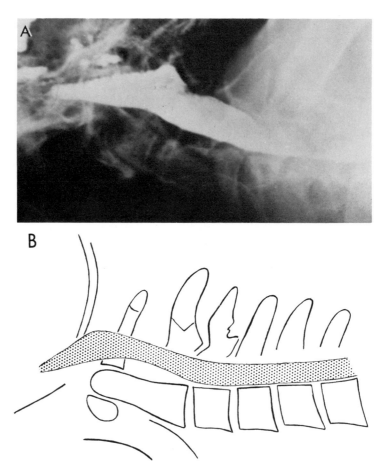

Fig 9–6.—A, prone lateral radiograph made during cervical myelography with the horizontal beam, showing the concavity on the ventral aspect of the Pantopaque column due to the transverse ligament. **B,** line drawing to illustrate the characteristic defect.

(Continued.)

Jirout has demonstrated significant mobility of the cervical and thoracic segments of the spinal cord. The cervical cord changes its position in the sagittal direction, i.e., in the prone position it shifts anteriorly and in the supine position it tends to shift posteriorly. Motion of the cervical cord is minimal at the level of C-3 and increases craniad and especially caudad to this level. The degree of mobility of the cervical cord is unrelated to the sagittal diameter of the spinal canal. According to Jirout, the thoracic cord moves in a similar fashion, the average mobility ranging slightly over 2 mm. Occasionally, the movement of the thoracic cord may exceed 4.5 mm and, rarely, 8–9 mm. Fixation of the spinal cord, i.e., absence of the normal physiologic mobility, has been used by Jirout to establish the diagnosis of caudad dislocation of the brain stem secondary to increased intracranial pressure. In the latter condition, there is also posterior displacement of the upper cervical cord against the posterior wall of the bony canal and widening of the anterior subarachnoid space extending over two or more vertebral segments. The changes are best visualized in the lateral projection with the spine in flexion. Caudad dislocation of the brain stem should not be confused with narrowing of the posterior subarach-

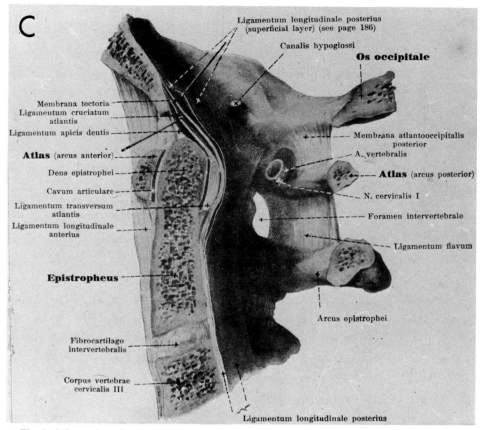

C

Ligamentum longitudinale posterius
(superficial layer) (see page 186)

Canalis hypoglossi

Os occipitale

Membrana tectoria
Ligamentum cruciatum
atlantis
Ligamentum apicis dentis

Membrana atlantooccipitalis
posterior

A. vertebralis

Atlas (arcus anterior)

Dens epistrophei

Atlas (arcus posterior)

Cavum articulare

N. cervicalis I

Ligamentum transversum
atlantis

Foramen intervertebrale

Ligamentum longitudinale
anterius

Ligamentum flavum

Epistropheus

Arcus epistrophei

Fibrocartilago
intervertebralis

Corpus vertebrae
cervicalis III

Ligamentum longitudinale posterius

Fig 9–6 (cont.).—C, sagittal section of anatomical specimen clearly demonstrating the relationship of the transverse ligament to the site of the defect. (After Spalteholtz.)

noid space due to anatomic constriction of the anteroposterior diameter of the spinal canal. This error can be avoided if the anteroposterior diameter of the bony canal is compared with the width of the spinal cord and with the width and shape of the anterior subarachnoid space.

THORACIC

In the upper thoracic region, the lateral band-like opacities enclosing the midline spinal cord are relatively wide in the frontal projection. They become progressively narrower down to the lower midthoracic region, distal to which they gradually increase in width again down to L-1. Below the point where the spinal cord terminates, there is a single, homogenous opacity through which the roots of the cauda equina may be seen to a varying degree. The latter parallels the lumbar enlargement of the cord. The ventrally convex curvature of the spinal cord from T-11 to approximately L-2 does not conform to the curvature of the vertebral column except in the first months of fetal life. The lower thoracic cord occupies a more dorsal position with respect to the meninges than the cervical or upper thoracic cord.

The nerve roots exit quite obliquely from the thoracic segment of the spinal cord.

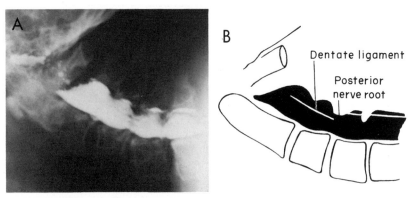

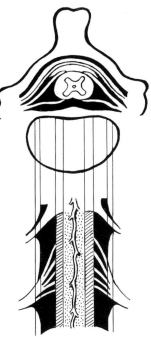

Fig 9–7.—Radiograph **(A)** and line drawing **(B)** of a patient with cervical spondylosis and a narrow bony canal, showing deep indentations on the posterior aspect of the Pantopaque column (prone lateral film with the horizontal beam and the neck in hyperextension). The indentations in this case probably are produced both by the posterior nerve roots and by the forward bulging of the ligamentum flavum. The dentate ligament is represented by the linear radiolucency immediately ventral to the posterior roots.

The axillary pouches in the thoracic region are not usually demonstrated in the frontal prone projection with Pantopaque because the oil in the ventral portion of the subarachnoid space does not reach the level of the nerve root sleeves. This is also true of metrizamide (Fig 9–16).

Irregularities of the Pantopaque column are quite frequent in the thoracic region (Fig 9–17). These may take the form of a round or oval radiolucency, an hourglass constriction, or a smooth unilateral concavity as the oil column passes over a normal

Fig 9–8.—Schematic representation of the anatomical factors responsible for the frontal roentgenogram in cervical myelography with Pantopaque. (After Wellauer.)

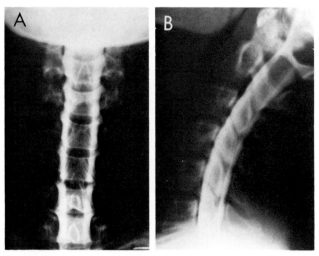

Fig 9–9.—Normal metrizamide cervical myelogram. **A,** frontal projection (cf. Fig 9–8). **B,** lateral shoot-through film of same patient.

bulging intervertebral disk. These defects are particularly accentuated in the thoracic region because of the shallowness of the Pantopaque column. The defects may be constant or inconstant. Because they occur so commonly in normal patients, a diagnosis of a herniated thoracic disk based on these findings alone usually will be erroneous. A defect is more significant if it produces some obstruction to the flow of Pantopaque, if it can be constantly demonstrated in the lateral prone shoot-

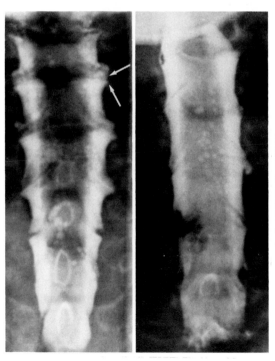

Fig 9–10.—Radiograph of a normal cervical myelogram with symmetric axillary pouches. **Left,** note the radiolucencies cast by the dorsal *(upper arrow)* and ventral *(lower arrow)* nerve roots as they enter the intervertebral foramen. **Right,** the deformed axillary pouch due to a herniated disk at C5-6 is evident.

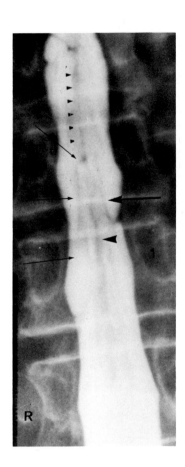
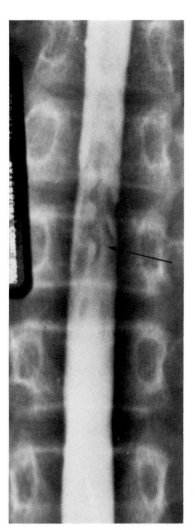

Fig 9–11.—Left, normal prone Pantopaque myelogram in the thoracolumbar region showing the arteria radicularis magna arising from the right first lumbar artery *(thin arrows)*. Note its characteristic course to the midline, the hairpin bend, and bifurcation into a smaller ascending *(small arrowheads)* and a larger descending *(broad arrowhead)* branch. Note also that the corresponding nerve root on the left *(thick arrow)* does not reach the midline. **Right,** prominent arteria radicularis magna in a 7-year-old child *(arrow)*. This is a normal finding in children and should not be mistaken for a vascular malformation.

through film, and if it correlates well with the clinical findings. Inconstant defects can be minimized or eliminated by using larger volumes of Pantopaque. The irregular defects on the posterior aspect of the cord produced by normal arachnoid folds at Pantopaque myelography are not seen with metrizamide.

LUMBAR

The normal lumbar myelogram is influenced by variations in the shape, width, depth, and termination of the subarachnoid space. It is also influenced by struc-

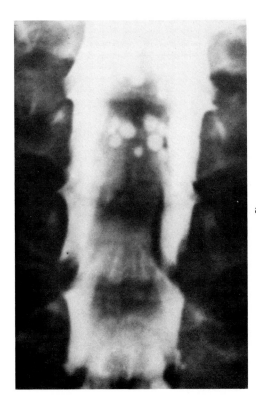

Fig 9–12.—Large radicular artery at C5-6 on the left.

tures contiguous to the subarachnoid space and by the arrangement of the individual nerve roots in the cauda equina.

In general, the column of contrast medium assumes one of two principal configurations with a number of intermediate gradations (Figs 9–18 and 9–19).

1. A more or less cylindric column in which the individual nerve roots are lined up across the width of the theca so that the root about to exit from the theca lies lateral to the other more medial roots arranged in numeric order.

2. A column with biconcave indentations at the level of the vertebral bodies between the points of emergence of the nerve roots. In this type, the roots are gathered into two large lateral bundles separated by a relatively wide subarachnoid space. Each root, loosely attached to its neighbors, lies posterior to the root cephalad to it.

The width of the contrast column in the frontal projection varies considerably, with no apparent correlation to the individual somatotype or the interpediculate distances. When the column is wide, it may be necessary to use a larger volume of contrast to obtain a completely satisfactory study. In the presence of spina bifida, the width of the subarachnoid space may exceed 3 cm. As the subarachnoid space continues caudad, it diminishes in width and eventually continues into the sacral canal to terminate at the level of the second sacral segment. Occasionally, there may be a short caudal sac with termination at the lumbosacral interspace. In the latter instance, a herniated lumbosacral disk may be missed. In this situation, the projection and the position of the patient are significant. If the caudal sac tapers abruptly, frontal or oblique views may show spurious foreshortening of the oil column. Similar spurious foreshortening may occur in patients with marked spondy-

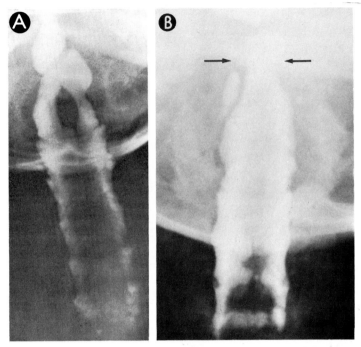

Fig 9–13.—**A,** oval-shaped radiolucency due to displacement of Pantopaque by the dens projecting into the anterior subarachnoid space. **B,** central constriction of the head of the Pantopaque column due to the flow of the oil into a small midline gutter in the presence of a shallow dens and a deep dorsolateral subarachnoid space.

lolisthesis. The true termination of the sac can be demonstrated only by taking a film in the erect position with the horizontal beam. The end of the sac may vary in shape from a conical pointed tip to a blunt, bulbous extremity and rarely to a bifid fork. Abrupt tapering of the normal short sac away from the ventral surface of the bony canal is common and should not be mistaken for the deformity produced by an extradural mass lesion (Figs 9–20 and 9–21).

The depth of the subarachnoid space may also vary to a lesser degree. This variation in depth influences the density of the contrast column. A deep subarachnoid space produces a more opaque column and a narrow space a less opaque column through which the nerve roots may be seen as radiolucent streaks (Figs 9–22 and 9–23).

Usually the anterior surface of the subarachnoid space is intimately related to the posterior margin of the intervertebral disk, separated only by the posterior longitudinal ligament and the dura. Consequently, in the prone lateral projection made with the horizontal beam, the anterior surface of the contrast column may be indented by the posterior margins of the intervertebral disks at the level of the interspaces. This tends to be diminished in flexion and accentuated in extension of the spine. The accentuated defects on the anterior aspect of the contrast column at the level of the interspaces are due to transverse infolding of the dura. Breig has shown that the spine elongates in flexion and shortens in extension by as much as 3 cm. The dura adapts to the shortened length of the bony canal by accordion-like pleating at the interspaces. The resulting transverse dural folds bulge into the subarach-

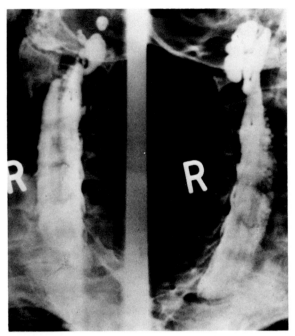

Fig 9–14.—Spot films demonstrating the oil column flowing around the dens toward the cisterna magna with the head extended and the chin turned first to the right and then to the left.

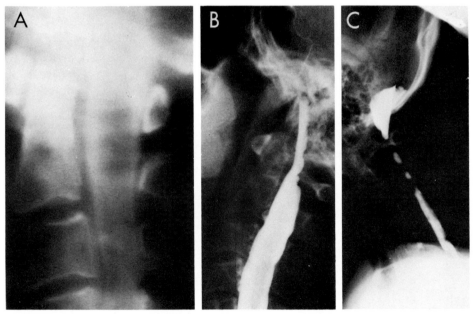

Fig 9–15.—**A,** midline tomographic cut of a cervical metrizamide myelogram, showing a normal foramen magnum. **B,** prone shoot-through Pantopaque study, demonstrating a normal anterior surface of the foramen magnum. **C,** supine film in same patient, showing a normal posterior rim of the foramen magnum.

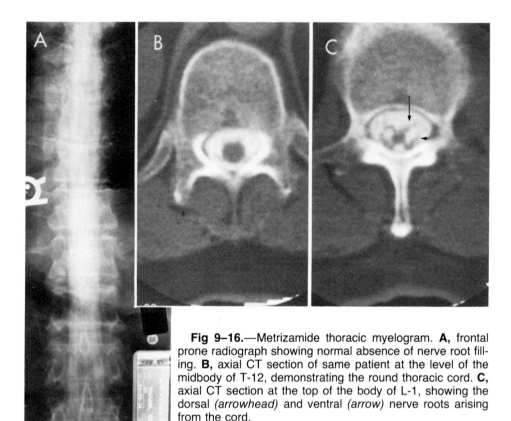

Fig 9–16.—Metrizamide thoracic myelogram. **A,** frontal prone radiograph showing normal absence of nerve root filling. **B,** axial CT section of same patient at the level of the midbody of T-12, demonstrating the round thoracic cord. **C,** axial CT section at the top of the body of L-1, showing the dorsal *(arrowhead)* and ventral *(arrow)* nerve roots arising from the cord.

noid space and produce anterior extradural defects that can simulate central disk herniations. At times, the ventral surface of the subarachnoid space lies several millimeters behind the posterior surface of the vertebra, particularly at the lumbosacral level. Under these circumstances, a central herniated disk may be completely missed at myelography (Fig 9–24).

Occasionally, also, the lumbar vertebral bodies present a markedly concave posterior surface. Under these circumstances, if a small-to-moderate quantity of Pantopaque is used, the opaque medium fills only the bony concavities, resulting in a bizarre appearance. Furthermore, such a study is most inadequate because the oil is not in contact with the intervertebral disks at the interspaces. In this situation, it may be necessary to use as much as 30–40 ml of Pantopaque so that the oil can spill over into the subarachnoid space beyond the vertebral concavities and make contact with the intervertebral disks (see Fig 4–8).

There are two common types of arrangement of the nerve roots in the cauda equina with intermediate gradations.

1. The individual roots may be recognizable as discrete separate structures on either side of the midline filum terminale. The root just about to leave the theca occupies the most lateral position, the remaining roots lying medial to this root in increasing numeric order (see Fig 9–21).

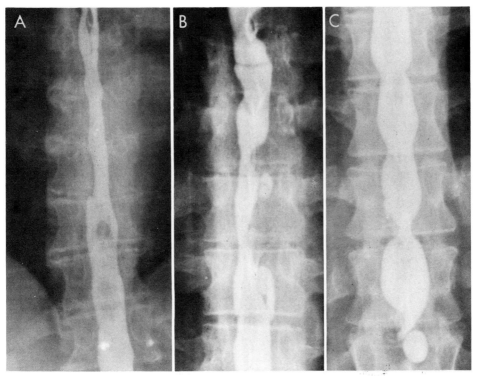

Fig 9–17.—Frontal myelographic spot films in three different patients **(A, B, C)** demonstrating defects in the Pantopaque column in the thoracic region due to inadequate oil and disk bulging.

2. The roots may be grouped together as a bundle on either side of a wide midline space.

As each root courses downward to leave the thecal sac, it lies against the lateral wall of the sac, thereby contributing to the outline of the contrast column. At the site of exit of each root from the thecal sac, there is a lateral and slightly inferior outpouching of the dura and arachnoid (axillary pouch), which may be visualized in profile in the oblique projections (Fig 9–25). Beyond this point, the dura and arachnoid continue for a varying distance as the root sheath. The prolongation of the subarachnoid space over each nerve root may be opacified to a varying degree, filling being more consistent and complete with aqueous contrast media. Under these circumstances, the nerve root itself may be visualized as a radiolucent streak within the opaque contrast medium. The lateral triangular outpouching of the meninges below the exit point of the nerve root from the thecal sac contains no anatomical structures and, therefore, fills with contrast material. The apex of the axillary pouch corresponds to the point where the root leaves the thecal sac. Normally, the nerve root passes inferiorly and laterally along the inner aspect of the vertebral pedicle to the intervertebral foramen and, therefore, exits above the intervertebral disk (Fig 9–26). At the site of the intervertebral foramen, the anterior and posterior roots unite just distal to the posterior ganglion to form the spinal nerve (Fig 9–27). With metrizamide myelography, the anterior (ventral) and posterior (dorsal) roots can often be clearly identified (Fig 9–28).

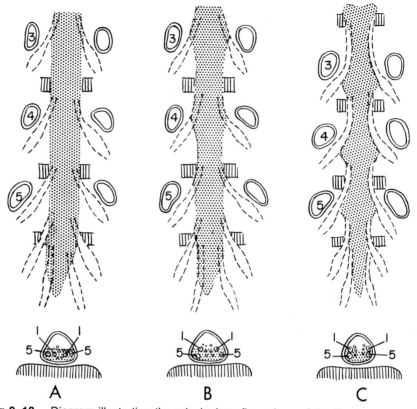

Fig 9–18.—Diagram illustrating the principal configurations of the Pantopaque column in the lumbar region: **A,** cylindric, **B,** intermediate, **C,** biconcave. *5,* fifth lumbar nerve; *1,* first sacral nerve. (Modified from Begg, Falconer, and McGeorge.)

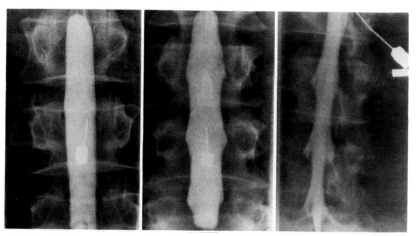

Fig 9–19.—Radiographs showing the principal configurations of the lumbar Pantopaque column in the frontal projection.

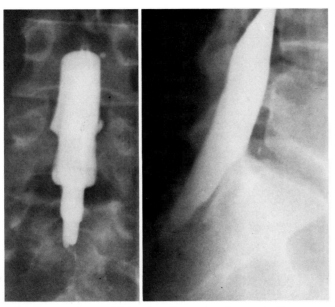

Fig 9–20.—Anteroposterior and lateral radiographs demonstrating normal termination of the caudal sac at S-2.

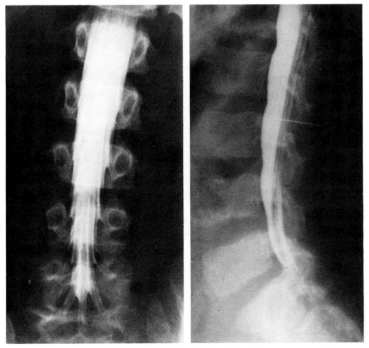

Fig 9–21.—Metrizamide lumbar myelogram (upright) in a patient with a caudal sac terminating at the L5-S1 interspace.

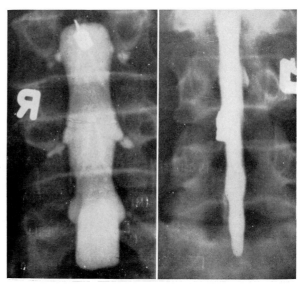

Fig 9–22.—Radiographs demonstrating the marked variability in the width of the lumbar subarachnoid space.

The axillary pouches at a given level tend to be symmetric, although filling of these pouches may vary. In general, the sacral pouches fill more completely than the lumbar pouches. Asymmetric filling of the axillary pouches at a single level is not abnormal per se. The pathologic pouch is characterized by distortion or deformity, for instance, elevation (Fig 9–29).

CEREBELLOPONTINE CISTERNS AND RELATED POSTERIOR FOSSA STRUCTURES

The pontine cistern lies on the clivus anterior to the pons. Its posterolateral extensions, the cerebellopontine cisterns, course around the brain stem along the

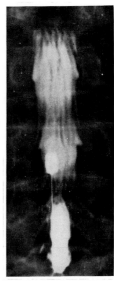

Fig 9–23.—Shallow subarachnoid space with the individual nerve roots of the cauda equina visualized as vertical radiolucent streaks.

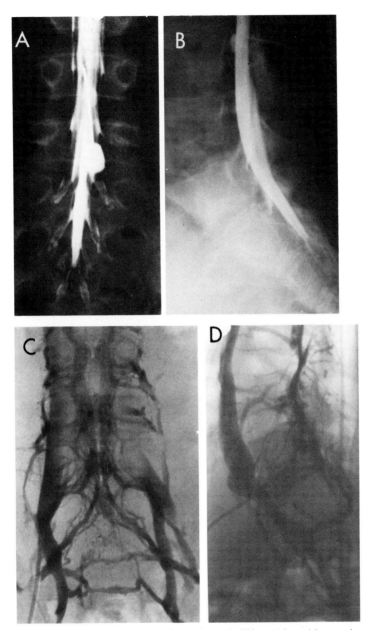

Fig 9–24.—AP **(A)** and lateral prone shoot-through **(B)** metrizamide myelograms in an 11-year-old girl with severe low back pain. Note the significant distance of the contrast column from the posterior aspect of the vertebral bodies. AP **(C)** and lateral **(D)** epidural venograms show no evidence of an intraspinal lesion (subtraction films).

posteromedial aspect of the petrous pyramids. Each cerebellopontine cistern is shaped like an equilateral triangle with its base parallel to the midline and the apex directed toward the internal auditory canal. A prolongation of the cistern extends into the internal auditory canal. Numerous vessels and nerves lying in the pontine and cerebellopontine cisterns are readily visualized as linear radiolucencies in the

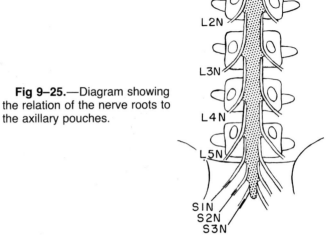

Fig 9–25.—Diagram showing the relation of the nerve roots to the axillary pouches.

opaque oil column (Fig 9–30). Structures frequently seen include the vertebral, basilar, anterior and posterior inferior cerebellar, internal auditory, pontine, superior cerebellar, and posterior cerebral arteries and cranial nerves V, VI, VII, VIII, and XI.

Although variations in the vascular pattern are common, the cranial nerves are constant in their course. The anterior and posterior inferior cerebellar arteries may have a reciprocal relationship in size. There is a danger of ligating a large anterior inferior cerebellar artery in the presence of a small posterior inferior cerebellar artery during the removal of an acoustic neurinoma. The former usually arises beyond the origin of the basilar artery and courses laterally and inferiorly to form a loop near (or at times within) the internal auditory canal; on its way toward the porus acusticus, it crosses cranial nerves VI, VII, and VIII. Just medial to the porus acusticus, the anterior inferior cerebellar artery gives off the internal auditory artery, which accompanies cranial nerves VII and VIII into the internal auditory

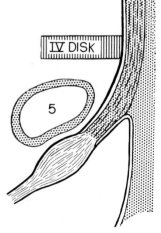

Fig 9–26.—Diagram showing the normal course of a lumbar nerve root after leaving the thecal sac. (After Begg, Falconer, and McGeorge.)

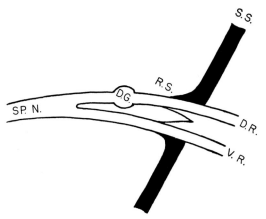

Fig 9–27.—Diagram showing the relationship of the arachnoid and dura to the dorsal and ventral roots of a spinal nerve. Abbreviations: *S.S.*, subarachnoid space filled with Pantopaque; *R.S.*, root (axillary) sleeve; *D.R.*, dorsal root; *V.R.*, ventral root; *D.G.*, dorsal ganglion; *SP.N.*, spinal nerve. (After Rexed.)

canal. Occasionally, the internal auditory artery arises directly from the basilar artery. The internal auditory artery (and the anterior inferior cerebellar artery when it loops in the meatus) may produce small filling defects in the oil-filled canal.

The largest neural impression in the oil column is made by the trigeminal nerve as it crosses the tentorium. This defect is readily recognizable as a discrete notch that interrupts the straight superior attachment of the cerebellopontine cistern to the petrous ridge (Fig 9–31, *A*). Cranial nerve VI is visualized as it courses in a craniad and lateral direction from the lower border of the pons roughly parallel to

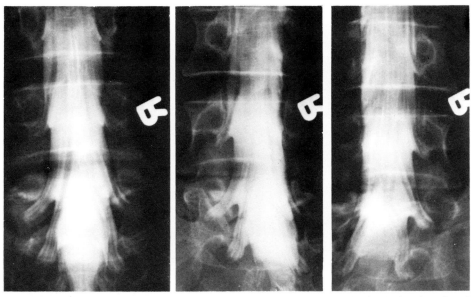

Fig 9–28.—Normal metrizamide lumbar myelogram, demonstrating both the dorsal and the ventral nerve roots at multiple levels.

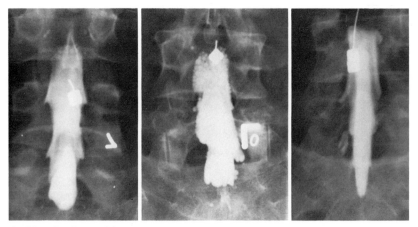

Fig 9–29.—Radiographic montage illustrating: **left,** symmetric filling of the lumbar axillary pouches; **center,** deformity of the axillary pouch at L5-S1 on the right due to a herniated disk; **right,** asymmetric filling of the axillary pouches at L5-S1 in a normal patient.

the basilar artery. Cranial nerves VII and VIII arise from the lower border of the pons near the flocculus and course laterally to enter the internal auditory canal. Although the diameter of the bony internal auditory canal varies widely from 2 mm to 10 mm (avg. 4.5–5.0 mm), the neurovascular bundle has a fairly constant diameter of 2.3 mm. The neural portion of this bundle consists of five nerves—the facial nerve, the nervus intermedius, the cochlear, the superior and inferior divisions of the vestibular nerve. The facial nerve and the nervus intermedius occupy the anterior superior portion of the internal auditory canal above the crista falciformis. The cochlear division of the acoustic nerve occupies the anterior inferior portion of

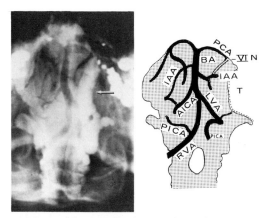

Fig 9–30.—Prone myelographic spot film in a patient with a large left cerebellopontine angle neurinoma (*arrow* points to the indentation on the cistern produced by the medial aspect of the tumor). Note the many vessels and nerves visualized as radiolucencies within the oil column. Abbreviations: *BA,* basilar artery; *RVA,* right vertebral artery; *LVA,* left vertebral artery; *PICA,* posterior inferior cerebellar artery; *AICA,* anterior inferior cerebellar artery; *PCA,* posterior cerebral artery; *IAA,* internal auditory artery; *VIN,* abducens nerve; *T,* tumor.

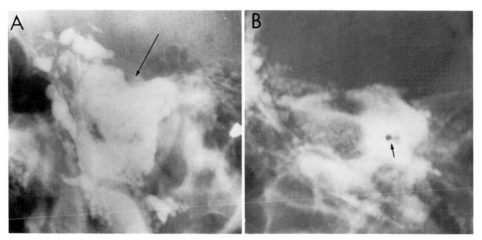

Fig 9–31.—**A,** normal right cerebellopontine cisternogram. Note the trigeminal nerve indenting the superior aspect of the oil column as it crosses the tentorium *(arrow).* **B,** normal right CP cisternogram in another patient. Note the sharply defined round radiolucency produced by the forward bend of the cochlear nerve *(arrow).*

the canal. The superior and inferior vestibular nerves occupy the posterior portion of the canal, above and below the crista falciformis, respectively. According to Valvassori, Pantopaque may be unable to enter the rare small canal (diameter 2.0–2.5 mm) because the latter is completely filled by the neurovascular bundle. In a slightly larger canal (2.5–3.0 mm), the oil may enter only above the crista falciformis and outline the facial nerve. In meati 2.0–4.5 mm in diameter, the oil normally fills the canal above and below the crista falciformis, outlining both the facial and auditory nerves as radiolucent streaks (Fig 9–32). In large canals (i.e., > 4.5 mm), there usually is complete filling of the canal with obscuration of the neurovascular bundle. Valvassori also points out that the lateral margins of the Pantopaque col-

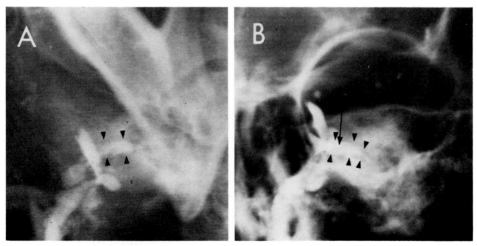

Fig 9–32.—Pantopaque study of a normal left internal auditory canal in a patient with a sensorineural hearing loss. **A,** base view. **B,** PA view. The arrowheads point to the oil in the internal auditory canal. Note the neurovascular bundle *(arrow).*

umn occasionally may be separated from the fundus of the canal by a thin crescentic radiolucency (1 mm) resulting from a short dural sac.

The facial nerve and nervus intermedius course in the superoanterior compartment of the internal auditory canal and exit from its lateral end via a foramen to enter the fallopian aqueduct. Nonfilling of the superoanterior compartment in canals with a diameter greater than 3 mm should be considered pathologic. The larger cochlear division of the acoustic nerve makes a sharp forward bend about 2–3 mm from the fundus of the canal to reach the modiolus. In so doing, the cochlear nerve may produce incomplete filling or a small round filling defect in the inferior compartment of the canal (see Fig 9–31, *B*). The smaller superior and inferior vestibular nerves run to the lateral end of the canal and exit via separate foramina to reach the vestibule.

Cranial nerve XI (accessory) arises from the posterolateral sulcus of the medulla and the lateral aspect of the upper cervical spinal cord. As the nerve courses laterally toward the hypoglossal canal, it may indent the inferolateral margin of the oil column.

In addition to the internal auditory canal, the jugular foramen and the hypoglossal canal also may fill with Pantopaque; if the oil spills over the tentorium into the middle fossa, Meckel's cave also may be opacified. The Pantopaque-filled hypoglossal canal should not be erroneously interpreted as a normal internal auditory canal in the prone oblique cross-table lateral projection when the latter is completely occluded by an intracanalicular neurinoma. A correct evaluation can be made by remembering that the oil-filled hypoglossal canal projects caudad to the petrous bone (Fig 9–33). This is best demonstrated in the cross-table base view made with the horizontal beam.

I have seen several patients with otherwise normal angle myelograms who demonstrated leakage of Pantopaque from the subarachnoid space along the lateral aspect of cerebellopontine cistern. Presumably this occurs through arachnoidal fenestrations (Fig 9–34).

Posteriorly, the variable-sized cisterna magna and cerebellar tonsils are always demonstrable. The fourth ventricle, aqueduct, and posterior third of the third ventricle are occasionally but not consistently opacified by contrast medium with the patient in the prone position. The posterior rim of the foramen margin usually

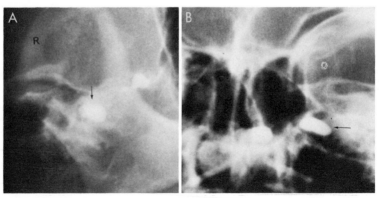

Fig 9–33.—Residual Pantopaque in the right internal auditory canal *(arrow)* **(A)** and in the left hypoglossal canal *(arrow)* **(B).**

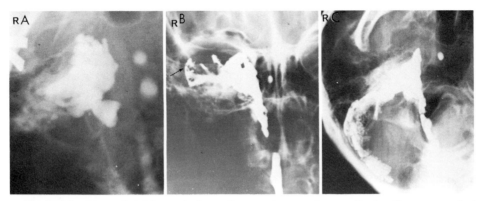

Fig 9–34.—Normal right cerebellopontine myelogram in a patient with a suspected eighth-nerve tumor and no previous operations. **A,** 45-degree oblique spot film taken at fluoroscopy shows filling of the internal auditory canal. **B,** frontal radiograph in the right lateral decubitus position shows early leakage of the oil laterally *(arrow)*. **C,** frontal sub-mentovertical projection with the patient in the right lateral decubitus position shows more extensive leakage of contrast medium laterally in the subarachnoid space around the right cerebellar hemisphere.

slants in a caudal direction. The inferior margins of the cerebellar tonsils do not usually (but may at times normally) project below the foramen magnum. Occasionally the caudal loop of the normal posterior inferior cerebellar artery dips below the posterior arch of the atlas. The tonsils are not always symmetric.

BIBLIOGRAPHY

Arnell S.: Myelography with water-soluble contrast. *Acta Radiol.* (Suppl. 75), 1948.

Begg A.C., Falconer M.A., McGeorge M.: Myelography in lumbar intervertebral disk lesions; correlation with operative findings. *Br. J. Surg.* 34:141, 1946.

Breig A.: *Biomechanics of the Central Nervous System. Some Basic Normal and Pathologic Phenomena* (Braxton, V., tr). Stockholm, Almqvist & Wiksell, 1960.

Breig A., Marions O.: Biomechanics of the lumbosacral nerve roots. *Acta Radiol.* 1(n.s.):1141, 1963.

Calabro A., Smaltino F.: Urea in positive contrast myelography. *Acta Radiol. (Diagn.)* 5:984, 1966.

Camp J.D.: Contrast myelography past and present. *Radiology* 54:477, 1950.

Capesius P., Babin E.: *Radiculosaccography with water-soluble contrast media.* Berlin-Heidelberg, Springer-Verlag, 1978.

Chin F.K., Anderson, W.B.: Improvement of root-sleeve filling in lumbar myelography with oil-soluble media. *Radiology* 96:668, 1970.

Davis D.O., Rumbaugh C.L.: Pantopaque myelography. *Semin. Radiol.* 7:197, 1972.

Decker K.: Mobility of the spinal cord in the vertebral canal. *Ann. de Radiol.* 4:515, 1961.

Epstein B.S.: The myelographic demonstration of the anterior spinal and radicular arteries. *Am. J. Roentgenol.* 91:427, 1964.

Epstein B.S.: Cinemyelographic examination of the cervical spinal canal and the craniovertebral junction. The dentate ligaments. *Br. J. Radiol.* 40:195, 1967.

Geilfuss G.J., Heriot L.: Demonstration of the hypoglossal canal at positive contrast posterior fossa myelography. The fickle finger sign. *Radiology* 102:363, 1972.

Gold L.H.A., Kieffer S.A.: Positive contrast evaluation of the posterior cranial fossa. *Radiology* 102:63, 1972.

Gold L.H.A., Leach C.G., Kieffer S.A., et al.: Large volume myelography: An aid in evaluation of curvatures of the spine. *Radiology* 97:531, 1970.

Goldman R.L., Heinz E.R.: Gas myelography. *Semin. Radiol.* 7:216, 1972.

Hampton A.O., Robinson J.M.: Rupture of the intervertebral disc into the spinal canal after the injection of Lipiodol. *Am. J. Roentgenol.* 36:782, 1936.

Harwood-Nash D.C.: Myelography in children. *Semin. Radiol.* 7:297, 1972.

Jirout J.: Pneumographic investigation of cervical spine. *Acta Radiol.* 50:221, 1958.

Jirout J.: Myelographic syndrome of caudad dislocation of brain stem. Changes in position, mobility and form of upper cervical spinal cord in cases of intracranial expanding lesions. *Br. J. Radiol.* 32:188, 1959.

Jirout J.: Mobility of cervical spinal cord under normal conditions. *Br. J. Radiol.* 32:744, 1959.

Jirout J.: Mobility of the thoracic spinal cord under normal conditions. *Acta Radiol.* 1(n.s.):729, 1963.

Jirout J.: Dynamics of the spinal dural sac under normal conditions. *Br. J. Radiol.* 40:209, 1967.

Khilnani M.T., Wolf B.S.: Transverse diameter of cervical spinal cord on Pantopaque myelography. *J. Neurosurg.* 20:660, 1963.

Lamont A.C., Zachary J., Sheldon P.W.E.: Cervical cord size in metrizamide myelography. *Clin. Radiol.* 32:409, 1981.

Langlotz M.: Lumbale myelographie mit wasserloslichen kontrastmitteln. Stuttgart, G. Thieme Verlag, 1981.

Liliequist B.: Gas myelography in the cervical region. *Acta Radiol.* 4(n.s.):79, 1966.

Long J.M., Kier E.L., Hilding D.A.: Pitfalls of posterior fossa cisternography using 2 ml of iophendylate (Pantopaque). *Radiology* 102:71, 1972.

Martins A.N., Kempe L.G., Pitkethly D.T., Ferry D.J.: Reappraisal of the cervical myelogram. *J. Neurosurg.* 27:27, 1967.

Narimatsu K.: Form and height of normal dural sac as observed in myelography. *Fukuoka-Ikwadaigaku Zasshi* 26:111, 1933.

Nordqvist L.: The sagittal diameter of the spinal cord and subarachnoid space in different age groups. *Acta Radiol.* (Suppl. 227), 1964.

Odin M., Runström G., Lindblom A.: Iodized oil as an aid to the diagnosis of lesions of the spinal cord and a contribution to the knowledge of adhesive circumscript meningitis. *Acta Radiol.* (Suppl. 7), 1929.

Paul L.W., Chandler A.: Myelography in expanding lesions of the cervical spinal cord. Exhibit at 45th Annual Meeting of the Radiological Society of North America, Chicago, Nov. 15–20, 1959.

Porter E.: Measurement of cervical spinal cord in Pantopaque myelography. *Am. J. Roentgenol.* 76:270, 1956.

Pribram H.F.W.: A simple biplane myelographic table. *Am. J. Roentgenol.* 105:411, 1969.

Rexed B.: Arachnoidal proliferation with cyst formation in human spinal nerve roots at their entry into the intervertebral foramen. *J. Neurosurg.* 4:414, 1947.

Sackett J.F., Strother C.M.: *New Techniques in Myelography.* Hagerstown, Md., Harper & Row, 1940.

Skalpe I.O., Sortland O.: *Myelography.* Oslo, Tanum-Nordi, 1978.

Smith C.G.: Changes in length and position of the segments of the spinal cord with changes in position in the monkey. *Radiology* 66:259, 1956.

Thibaut A.: Myélographie gazeuse selective totale. Une amélioration technique. *Acta Radiol.* (Diagn.) 9:754, 1969.

Valvassori G.E.: Myelography of the internal auditory canal. *Am. J. Roentgenol.* 115:578, 1972.

Wellauer J.: Die myelographie mit positiven Kontrastmitteln. Stuttgart, G. Thieme Verlag, 1961.

Wendth A.J., Jr., Moriarty D.J.: A simplified method for the rapid removal of myelographic contrast medium. *Radiology* 93:1092, 1969.

10

Artifacts

SATISFACTORY MYELOGRAPHY depends on precise injection of the contrast medium into the subarachnoid space. Meticulous care in achieving an atraumatic puncture and time spent in fluoroscopically checking the injection of the contrast medium are amply rewarded. Multiple punctures frequently lead to leakage of cerebrospinal fluid and an increased probability of introducing the contrast material outside the subarachnoid space. It is well to remember that, if feasible, myelography should not be performed less than 10–14 days after prior lumbar puncture. Although successful injection of contrast medium into the subarachnoid space is often possible shortly after a diagnostic lumbar puncture, defects may be seen that are difficult to interpret with certainty. Thus, there may be a constriction of the contrast column at the site of previous puncture resembling an extradural mass lesion or compression of the column due to a dorsal extra-arachnoid collection of cerebrospinal fluid. Introduction of the contrast medium beyond the confines of the subarachnoid space may result in findings that are either inconclusive or quite misleading.

It is possible to introduce contrast material inadvertently into the subdural or extradural spaces or into any combination of the subarachnoid, subdural and extradural spaces.

SUBDURAL PANTOPAQUE

When Pantopaque is injected into the subdural space, it separates the arachnoid from the dura and flows to the dependent portion of the spinal canal. Contrary to some opinions, subdural Pantopaque does move, albeit more slowly than subarachnoid oil. It also responds less promptly to changes in CSF pressure and to tilting of the table. Unlike subarachnoid Pantopaque, subdural oil does not present the appearance of a uniform, continuous column. It tends to be distributed irregularly and to remain relatively fixed in isolated collections in the upright position. Both the proximal and distal ends of the oil column tend to be sharply angulated (Fig 10–1, A and B). In the frontal projection, subdural Pantopaque has only a superficial resemblance to subarachnoid oil. Closer inspection reveals a bizarre angular configuration laterally in the region of the cervical nerve roots and a concavity of the column between the roots. A prone lateral radiograph with the horizontal beam

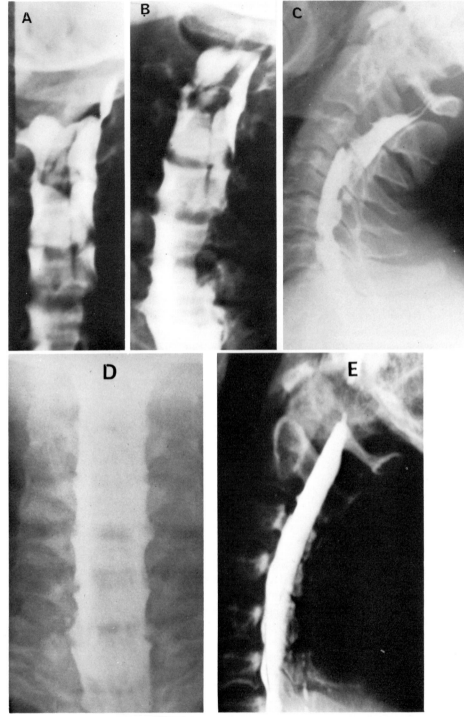

Fig 10–1.—Subdural Pantopaque cervical myelogram in a 33-year-old woman, demonstrating angularity of the margins of the oil column and a nonuniform appearance (**A,** frontal; **B,** oblique). The lateral film **(C)** shows the characteristic posterior defect at C1-2. A repeat subarachnoid study one month later **(D, E)** is entirely normal.

clearly demonstrates the posterior location of the oil, which does not gravitate to the normal ventral aspect of the subarachnoid space. With the patient upright, the normal termination of the caudal sac is grossly distorted, and the nerve roots themselves cannot be identified.

Azar-Kia et al. have pointed out the characteristic appearance of subdural Pantopaque in the upper cervical area. Lateral radiographs of this region demonstrate a prominent posterior defect in the oil column between C-1 and C-2 (Fig 10–1, C). This is produced by collapse of the arachnoid over the dentate ligament and the large posterior root and ganglion of the second cervical nerve.

Because the posterior subdural space has the larger sagittal diameter, Panto-

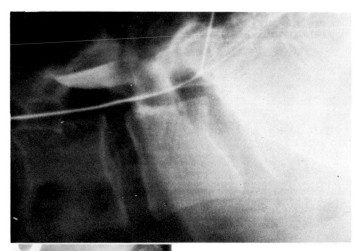

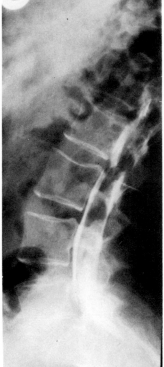

Fig 10–2.—Top, prone lateral shoot-through film, showing Pantopaque in the anterior and posterior subdural spaces. None of the oil is in the subarachnoid space. **Bottom,** lateral shoot-through radiograph during lumbar metrizamide myelography, showing contrast in the anterior and posterior subdural spaces.

paque preferentially collects there. Contrast medium in the smaller anterior sub-dural space has the appearance of a thin streak (Fig 10–2). The oil cannot collect laterally in the cervical and thoracic regions because the arachnoid is fixed laterally to the dura by the dentate ligaments and the nerve roots. Since the anteroposterior position of the spinal cord varies with gravity, the anterior subdural space may be further narrowed with the patient in the prone position. It is possible for a small amount of oil to pass from the posterior to the anterior compartment through the openings between the dentate ligaments and the nerve roots.

Frequently, there is a mixed injection with oil in both the subdural and sub-arachnoid spaces. This should be readily apparent on a prone lateral film with the horizontal beam (Figs 10–3, 10–4, 10–5). It is also obvious in the frontal view because the subdural Pantopaque tends to produce peculiar angular opacities that do not correspond to any anatomical structures in the subarachnoid space. In such cases, the subarachnoid oil moves freely, while the subdural oil tends to lag behind. Furthermore, the two opacities cannot be fused into a single column.

Subdural oil is difficult to remove, although at times it is possible to recover varying amounts by careful, patient manipulation of the needle. On the other hand, if the introductory 0.5 ml. of Pantopaque proves to be subdural at check fluoros-copy, it often can be removed completely at that time.

EXTRADURAL PANTOPAQUE

Pantopaque in the extradural tissues tends to coat the periphery of the spinal cord and roots in an irregular, confluent, streaky fashion. Extradural Pantopaque

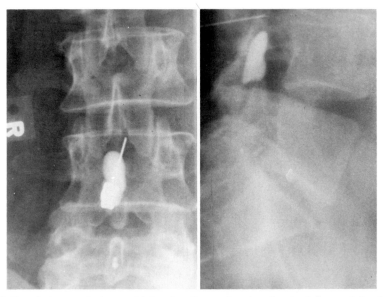

Fig 10–3.—Anteroposterior and lateral radiographs showing test dose of 1 ml of Pan-topaque in the subdural space. In the frontal projection, the appearance is similar to that of subarachnoid oil. At fluoroscopy, however, the movement of the oil was sluggish. In the lateral view, the characteristic posterior position of the Pantopaque confirms its subdural location.

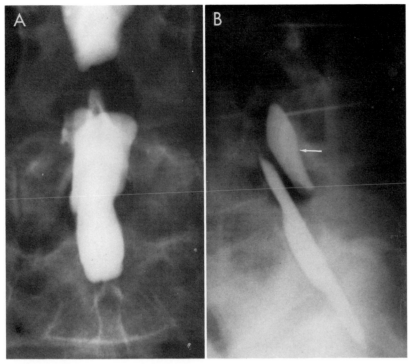

Fig 10–4.—Combined subdural-subarachnoid injection showing a spurious defect in the frontal projection. Note the complete separation of the two columns of oil in the lateral projection. The subdural Pantopaque lies more dorsally *(arrow)*.

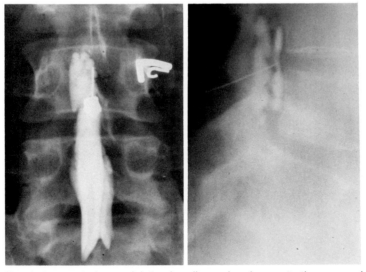

Fig 10–5.—Anteroposterior and lateral radiographs demonstrating a combined subdural-subarachnoid injection of Pantopaque. In the frontal projection, the bizarre streaky appearance of the superimposed dual columns of oil, which cannot be fused, is typical of a mixed injection. On the lateral shoot-through film, the ventrally placed oil is subarachnoid, and the more dorsal oil is subdural.

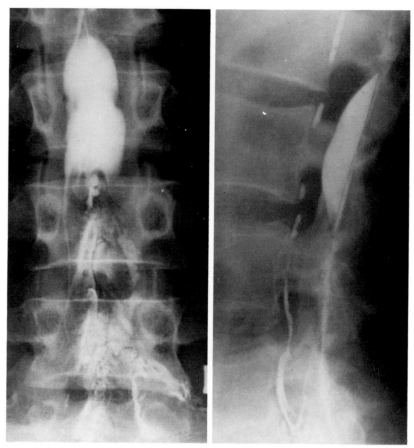

Fig 10–6.—Anteroposterior and lateral radiographs of a mixed subdural-extradural injection. The extradural Pantopaque appears smudgy and streaky, extending along a lower nerve root in the frontal projection. In the lateral view, the extradural oil can be seen coating the surface of the cauda equina.

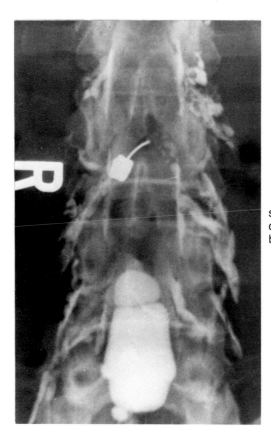

Fig 10–7.—Combined extradural-subarachnoid injection. The extradural oil extends along the nerve roots bilaterally in a characteristic manner.

also has a proclivity for spreading along the nerve roots in a characteristic bizarre, streaky pattern, often beyond the intervertebral foramina (Figs 10–6, 10–7). Occasionally, when subarachnoid Pantopaque is not adequately removed, a film made several days after myelography may show extradural extension of the oil along the nerve roots, even though the original films failed to demonstrate oil outside the subarachnoid space. Usually, this occurs after a traumatic tap that produced a small tear in the dura. Extradural Pantopaque does not flow craniad for any distance, nor does it sustain the appearance of a unified column when the table is tilted with the head down. It usually is absorbed extremely slowly. Occasionally, however, significant quantities of Pantopaque may be absorbed from the extradural space within a few years (Fig 10–8).

INTRAVENOUS PANTOPAQUE

Subsequent to traumatic lumbar puncture and extra-arachnoid injection of Pantopaque, the oil may intravasate into the spinal veins (Figs 10–9, 10–10). It results in transient venous opacification and fairly rapid disappearance of the oil from the lumbar region. The patient may complain of chest pain and cough due to multiple small pulmonary emboli. If a roentgenogram of the chest is made at this time, many small irregular densities can be seen in both lungs.

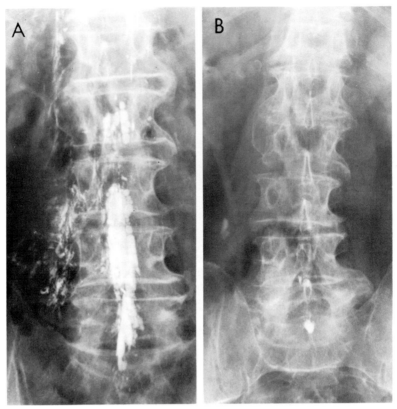

Fig 10–8.—**A,** mixed injection of Pantopaque with considerable oil in the extradural space on April 27, 1968. Re-examination 3 years later **(B)** shows resorption of all the extradural oil—a droplet remains in the subarachnoid caudal sac.

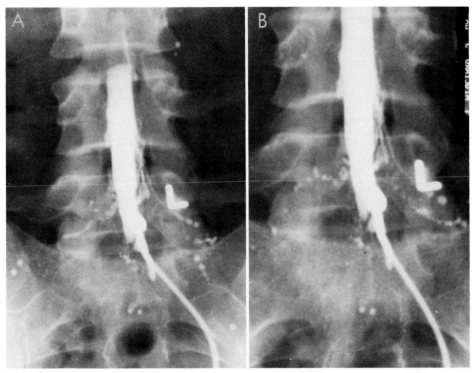

Fig 10–9.—Frontal spot films in a patient after a bloody spinal tap. Although most of the Pantopaque is in the subarachnoid space, small globules are in the external vertebral plexus and quickly disappeared. Note the change in position of several globules on the two successive films made as rapidly as possible.

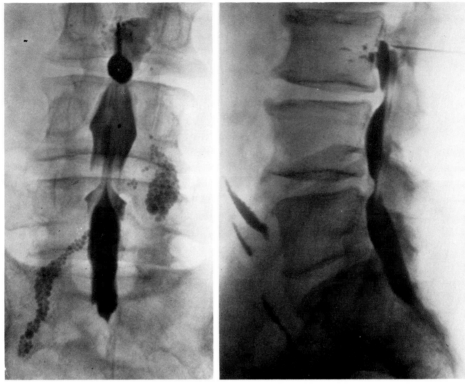

Fig 10–10.—Direct traumatic injection of Pantopaque into extradural vertebral venous plexus (image reversal).

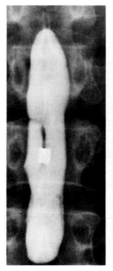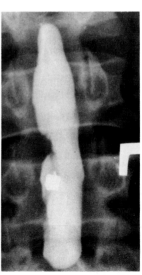

Fig 10–11.—Spot film demonstrating transfixation of the meninges by the lumbar puncture needle.

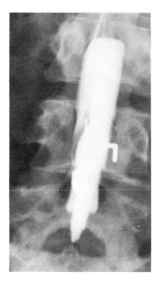

Fig 10–12.—Medial displacement of nerve root at L3-4 on the right by a lateral puncture.

Rarely, nontraumatic venous extravasation may occur via direct arachnoid-venous communications.

FAULTY INSERTION OF NEEDLE

It is always preferable to insert the needle at an interspace not under investigation because the needle itself may produce a defect. As a rule, such a defect is due

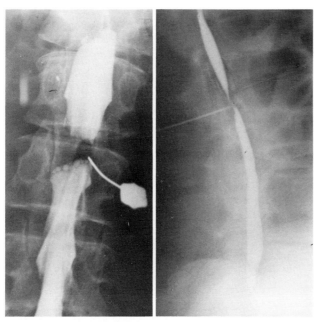

Fig 10–13.—Needle defect due either to a localized subdural collection of cerebrospinal fluid or to an extradural hematoma.

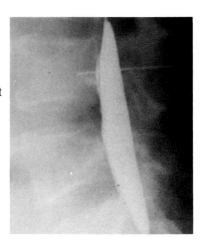

Fig 10–14.—The fluoroscopic spot film device was inadvertently not locked in place. During the examination, it came down on the needle and impaled the latter in the body of L-4.

to a lateral traumatic tap and is less likely to occur when a careful midline puncture is done. The needle may (1) push the meninges ahead of it (Fig 10–11), (2) puncture the lateral aspect of the dural sheath and displace a nerve root medially (Fig 10–12), (3) perforate the arachnoid, with resultant formation of a localized subdural collection of cerebrospinal fluid, which compresses the cauda equina (Fig 10–13), or (4) traumatize extradural veins and produce a localized hematoma that deforms the cauda equina.

Overzealous advancement of the needle without attention to "feel" may rarely

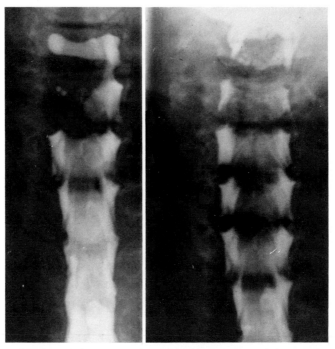

Fig 10–15.—Spurious defect along the right lateral aspect of the cervical Pantopaque column due to insufficient oil *(left);* disappearance of the defect when more oil was brought up *(right).*

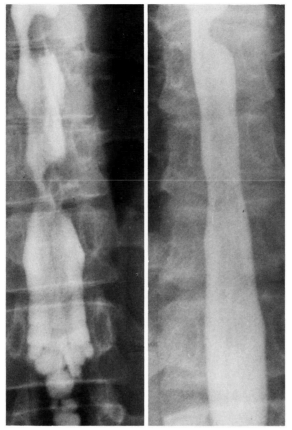

Fig 10–16.—Multiple constrictions of Pantopaque column in the interspaces in the thoracic region due to insufficient oil *(left)*; normal appearance with a full column of oil *(right)*.

result in insertion of the needle into the vertebral body or intervertebral disk space (Fig 10–14). This can also occur if the fluoroscopic spot film device is not locked or the patient is not forewarned about raising his back from the table.

DEFECTS DUE TO INSUFFICIENT CONTRAST MEDIUM AND GLOBULATION

Peculiar, striking artifacts may arise anywhere in the spinal canal due to the use of an inadequate amount of Pantopaque (Fig 10–15). Similar pseudodefects occur when the oil column breaks up into globules, particularly in the thoracic and, to a lesser extent, in the cervical regions. A common artifact resulting from the use of insufficient Pantopaque is the hourglass, waist-like constriction seen at one or more interspaces (Fig 10–16). This is particularly prone to occur in the presence of generalized bulging of the intervertebral disks. Similar defects occur when the oil pools in deep concavities on the posterior surface of the vertebral bodies. When the concave excavations are unusually deep, the oil column may be completely interrupted at the interspaces. These defects can be eliminated by using sufficient Pantopaque to fill the subarachnoid space adequately.

BIBLIOGRAPHY

Azar-Kia B., Batnitzky S., Liebeskind A., Schechter M.M.: Subdural Pantopaque: A radiologist's dilemma. *Radiology* 112:623, 1974.

Fullenlove T.M.: Venous intravasation during myelography. *Radiology* 53:410, 1949.

Ginsberg L.B., Skorneck A.B.: Pantopaque pulmonary embolism. Complication of myelography. *Am. J. Roentgenol.* 73:27, 1950.

Hinkel C.L.: The entrance of Pantopaque into the venous system during myelography. *Am. J. Roentgenol.* 54:230, 1945.

Jones M.D., Newton T.H.: Inadvertent extra-arachnoid injections in myelography. *Radiology* 80:818, 1963.

Keats T.E.: Pantopaque pulmonary embolism. *Radiology* 67:748, 1956.

Lewitan S., Gilbert S., Karvounis P.: Twenty-four-hour film as aid in recognition of mixed injections (subarachnoid, subdural and epidural) in Pantopaque myelography. *Radiology* 93:177, 1969.

11

The Pathologic Myelogram

THE PATHOLOGIC MYELOGRAM can best be understood by analyzing the relationship of various intraspinal lesions to the structures outlined by the contrast-filled subarachnoid space. The location of intraspinal lesions may be conveniently classified as intramedullary and extramedullary, and the latter as intradural and extradural. At first glance, one might think that myelography should consistently be able to distinguish these various locations. In practice, however, this is not the case. Myelography can accurately establish the relationship of an intraspinal lesion to the investing membranes in most, but not all, cases. Analysis of the incorrect localizations points up the limitations of myelography in this regard and the factors responsible for such errors.

1. PROJECTION.—It is important to have multiple projections so that a concise representation of the lesion can be established. Depending on the particular situation, this may require oblique, frontal, and lateral films made with the horizontal beam in both the supine and prone positions (Figs 11–1 to 11–3). An inadequate number of projections may lead to incomplete delineation of a lesion and, hence, to an erroneous conclusion.

2. SHAPE.—It is customary to idealize the shape of a mass lesion diagrammatically, e.g., most frequently, a round tumor is depicted. In truth, however, many intraspinal tumors are not round but irregular in shape. Therefore, it is essential to visualize as much of the surface of a lesion as possible in order to be able to reconstruct and localize it in relation to the meninges and the spinal canal. The more irregular the shape of a tumor the more difficult it is to determine its exact compartment within the spinal canal.

3. SIZE.—There is a minimal threshold below which the exact relationship of a tumor to the theca cannot be established by myelography. By the same token, there is an upper threshold beyond which excessive distortion of anatomical landmarks interferes with accurate localization.

4. SITE OF LESION WITH RESPECT TO VERTICAL AXIS.—The specific localization of tumors involving the spinal cord usually can be determined accurately in the absence of complete obstruction. This is not quite so true in the region of the cauda equina. In the former instance, the cord provides an additional anatomical landmark that significantly enhances the accuracy of localization.

183

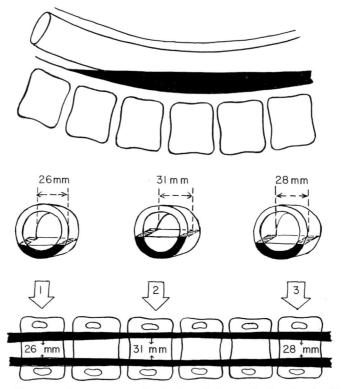

Fig 11–1.—Diagram of a segment of spinal cord demonstrating the factitious appearance of widening of the cord in the frontal projection during myelography (patient prone). This illustrates the necessity for multiple projections and the possibility of making an erroneous diagnosis of cord widening on the basis of a single projection. If one assumes a constant diameter for a given segment of spinal cord deeply submerged in the concavity of the Pantopaque pool (due to the cervical lordosis), the entire diameter will be outlined by the oil. However, as the cord emerges from the Pantopaque pool, the oil outlines a secant that is less than the true diameter of the spinal cord.

5. ADHESIONS.—The presence of adhesions with resultant loculation of CSF may not permit the contrast medium to come in contact with, and delineate, the lesion. This is responsible, at times, for false localization.

6. CONTRAST MEDIUM.—It is necessary to use sufficient contrast medium to outline a lesion in its entirety. An insufficient quantity of contrast medium may lead to artifacts and incomplete depiction of the intraspinal disease.

INTRAMEDULLARY LESIONS

Since intramedullary lesions arise within the substance of the cord, they necessarily expand the cord as they grow (Fig 11–4). The enlarged segment of cord tends to fade off gradually at either end because most intramedullary tumors are invasive gliomas that infiltrate the cord in a diffuse, fusiform fashion. Similarly, the involved segment is usually fairly long because intramedullary gliomas commonly involve a considerable length of spinal cord and occasionally the entire cord.

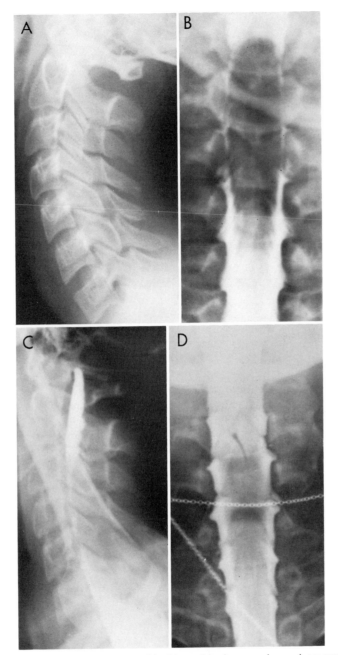

Fig 11–2.—The patient, a 14-year-old girl, suddenly experienced severe pain in the posterior cervical region associated with numbness of both arms and legs. There was no history of a previous injury, and the patient's hematologic status was normal. Physical examination revealed a flaccid quadriparesis. **A,** the plain lateral radiograph of the cervical spine was negative. **B** and **C,** myelography limited to the prone position was thought to indicate an intramedullary lesion. Note the apparent widening of the cord in the frontal projection, **B.** Had the patient been examined in the supine position as well, the correct diagnosis would have been established preoperatively. At surgery, a large extradural hematoma extending from the lower border of C-2 to C-5 was found. The cord appeared normal and pulsated freely after evacuation of the hematoma. A complete clinical recovery occurred in 24 hours. Repeat myelography 2 months postoperatively **(D)** was normal. (Courtesy of D.W. Cooper and P.M. Molloy.)

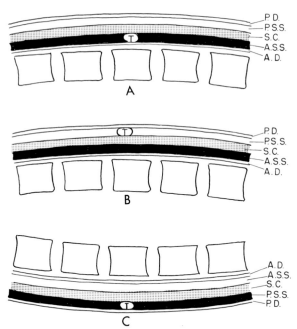

Fig 11–3.—An anterior extramedullary intradural tumor is readily demonstrable in the lateral projection, **A,** using the horizontal beam with the patient prone. On the other hand, a similar tumor on the posterior surface of the spinal cord is not visualized in the same projection, **B,** because the Pantopaque collects anteriorly due to gravity and does not come in contact with the tumor. However, the latter is readily demonstrable with the patient in the supine position, **C.**

The dilated, fusiform cord narrows the bands of contrast medium lateral to it (Fig 11–5). The narrowing is often pronounced, so that the contrast medium lateral to the distended cord appears as a thin streak along the inner margin of the vertebral pedicles. These streaks are constant and extend over several vertebral segments. In addition, the axillary pouches between adjacent pedicles may also be visualized as small triangular opacities projecting out from the lateral streaks. If the lesion

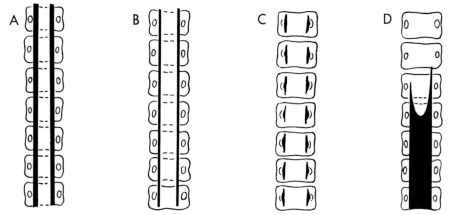

Fig 11–4.—Diagram demonstrating the normal appearance, **A,** and progressive enlargement of the spinal cord in intramedullary lesions, **B, C, D,** culminating in complete obstruction, **D.**

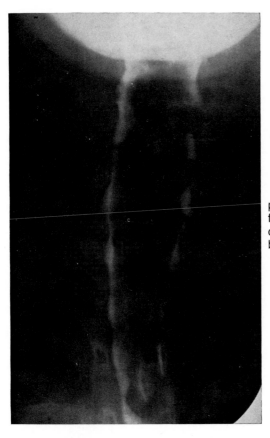

Fig 11–5.—Myelogram in a patient with syringomyelia, showing fusiform swelling of a long segment of cord with narrowing of the lateral bands of contrast medium.

involves the entire circumference of the cord uniformly, the lateral streaks are bilaterally symmetric. If, however, the lesion involves one half of the cord more extensively, the cord expands unequally, narrowing the lateral band of contrast material on the involved side to a greater extent or even obliterating it. As a result, only the streak of contrast material on the contralateral side may be visualized.

It is important to realize that enlargement of the cord is not pathognomonic of an intramedullary neoplasm. Similar enlargement may occur in myelitis, granuloma, abscess, cyst and syringomyelia. Although exact roentgen differential diagnosis may not be possible, the associated presence of atrophy of the thoracic cord is strongly suggestive of syringomyelia. This finding can best be demonstrated by CT or by air myelography with tomography. Occasionally, a midline extradural mass, i.e., a herniated cervical disk, may flatten the cord in its sagittal diameter and thus give the appearance of a widened cord in the frontal projection. Differentiation can readily be made by lateral decubitus films with the horizontal beam, which clearly demonstrate the anterior extradural location of the lesion (Fig 11–6). In addition, whereas most intramedullary gliomas extend over several segments, the pseudoexpansion of the cord due to a herniated disk characteristically involves a short segment (Fig 11–7).

Intramedullary lesions frequently produce only a partial block. Under these circumstances, they can usually be identified properly. In the presence of complete obstruction (Fig 11–8), however, recognition of the intramedullary nature of a lesion may be difficult or, at times, impossible. This is particularly true in the region

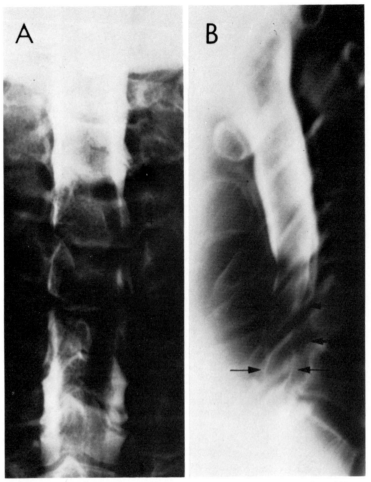

Fig 11–6.—Metrizamide cervical myelogram. The posteroanterior film **(A)** suggests an intramedullary mass. However, the lateral radiograph **(B)** clearly shows that the pseudo-widening of the cord is due to an anterior extradural lesion at C4-5, i.e., a herniated disk *(arrows)*. (Courtesy of G.B. Bradec and A. Kaernbach.)

of the conus medullaris and cauda equina. Gliomas (particularly ependymomas) of the conus medullaris may grow large enough to obliterate the subarachnoid space. The resultant complete obstruction cannot be differentiated from any other intra-dural tumor. If contrast medium is injected below the level of such a tumor, the smooth inferior surface of the tumor may simulate an intradural extramedullary lesion, i.e., neurilemoma (Fig 11–9).

EXTRAMEDULLARY LESIONS

Intradural Lesions

For all practical purposes, these lesions lie within the subarachnoid space, thereby coming into direct contact with the contrast medium. Consequently, they

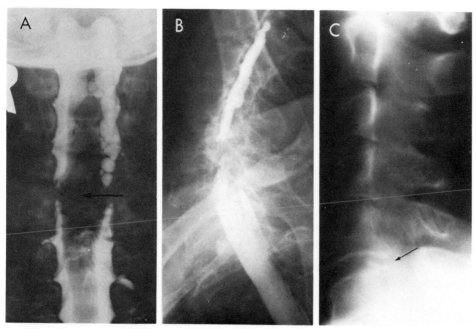

Fig 11–7.—Frontal view **(A)**, swimmer's view **(B)** made during Pantopaque myelography, and lateral tomogram **(C)** in a 63-year-old woman with long tract signs and C-6 nerve-root involvement. Note that the pseudo-widening of the cord on the frontal film is limited to a short segment *(arrow)*. The swimmer's view clearly shows the lesion to be extradural rather than intramedullary; the tomogram points up the prominent osteophyte at C5-6 *(arrow)* responsible for the defect.

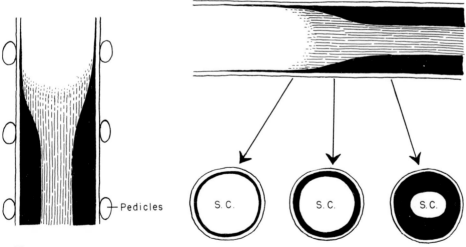

Fig 11–8.—Diagram of the myelographic appearance in complete obstruction due to an intramedullary lesion with serial cross-sections of the cord at various levels near the tumor.

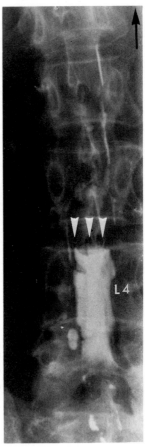

Fig 11–9.—Ependymoma of the conus medullaris and cauda equina, resulting in a complete obstruction at the level of L3-4. Note the "cap" defect *(arrowheads)* produced by the inferior margin of the tumor, which has the appearance of an intradural extramedullary lesion. Some of the Pantopaque is extra-arachnoid.

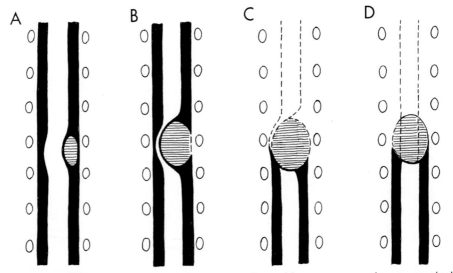

Fig 11–10.—Diagram demonstrating the myelographic appearance in progressively larger symmetric, lateral-lying, extramedullary intradural tumors, **A, B, C,** and in a similar midline tumor, **D.**

produce a sharply defined, rounded defect at the interface between the tumor and the contrast medium. If the tumor produces a complete block, the margin of the tumor abutting on the contrast medium is outlined as a clear-cut "cap" defect.

Unlike intramedullary tumors, which usually enlarge the cord without displacing it, extramedullary intradural tumors always displace the cord. If the tumor is anterior, the cord is displaced posteriorly; a posterior tumor displaces the cord anteriorly. A lateral-lying tumor displaces the spinal cord toward the opposite side against the inner surface of the spinal canal. In so doing, the subarachnoid space on the side of the tumor is usually widened, whereas the contralateral subarachnoid space is narrowed or obliterated. On the side of the tumor, the widened subarachnoid space frequently takes the configuration of a triangle. This differs from an extradural mass, which, in displacing the cord, indents but does not expand the theca. The fundamental myelographic differences between an extramedullary intradural mass

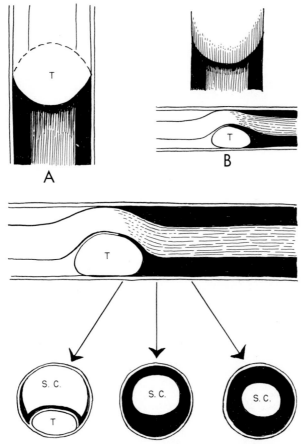

Fig 11–11.—Diagram of the myelographic appearance in complete obstruction due to a symmetric extramedullary intradural tumor on the anterior aspect of the spinal cord. In **A,** the Pantopaque column is arrested at the same level anteriorly and posteriorly in the prone lateral projection. Therefore, one sees a sharp, well-defined "cap" defect. In **B,** the Pantopaque is arrested at a higher level posteriorly, thus resulting in a somewhat unsharp interface that resembles an extradural tumor in the frontal projection. The correct localization can be made from the lateral prone projection.

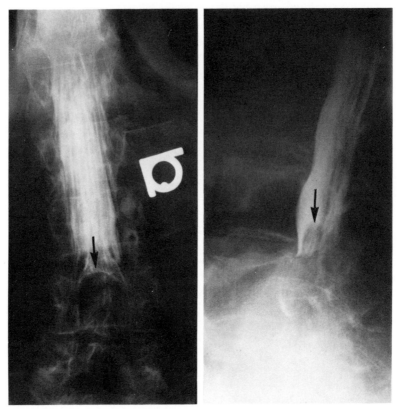

Fig 11–12.—Frontal and lateral films taken during metrizamide myelography (C1-2 puncture) in a 65-year-old woman with a complete block at the superior aspect of L-3. Note the classic "cap" defect *(arrow),* indicative of an intradural lesion. At surgery, a neurilemoma was removed.

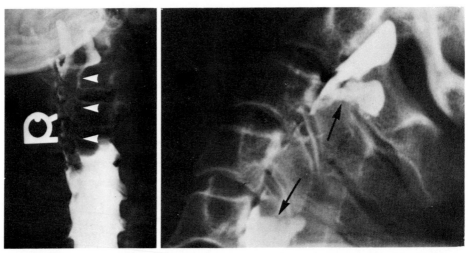

Fig 11–13.—AP and lateral films of an extramedullary intradural neurilemoma on the left posterolateral aspect of the cord, extending from the lower border of C-3 down to C-5 *(arrows).* Note the contrast medium capping the sharply defined lobulated tumor and the clear delineation of the displaced spinal cord *(arrowheads).*

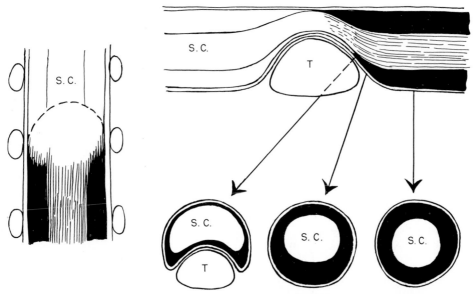

Fig 11–14.—Diagram of the myelographic appearance of a symmetric midline (anterior) extradural lesion causing complete obstruction, with multiple cross-sections of the cord in the region of the lesion. The frontal projection would have a similar appearance if the lesion were situated posteriorly.

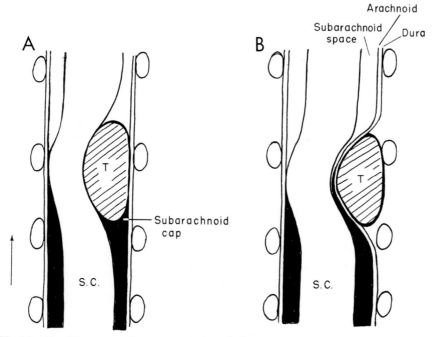

Fig 11–15.—Diagrammatic representation of, **A,** a symmetric, lateral-lying extramedullary intradural tumor and, **B,** extradural tumor. Note the subarachnoid cap in the former due to stripping of the dura away from the tumor with widening of the ipsilateral subarachnoid space contiguous to the tumor.

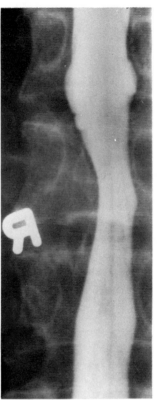

Fig 11–16.—Extradural metastasis along the right side of the cord at T-11 and T-12, displacing the cord to the left away from the pedicles. Note the unsharp interface between the lesion and the contrast medium and the absence of a "cap."

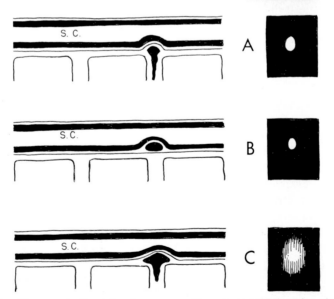

Fig 11–17.—Diagram in the lateral prone position demonstrating the similar appearance produced by, **A,** small, round, well-defined extradural and, **B,** intradural lesions. A larger extradural lesion, i.e., a large herniated disk, **C,** can be readily recognized because of the steep declivity of the defect and the fact that the dura is not stripped away from the spinal cord.

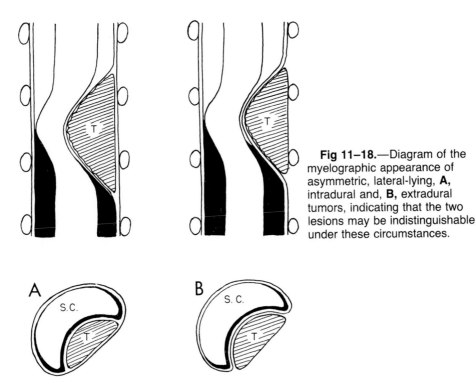

Fig 11–18.—Diagram of the myelographic appearance of asymmetric, lateral-lying, **A,** intradural and, **B,** extradural tumors, indicating that the two lesions may be indistinguishable under these circumstances.

and an extradural mass are (1) the interface between the lesion and the contrast medium is more sharply defined in the former since only the arachnoid separates the mass from the contrast medium (this can more readily be appreciated in the region of the cord), and (2) the dura is not stripped away from the extradural mass even though the cord is shifted (Figs 11–10 to 11–15).

Extradural Lesions

Since extradural lesions (Figs 11–16 to 11–20) lie outside the subarachnoid space, they do not come into intimate contact with the contrast medium. Consequently, the interface between the lesion and the contrast medium tends to be somewhat unsharp. In all other respects, particularly in the cauda equina, the appearance of an extradural lesion may be indistinguishable from that of an intradural lesion. The typical benign, laterally placed extradural tumor indents one side of the contrast column. The resulting defect is usually confined to one or two vertebral bodies and tends to be maximal at its center. If the tumor is very large, it may compress the dura and the subarachnoid space and produce a complete block with tapering of the leading edge of the contrast column. Occasionally, the tumor may angulate the spinal cord and produce a complete obstruction without tapering. In the presence of a complete block below the level of the conus medullaris, an extradural lesion can often be identified by its feathered, serrated interface. The latter is due to the fact that the opacified subarachnoid space over the nerve roots is not in direct contact with the extradural lesion (Fig 11–21).

At times, particularly in the presence of a complete block, it may not be possible to determine the exact location of a spinal lesion from its myelographic appearance.

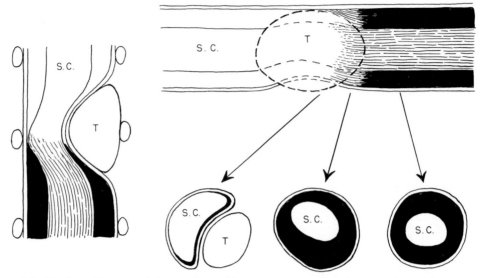

Fig 11–19.—Diagram of the myelographic appearance of a symmetric, lateral-lying extradural lesion producing a complete block, with serial cross-sections of the cord in the region of the tumor.

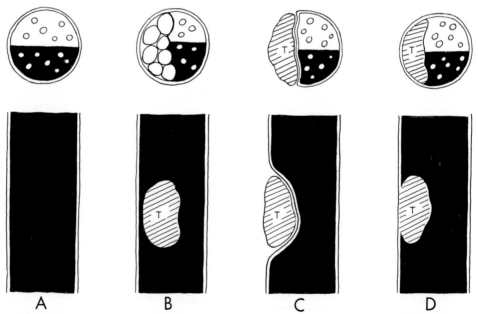

Fig 11–20.—Diagram of the myelographic appearance of: **A,** the normal cauda equina; **B,** intrinsic tumor of the cauda; **C,** extradural tumor; and **D,** intradural tumor. Note that the extradural mass does not strip the dura away from the cauda equina. Note also the resemblance between the expanding intrinsic tumor of the cauda and the intradural tumor.

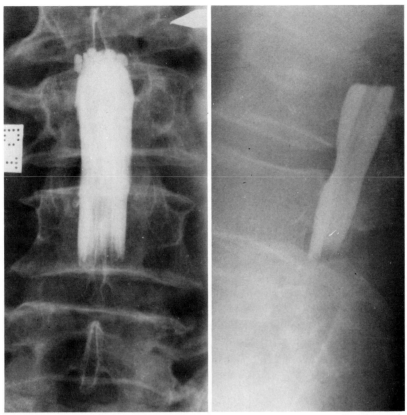

Fig 11–21.—Herniated disk at L4-5 producing paraplegia and a complete block. Note the feathered interface at the site of obstruction, indicating the extradural location of the lesion.

This is particularly true late in the course of a tumor that has grown large enough to produce marked displacement and compression of the cord and the subarachnoid space. Thus, an intradural or an extradural tumor may mimic the appearance of an intramedullary lesion by compressing and widening the spinal cord (see Figs 11–6, 11–7). Similarly, an extramedullary intradural lesion may mimic an extradural lesion. As the former grows, it fills the ipsilateral subarachnoid space, displacing the cord to the opposite side. Progressive displacement of the cord eventually obliterates the subarachnoid space on the side away from the tumor. If the contrast material does not come in contact with the tumor because of angulation of the cord, the intradural location of the tumor is not appreciated.

BIBLIOGRAPHY

Borrelli F.J., Maglione A.A.: The importance of myelography in spinal pathology. Analytical study of 150 cases. *Am. J. Roentgenol.* 76:273, 1956.

Camp J.D.: Contrast myelography past and present. *Radiology* 54:477, 1950.

Lindgren E.: In Schinz H.R., et al. (eds.): *Roentgen-Diagnostics*, vol. 2. New York: Grune & Stratton, 1952, p. 1565.

Tucker A.S.: Myelography of complete spinal obstruction. *Am. J. Roentgenol.* 76:248, 1956.

Walker A., Jessico C.M., Marcovich A.W.: Myelographic diagnosis of intramedullary spinal cord tumors. *Am. J. Roentgenol.* 45:321, 1941.

12

Congenital Lesions

Early in embryonic life, three primary germ layers can be identified—the ectoderm, which forms the neural plate, the entoderm, which forms the primitive gut, and the mesoderm, which gives rise to the musculoskeletal and circulatory systems. The central nervous system is derived from the neural plate, which deepens into a groove that fuses posteriorly. The fusion begins in the cervical area and proceeds cranially and caudally to form the neural tube containing the ventricles and central canal of the spinal cord (the latter actually is a continuation of the fourth ventricle). Closure of the neural tube is normally complete by the fourth week. The meninges probably develop from a mesodermal anlage and the spine from a condensation of scleroderm around the notochord. The notochord and the spinal cord become enclosed within the vertebral body by fusion of the mesodermal mass ventral to the notochord and dorsal to the primitive gut. At the cephalic end of the embryo, the ectodermal neural plate and the entoderm are intimately connected by the neurenteric and accessory neurenteric canals, which normally atrophy and disappear. The notochord, neural tube, and the primitive mesodermal substrate significantly influence the growing axial skeleton.

According to von Recklinghausen, malformations of the spinal cord and meninges and other dysraphic states are due to failure of closure of the neural tube. If the neurenteric canal remains widely patent, complete rachischisis occurs. If the neurenteric canal persists in part, local rachischisis with alimentary dorsal herniation results. Persistence of remnants of the canal may produce diastematomyelia or adhesions between the spinal cord and the intestinal tract, which draw out diverticula from the gut or glial tissue from the spinal cord. The adhesions also interfere with midline cephalic development of the notochord, dividing the latter into halves. Absorption of either half of the notochord or of the adhesions may result in various anomalies, such as hemivertebra, anterior meningocele, or spinal enteric cyst (Fig 12–1). With regard to the latter, the notochord plate is in intimate contact with the entoderm during the third month of gestation. Normally, the notochord separates from the entoderm and becomes completely enveloped by paraxial mesodermal cells, which undergo segmentation to form the spinal column. If the foregut and notochord do not separate normally, a cyst or diverticulum may result, along with failure of ventral fusion of the mesodermal anlage of the spine. This explains why

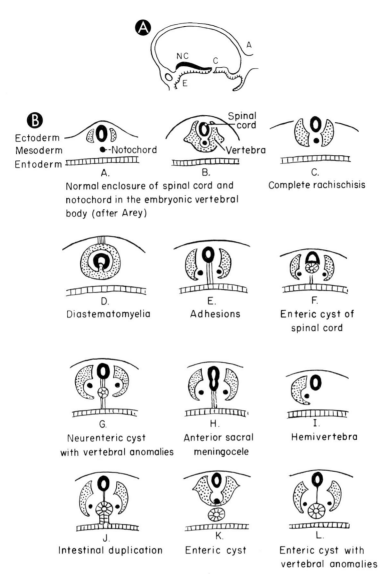

Fig 12–1.—A, diagrammatic cross-section of presomite human embryo demonstrating the intimate connection of the ectodermal neural plate and the entoderm by the neurenteric canal. Abbreviations: *A,* amnion; *C,* neurenteric canal; *E,* entoderm; *NC,* neural crest. **B,** cross-section diagrams illustrating the normal process of enclosure of the spinal cord and notochord in the vertebral body and various developmental anomalies resulting from persistence of the neurenteric canal.

congenital anomalies of the foregut are frequently associated with bony vertebral defects. The foregut malformation occasionally may be several segments away from the vertebral defect because of unequal growth of various fetal organs. Established causes of persistent posterior cleavage include viral infections, vitamin deficiencies, mechanical and metabolic intrauterine damage in the first 6 weeks of pregnancy, and genetic abnormalities.

RACHISCHISIS

The term rachischisis literally means cleft spine (Gr. *rachi*, spine + *schisis*, cleft). A commonly accepted classification includes:

1. Spina bifida occulta—a simple bone defect, with the spinal cord and cauda equina inside the bony canal.

2. Meningocele—a dural outpouching through a bone defect containing no neural elements.

3. Meningomyelocele—a protrusion of the spinal cord and meninges through a bone defect.

4. Myelocele—exposure of a portion of the spinal cord to the posterior body surface.

Spina Bifida Occulta

In its simplest form, this defect consists of failure of fusion of the posterior neural arch of one or more vertebrae, most often L-5 and S1-2. It is so common at the latter location that it may be regarded as a normal variant in an asymptomatic patient. However, it is important to remember that spina bifida occulta may be part of the syndrome of occult spinal dysraphism. A hairy patch of skin, lipoma, dimple, sinus tract, or nevus overlying the spina bifida should raise the suspicion of occult dysraphism.

Meningocele

This relatively uncommon lesion has a proclivity for the occipital (33%) and the proximal and distal lumbar areas. There usually is an intact skin and no significant neurologic deficit. However, there may be evidence of cord compression in patients with large cysts under pressure. The spinal cord and cauda equina occupy a normal position in the bony canal, whereas the arachnoid and dura balloon out through the bone defect. Frontal films of the spine usually demonstrate widening of the spinal canal and an increased interpediculate distance. The laminae may be rudimentary, with a downward, lateral slant. The lateral radiographs often show underdevelopment of the spinous processes and a posterior soft tissue mass. In some cases, the bone defect is small (i.e., a narrow slit in one spinous process) and, therefore, difficult to visualize on routine films.

Howieson, Norrell, and Wilson have pointed out that expansion of the subarachnoid space within the spinal canal does not constitute a meningocele, since there is no meningeal herniation through a bone defect. Hence, the diffuse dilatation of the subarachnoid space associated with scalloping of the posterior surface of the vertebral bodies in neurofibromatosis, Marfan's syndrome, Ehlers-Danlos syndrome, and various bone dysplasias does not represent a true meningocele (Fig 12–2). Although this reservation also applies to occult intrasacral meningocele, I consider the latter to fall within the spectrum of anterior sacral meningocele.

Anterior Sacral Meningocele

This uncommon anomaly may have a familial incidence, possibly associated with an X-linked dominant gene. It may be totally confined to the sacrum and expand

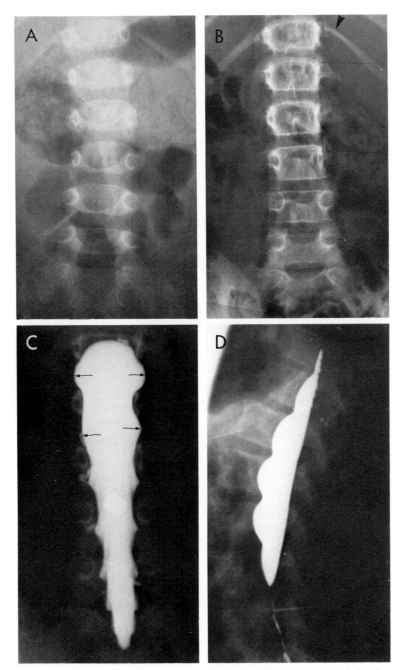

Fig 12–2.—Four-year-old girl with generalized neurofibromatosis and dural ectasia. **A,** frontal radiograph of lumbar spine on March 23, 1965. **B,** re-examination on November 23, 1970. Note the marked thinning of the pedicles and the "waisting" of the left 12th rib *(arrowhead)* that have occurred during the five-year interval. **C,** frontal and, **D,** lateral shoot-through films made during Pantopaque myelography demonstrating widening of the thecal sac, dural ectasia *(arrows),* and excavation of the posterior surface of the lumbar vertebral bodies.

the anterior and posterior sacral walls, i.e., occult intrasacral meningocele (Fig 12–3), or erode the anterior sacral wall and protrude into the pelvis (Fig 12–4). It is accompanied by partial or, rarely, by total sacral agenesis. Partial sacral agenesis usually involves the lower half of the sacrum unilaterally or bilaterally.

The bony deformity consists of a scimitar-shaped defect involving one side of the lower sacrum (Fig 12–5). Unlike the more common posterior sacral meningocele, there are no external manifestations of the anterior sacral meningocele. The latter usually presents as a pelvic mass palpable on rectal examination. An important clinical sign is increased tenseness of the mass following straining, coughing, or any effort that raises cerebrospinal fluid pressure. The rectum may be displaced anteriorly or laterally. The communication of the meningocele with the general subarachnoid space can be demonstrated by metrizamide or Pantopaque myelography. At times, the communication may be difficult or impossible to demonstrate by the more viscid Pantopaque. In these circumstances, it is wise to leave some of the oil in and take a delayed film 24–48 hours later. Anterior sacral meningocele may be associated with tethering of the conus and intraspinal lipoma.

Total sacral agenesis is usually associated with the caudal regression syndrome and an increased incidence in the offspring of diabetic mothers. Although only 1%

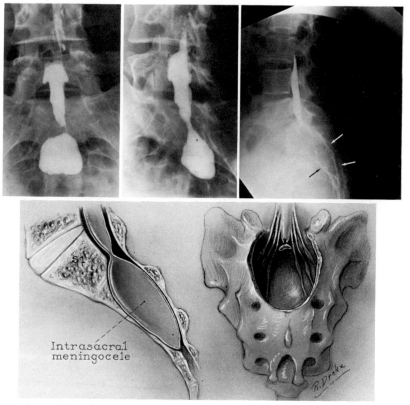

Fig 12–3.—Top, anteroposterior, oblique, and lateral radiographs of a case of localized dilatation of the caudal subarachnoid space. The erosion of the sacrum is outlined by arrows. **Bottom,** operative findings following resection of the dilated sac. (Reprinted, with permission, from Baker B., Webb J.H., *Proc. Staff Meet. Mayo Clin.* 27:231, 1952.)

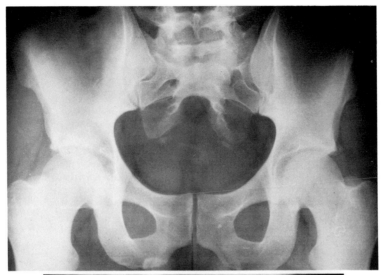

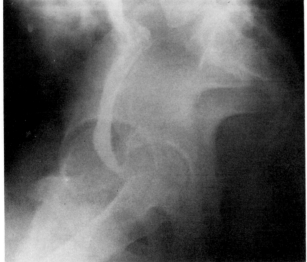

Fig 12–4.—Top, anteroposterior radiograph of a large anterior sacral meningocele in a 26-year-old male student whose presenting complaint was marked constipation. Note the large, smoothly marginated, sharply defined bone defect involving the lower sacrum; **bottom,** lateral postevacuation film following a barium enema, demonstrating marked anterior displacement of the rectum by the meningocele.

of the latter infants have the syndrome, approximately 15% of children with the caudal regression syndrome have diabetic mothers. The syndrome probably represents one aspect of a spectrum of midline dorsal closure defects. It consists of various abnormalities involving the urinary tract, anorectal region, lower limbs, and spine. The more benign end of the spectrum includes varying degrees of neurogenic bladder (Fig 12–6), while the extreme lethal form is represented by symmelia (mermaid syndrome) with fusion of the lower limbs, lumbosacral spine anomalies, imperforate anus, and agenesis of the genitourinary tract (exclusive of the gonads).

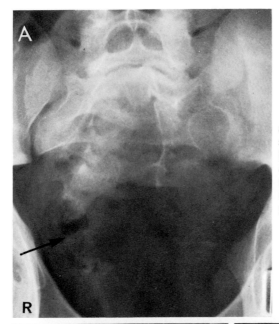

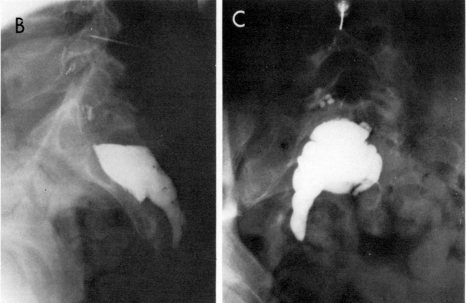

Fig 12–5.—Partial sacral agenesis characterized by a scimitar- or sickle-shaped right lower hemisacrum **(A)** *(arrow)*, associated with an intrasacral meningocele **(B** and **C)**. There was no anterior sacral meningocele present.

Brooks et al. have reported that the myelographic findings in these patients can be divided into two groups: (1) a high termination of the subarachnoid space with dural sac stenosis; (2) a normal or widened subarachnoid space with tethering of a low-lying spinal cord frequently associated with intra- or extrathecal masses, i.e., lipoma, teratoma, cauda equina cyst. Surgical treatment of the dural sac, stenosis, tethered cord, and associated masses may significantly benefit the patient. The termination of the dural sac usually corresponds to the level of bony aplasia.

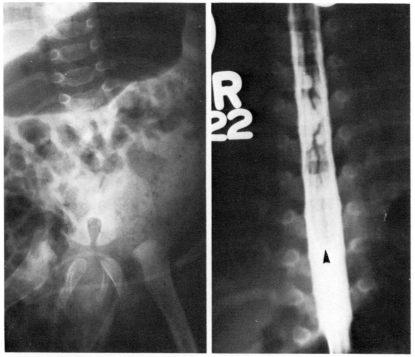

Fig 12–6.—Sacral and lumbar agenesis in a 6-year-old male with a high conus terminating at T9-10 *(arrowhead);* the caudal sac terminated at T-12. There was also an associated meningocele, which could only be filled in the supine position (not shown). The patient presented with a soft tissue mass overlying the lower spine, a neurogenic bladder, and weakness of both lower extremities.

Lateral Meningocele

A lateral meningocele is a protrusion of the arachnoid and dura through an enlarged intervertebral foramen into the paravertebral gutter. The majority of cases occur in the thoracic region, possibly related to the pressure gradient between the subarachnoid and pleural spaces. However, a small number of lateral meningoceles in the lumbar area have been reported. Approximately 70% of all patients with lateral meningocele have generalized neurofibromatosis. Indeed, a lateral meningocele is the most common posterior mediastinal mass associated with von Recklinghausen's disease. Although lateral meningoceles are commonly asymptomatic, they may produce pain by pressure on adjacent structures or traction on spinal nerves. The classic roentgenographic appearance is that of a single spherical posterior mediastinal mass, more often on the right side (Fig 12–7). At times, however, the meningeal sac may be multiple and polycyclic (Fig 12–8). At fluoroscopy, one usually (though not always, perhaps due to peripheral fibrosis) sees pulsations and a changing shape in response to the Valsalva maneuver. Lateral intrathoracic meningoceles are almost always associated with characteristic abnormalities in the adjacent ribs and vertebrae, i.e., kyphoscoliosis, excavation of the posterior surface of the vertebral body or bodies, enlargement of the intervertebral foramen at the level of the meningocele, pedicular erosion, thinning of the adjacent surfaces of the head

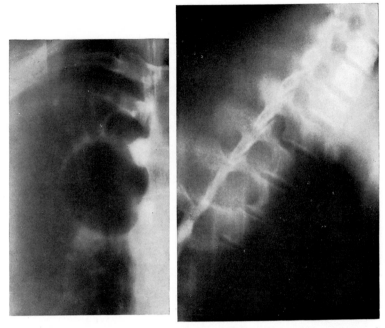

Fig 12–7.—Anteroposterior **(left)** and lateral **(right)** tomographic sections of a patient with a classic lateral thoracic meningocele in the right posterior mediastinal gutter. Note the air in the meningeal sac and the erosion of the posterior surfaces of the contiguous vertebral bodies (Reprinted, with permission, from Hillenius L., *Acta Med. Scandinav.* 163:15, 1959.)

and neck of the involved ribs along with splaying and a widened intercostal space. Myelography plays a key role in the diagnosis of intrathoracic meningocele, demonstrating flow of the contrast medium from the spinal subarachnoid space into the meningeal sac. Occasionally, a pronounced kyphoscoliosis may impede the craniad flow of oily contrast medium in the prone position. In this circumstance, the patient should be examined in the supine position. Actually, if lateral intrathoracic meningocele is suspected on the basis of clinical and conventional roentgenographic findings, gas myelography may well be the technique of choice.

Meningomyelocele and Myelocele

Many so-called meningoceles are epithelialized myeloceles, the most common, serious malformation of the spinal canal. Although usually cystic, at times they may be "dry," i.e., without a cyst. These patients often have hydrocephalus due to an associated Arnold-Chiari malformation or aqueductal stenosis. Uncommonly, meningomyelocele may be associated with a congenital benign intraspinal neoplasm, i.e., dermoid, teratoma.

OCCULT SPINAL DYSRAPHISM

This syndrome has a variety of names: tethered cord, cord tract syndrome, tethered conus, low conus, tethered filum, tight filum. The term spinal dysraphism was

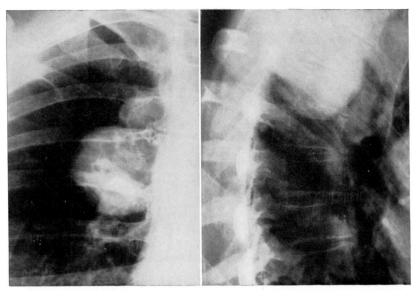

Fig 12–8.—Anteroposterior **(left)** and lateral **(right)** chest roentgenograms of a polycyclic intrathoracic meningocele. (Reprinted, with permission, from Hillenius L., *Acta Med. Scandinav.* 163:15, 1959.)

introduced by Lichtenstein to describe incomplete fusion of the posterior midline structures. It was used by James and Lassman to characterize a symptom complex with progressive deformities of the feet in children due to congenital lesions of the conus and cauda equina associated with spina bifida occulta. Occasionally, the symptoms may not develop until adulthood.

The history is often one of slowness in learning to walk or walking with a limp; a pes cavovarus deformity is commonly present. The neurologic findings include unilateral or (less commonly) bilateral lower limb muscle atrophy, abnormal tendon reflexes (usually exaggerated but sometimes diminished), sensory loss, trophic ulceration of the foot or leg, bowel and bladder dysfunction. Inspection of the skin of the back shows an abnormality in approximately half of the patients, e.g., focal hypertrichosis, nevus, lumbosacral dimple or lipoma, dermoid, sinus tract. Similar clinical findings may occur in other types of spinal dysraphism such as meningocele and diastematomyelia. In fact, spinal dysraphism represents a spectrum of abnormalities, ranging from the mildest form with a wide dural sac and spina bifida occulta to the most severe form with an epithelialized myelocele. The latter patients often have hydrocephalus due to associated aqueductal stenosis or an Arnold-Chiari malformation. I know of no report of an associated Arnold-Chiari malformation in a patient with a tethered conus. On the other hand, this association has occasionally been found in diastematomyelia. It is noteworthy that some patients with a tethered conus also have a benign intradural congenital tumor, i.e., lipoma, dermoid, as do patients with diastematomyelia.

Plain films of the spine demonstrate varying degrees of spina bifida occulta in all patients. Other findings may include abnormal vertebral segmentation, vertebral scalloping, scoliosis, midline bony spur (diastematomyelia), widening of the spinal canal. A wide spinal canal with an increased interpediculate distance per se is not necessarily indicative of an intraspinal mass lesion.

The tail bud in the embryo slowly regresses and is no longer evident externally by 9 weeks of gestation (30–35-mm stage). At this time, the conus and the filum terminale, which develop from the tail bud, lie at the lower end of the spinal canal. According to Barson, the spinal cord and the vertebral column have a parallel growth rate until 12 weeks of gestation. At that time, caudal growth of the vertebral column accelerates, resulting in rapid ascent of the conus until 20 weeks of gestation. Thereafter, ascent continues slowly until the adult level of L1-2 is reached, on the average by the age of 2 months postnatally. In some fetuses, the adult level may be reached as early as 31 weeks of gestation. A conus below the L2-3 interspace after the age of 5 years is definitely abnormal. The normal tip of the conus should lie at the level of the mid body of L-2 by the age of 12 years (see Fig 7–5). The normal filum terminale should not exceed 2 mm in width at myelography (uncorrected measurement).

Gryspeerdt reported the myelographic findings in these patients in some detail, utilizing Pantopaque injected by cisternal or lateral C1-2 puncture. Since that time, Fitz and Harwood-Nash have added their experience with air, metrizamide, and metrizamide-CT, as well as with Pantopaque. They utilize lumbar puncture rather than the cisternal or C1-2 approach. The puncture is preferably made slightly to one side of the midline. General anesthesia is usually employed in children. If Pantopaque is used, the amount of oil should be individualized according to the age of the patient and the capacity of the dural sac. Sufficient contrast material should be used to fill the dural sac adequately so that small posterior-lying lesions and the conus medullaris can be visualized. The entire subarachnoid space, from the caudal sac to the posterior fossa, should first be studied in the prone position to rule out other abnormalities. The patient should then be placed in the supine position, which is crucial for making the diagnosis of a tethered conus since the latter lies posteriorly.

Although air myelography is used by some to study patients with tethered conus, the filum terminale and the nerve roots are better visualized by positive contrast medium. Presently, I believe that metrizamide augmented by CT is the technique of choice because it elegantly delineates the anatomical findings, does not require examination in both the prone and supine positions, and does not have to be removed.

The key to the diagnosis is the demonstration of the anterior spinal artery and the conus tip at an abnormally low level (Figs 12–9 to 12–13). Although the anterior spinal artery ends at the tip of the conus, it may not appear to lie at that level in the prone position because of the posterior position of the tethered conus. Furthermore, if Pantopaque is used, the large amount of oil necessary for a complete study may obscure the artery. Hence, the supine position is crucial for visualizing the conus, the filum, the nerve roots, and various masses that may be present, i.e., lipomas, cysts.

When the conus is tethered, the nerve roots lose their normal course parallel to the conus and become considerably angulated. Occasionally, they may even assume the upward course of the roots in the Arnold-Chiari malformation. The abnormal position of the nerve roots does not involve the entire spinal cord; it is limited to multiple segments adjacent to the tethered conus. The conus may be low in position but normal in configuration, with a thickened filum terminale. On the other hand, the conus may not have a clear-cut termination, tapering imperceptibly to an

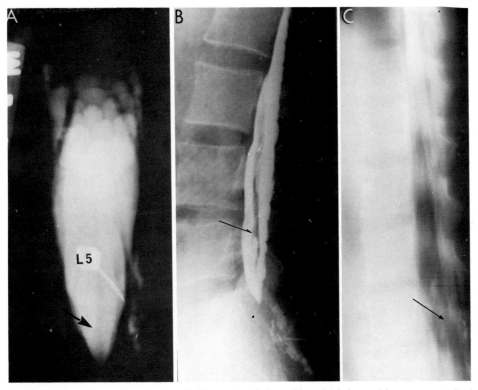

Fig 12–9.—The patient, a man in his early thirties with spinal dysraphism, was studied by both Pantopaque and gas myelography. The prone Pantopaque myelographic spot film **(A)** clearly shows the low position of the anterior spinal artery *(arrow);* the lateral cross-table file **(B)** outlines the low position of the conus medullaris *(arrow);* the lateral radiograph during pneumomyelography **(C)** graphically demonstrates the dorsal fixation of the cord *(arrow).*

abnormally thickened, fibrous filum. Occasionally, the conus may lie within the sac of a lumbar meningocele to which it is tethered by a lipoma. Traction bands are visualized as radiolucent defects within the contrast column in the supine position. This differentiates them from a midline septum, which is demonstrable in both the supine and prone positions.

In my opinion, the lipomas associated with a tethered conus are hamartomas rather than true neoplasms of fat. An associated subcutaneous lipoma may extend through the posterior midline bone defect into the spinal extradural space and invade intradurally, with involvement of the conus medullaris and/or the cauda. In some patients, the intrathecal lipomas present as large filling defects within a wide dural sac. The combination of a distorted, compressed large dural sac in a patient with a low-lying conus should suggest the presence of an associated lipoma.

There is no consensus concerning the etiology of the neurologic findings. Perhaps stretching of the cord during periods of rapid growth or secondary to the scoliosis may compromise the blood supply. Possibly the dural bands attached to the conus or filum produce traction on the cord. Possibly there is traction upon the neural fibers in the corticospinal tracts.

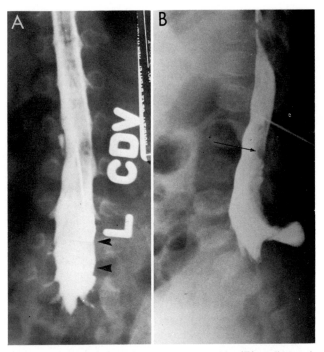

Fig 12–10.—Anteroposterior **(A)** and lateral cross-table **(B)** radiographs taken during myelography in a 16-month-old girl with spinal dysraphism. The patient had a posterior dimple and a spina bifida occulta. At operation, in addition to the meningocele, there was an extensive extradural lipoma with intradural extension through a dural defect. The extradural lipoma deforms the left lateral aspect of the Pantopaque column caudally *(arrowheads)*. Note the low-lying cord *(arrow)* and tapering of the conus dorsally as it attaches to the meningocele.

DIASTEMATOMYELIA

Diastematomyelia (Gr. *diastema,* fissure + *myelos,* spinal cord) is a malformation of the neural axis characterized by segmental midline cleavage of the spinal cord or cauda equina. The cord or cauda is divided into halves by a bony, fibrocartilaginous, or fibrous spur projecting from the posterior surface of the vertebral body through the middle of the spinal canal (Fig 12–14). This malformation, most common in the lower thoracic and lumbar regions, is always associated with body and/or arch anomalies of one or more vertebrae in the vicinity of the lesion. Rarely, there may be double diastematomyelia (two spurs) or diastematomyelia without a septum and an unusual termination of both halves of the spinal cord, i.e., one half of the cord terminating in the neural plate and the other half entering the distal sacral canal. Plain spine films may show widening of the spinal canal with an increased interpediculate distance extending over a varying number of segments. The pedicles are usually not narrowed or eroded unless there is an associated intraspinal lipoma or dermoid cyst. Other associated skeletal abnormalities may include hemivertebrae, butterfly vertebra, unsegmented or hypoplastic vertebral bodies, narrowed intervertebral disks, scoliosis, kyphosis, and deformities of the neural arches. Various cutaneous defects, such as hair tufts, dimpling of the skin, and subcuta-

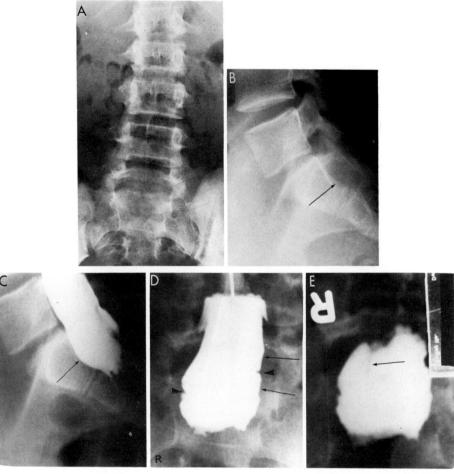

Fig 12–11.—Radiographs of a 13-year-old boy with spinal dysraphism. The anteroposterior radiograph **(A)** shows an increased interpediculate distance and occult spina bifida; the lateral projections **(B** and **C)** demonstrate localized erosion of the sacrum *(arrow)* produced by the dilated subarachnoid space; the prone myelographic spot film **(D)** shows the irregular bizarre roots *(arrowheads)* and extrinsic pressure on the left lateral aspect of the oil column by the lipoma *(arrows);* the supine film **(E)** clearly outlines the apex of the low-lying conus medullaris and the filum terminale *(arrow)* at the level of L-5.

neous fatty tumors may also be present in or close to the midline in the same segment as the vertebral abnormality.

When the septum dividing the spinal cord is ossified, it may be seen on the routine frontal projection as a small, oval density within a widened vetebral canal. Body section radiography may be helpful in demonstrating the bony septum. If the midline spur is fibrocartilaginous, it is not visible on ordinary films. In this circumstance, myelography can provide the correct differential diagnosis, since similar vertebral anomalies may also occur with other lesions, such as meningocele, congenital dermoids, and lipoma. The myelogram classically demonstrates a midline filling defect in the contrast column that may be elongated or small and rounded, depending on the size and shape of the osseous or fibrocartilaginous spur (Figs 12–

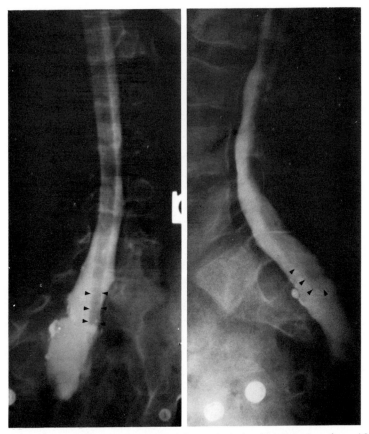

Fig 12–12.—Metrizamide myelogram performed via lumbar puncture in a 12-year-old boy with weakness of the lower extremities and bowel and bladder incontinence. At surgery, there was tethering of the cord with lipomyelomeningocele. The patient had had a previous Pantopaque myelogram. Note the low position of the cord *(arrows)* and the dilated caudal sac. The patient also had basilar invagination and failure of segmentation of C-2 and C-3.

15, 12–16). The contrast column is split into two columns at the level of the spur. The association of a midline filling defect and segmental anomalies of the spine clinches the diagnosis of diastematomyelia, although either one of these findings may occur separately in other lesions. When the septum occurs below L-2, it usually transfixes the low-lying conus. The septum can be readily demonstrated at myelography with the patient in the prone position, whereas the conus is best demonstrated caudad to the septum with the patient supine. Metrizamide-CT myelography is presently the technique of choice for diagnosing this lesion.

CONGENITAL DERMAL SINUS

These tracts occur along the cerebrospinal axis in or near the midline posteriorly. Dermal sinuses are rare in the cervical region, somewhat more common in the thoracic area, and most common in the lumbosacral area. The dermal sinus enters

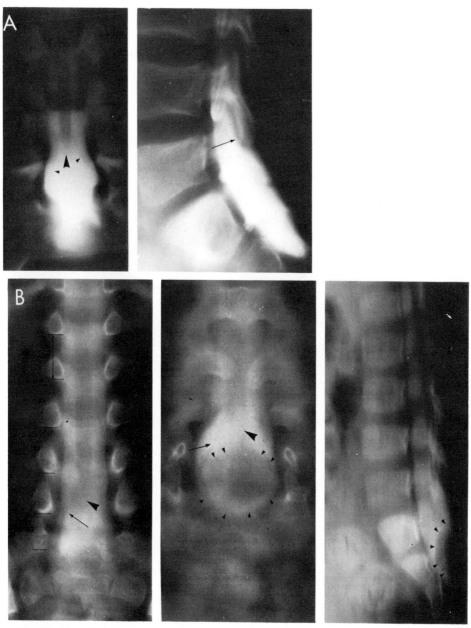

Fig 12–13.—A, frontal and lateral tomograms made during metrizamide myelography in a 12-year-old boy with tethering of the cord. Note the low position of the cord *(large arrowhead),* the abnormal nerve roots *(small arrowhead),* and the posterior tethering *(arrow).* **B,** tomographic sections of a metrizamide myelogram in a 5-year-old boy who had had a meningocele repair at an early age. There is obvious tethering of the cord as evidenced by the low position of the conus at L4-5 *(thick arrowhead).* Note also the abnormal nerve roots *(thin arrow)* and the spina bifida. The large, rounded defect at the inferior aspect of the contrast column *(arrowheads)* was an epidermal inclusion cyst. Congenital vs. acquired?

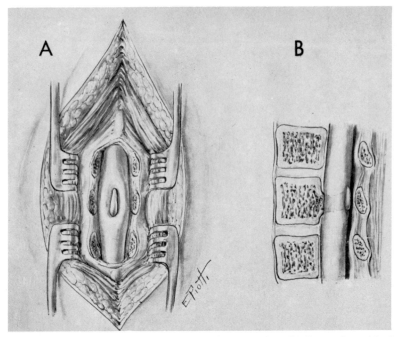

Fig 12–14.—Operative findings in a case of diastematomyelia illustrating widening and bifurcation of the spinal cord by a bony spicule. (Reprinted, with permission, from Neuhauser E.B.D., et al.: *Radiology* 54:659, 1950.)

the spinal canal through a defect in the neural arch or in the interspinous ligament. In a review of 12 thoracic dermal sinuses by Wright, the opening of the sinus on the skin was found between T-1 and T-4 in 10 cases and in the lower thoracic area in two cases. In the upper thoracic region, the sinus usually enters the spinal canal 1–2 vertebrae caudal to its cutaneous opening; in the lumbosacral area, the entrance usually is 1–2 vertebral segments above the cutaneous opening. In the experience cited above, the sinus terminated, respectively, in an intradural epidermoid, a teratoma, and an intramedullary abscess in three patients and in a dermoid cyst in nine patients (Fig 12–17). Infection in the form of meningitis or intraspinal abscess is relatively common in lumbosacral dermal sinuses.

CONGENITAL FISTULA

Rockett and his co-workers reported an unusual case of intermittent otorrhea and rhinorrhea in a child with meningitis due to a congenital fistula between the lateral cerebellopontine cistern and the middle ear. After multiple surgical explorations failed to show a fistula, the latter was demonstrated by Pantopaque instilled into the cisterna magna.

ARNOLD-CHIARI MALFORMATION

The Arnold-Chiari malformation is a congenital anomaly of the hindbrain characterized by downward displacement of the cerebellum and medulla through the

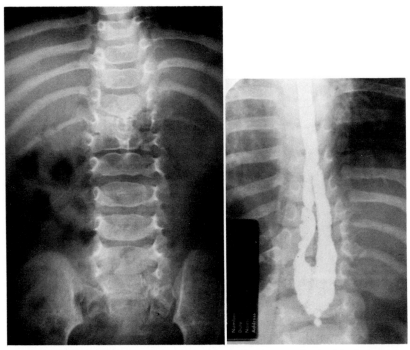

Fig 12–15.—Left, anteroposterior view of the spine in a patient with diastematomyelia of the lower thoracic cord showing interpediculate widening and bony anomalies of T-11, T-12, and L-1. **Right,** myelogram showing the central defect of the Pantopaque column produced by a fibrous septum. (Reprinted, with permission, from Perret G., *Surg., Gynecol. Obstet.* 105:69, 1957.)

foramen magnum into the cervical spinal canal. The anomaly was first mentioned by Cleland in 1883 in a description of a case of thoracolumbosacral myelomeningocele with hydrocephalus. The medullary component was described by Chiari in 1891 and again more fully in 1895.

Chiari described three types of hindbrain malformations:

Type I—downward displacement of the cerebellar tonsils into the vertebral canal with a normal position of the medulla and fourth ventricle.

Type II—in addition to downward displacement of the tonsils, there is associated caudal displacement of the lower pons, medulla, and an elongated fourth ventricle into the vertebral canal. This is the most common form of the malformation and is associated with a myelomeningocele and some form of spinal dysraphism.

Type III—displacement of the medulla, fourth ventricle, and most of the cerebellum into a high cervical and occipital meningocele.

The cerebellar component of the malformation was noted briefly by Arnold in a case reported in 1894. The kinking of the medulla on the cervical cord in the more common type II malformation is associated with elongation and upward obliquity of the cervical roots as they ascend to exit through the intervertebral foramina. The Arnold-Chiari defect may be associated with spina bifida or with a variety of other bony anomalies of the basiocciput and cervical spine, e.g., occipitalization of the atlas, basilar impression, Klippel-Feil syndrome. Hydrocephalus is said to occur in 50%–90% of patients with the Arnold-Chiari malformation and myelomeningocele.

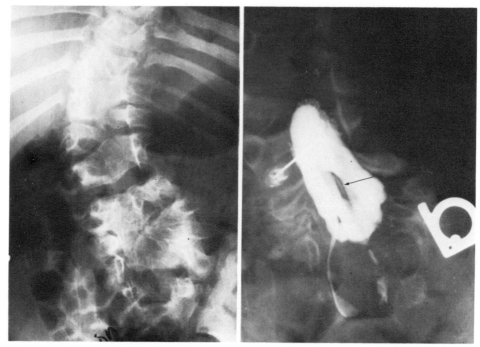

Fig 12–16.—Gross osseous abnormalities in the lower thoracic and lumbar spine of a 7-year-old girl with diastematomyelia. The bony spur *(arrow)* is clearly shown at L-2 on the Pantopaque myelogram.

The hydrocephalus usually is due to aqueductal stenosis or to constriction or obliteration of the cisterna magna and outlet foramina of the fourth ventricle.

Clinically, the Arnold-Chiari malformation may produce cerebellar signs, manifestations of brain stem and cord compression, and hydrocephalus. Because of the multiplicity of neurologic findings, the clinical picture may simulate disseminated sclerosis; basilar arachnoiditis; tumor of the cerebellum, brain stem, or cervical cord; or syringomyelia. In the latter connection, the Arnold-Chiari malformation may be associated with hydromyelia, as illustrated in Figure 12–18, *C*.

Positive contrast myelography, particularly in the supine position, is helpful in the diagnosis of this anomaly by demonstrating an obstructive high cervical lesion. Characteristically, the lower margin of the lesion has a bifid, lobulated border produced by the inferior surface of the herniated cerebellar tonsils, the central incisura corresponding to the space between the cerebellar tonsils. The defect may be symmetric when both cerebellar tonsils are herniated to the same degree or asymmetric when one tonsil is lower than the other. The central incisura may be obliterated by adhesions or cerebellar edema, thereby producing a semilunar defect commonly associated with intradural tumors. On the other hand, a lobulated extramedullary intradural tumor may present a bilobate appearance with a central incisura (Fig 12–19). Consequently, the myelographic picture is not pathognomonic (Fig 12–20). However, the demonstration of cervical roots passing obliquely upward is a helpful diagnostic sign, as is the presence of hydromyelia. Also, if sufficient contrast passes craniad to delineate an ill-defined superior border and a deformed cisterna magna,

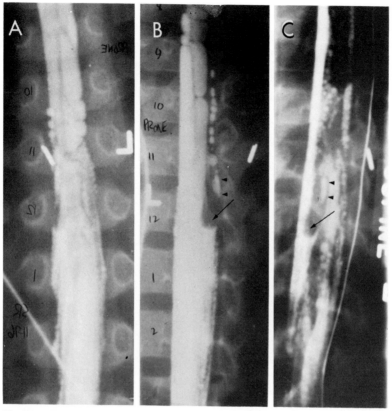

Fig 12–17.—The patient was an 18-month-old male child who had a subcutaneous mass resected from his back in the region of T10-11. Note metallic clips. The pathologic diagnosis was a dermoid cyst. The plain films of the spine demonstrated an abnormal lamina at T-10 (and ? T-11). Pantopaque myelography and subsequent operation revealed a dermoid in the T-10 lamina with epidural extension. A sinus tract from the latter entered the dura at this level and connected with an extramedullary intra-arachnoid dermoid at T11-12 *(arrowhead)*. The cord and nerve roots were not involved. The prone frontal **(A)**, the lateral prone **(B)**, and the supine **(C)** shoot-through films show the intra-arachnoid dermoid *(arrowheads)*. A portion of the connecting tract is demonstrated on the lateral shoot-through films *(arrowheads)*.

the likelihood of an Arnold-Chiari malformation is great. It is important to remember that the inferior limit of the filling defect occasionally may extend as low as C-6.

If pneumomyelography is employed, the cerebellar tonsils may be demonstrated in the air-filled cervical subarachnoid space as narrow, elongated, pointed densities. Frequently, the fourth ventricle is also displaced caudad below the foramen magnum. Because the cerebellar tonsils may be adherent to the medulla anteriorly, it may be difficult to differentiate an Arnold-Chiari malformation from an intramedullary tumor or syrinx unless air either dissects between the tonsils and the posterior surface of the medulla or passes up into the foramen of Magendie. In the latter instance, the foramen is visualized as a radiolucent vertical channel anterior to the tonsils, thereby identifying the latter. If the fourth ventricle is not displaced caudad

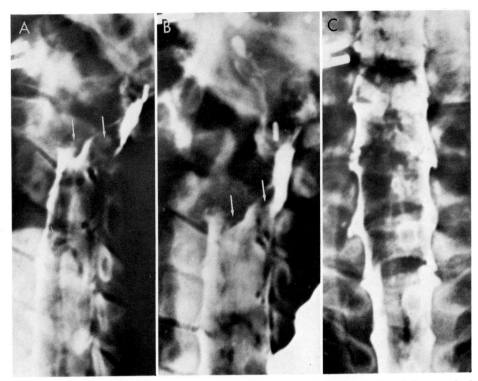

Fig 12–18.—Arnold-Chiari malformation associated with hydromyelia of the cervical cord. The patient, a 39-year-old female, complained of unsteadiness of gait, stiffness, and numbness of the hands and arms of 8 months' duration. At operation, an Arnold-Chiari malformation was found with the tonsils at C2-3, kinking of the medulla on the cervical cord, and extensive dural adhesions. In **A** and **B**, note the low position of the tonsils in the oblique projections *(arrows)* and, **C**, widening of the lower cervical cord due to hydromyelia.

and lies in its normal position, it may not be possible to differentiate between an intramedullary tumor and an Arnold-Chiari malformation. A further difficulty is presented by herniated cerebellar tonsils due to increased intracranial pressure. The herniated tonsils usually present rounded inferior margins that more or less completely fill the subarachnoid space below the foramen magnum. In the more chronic types of tonsillar herniation due to slowly growing tumors, the tonsils may become quite flattened and resemble the appearance of the tonsils in the Arnold-Chiari malformation. Hence, it may not be possible to make the correct differential diagnosis safely from the appearance of the tonsils.

HYDROMYELIA

Hydromyelia refers to dilatation of the central canal, which communicates with the fourth ventricle at its obex. According to Gardner, there is normally a connection between the fourth ventricle and the central canal of the spinal cord during the fifth week of gestation. Increasing pressure within the primitive ventricles and central canal ruptures the rhombic roof and opens the foramina of Luschka and

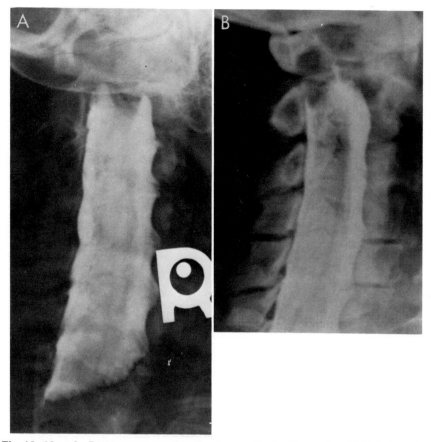

Fig 12–19.—A, Pantopaque myelogram in a patient with an Arnold-Chiari malformation with a central "cap" defect commonly associated with intradural tumors. Note absence of a central incisura. **B,** intradural meningioma presenting as a bilobate defect with a central incisura, simulating an Arnold-Chiari malformation. (Reprinted, with permission, from Shapiro R., Robinson F., *Am. J. Roentgenol.* 73:390, 1955.)

Magendie, thereby creating the subarachnoid space. Further distention of the neural tube is prevented by the absorption of cerebrospinal fluid. Incomplete or absent perforation of the rhombic roof results in dilatation of the ventricles and the central canal. Hydromyelia may occur as an isolated developmental anomaly or in association with the Arnold-Chiari malformation. In the latter instance, the cervical roots have a horizontal or upward course.

Positive contrast myelography demonstrates diffuse enlargement of the spinal cord, which may be indistinguishable from the appearance produced by syringomyelia or intramedullary tumor (Fig 12–21). If the contrast medium enters the dilated central canal, a definite diagnosis of hydromyelia can be established. At times, Pantopaque in the dilated central canal has a destructive globulated, corkscrew appearance (Fig 12–22).

It is important to visualize the fourth ventricle at myelography because it may demonstrate abnormalities in the region of the foramen magnum and posterior fossa, i.e., Arnold-Chiari malformation, lack of ventricular filling, hydrocephalus.

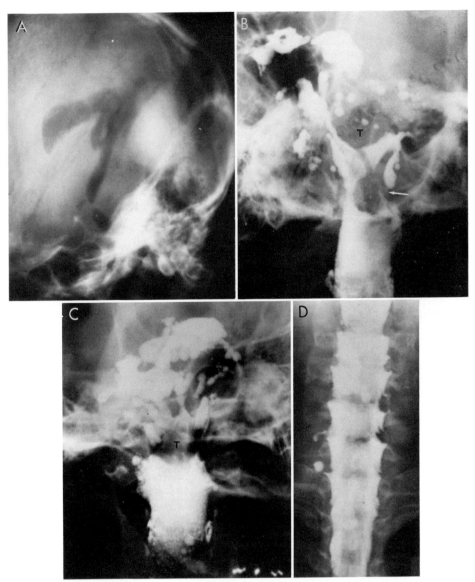

Fig 12–20.—The patient, a young woman, complained of vertigo, nystagmus, ataxia, and postural difficulty in the upper extremities for some time. A posterior fossa lesion was suspected on clinical grounds. **A,** pneumoencephalography demonstrated a low position of the fourth ventricle. Myelography was then performed. **B,** oblique spot films demonstrate the left tonsil *(T)* lying at the level of the foramen magnum and suggestive aneurysm (unconfirmed) of the left vertebral artery *(arrow)*. **C,** the right tonsil is at the level of C1-2. **D,** note the horizontal position of the cervical roots. At operation, the vallecula was obliterated by adhesions, which also occluded the outlet of the fourth ventricle. The left cerebellar tonsil was situated normally, at the level of the foramen magnum, but the right tonsil was found at the level of C1-2 firmly bound down by adhesions. No evidence of tumor was present.

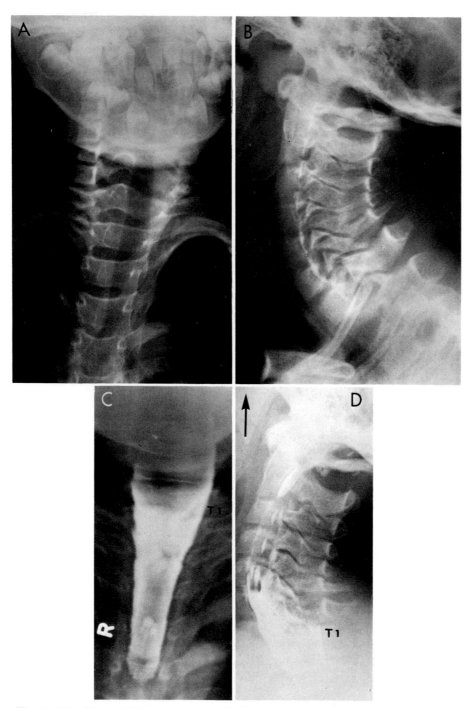

Fig 12–21.—Dandy-Walker syndrome with hydromyelia of the cervical cord (confirmed at surgery). The plain films, **A** and **B,** demonstrate an exaggerated lordotic curve, an increased interpediculate distance, and a wide sagittal diameter of the spinal canal; anteroposterior and lateral myelograms, **C** and **D,** show marked enlargement of the entire cervical cord down to T-1.

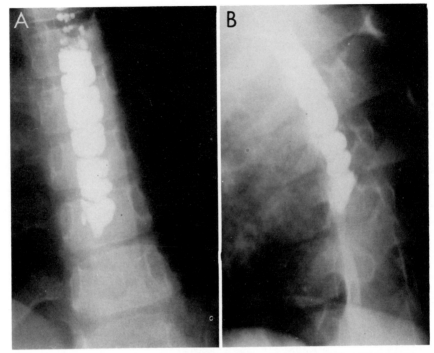

Fig 12–22.—Anteroposterior **(A)** and lateral **(B)** radiographs during Pantopaque myelography in a young male with hydromyelia. Note the continuous, corkscrew appearance of the oil in the dilated central canal. Note also the widening of the thoracolumbar interpediculate spaces.

Syringomyelia refers to an outpouching of the central canal resulting from rupture of the canal with dissection of CSF into the cord. Unlike hydromyelia, the wall of the canal is not lined by ependymal cells. Williams applied the term communicating syringomyelia to both hydromyelia and syringomyelia to distinguish these lesions from the acquired, noncommunicating cysts secondary to tumor, trauma, or degenerative disease. Since congenital cysts of the central canal and acquired cysts of the cord have a similar myelographic appearance, Ballantine et al. and Gardner suggested the term syringohydromyelia, which will be discussed in detail in Chapter 16.

CONGENITAL SPINAL EXTRADURAL CYST

The congenital spinal extradural cyst probably arises as an arachnoidal herniation through a small dural defect. The result is a thin-walled cyst containing cerebrospinal fluid attached to the dura by a narrow stalk posteriorly or posterolaterally. The cyst may or may not communicate with the subarachnoid space. The term congenital is used in contradistinction to the acquired cyst, which develops secondary to trauma, laminectomy, or lumbar puncture. The congenital extradural cyst is a rare lesion. In a review of the literature in 1963, Gortvai found 56 cases to which he added five of his own. Most of the cases occur in the second and third decades of life, with a male preponderance of 2:1. Unlike the acquired cysts, which are usually

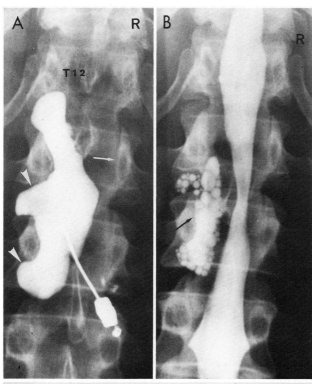

Fig 12–23.—A, frontal myelogram in a patient with a lumbar extradural cyst. Note the erosion of the right pedicle of L-1 *(arrow)* and the projection of the cyst through the intervertebral foramina at L1-2 and L2-3 on the left side *(arrowheads)*. **B,** frontal myelogram demonstrating Pantopaque within the lumen of the cyst *(arrow)*. **C,** operative sketch of the cyst in relationship to the vertebrae. (Reprinted, with permission from Smith G.W., Chavez M., *A.M.A. Arch. Neurol. Psychiatr.* 80:436, 1958.)

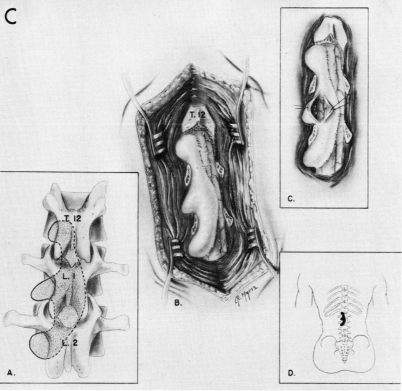

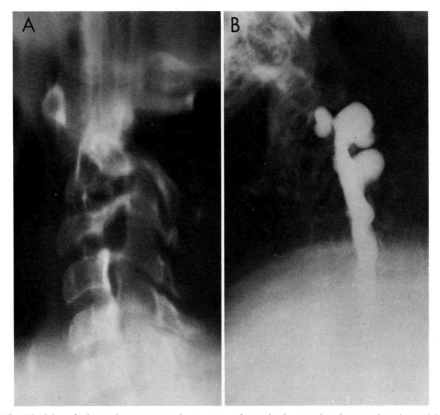

Fig 12–24.—A, lateral tomogram in a case of cervical extradural cyst showing widening of the upper spinal canal with bony erosion at C2-3 and marked separation between the anterior arch of the atlas and the dens. **B,** lateral myelogram (the patient's chin is to the reader's right) in the same patient, demonstrating communication between the cyst and the subarachnoid space, together with diverticula projecting into the left second and third cervical foramina. (Reprinted, with permission, from Gortvai P., *J. Neurol., Neurosurg. Psychiatr.* 26:223, 1963.)

lumbar in location, the predominant site of involvement is the mid and lower thoracic spine; rarely, the cyst is situated in the lumbar (Fig 12–23) and, very rarely, in the cervical region (Fig 12–24).

The syndrome of congenital spinal extradural cyst originally was described by Elsberg et al. in 1934. The typical patient is an adolescent or in the early twenties, with symptoms and signs of progressive spastic paraplegia. Pain and objective sensory signs usually (but not always) are minimal. Remission of symptoms may occur spontaneously or after some orthopedic procedure. The remission probably is related to a decrease in the cyst volume and pressure. Partial or complete block with elevation of the CSF protein level is present in approximately half of the patients.

Plain-film findings include kyphosis (with or without Scheuermann's disease) or kyphoscoliosis, erosion of the pedicles, widening of the interpediculate distance, enlargement of the spinal canal, and excavation of the posterior surface of the involved vertebrae (Fig 12–25). Myelography can establish the correct diagnosis if the examination is carried out properly. Because the cyst and its opening into the

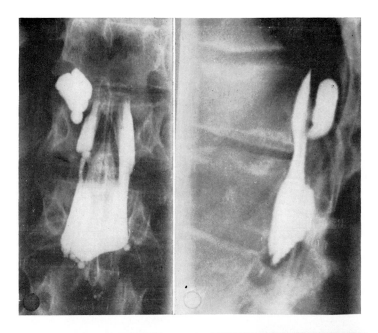

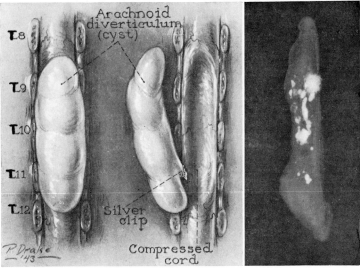

Fig 12–25.—**Top,** posteroanterior and lateral roentgenograms with the table tilted craniad, demonstrating a block at T-11 with an extradural collection of Pantopaque. Note the pedicle erosion of T-11 and T-12 and the wedging of the lower thoracic and upper lumbar vertebrae. **Bottom left,** relationship of the cyst to the dorsal surface of the spine. **Bottom right,** roentgenogram of the specimen after surgical removal showing residual Pantopaque contained within the somewhat collapsed cyst. (Reprinted, with permission, from Good, C.A., et al., *Am. J. Roentgenol.* 52:53, 1954.)

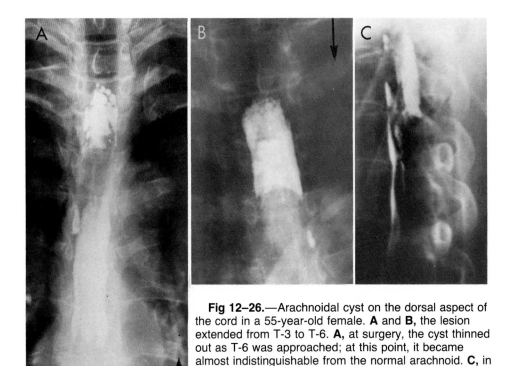

Fig 12–26.—Arachnoidal cyst on the dorsal aspect of the cord in a 55-year-old female. **A** and **B,** the lesion extended from T-3 to T-6. **A,** at surgery, the cyst thinned out as T-6 was approached; at this point, it became almost indistinguishable from the normal arachnoid. **C,** in the lateral film, the cord is thinned and displaced anteriorly by the cyst.

subarachnoid space lie on the dorsal surface of the spinal cord, it usually fails to fill in the prone position. In the latter position, one sees a nonspecific partial or complete extradural block. Therefore, the patient should also be examined in the supine position as well. If Pantopaque is used, the superior and inferior limits of the cyst can be defined by taking appropriate films with the table tilted craniad and caudad (Figs 12–26 and 12–27). The cyst is usually pear-shaped, with a single connection to the subarachnoid space. However, occasionally it may be multiple, with more than one orifice.

CONGENITAL SPINAL INTRADURAL CYST

The congenital variety has been described in the literature by a variety of names—spinal arachnoid cyst, leptomeningeal cyst, spinal arachnoid diverticulum. This should be differentiated from acquired intradural arachnoid cysts, which occur secondary to adhesive arachnoiditis. According to Perrett, the congenital cyst arises within the septum posticum in the posterior subarachnoid space, usually in the thoracic region (Fig 12–28). Plain radiographs are usually negative. At myelography, contrast medium usually enters the cyst cavity. In order to demonstrate the cyst completely with Pantopaque, it may be necessary to examine the patient in the supine and erect positions as well as in the prone position. If the examination

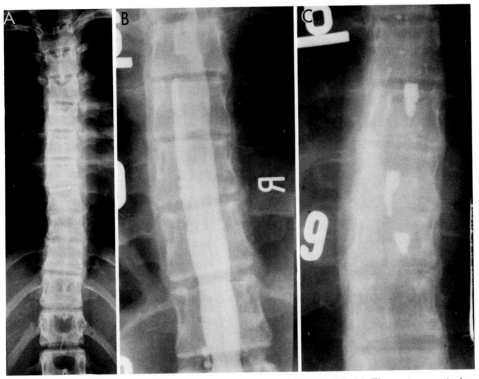

Fig 12–27.—Congenital spinal extradural cyst in a 16-year-old girl. The anteroposterior radiograph **(A)** shows a slight scoliosis and extensive erosion of the pedicles, beginning at T-3. In the prone position **(B)**, the Pantopaque did not enter the cyst. The needle was removed and the patient was placed in the supine position. The erect film made thereafter **(C)** shows several collections of Pantopaque in the cyst. At operation, and extensive elongated extradural cyst was resected.

is limited to the routine prone position, the diverticula may not fill. This demonstrates the need for including a supine study in patients with good neurologic findings and a negative myelogram in the prone position.

Vonafakos et al. reported a 38-year-old woman with multiple communicating thoracic arachnoid cysts which were not demonstrated on a metrizamide myelogram but were shown by Pantopaque myelography. Apparently, the metrizamide promptly entered the cysts, mixing uniformly with the CSF in and outside the cysts so that no fluid levels were present. Furthermore, the thin cyst walls could not be identified. It seems to me that a patient presenting with an episodic relapsing history of back pain, difficulty in walking, sphincter disturbances, and a thoracic sensory level should receive special attention. Such a patient should either have a Pantopaque myelogram at the outset or have a metrizamide myelogram followed by Pantopaque myelography if the first study is negative.

Teng and Papatheodoru have described a group of patients with so-called multiple arachnoidal diverticula that belong in the category of congenital spinal intradural cysts. The typical patient is likely to be a woman in the late thirties or forties without plain-film changes. The symptoms tend to be gradual in onset and quite

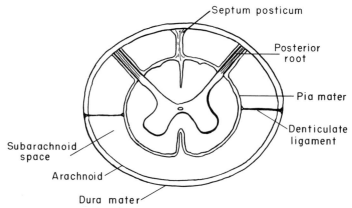

Fig 12–28.—Diagram demonstrating the relationship of the septum posticum and the posterior portion of the subarachnoid space. (After Key and Retzius.)

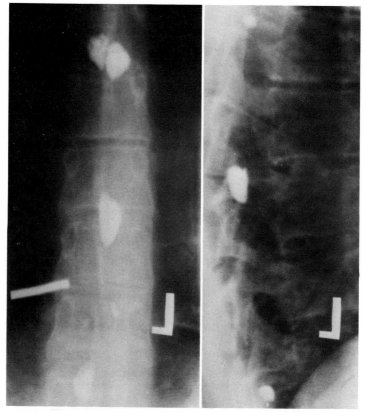

Fig 12–29.—Anteroposterior and lateral radiographs during Pantopaque myelography in a young female with syringohydromyelia. Note the corkscrew appearance of the oil in the dilated central canal due to loculations produced by circumferential glial septae. Note also the widening of the thoracolumbar interpediculate spaces.

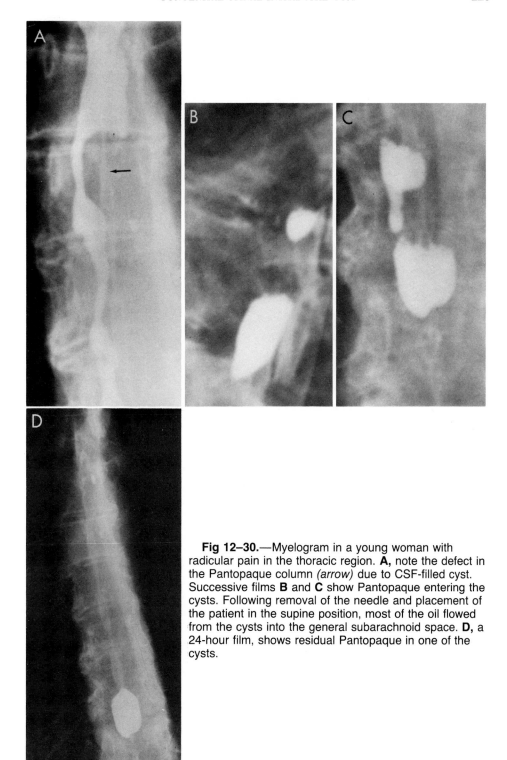

Fig 12–30.—Myelogram in a young woman with radicular pain in the thoracic region. **A,** note the defect in the Pantopaque column *(arrow)* due to CSF-filled cyst. Successive films **B** and **C** show Pantopaque entering the cysts. Following removal of the needle and placement of the patient in the supine position, most of the oil flowed from the cysts into the general subarachnoid space. **D,** a 24-hour film, shows residual Pantopaque in one of the cysts.

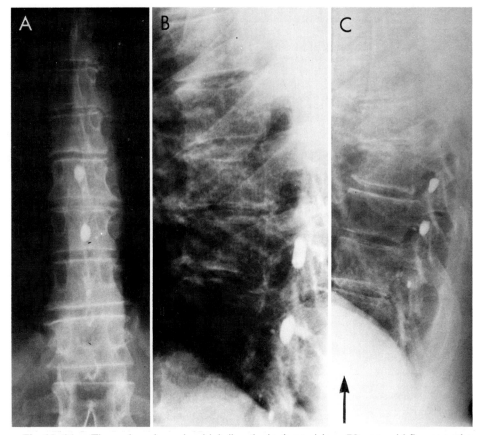

Fig 12–31.—Three dorsal arachnoidal diverticula *(arrow)* in a 50-year-old fireman who had a cervical myelogram for a herniated disk at C5-6 2 years previously. The patient came in for a chest examination and had no symptoms referable to the thoracic region. Note the characteristic midline posterior position of the residual Pantopaque in the arachnoidal diverticula. Films labeled **A** and **B** were made with the patient in the recumbent and **C** in the erect position.

variable, with dysesthesia, backache, radicular pain, and tenderness over the involved spinous processes. There may or may not be motor weakness in the lower extremities and urinary difficulty. There may be a distinct relationship of symptoms to posture, with exacerbation in the erect and relief in the supine position. This is readily understandable, because the diverticula present on the dorsal aspect of the cord. Consequently, they tend to become distended with CSF and exert traction on the cord in the erect position; in the supine position, they empty into the subarachnoid space. The diverticula are visualized as single or multiple collections of contrast medium of varying size, usually in the thoracic region; rarely, they may occur in the cervical or upper lumbar areas. Some of the patients also have associated perineurial sacral cysts. In addition to three cases in symptomatic young females proved at operation (Figs 12–29 and 12–30), I have observed a number of patients with asymptomatic small thoracic cysts (Figs 12–31 and 12–32). Some of the latter patients also had cervical diverticula (perineurial cysts).

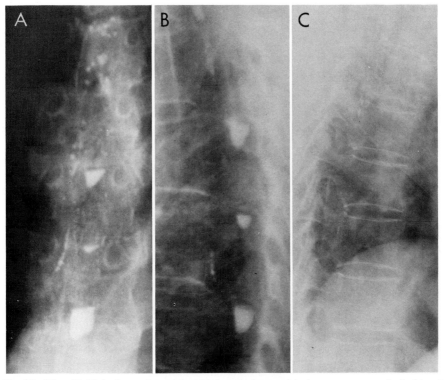

Fig 12–32.—Multiple thoracic arachnoidal cysts in an elderly nurse suspected of having a foramen magnum tumor. The posterior fossa myelogram was negative. Incidentally, the thoracic diverticula were noted on **A,** the upright frontal, and, **B,** the lateral spot films. When the needle was withdrawn and the patient placed in the supine position, a later film, **C,** demonstrated emptying of the cysts.

PERINEURIAL SACRAL CYSTS

In a study of autopsy material in 1938, Tarlov reported the presence of cysts on the posterior sacral roots. Ten years later, he published his observations on the role played by these cysts in the production of sciatic pain. Since that time, a number of reports dealing with similar lesions have appeared in the literature under various headings, i.e., Rexed cysts, meningeal diverticula.

Perineurial cysts usually occur at the junction of the posterior root and the dorsal ganglion. Although they may be found on any of the sacral and coccygeal roots and on the dorsal ganglia of thoracic nerves, they are most common on the second and third sacral roots. The cysts are frequently multiple and may either be asymptomatic or produce sciatic pain. Presumably, the latter is due to stretching and compression of sensory nerve fibers. The etiology and the pathogenesis of perineurial cysts are obscure. Tarlov believes that they are the result of splitting of the nerve root sheath with formation of a space between the pia-derived endoneurium and the arachnoid-derived perineurium. Schreiber and Haddad, however, think that they are a sequel of trauma with intraneural hemorrhage, whereas Strully considers them to be congenital arachnoidal diverticula of the nerve roots. These cysts are quite different from the extradural cysts described by Elsberg, Dyke, and

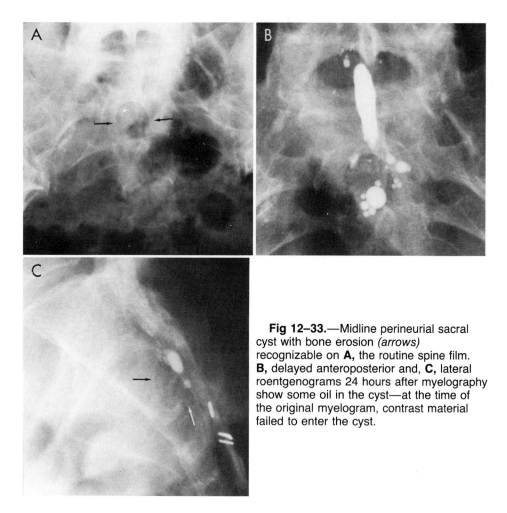

Fig 12–33.—Midline perineurial sacral cyst with bone erosion *(arrows)* recognizable on **A,** the routine spine film. **B,** delayed anteroposterior and, **C,** lateral roentgenograms 24 hours after myelography show some oil in the cyst—at the time of the original myelogram, contrast material failed to enter the cyst.

Brewer. Regardless of the specific etiology of the cysts, they present similar clinical and radiologic pictures.

The plain roentgenograms may be negative or demonstrate localized thinning and erosion of the sacrum, usually involving the second, third, or fourth segments. These changes are seen best in the lateral projection (Figs 12–33 and 12–34). Myelography may reveal a free communication between the subarachnoid space and the cysts (Figs 12–35 to 12–37). In this circumstance, Pantopaque can be visualized passing in and out of the cyst at fluoroscopy. This is in contradistinction to Tarlov's early experience, which denied any communication with the subarachnoid space. In some cases, there is only a partial communication or none at all. In the former instance, although Pantopaque may not enter the cyst at myelography, it may do so hours or days later if some oil is left behind. Hence, a film taken at 24 or 48 hours may be quite helpful (see Fig 12–34). In the absence of communication, the presence of a perineurial cyst may be inferred by lateral displacement of the caudal sac associated with localized erosion of the sacrum. On a few occasions, I have seen sacral perineurial cysts in conjunction with cervical diverticula (perineurial cysts).

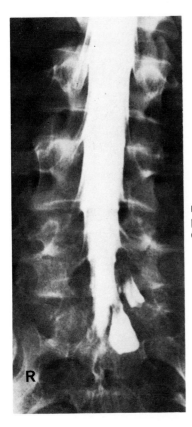

Fig 12–34.—Metrizamide myelogram demonstrating two prominent left perineurial diverticula.

Anomalous Lumbar Spinal Roots

Anomalies of the lower lumbar spinal roots have been reported by a number of authors. These anomalies were more difficult to demonstrate with Pantopaque myelography because the relatively high viscosity of the oil mitigated against filling of the subarachnoid extensions along the nerve root sleeves. The use of metrizamide and CT has facilitated demonstration of these anatomical variants.

Cannon classified these anomalies into three types (Fig 12–38):

1. The conjoint or fused type, in which two roots share a common dural sleeve. Because the parallel course of the emerging two fused roots resembles a rifle barrel, this has been termed by Pecker et al. "rifle barrel" fusion of the spinal roots (Fig 12–39). The fused roots may emerge together at the appropriate level for the lowermost root or midway between the normal levels for each root.

2. The anastomotic type, in which a normal root bifurcates after it emerges from the dura and anastomoses with the root immediately caudal to it.

3. The transverse type, in which the origin is normal but the course is horizontal instead of obliquely downward.

To date, all of the cases of anomalous roots with one exception (S-1, S-2) have involved the L-4 and L-5 roots emerging at the level of L-5, or the L-5 and S-1 roots exiting at the level of S-1. One must remember, however, that most herniated disks and most laminectomies occur at these levels. Association of a disk herniation

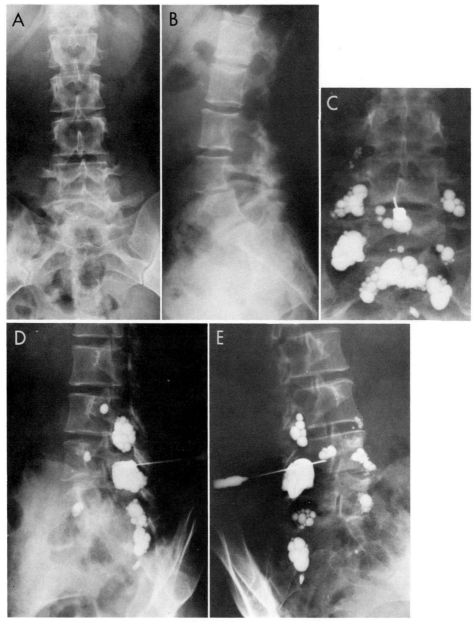

Fig 12–35.—Multiple large bilateral perineurial lumbar and sacral cysts in a 31-year-old woman with neurofibromatosis and dural ectasia. Radiographs made 9 years previously demonstrated changes in the lumbar spine characterized by thinning of the pedicles and scalloping of the posterior aspect of the last three lumbar vertebral bodies. These abnormalities may be found in generalized neurofibromatosis as part of a diffuse congenital dysplasia and should not be mistaken for erosive changes produced by intraspinal neurilemomas. (The reader will also recall the association of neurofibromatosis with lateral meningoceles, discussed in this chapter.) Present films **A** and **B** of the lumbar spine show erosion of the medial inferior aspect of the pedicles at L-2, more marked pedicle changes at L-3 and loss of the pedicle outline at L-4 and L-5. In addition, there is scalloping of the posterior margins of L-3, L-4, and L-5, with marked enlargement of the corresponding intervertebral foramina. At myelography **(C, D,** and **E),** the multiple large bilateral perineurial cysts at L-4, L-5, and S-1 are clearly visible. (Courtesy of A. Grugan, Springfield, Mass.)

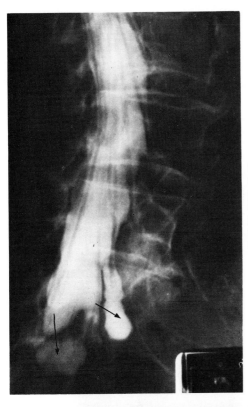

Fig 12–36.—Metrizamide myelogram in a 72-year-old woman with a history of trauma one year previously and backache radiating to the left lower extremity. The study was negative except for the incidental finding of perineurial diverticula of the S-1 and S-2 roots *(arrows)*.

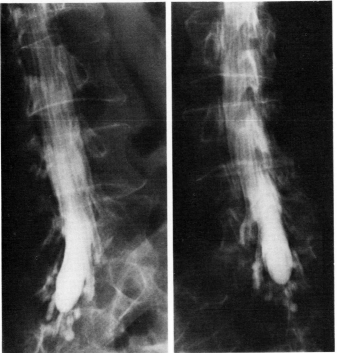

Fig 12–37.—Metrizamide myelogram demonstrating multiple small perineurial diverticula of the proximal sacral roots.

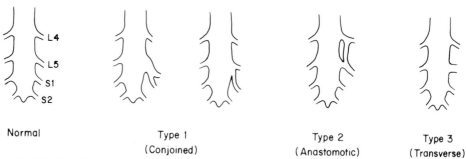

Normal   Type 1   Type 2   Type 3
              (Conjoined)   (Anastomotic)   (Transverse)

Fig 12–38.—Diagram of normal lower lumbar and lumbosacral nerve roots and various nerve root anomalies. (After Cannon.)

at the junction of a pair of fused nerves produces biradicular pain. Conversely, if the herniated disk is located at the level where there is no root, only severe lumbar pain is present. In some patients with this anomaly, sciatic pain has been reported in the absence of a herniated disk. At myelography with metrizamide, a separate subarachnoid space is visualized within the common dural sleeve covering the two nerves. The diagnosis may or may not be made when Pantopaque is used.

ABSENT CERVICAL PEDICLE SYNDROME

Oestreich and Young have reviewed the literature on the absent cervical pedicle syndrome. In this condition, there is unilateral agenesis of a pedicle, resulting in a large common orifice consisting.of two adjacent foramina. In addition, there is absence of the posterior portion of the ipsilateral transverse process normally associated with the pedicle, and an abnormality of the lateral mass containing the superior and inferior articulating facets. Most often, the latter is displaced posteriorly; however, one or both articulating facets may articulate abnormally or be absent.

In the reported cases, the age has ranged from 13 to 56 years. Approximately 70% of the patients have been symptomatic, i.e., pain in the neck, scapula or arm, numbness of fingers, stiff neck on flexion. However, I have seen a patient with no symptoms referable to the cervical spine. Myelography shows two roots leaving the cervical cord (usually but not always to a common dural outpouching) at the level of the bony anomaly. There also may be a concavity of the contrast column on the side opposite the dural outpouching (Fig 12–40). The exact explanation for this finding is not obvious. Oestreich and Young suggest that it may be due to compensatory retraction of the contralateral dura. It is interesting that Luoyot et al. reported a case with a large posterior disk herniation at the level of the absent pedicle. Absence of a pedicle in the thoracic region is extremely rare.

It is important to distinguish this entity from erosion of the intervertebral foramen by neurilemoma and a tortuous vertebral artery. Although a neurogenic tumor can erode the body, lamina, and articulating mass of a vertebra, the residual articulating pillar is not deranged. Hence, a normal chain of facet articulations on oblique roentgenograms excludes agenesis of a cervical pedicle. A tortuous vertebral artery may also erode a pedicle. However, the foraminal enlargement usually is in an anteromedial and superior direction because of the looping of the vertebral

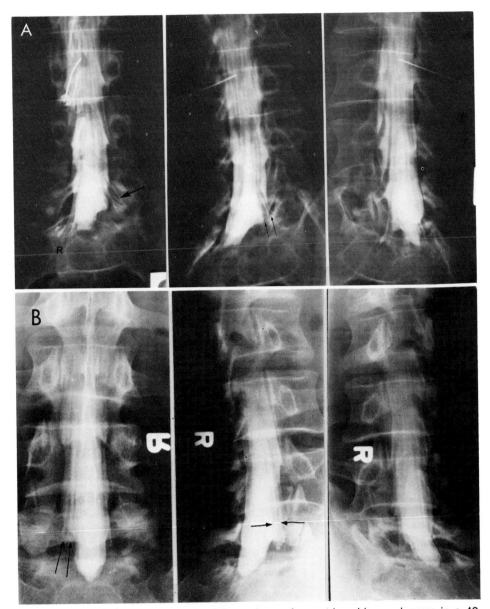

Fig 12–39.—A, frontal and both oblique views of a metrizamide myelogram in a 49-year-old woman, showing the left L-5 and S-1 roots emerging together *(arrows).* **B,** similar findings on the right in a 50-year-old man *(arrows).*

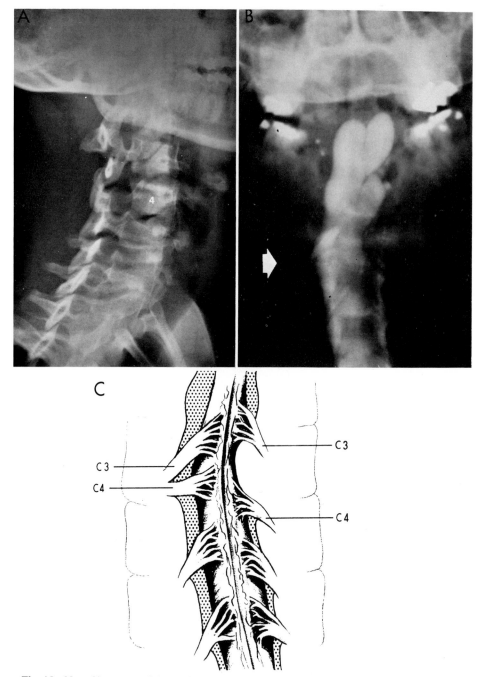

Fig 12–40.—Absent pedicle at C-4 on the right. The left posterior oblique radiograph of the cervical spine **(A)** shows the anomalous large foramen between C-3 and C-4, with posterior displacement of the fourth right articular pillar. The frontal myelographic film **(B)** demonstrates the common outpouching at C3-4 on the right, with two roots exiting together *(arrow).* Note also the concavity on the contralateral normal right side—cause? Artist's drawing of the operative findings **(C).** (Reprinted, with permission, from Oestreich A.E., Young L.W., *Am. J. Roentgenol.* 107:505, 1969.)

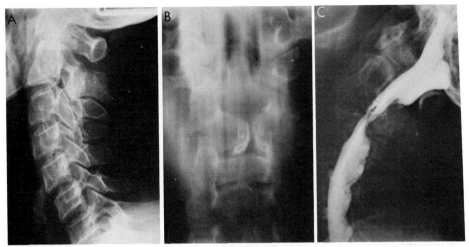

Fig 12–41.—Congenital duplication of the bony posterior vertebral arch at C-2 producing compression of the cervical cord. Lateral plain radiograph **(A)** and anteroposterior tomogram **(B)** demonstrate the bony anomaly. The lateral cross-table radiograph during myelography **(C)** shows the extradural defect produced by the anomalous bony mass.

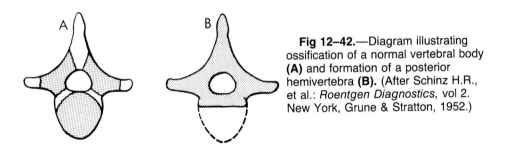

Fig 12–42.—Diagram illustrating ossification of a normal vertebral body **(A)** and formation of a posterior hemivertebra **(B).** (After Schinz H.R., et al.: *Roentgen Diagnostics,* vol 2. New York, Grune & Stratton, 1952.)

artery. In addition, the articulating pillar is normal. CT has simplified the diagnosis of an absent cervical pedicle.

DUPLICATION OF POSTERIOR VERTEBRAL ARCH

I have seen a single case of extradural compression of the cervical cord by a congenital double posterior neural arch (Fig 12–41).

POSTERIOR (DORSAL) HEMIVERTEBRA

This rare malformation is characterized by rudimentary development or absence of the anterior (ventral) half of the vertebral body (Fig 12–42). Following weight-bearing, the vertebra becomes wedge-shaped with a resultant kyphosis (Fig 12–43). Although the kyphos produces compression of the spinal cord, a neurologic deficit is not always present.

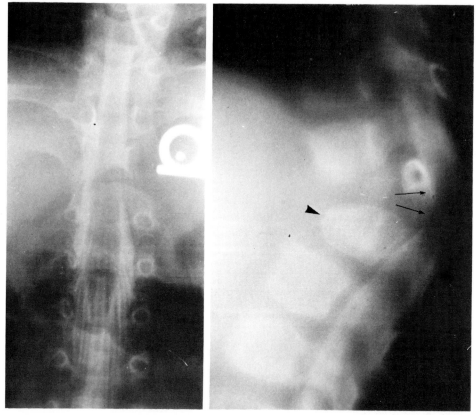

Fig 12–43.—AP and lateral views of a metrizamide myelogram in a 3-year-old boy, showing posterior displacement and compression of the spinal cord by a dorsal hemivertebra *(arrows)*. Note the rudimentary development of T-12 *(arrowhead)*.

BIBLIOGRAPHY

Adams R.D., Schatzki R., Scoville W.B.: The Arnold-Chiari malformation. Diagnosis. Demonstration by intraspinal Lipiodol and successful surgical treatment. *N. Engl. J. Med.* 225:125, 1941.

Adams R.D., Wegner W.: Congenital cyst of the spinal meninges as cause of intermittent compression of the spinal cord. *Arch. Neurol. Psychiatr.* 58:57, 1947.

Agnoli A.L.: Anomale wurzelabgänge im lumbosacralen Bereich und ihre klinische Bedentung. *J. Neurol.* 211:217, 1976.

Archer V.W., Cooper G., Jr., Cimmino C.V.: Occult meningocele of the sacrum. *Radiology* 51:691, 1948.

Arnold J.: Myelocyste. Transposition von Gewebskeimen und Sympodie. *Beitr. Path. Anat.* 16:1, 1894.

Ballantine H.R., Jr., Ojemann R.G., Drew J.H.: Syringohydromyelia. *Prog. Neurol. Surg.* 4:227, 1971.

Barnett H.J.M., Faster J.G., Hudgson P.: *Syringomyelia.* Philadelphia, W.B. Saunders Co., 1973.

Barson A.J.: Radiological studies of spina bifida cystica. *Br. J. Radiol.* 38:294, 1965.

Barson A.J.: Vertebral level of termination of spinal cord during normal and abnormal development. *J. Anat.* 106:489, 1969.

Barson A.J., Cole F.M.: Neurofibromatosis with congenital malformation of the spinal cord. *J. Neurol., Neurosurg. Psychiatr.* 30:71, 1967.

Beardmore H.E., Wiglesworth F.W.: Vertebral anomalies and alimentary duplications. *Pediatr. Clin. North Am.* 5:457, 1958.

Bennett A.E., Keegan J.J.: Circumscribed suppurations of the spinal cord and meninges: Report of a case of subdural abscess with functional recovery following operation. *A.M.A. Neurol. Psychiatr.* 19:329, 1928.

Benstead J.G.: A case of diastematomyelia. *J. Pathol. Bacteriol.* 66:553, 1953.

Bentson J.R.: Comparison of myelographic agents for studying spinal dysraphism. *Clin. Orthop.* 134:204, 1978.

Berglund R.M.: Congenital intraspinal extradural cyst. Report of three cases in one family. *J. Neurosurg.* 28:495, 1968.

Bernini P.M., Wiesel S.W., Rothman R.H.: Metrizamide myelography and the identification of anomalous lumbosacral nerve roots: Report of two cases and review of the literature. *J. Bone Joint Surg.* 62A:1203, 1980.

Bligh A.S.: Diastematomyelia. *Clin. Radiol.* 12:158, 1961.

Booth A.E.: Lateral thoracic meningocele. *J. Neurol., Neurosurg. Psychiatr.* 32:111, 1969.

Bouchard J.M., Copty M., Langelier R.: Preoperative diagnosis of conjoined root anomaly with herniated lumbar disks. *Surg. Neurol.* 10:229, 1978.

Bremer J.L.: Dorsal intestinal fistula; accessory neurenteric canal: Diastematomyelia. *A.M.A. Arch. Path.* 54:132, 1952.

Brooks B.S., El Gammal T., Hartlage P., Beveridge W.: Myelography of sacral agenesis. *A.J.N.R.* 2:319,1981.

Brunner S.: Lateral intrathoracic meningocele. *Acta Radiol.* 51:1, 1959.

Burrows F.G.O.: Some aspects of occult spinal dysraphism. A study of 90 cases. *Br. J. Radiol.* 41:496, 1968.

Cabot Case 46122. *N. Engl. J. Med.* 262:623, 1960.

Calihan R.J.: Anterior sacral meningocele. *Radiology* 58:104, 1952.

Cameron A.H.: The spinal cord lesion in spina bifida cystica. *Lancet* 2:171, 1956.

Cannon B.W., Hunter S.E., Picaza J.A.: Nerve-root anomalies in lumbar disc surgery. *J. Neurosurg.* 19:208, 1961.

Chambers W.R.: Diastematomyelia: Report of case diagnosed preoperatively. *J. Pediatr.* 45:668, 1954.

Chandler A., Herzberger E.F.: Lateral intrathoracic meningocele. Case report with preoperative diagnosis. *Am. J. Roentgenol.* 90:1216, 1963.

Chiari H.: Über Veränderungen des Kleinhirns in Folge von Hydrocephalie des Grosshirns. *Deutsch. Med. Wschr.* 17:1172, 1891.

Chiari H.: Über die Veränderungen des Kleinhirns, des Pons under der Medulla oblongata in Folge von congenitaler Hydrocephalie des Grosshirns. *Denschr. Akad. Wissensch. Math. Naturw. Kl.* 63:71, 1895.

Cleland J.: Quoted by Doran P.A., Guthkelch A.N.: Studies in spina bifida cystica. *J. Neurol., Neurosurg. Psychiatr.* 24:331, 1961.

Cliffton E.E., Rydell J.R.: Congenital dermal (pilonidal) sinus with dural connection. Case report and discussion. *J. Neurosurg.* 4:276, 1947.

Cohn J., Bay-Nielsen, E.: Hereditary defect of the sacrum and coccyx with anterior sacral meningocele. *Acta Paediatr. Scandinav.* 58:268, 1969.

Cowie T.N.: Diastematomyelia: Tomography in diagnosis. *Br. J. Radiol.* 25:263, 1952.

Curtis B.H., Fisher R.L., Butterfield W.L., Saunders F.P.: Neurofibromatosis with paraplegia. Report of eight cases. *J. Bone Joint Surg.* 51A:843, 1969.

Dale A.J.D.: Diastematomyelia. *Arch. Neurol.* 20:309, 1969.

Dasturi H.M.: Radiological appearance of spinal extradural cysts. *J. Neurol., Neurosurg. Psychiatr.* 26:231, 1963.

Davies H.W.: Radiological changes associated with Arnold-Chiari malformation. *Br. J. Radiol.* 40:262, 1967.

Doran P.A., Gutkelch A.N.: Studies in spina bifida cystica. I. General survey and reassessment of the problem. *J. Neurol., Neurosurg. Psychiatr.* 24:331, 1961.

Duncan A.W., Hoare G.T.: Spinal subarachnoid cysts in children. *Radiology* 126:423, 1978.

Dzenitis A.J.: Spontaneous atlanto-axial dislocation in mongoloid child with spinal cord compression. *J. Neurosurg.* 25:458, 1966.

Edeiken J., Lee K.F., Libshitz H.: Intrathoracic meningocele. *Am. J. Roentgenol.* 106:381, 1969.

Eder D.: Anterior sacral meningocele: Survey of the literature and report of a case. *Bull. Los Angeles Neurol. Soc.* 14:104, 1949.

Elsberg C.A., Dyke C.G., Brewer E.D.: The symptoms and diagnosis of extradural cysts. *Bull. Neurol. Inst. New York* 3:395, 1934.

Emery J.L., Naik D.: Spinal cord segment lengths in children with meningomyelocele and the "Cleland-Arnold-Chiari" deformity. *Br. J. Radiol.* 41:287, 1968.

Enderle C.: Occulta intrasacral meningocele revealed by myelography. *Riv. Neurol.* 5:418, 1942.

English W.J., Maltby G.L.: Diastematomyelia in adults. *J. Neurosurg.* 27:260, 1967.

Epstein B.S.: Pantopaque myelography in the diagnosis of the Arnold-Chiari malformation without concomitant skeletal or central nervous system defects. *Am. J. Roentgenol.* 59:359, 1948.

Epstein J.A., Carras R., Ferrar J., et al: Conjoined lumbosacral nerve roots. *J. Neurosurg.* 55:585, 1981.

Ethelberg S., Riishide J.: Malformation of lumbar spinal roots and sheaths in the causation of low backache and sciatica. *J. Bone Joint Surg.* 34B:442, 1952.

Fahrenkrug A., Højgaard K.: Multiple paravertebral lumbar meningocele. *Br. J. Radiol.* 36:574, 1963.

Fitz C.R., Harwood-Nash D.: The tethered conus. *Am. J. Roentgenol.* 125:515, 1975.

Gardner W.J.: Anatomic anomalies common to myelomeningocele of infancy and syringomyelia of adulthood suggesting a common origin. *Cleveland Clin. Quart.* 26:118, 1959.

Gardner W.J.: Myelomeningocele, the result of rupture of the embryonic neural tube. *Cleveland Clin. Quart.* 27:88, 1960.

Gardner W.J.: Diastematomyelia and the Klippel-Feil syndrome. Relationship to hydrocephalus, syringomyelia, meningocele, meningomyelocele, and iniencephalus. *Cleveland Clin. Quart.* 31:19, 1964.

Ghouralal S., Myers P.W., Campbell E.: Persistent cerebrospinal rhinorrhea originating in fracture through petrous bone and cured by muscle graft: Report of case. *J. Neurosurg.* 13:205, 1956.

Gleeson J.A., Stovin P.G.I.: Mediastinal enterogenous cysts associated with vertebral anomalies. *Clin. Radiol.* 12:41, 1961.

Gold L.H.A., Kieffer S.A., Peterson H.O.: Lipomatous invasion of the spinal cord associated with spinal dysraphism: Myelographic evaluation. *Am. J. Roentgenol.* 107:479, 1969.

Gortvai P.: Extradural cysts of the spinal canal. *J. Neurol., Neurosurg. Psychiatr.* 26:223, 1963.

Gortvai P., El-Gindi S.: Spinal extradural cyst. Case report. *J. Neurosurg.* 26:432, 1967.

Govoni A.F.: Developmental stenosis of a thoracic vertebra resulting in narrowing of the spinal canal. *Am. J. Roentgenol.* 112:401, 1972.

Gryspeerdt G.L.: Myelographic assessment of occult forms of spinal dysraphism. *Acta. Radiol. (Diagn.)* 1:702, 1963.

Hackensellner H.A., Paper R.: Meningocele associated with Recklinghausen's neurofibromatosis. *Fortschr. Geb. Röntgenstrahlen* 81:66, 1954.

Haddad F.S.: Anterior sacral meningocele: Report of two cases and review of the literature. *Can. J. Surg.* 1:230, 1958.

Hadley L.A.: Congenital absence of pedicle from cervical vertebra. *Am. J. Roentgenol.* 80:306, 1958.

Hamby W.B.: Pilonidal cyst, spina bifida occulta and bifid spinal cord. Report of case with review of literature. *Arch. Pathol.* 21:831, 1936.

Harwood-Nash D.C., Fitz C.R.: Myelography and syringomyelia in infancy and childhood. *Radiology* 113:661, 1974.

Harwood-Nash D.C., Fitz C.R., Resjo I.M., Chuang S.: Congenital spinal and cord lesions in children and computed tomographic metrizamide myelography. *Neuroradiology* 16:69, 1978.

Hauge T.: Myelography in a case of the occult form of spinal dysraphism. *Acta Radiol. (Diagn.)* 1:718, 1963.

Heard G., Payne E.E.: Scalloping of the vertebral bodies in von Recklinghausen's disease of the nervous system (neurofibromatosis). *J. Neurol., Neurosurg. Psychiatr.* 25:345, 1962.

Heinz E.R., Rosenbaum A.S., Scarff T.B., et al.: Tethered spinal cord following meningo-myelocele repair. *Radiology* 131:153, 1979.

Heinz E.R., Schlesinger E.B., Potts D.G.: Radiologic signs of hydromyelia. *Radiology* 86:311, 1966.

Herren R.Y., Edwards J.E.: Diplomyelia (duplication of the spinal cord). *Arch. Pathol.* 30:1203, 1940.

Hillenius L.: Intrathoracic meningocele. *Acta Med. Scandinav.* 163:15, 1959.

Hoefnagel D., Benirschke K., Duarte J.: Teratomatous cysts within the vertebral canal. Observations on the occurrence of sex chromatin. *J. Neurol., Neurosurg. Psychiatr.* 25:159, 1962.

Hoffman G.T.: Cervical arachnoid cyst. Report of a 6-year-old Negro male with recovery from quadriplegia. *J. Neurosurg.* 17:327, 1960.

Holcomb G.W., Jr., Matson D.D.: Thoracic neurenteric cyst. *Surgery* 35:115, 1954.

Holman C.B., et al: Diastematomyelia. *Pediatrics* 15:191, 1955.

Hoppenfield S.: Congenital kyphosis in myelomeningocele. *J. Bone Joint Surg.* 49B:276, 1967.

Howieson J., Norrell H.A., Wilson C.B.: Expansion of subarachnoid space in lumbosacral region. *Radiology* 90:488, 1968.

Hoy R.J., Faulder K.C.: Spinal arachnoid cysts. *Australasian Radiol.* 12:344, 1968.

Hunt P.T., Davidson K.C., Ashcraft K.W., Holder T.M.: Radiography of hereditary presa-cral teratoma. *Radiology* 122:187, 1977.

James C.C.M., Lassman L.P.: Spinal dysraphism. *Arch. Dis. Child.* 35:315, 1960.

James C.C.M., Lassman L.P.: Spinal dysraphism. The diagnosis and treatment of progres-sive lesions in spina bifida occulta. *J. Bone Joint Surg.* 44B:828, 1962.

James C.C.M., Lassman L.P.: Diastematomyelia and tight filum terminale. *J. Neurol. Sci.* 10:193, 1970.

Janecki C.J., Nelson C.L., Dohn D.F.: Intrasacral cyst. Report of a case and review of the literature. *J. Bone Joint Surg.* 54A:423, 1972.

Joseph R.A., McKenzie T.: Occult intrasacral meningocele. *J. Neurol., Neurosurg. Psy-chiatr.* 33:493, 1970.

Kendall B.E., Valentine A.R., Keis B.: Spinal arachnoid cysts: Clinical and radiological cor-relation with prognosis. *Neuroradiology* 22:225, 1982.

Keon-Cohen B.: Abnormal arrangement of the lower lumbar and first sacral nerves within the spinal canal. *J. Bone Joint Surg.* 50B:261, 1968.

Key E.A.H., Retzius M.G.: *Studien in der Anatomie des Nervensystems und des Bindegew-ebes.* Stockholm, Samson & Wallin, 1875.

Krieger A.J., Rosomoff H.L., Kuperman A.S., Zingesser L.H.: Occult respiratory dysfunc-tion in a craniovertebral abnormality. *J. Neurosurg.* 31:15, 1969.

Kunitomo K.: Development and reduction of tail and of caudal end of spinal cord. *Contrib. Embryol.* 8:161, 1918.

Larson J.L., Smith D., Fossan G.: Arachnoidal diverticula and cyst-like dilatations of the nerve-root sheaths in lumbar myelography. *Acta Radiol. (Diagn.)* 21:141, 1980.

Lassman L.P., James C.C.M.: Lumbosacral lipomas: Critical survey of 26 cases submitted to laminectomy. *J. Neurol., Neurosurg. Psychiatr.* 30:174, 1967.

LaViele C.J., Campbell D.A.: Neurofibromatosis and intrathoracic meningocele. *Radiology* 70:62, 1958.

Leeds N.E., Jacobson H.G.: Spinal neurofibromatosis. *Am. J. Roentgenol.* 126:617, 1976.

Leigh T.F., Rogers J.V., Jr.: Anterior sacral meningocele. *Am. J. Roentgenol.* 71:808, 1954.

Lewin J.R., Wycis H.T., Young B.R.: Roentgen diagnosis of herniation of brain into spinal canal (Arnold-Chiari deformity) by Pantopaque myelography. *Radiology* 54:591, 1950.

Lichtenstein B.W.: "Spinal dysraphism," spina bifida and myelodysplasia. *Arch. Neurol. Psychiatr.* 44:792, 1940.

Lombardi G., Morello G.: Congenital cysts of the spinal membranes and roots. *Br. J. Radiol.* 36:197, 1963.

Luoyot P., Gaucher A., Laxenaire M., Combebias J.F.: Agénésie du pédicle droit de la sixième vertèbre cervicale et syndrome radiculaire C7 par hernie discale. *Rev. Rhumatisme* 34:276, 1966.

Malis L.I., Cohen I., Gross S.W.: Arnold-Chiari malformation. *A.M.A. Arch. Surg.* 63:783, 1951.

Marano G.D., Elyaderani M.K.: Lateral lumbar meningocele: A possible pitfall in renal sonography. *J. Clin. Ultrasound* 9:334, 1981.

Margolis G., Kilham L.: Experimental virus-induced hydrocephalus. Relation to pathogenesis of Arnold-Chiari malformation. *J. Neurosurg.* 31:1, 1969.

Marks J.H., Livingston K.E.: Cervical subarachnoid space with particular reference to syringomyelia and Arnold-Chiari deformity. *Radiology* 52:63, 1948.

Marr G.E., Uihlein A.: Diplomyelia and compression of the spinal cord and not of the cauda equina by a congenital anomaly of the third lumbar vertebra. *Surg. Clin. North Am.* 24:963, 1944.

Martel W., Uyham R., Stimson C.W.: Subluxation of the atlas causing spinal cord compression in a case of Down's syndrome with a "manifestation of an occipital vertebra." *Radiology* 93:838, 1969.

Maxwell H.P., Bucy P.R.: Diastematomyelia. Report of a clinical case. *J. Neuropath. Exper. Neurol.* 5:165, 1946.

McAllister V.L.: Myelography with metrizamide in occult spinal dysraphism. *Acta Radiol.* (Suppl.) 355:200, 1977.

McCormick C.C.: Developmental asymmetry of roots of the cauda equina at metrizamide myelography: Report of seven cases with a review of the literature. *Clin. Radiol.* 33:427, 1982.

McCrae D.L., Stander J.: Roentgenologic findings in syringomyelia and hydromyelia. *Am. J. Roentgenol.* 98:695, 1966.

McElvenny R.T.: Anomalies of the lumbar spinal cord and nerve roots. *Clin. Orthop.* 8:61, 1956.

Miles J., Pennybacker J., Sheldon P.: Intrathoracic meningocele. *J. Neurol., Neurosurg. Psychiatr.* 32:99, 1969.

Nathan H., Rosner S.: Multiple meningeal diverticula and cysts associated with duplications of the sheaths of spinal nerve posterior roots. *J. Neurosurg.* 47:68, 1977.

Nelson J.D.: The Marfan syndrome with special reference to congenital enlargement of the spinal canal. *Br. J. Radiol.* 31:561, 1958.

Neuhauser E.B.D., Harris G.B.C., Berrett A.: Roentgenographic features of neurenteric cysts. *Am. J. Roentgenol.* 79:235, 1958.

Neuhauser E.B.D., Wittenborg M.H., Dehlinger K.: Diastematomyelia: Transfixation of the cord or cauda equina with congenital anomalies of the spine. *Radiology* 54:659, 1950.

Oestreich A.E., Young L.W.: The absent cervical pedicle syndrome: A case in childhood. *Am. J. Roentgenol.* 107:505, 1969.

Oliver L.C.: Primary arachnoid cysts. *Br. Med. J.* 1:1147, 1958.

Palmer J.J.: Spinal subarachnoid cysts. Report of six cases. *J. Neurosurg.* 41:728, 1974.

Pecker J., Simon J., Bou-Salah A., Pivault C.: Rifle barrel fusion of spinal roots as a source of diagnostic error. *Nouv. Presse Med.* 3:1155, 1974.

Pendergrass E.P., Schaeffer J.P., Hodes P.J.: *The Head and Neck in Roentgen Diagnosis*, ed. 2. Springfield, Ill.: Charles C Thomas, Publisher, 1956.

Pendergrass R.C., Walker A.E., Bond J.P.: Extraspinal lumbar meningocele. *J. Neurosurg.* 4:80, 1947.

Perrett G.: Diagnosis and treatment of diastematomyelia. *Surg., Gynecol. Obstet.* 105:69, 1957.

Perrett G., Green D., Keller J.: Diagnosis and treatment of intradural arachnoid cysts of thoracic spine. *Radiology* 79:425, 1962.

Raja I.A., Hankinson J.: Congenital spinal arachnoid cysts. Report of two cases and review of the literature. *J. Neurol., Neurosurg. Psychiatr.* 33:105, 1970.

Rask M.R.: Anomalous lumbosacral nerve roots associated with spondylolisthesis. *Surg. Neurol.* 8:139, 1977.

Ritchie J.W., Flanagan M.N.: Diastematomyelia. *Can. Med. Assoc. J.* 100:428, 1969.

Rockett F.X., Wittenborg M.H., Shillito J., Jr., Matson D.D.: Pantopaque investigation of a congenital dural defect of the internal auditory meatus causing rhinorrhea. Report of a case. *Am. J. Roentgenol.* 91:640, 1964.

Rosenbloom D.J., Derow J.R.: Spinal extradural cysts with report of an ossified spinal extradural cyst. *Am. J. Roentgenol.* 90:1227, 1963.

Ruscalleda J., Guardia E., dos Santos F.M., Carvajal A.: Dynamic study of arachnoid cysts with metrizamide. *Neuroradiology* 20:185, 1980.

Sammons B.P., Thomas D.F.: Extensive lumbar meningocele associated with neurofibromatosis. *Am. J. Roentgenol.* 81:1021, 1959.

Sands W.W., Clark W.K.: Diastematomyelia. *Am. J. Roentgenol.* 72:64, 1954.

Saunders, R.L.: Intramedullary epidermoid cyst associated with a dermal sinus. Case report. *J. Neurosurg.* 31:83, 1969.

Say B., Coldwell J.G.: Hereditary defect of the sacrum. *Hum. Genet.* 27:231, 1975.

Schreiber F., Haddad B.: Lumbar and sacral cysts causing pain. *J. Neurosurg.* 8:504, 1951.

Scotti G., Harwood-Nash D.C., Hoffman H.J.: Congenital thoracic dermal sinus: Diagnosis by computer-assisted metrizamide myelography. *J. Comput. Assist. Tomogr.* 4:675, 1980.

Seaman W., Schwartz H.G.: Diastematomyelia in adults. *Radiology* 70:692, 1958.

Sengpiel G.W., Ruzicka F.F., Lodmell E.A.: Lateral intrathoracic meningocele. *Radiology* 50:515, 1949.

Shapiro R., Robin'son F.: The roentgenographic diagnosis of the Arnold-Chiari malformation. *Am. J. Roentgenol.* 73:390, 1955.

Shealy C.N., LeMay M.: Intrathoracic meningocele. Two additional cases of this rare entity. *J. Neurosurg.* 21:880, 1964.

Shorey W.D.: Diastematomyelia associated with dorsal kyphosis producing paraplegia. *J. Neurosurg.* 12:300, 1955.

Silvernail W.I., Brown R.B.: Intramedullary enterogenous cyst. Case report. *J. Neurosurg.* 36:235, 1972.

Skoog A.L.: Spinal cord compression from leptomeningeal cysts with report of two cases. *J.A.M.A.* 65:394, 1915.

Smith G.W., Chavez M.: Lumbar extradural cysts—congenital: Their proper classification. *A.M.A. Arch. Neurol. Psychiatr.* 80:436, 1958.

Sogani K.C., Kalani B.P.: Paravertebral lumbar meningomyelocele. *J. Neurosurg.* 37:746, 1972.

Steinbach H.L., Boldrey E.B., Sooy F.A.: Congenital absence of pedicle and superior facet from cervical vertebra. *Radiology* 59:838, 1952.

Strand R.D., Eisenberg H.M.: Anterior sacral meningocele in association with Marfan's syndrome. *Radiology* 99:653, 1971.

Strully K.J.: Meningeal diverticula of sacral nerve roots (perineurial cysts). *J.A.M.A.* 161:1147, 1956.

Sutton D.: Sacral cysts. *Acta. Radiol. (Diagn.)* 1:787, 1963.

Swedberg M.: Meningo- and myelomeningocele studied by gas myelography. *Acta Radiol. (Diagn.)* 1:796, 1963.

Talwalker V.C., Dastur D.K.: "Meningoceles" and "meningomyeloceles" (ectopic spinal cord). Clinicopathological basis of a new classification. *J. Neurol., Neurosurg. Psychiatr.* 33:251, 1970.

Tarlov I.M.: Perineural cyst of the spinal nerve roots. *Arch. Neurol. Psychiatr.* 40:1067, 1938.

Tarlov I.M.: Cysts (perineurial) of sacral roots. Another cause (removable) of sciatic pain. *J.A.M.A.* 138:740, 1948.

Tarlov I.M.: *Sacral Nerve-Root Cysts: Another Cause of the Sciatic or Cauda Equina Syndrome.* Springfield, Ill. Charles C Thomas, Publisher, 1953.

Teng P., Papatheodoru C.: Spinal arachnoidal diverticula. *Br. J. Radiol.* 39:249, 1966.

Thorp R.H.: Carcinoma associated with myelomeningocele. Case report. *J. Neurosurg.* 27:446, 1967.

Till K.: Spinal dysraphism. A study of congenital malformations of the lower back. *J. Bone Joint Surg.* 51B:415, 1969.

Tomsick T.A., Lebowitz M.E., Campbell C.: The congenital absence of pedicles in the thoracic spine: Report of two cases. *Radiology* 111:587, 1974.

Vonafakos D., Grau H., Stendel W.: Multiple spinal arachnoid cysts: The role of oily contrast medium. *Surg. Neurol.* 15:125, 1981.

von Recklinghausen F.E.: *Über die multiplen Fibrome der Haut und ihre Beziehung zu den multiplen Neuromen.* Berlin, A. Hirschwald, 1882.

Wackenheim A.: Diagnostic radiologique des formes congénitales des formes intermittentes et des formes progressives de stenose du canal rachidién au niveau de l'atlas. *Acta Radiol. (Diagn.)* 9:759, 1969.

Wadia N.H.: Myelopathy complicating congenital atlanto-axial dislocation (a study of 28 cases). *Brain* 90:449, 1967.

Walker A.E.: Dilatation of the vertebral canal with congenital anomalies of spinal cord. *Am. J. Roentgenol.* 52:571, 1944.

Wickbom I., Hanafee W.: Soft tissue masses immediately below the foramen magnum. *Acta Radiol. (Diagn.)* 1:647, 1963.

Wiedenmann O.: Perineurial cysts of the lumbar and sacral roots. *Fortschr. Geb. Röntgenstrahlen* 88:662, 1958.

Willis R.A.: *The Borderland of Embryology and Pathology,* ed. 2. London, Butterworth, 1962, p. 154.

Wilson C.B., Norrell H.A., Jr.: Congenital absence of pedicle in cervical spine. *Am. J. Roentgenol.* 97:639, 1966.

Wilson S.A.K., Walker C.P.G.: Occult lumbosacral meningocele. *J. Neurol. Psychopathol.* 13:45, 1932.

Wöber G., Böck F.: Lumbale Nervenwurzel-anomalien bei Ischalgie. *Nervenarzt* 42:552, 1971.

Wollen D.G., Elliott G.B.: Coronal cleft vertebrae and persistent notochordal derivatives of infancy. *J. Can. Assoc. Radiol.* 12:78, 1961.

Wright R.L.: Congenital Dermal Sinuses, in Krayenbühl, H., et al. (eds.): *Progress in Neurological Surgery.* Basel, S. Karger A.G., 1971, vol. 4, pp. 175–191.

Wyler A.R., Loeser J.D., Killien F.C.: Septum posticum cysts: An uncommon cause of chronic back pain. *Pain* 1:271, 1975.

Young I.S., Brewer A.J.: The occult intrasacral meningocele. *Am. J. Roentgenol.* 105:390, 1969.

Zacks A.: Atlanto-occipital fusion, basilar impression and block vertebrae associated with intraspinal neurofibroma, meningocele and von Recklinghausen's disease. *Radiology* 75:223, 1960.

13

Trauma to the Spinal Cord and Nerve Roots

CHATRACHI VIRAPONGSE, M.D.

E. LEON KIER, M.D.

THERE ARE APPROXIMATELY 5,000–10,000 new cases of spinal cord injury in the United States each year (Leo, Cloward). Of these, 2,500–3,000 require long-term hospitalization (Collins and Cherazi, Carter, Krause et al.). Eighty percent of the injuries involve the cervical cord, with motor vehicle accidents accounting for half of these cases. The average patient age in a recent study was 33 years (Wagner and Cherazi). Because these frequently devastating injuries tend to involve young, healthy adults in the prime of life, early correct diagnosis and treatment is imperative.

Radiology plays a key role not only in diagnosing the bone abnormalities but also in assessing the status of the spinal cord, which, compared with the spinal column, has received little consideration in the radiologic literature. This may be due in part to the fact that the cord is not visible on routine films, and in part to our imperfect knowledge about proper management of spinal cord injuries, compared with our experience in treating spine fractures.

INDICATIONS

Physicians often disagree on the indications for myelography in spinal trauma. We believe that the procedure adds little useful information in the following cases:

1. Complete transection of the cord.—The neurologic damage is irreversible; hence, therapy should be directed toward reducing the fracture-dislocation and stabilizing the spine.

2. Obliteration of, or severe bone encroachment upon, the spinal canal seen on plain films.—Myelography inevitably reveals a block and/or rupture of the thecal sac.

Traditionally, the use of myelography to diagnose spinal cord compression or impingement has been based on the premise that surgical removal of blood, bone, or disk material will restore neurologic function. In fact, however, Wagner and Cherazi have shown that such aggressive treatment (freeing the spinal cord within 48 hours after injury) has little bearing on the neurologic outcome. It is difficult to evaluate the modes of therapy because patients with spinal cord dysfunction do not usually have symptoms that conform precisely to the classic syndromes (e.g., Brown-Séquard, anterior cord, etc.); they tend to exhibit a mixed neurologic pattern. Although Cherazi et al. have proposed a scale for evaluating neurologic signs, subtle changes in neurologic function make it difficult to determine whether a patient has benefited from a particular treatment protocol.

At Yale-New Haven Hospital, the two objectives in managing patients with cord trauma are: (1) to relieve compression on the spinal cord, and (2) to prevent further injury to the cord. Conscious patients with neck and back pain and clinical evidence of paralysis, or unconscious patients with head injury are presumed to have spinal cord injury as well (Wagner and Cherazi). If a cervical cord injury is suspected and plain films demonstrate a cervical vertebral fracture, the patient is transferred to a body-length radiolucent frame and put in skeletal traction. If radiographs are negative, the patient is placed in a cervical collar. If a patient with a fracture but no dislocation has an incomplete neurologic deficit that is not improving, a myelogram is performed (Table 13–1). Fracture-dislocations are reduced by skull traction. If laminagraphy shows incomplete reduction, with residual encroachment on the spinal canal equal to or greater than one third its normal sagittal diameter, myelography is not indicated because a block by osseous structures is usually found. If reduction decreases encroachment on the spinal canal to less than a third of its normal sagittal diameter and the patient is not improving neurologically, myelography is performed (see Table 13–1).

Plain films and laminagraphy or CT should always precede myelography because laminagraphy and CT both depict bone distortion more accurately and help to localize bone fragments within the spinal canal that might be obscured by positive-contrast myelography. We believe laminagrams to be the most useful. In our opinion, myelography should facilitate more aggressive treatment of a spinal cord injury.

RADIOGRAPHIC FINDINGS (Figs 13–1 to 13–16)

In patients with spinal injury, a complete block is commonly caused by severe vertebral dislocation. Other causes of complete block are cord swelling (Figs 13–1 and 13–3), disk herniation (Figs 13–4 and 13–5), bone fragments (Figs 13–2, 13–6 to 13–9, 13–12, 13–14), extradural hematoma (Figs 13–5, *B* and 13–10), intradural hematoma (Figs 13–11 and 13–13), and arachnoiditis secondary to penetrating injury (Fig 13–15). Cord swelling at the level of the block may be due to edema, intramedullary hematoma, or abscess (Fig 13–16). Myelographically, it is impossible to distinguish among these conditions. However, it should be possible to make the distinction with high-resolution CT. This is important because surgical evacuation can improve the neurologic status in patients with an intramedullary hematoma (Fig 13–17). The myelographic appearance of cord swelling is that of focal enlargement of the spinal cord (Fig 13–3, *C*). More commonly, the swelling produces a partial block. Other lesions produce extradural defects (Fig 13–1). Unless conventional tomograms are obtained beforehand, a bone fragment impinging on the

TABLE 13–1.—INDICATIONS FOR MYELOGRAPHY IN PATIENTS WITH CERVICAL
AND THORACIC SPINE TRAUMA*

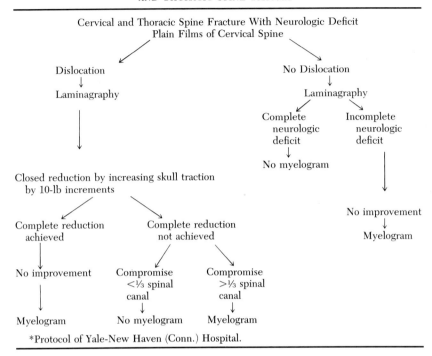

Cervical and Thoracic Spine Fracture With Neurologic Deficit
Plain Films of Cervical Spine

Dislocation

↓

Laminagraphy

Closed reduction by increasing skull traction
by 10-lb increments

Complete reduction   Complete reduction
achieved   not achieved

No improvement   Compromise   Compromise
                   <⅓ spinal   >⅓ spinal
                   canal   canal

Myelogram   No myelogram   Myelogram

No Dislocation

↓

Laminagraphy

Complete   Incomplete
neurologic   neurologic
deficit   deficit

↓

No myelogram

No improvement

↓

Myelogram

*Protocol of Yale-New Haven (Conn.) Hospital.

spinal cord can be missed on positive-contrast myelography because of obscuration by the contrast agent. In our experience, such bone fragments are rare in the cervical region and more common in the thoracolumbar area, where the vertebral body is frequently crushed into several fragments that are displaced posteriorly into the spinal canal (Figs 13–8 to 13–10, 13–12). Disk herniation is a common cause of spinal cord compression in the cervical region but is rare in the thoracolumbar area (Figs 13–4 and 13–5). The herniation appears as a localized extradural bulge at the vertebral interspace, impinging upon, and frequently compressing, the spinal cord.

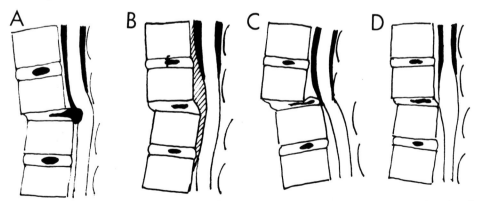

Fig 13–1.—Diagram of various pathologic entities in blunt spinal trauma. **A,** herniated disk. **B,** extradural hematoma *(diagonal lines).* **C,** subluxation with osseous compression of the spinal cord. **D,** cord swelling. The dark area surrounding the cord represents contrast material in the subarachnoid space.

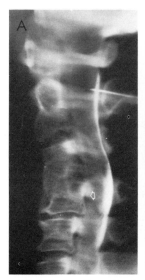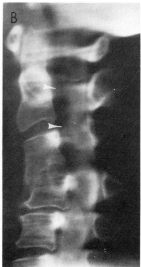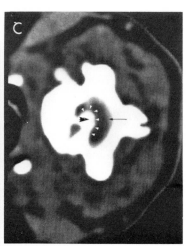

Fig 13–2.—Bone impingement on the anterior aspect of the spinal cord in a 44-year-old female. **A,** anterolisthesis of C-3 on C-4. Laminagrams after the introduction of metrizamide via a C1-2 puncture. The canal is still patent; however, the contrast column is interrupted at C-4 ventrally due to compression by the C-4 vertebral body *(arrow)*. **B,** the finding of bone impingement is confirmed with gas. Note the tendency for the gas to fill the ventral subarachnoid space *(arrows)*. **C,** CT immediately following the metrizamide myelography demonstrates the severity of canal narrowing and the bone impingement on the spinal cord *(large arrowhead)*. Note the complete obliteration of the ventral subarachnoid space; dorsally it is patent *(arrow)*. The cord is flattened and biconcave *(small arrowheads)*.

Hematomas arising from disrupted epidural veins rarely cause spinal cord compression (Figs 13–5 and 13–10). This subject is discussed in detail on pages 269–272.

Partial Block

After the cervical spine has been straightened by traction, lesions producing a partial block are more difficult to detect by myelography because contrast cannot pool readily, as it does in the concavity of the normal cervical spine. This problem is accentuated with metrizamide, which quickly flows caudad after a C1-2 puncture (Fig 13–4). Rapid sequential midline lateral tomograms are therefore crucial for correct diagnosis. Lesions causing a complete block may also give rise to a second, partial block, depending on the size of the lesion and the degree of spinal canal encroachment. In the presence of a partial block, the abnormality and its relationship to the spinal cord can be visualized above and below the lesion (Figs 13–2 and 13–4).

Hematomyelia

Bleeding into the spinal cord may occur immediately or days after injury. Clues to its pathogenesis are suggested by the microangiographic studies of feline spinal

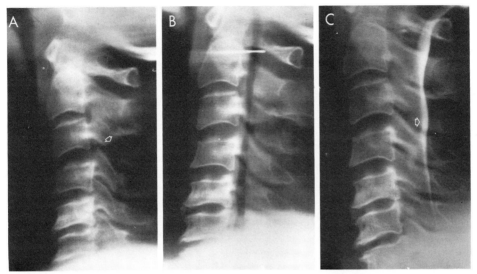

Fig 13–3.—51-year-old male with cord swelling who presented with Brown-Séquard syndrome. **A,** lateral tomographic projection (Mimer biplane fluoroscopic unit) with the patient supine in skull traction demonstrates minimal C3-4 subluxation and distraction of the disk space. The lamina is fractured *(arrow)*. **B,** gas myelogram shows a normal, patent ventral subarachnoid space, except for slight encroachment at C3-4 due to posterior bulging of the posterior longitudinal ligament from a traumatized disk. The anterior aspect of the cord is normal. **C,** since gas failed to demonstrate the posterior aspect of the cord, metrizamide myelography was performed. Note the almost imperceptible bulge of the cord at this level *(arrow),* suggesting cord swelling.

cords by Dohrmann and Allen. These investigators found that a blunt impact of 300 gm/cm to the spinal cord immediately decreased perfusion of both the white and gray matter. Within minutes after impact, multiple hemorrhages occurred in the gray matter, which coalesced to form larger hematomas. The lesions were probably due to direct trauma to vessels rather than to hemorrhagic necrosis secondary to vascular spasm. An impact that produces permanent paraplegia causes larger hematomas more frequently than does trauma that produces transient paraplegia. Dohrmann and Allen also found more severe prolonged vasospasm in vessels supplying the white matter. Hematomyelia may also occur in the absence of trauma, e.g., in patients with blood dyscrasias or hemophilia or in patients on anticoagulant therapy.

Like edema, hematomyelia produces cord enlargement that may be severe enough to cause a complete block (Fig 13–17). On a myelogram, this lesion can be easily differentiated from those producing extradural compression by noting the true widening of the cord shadow; this requires visualization of both the anterior and the posterior surfaces of the cord. The widening may be difficult to see with air or Pantopaque via a C1-2 puncture because air tends to coat the anterior aspect of the cord and Pantopaque, the posterior aspect. Unless both cord surfaces are visualized, the examiner may be misled by spurious cord widening on the anteroposterior film due to flattening of the cord by an extradural mass. Metrizamide allows visualization of both the anterior and posterior surfaces of the cord with metrizamide in most patients.

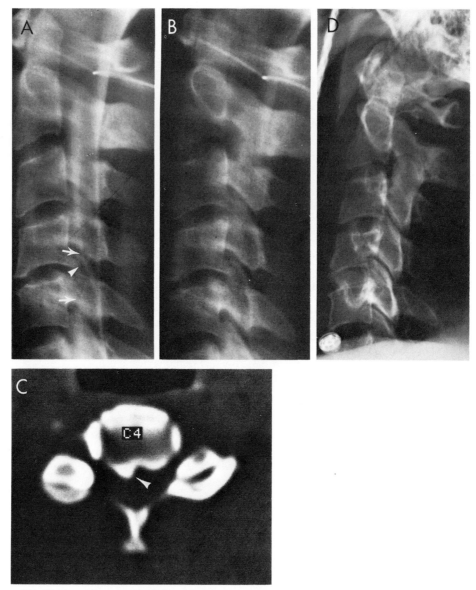

Fig 13–4.—27-year-old male with disk herniation who presented with central cord syndrome after a motor vehicle accident. **A,** metrizamide myelogram (lateral tomographic projection), showing minimal subluxation at C4-5. A large osteophyte at the posteroinferior aspect of C-4 projects into the canal *(arrowhead),* and a convex extradural defect *(arrows)* impinges on the anterior aspect of the spinal cord, suggesting disk herniation. **B,** lateral tomographic film 3 minutes later. All but a small amount of metrizamide around the needle has disappeared caudally, indicating the importance of rapid sequential tomographic filming. **C,** CT immediately following the myelogram shows no evidence of contrast in the subarachnoid space. Note the osteophyte at C-4 *(arrow).* **D,** after disk and osteophyte removal, an interbody fusion resulted in marked neurologic improvement.

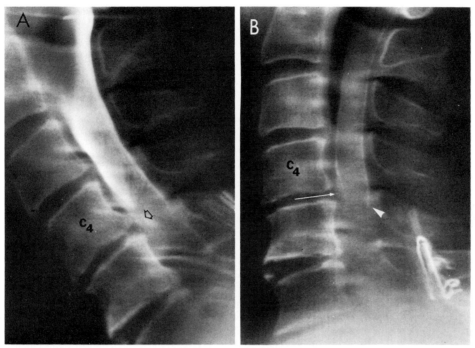

Fig 13–5.—78-year-old female with a central cord syndrome and a complete block at myelography. **A,** metrizamide myelogram, showing complete block at C4-5. There is a suggestion of a small anterior extradural defect *(arrow)*. **B,** with the patient tilted head down, gas was added as metrizamide filled the cisterna magna. A thin coat of metrizamide covers the surface of the cord, outlined by overlying gas, giving an excellent delineation of the cord surface. Now both anterior and posterior extradural defects can be seen compressing the spinal cord, the former *(arrow)* a herniated disk and the latter *(arrowhead),* an extradural hematoma. This double-contrast technique is similar to that employed in gastrointestinal studies.

AVULSION OF NERVE ROOTS

Brachial Plexus

Avulsion of one or more roots of the brachial plexus (Figs 13–18 to 13–24) results from severe trauma that forcibly separates the arm from the shoulder. Knowing the position of the arm at impact is important in determining the type of injury. With the arm in marked adduction, maximal stretch is placed on the upper roots (C-5 and C-6), producing the Erb-Duchenne form of paralysis. With the arm in marked abduction, the lower roots (C-7, C-8, T-1) are more likely to be injured, resulting in Klumpke's paralysis involving the small muscles of the hand and flexors of the wrist, and an ulnar distribution of sensory loss. If the first thoracic root is injured, Horner's syndrome may be present as well, because the sympathetic fibers to the stellate ganglion are involved.

To understand the myelographic findings, it is important to review the anatomy of the nerve root and the mechanism of injury. As the anterior and posterior roots leave the spinal cord, they carry with them an extension of the arachnoid and dura,

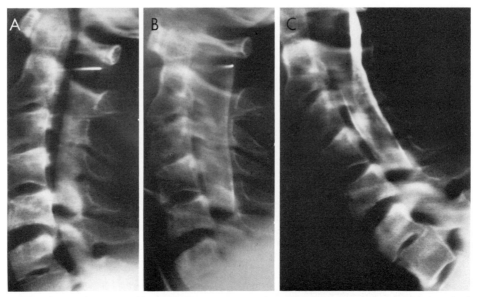

Fig 13–6.—Complete block by bone compression. **A,** gas myelogram shows a patent canal and minimal subluxation of C-5 on C-6. **B,** metrizamide myelogram. Further dislocation has occurred; compression by the posterior aspect of the C-5 vertebral body and the lamina of C-6 produces a complete block. **C,** Pantopaque myelogram confirms the finding.

forming the root sleeve, which usually does not extend beyond the intervertebral foramen. The arachnoid and dura then become the epineurium and perineurium, covering the roots as they leave the intervertebral foramen (Fig 13–18). The pia mater invests each nerve root within the subarachnoid space, forming the endoneural sheath. The presence of epineural and perineural sheaths gives a certain elastic strength to the nerve roots so that unsupported roots within the subarachnoid space will tear when stretched abruptly. In trauma, a series of protective mechanisms are activated. First, with traction on nerve roots, their fibrous attachments to the respective transverse processes are stretched and may be the first to tear (Fig 13–19). At the same time, the root sleeve covered with the dura and arachnoid is pulled into the intervertebral foramen and may be torn before the nerve roots rupture. (This explains why a traumatic meningocele may exist without nerve root rupture, but nerve root rupture is usually accompanied by a meningocele.) Since the spinal cord is pulled in the direction of the force by its attachment (the dentate ligament) to the dura, simultaneous cord injury often occurs. When these compensatory mechanisms fail to absorb the traction force and the elastic tolerance of the nerve root is exceeded, the nerve root snaps—usually at its junction with the spinal cord. CSF then leaks from the meningeal tear into the surrounding soft tissues and down the axillary sheath, i.e., the continuation of the deep cervical fascia enveloping the brachial plexus. Myelography performed at this point may show contrast extending beyond the rent in the dura, down into the axillary sheath. Frequently, an axillary sheath tear allows contrast to collect within the adipose tissue in the apex of the axilla (Fig 13–20). Since the contents of the axillary sheath offer considerable resistance to the flow of a viscous contrast me-

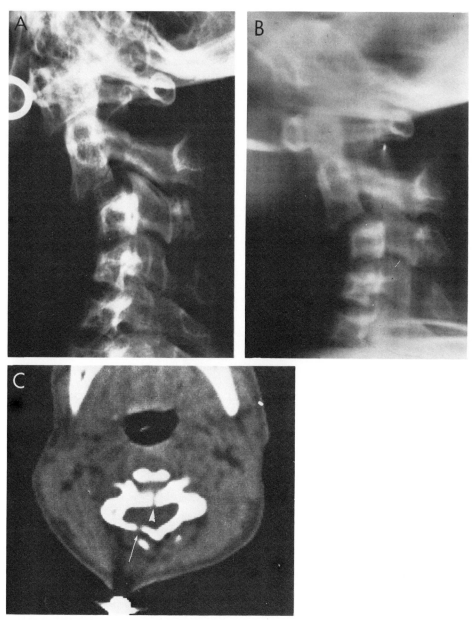

Fig 13–7.—8-year-old male with a family history of neurofibromatosis who fell off a bicycle and became monoplegic. **A,** plain film, lateral projection, of the cervical spine demonstrates numerous biconcave vertebral bodies typical of neurofibromatosis. Note marked subluxation between C-2 and C-3. The possibility of a congenital etiology cannot be ruled out. No fractures are seen. **B,** metrizamide myelogram demonstrates impingement and posterior displacement of the spinal cord by the subluxated C-3 vertebral body. **C,** CT shows fractures through the body of C-3 *(arrowhead)* and right lamina *(arrow)*, indicating acute injury.

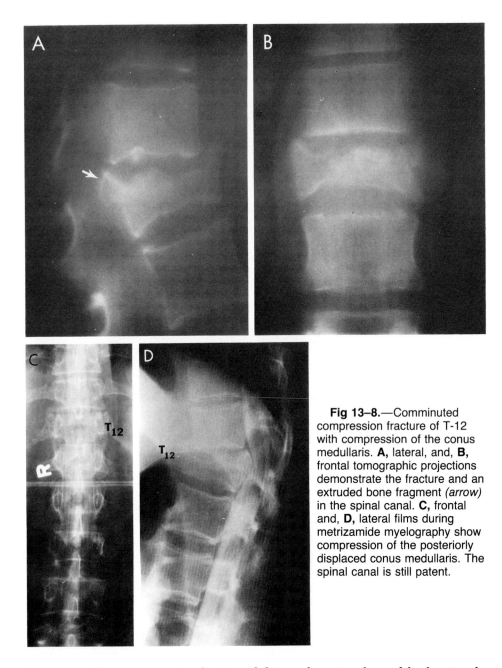

Fig 13–8.—Comminuted compression fracture of T-12 with compression of the conus medullaris. **A,** lateral, and, **B,** frontal tomographic projections demonstrate the fracture and an extruded bone fragment *(arrow)* in the spinal canal. **C,** frontal and, **D,** lateral films during metrizamide myelography show compression of the posteriorly displaced conus medullaris. The spinal canal is still patent.

dium—i.e., Pantopaque—visualization of this tracking is enhanced by leaving the patient with the affected side down for several minutes. Shortly after the dura is torn, meningeal cells and surrounding fibroblasts begin to proliferate. Within hours or days, depending on the size of the tear, the opening in the dura and arachnoid is closed, leaving a pouch-like extension of the root sleeve. The cellular proliferation may obliterate the meningocele entirely, resulting in an apparently normal axillary sheath. This accounts for the failure to visualize abnormalities on myelo-

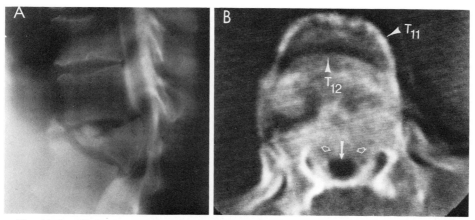

Fig 13–9.—Severely wedged compression fracture of T-12, with compression of the conus medullaris. **A,** lateral tomographic projection during metrizamide myelography. **B,** CT shows marked encroachment on the spinal canal by the posterior aspect of T-12 *(open arrows)* and impingement on the ventral surface of the conus medullaris *(closed arrow).*

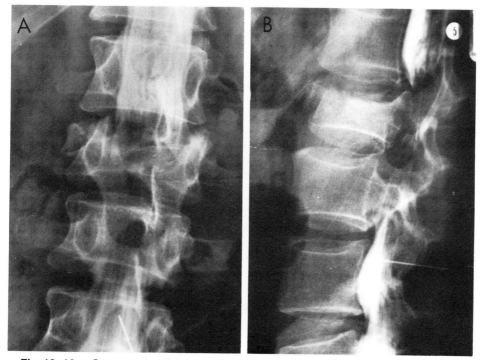

Fig 13–10.—Compression fracture associated with a large extradural hematoma. **A,** metrizamide myelogram (AP projection), showing a poorly defined defect in the contrast column at L-2 and L-3. **B,** lateral projection discloses a large anterior extradural defect suggestive of a hematoma extending from L-2 to the lower border of L-3.

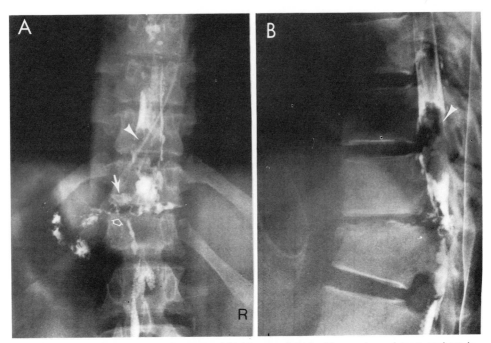

Fig 13–11.—Compression fracture of T-12 associated with meningeal tear and an intradural hematoma. **A,** AP Pantopaque myelogram. Note the complete obstruction of the oil column at T11-12. A track of contrast extends laterally into the paraspinal tissues, indicating a meningeal tear *(closed arrow)*. Some contrast has re-entered the spinal canal *(open arrow)*. More cephalad, an intradural mass (hematoma) is present *(arrowhead)*. **B,** lateral projection demonstrates the ovoid configuration of the hematoma *(arrowhead)*.

grams of patients with clinically obvious root avulsions. Metrizamide, which provides better visualization of the root sleeves than Pantopaque, probably demonstrates these irregularities more accurately.

In 1947, Murphy described the myelographic findings in brachial root avulsion injury. Since then, a large body of literature has accumulated on the subject. The abnormal findings (Figs 13–20 to 13–25) consist of: (1) a pouch-like appearance of the root sleeve, extending for a variable distance into the intervertebral foramen; (2) blunting and distortion of the normal root sheath; (3) cystic accumulation of CSF within the spinal canal, which may or may not fill with contrast; (4) nerve root abnormalities, i.e., absence or decreased size compared with the normal counterpart; (5) tracking of contrast down the axillary sheath to collect in the axilla.

Nerve root avulsions can be readily differentiated from diverticula of the subarachnoid space. Diverticula have smooth, delicately rounded contours and exhibit the normal radiolucent outlines of intact nerve roots in contrast to the opaque, contrast-filled pocket. Also, nontraumatic meningoceles usually have a neck, while traumatic meningoceles frequently do not. An abnormal axillary sleeve does not necessarily mean root avulsion; it simply indicates a meningeal tear. On the other hand, a normal axillary sleeve on a myelogram done immediately after trauma decreases the likelihood of brachial plexus avulsion.

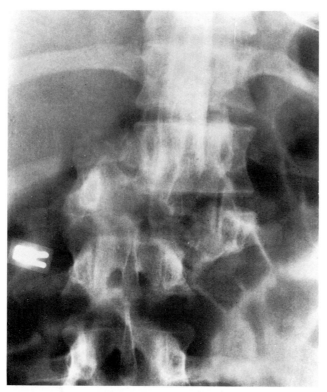

Fig 13–12.—Transverse (Chance) fracture of L-1 with complete block of the metriza-mide column due to an anteroposterior dislocation of L-1 (C1-2 puncture). The spinal canal is completely obliterated. Because the L-1 vertebral body blocks the spinal canal, a concomitant caudal meningeal tear, which probably exists, cannot be seen.

Lumbar Plexus

Although avulsion of the brachial plexus is not uncommon, avulsion of lumbosa-cral nerve roots is rare. Pelvic trauma severe enough to produce traction on the lumbosacral plexus usually fractures the pelvis or separates the sacroiliac joint or symphysis pubis. The reverse is true in the shoulder joint, where marked mobility is achieved at the cost of stability. Here, there is little protection for the brachial plexus roots against marked traction. All documented cases of lumbosacral nerve root avulsion have occurred in young males involved in auto accidents. Most pa-tients had one or more pelvic fractures; only one case of nerve root avulsion was secondary to a posterior hip dislocation. All patients had motor and sensory deficits of the corresponding lower extremity (Fig 13–26).

Meningeal Tear

In nonpenetrating trauma, a meningeal tear results from severe vertebral dis-placement. The thecal sac is stretched and torn by sharp edges of intact bone or bone fragments. Usually the dislocation does not reduce spontaneously; without prior closed reduction, a block above the tear is demonstrated myelographically,

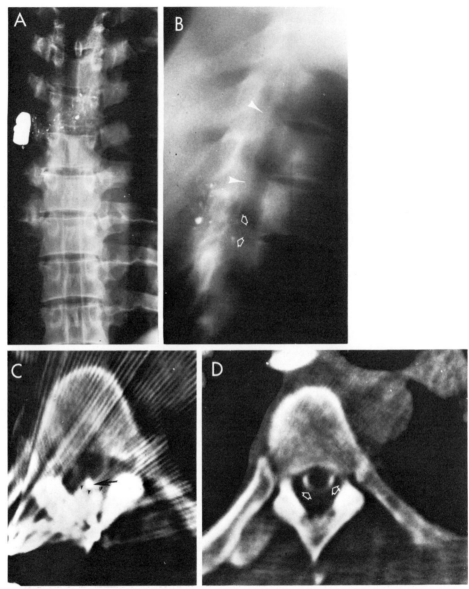

Fig 13–13.—Young male with a bullet wound of the thoracic spine and paraplegia. **A,** plain AP roentgenogram, demonstrating bullet lodged in the right paraspinal soft tissues. Numerous small bullet fragments are scattered along the bullets trajectory through T-4. **B,** metrizamide myelogram (lateral tomographic projection), disclosing two small fragments *(open arrows)* close to the dorsal aspect of the cord. The posterior thecal sac is uniformly displaced anteriorly *(closed arrows)*. **C,** CT at T-4 demonstrates the proximity of the bullet fragments *(arrows)* to the spinal cord *(arrowheads)*. The picture is obscured by streak artifacts from the large bullet fragment. **D,** CT at a higher level, showing the anteriorly displaced thecal sac from a subdural hematoma *(arrows)*. These findings were confirmed at surgery.

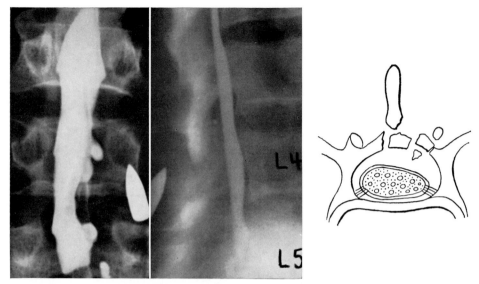

Fig 13–14.—Penetrating injury resulting in intraspinal bone fragments. **Left,** antero-posterior and lateral roentgenograms show a clear-cut, sharply marginated indentation due to pressure from a fractured spinous process and left lamina following a bullet wound. **Right,** cross-sectional diagram shows indentation of the dura-arachnoid and crowding of the caudal filaments by the bone fragments. (Reprinted, with permission, from Hinkel C.L., Nichols R.L.: *Am. J. Roentgenol.* 55:689, 1946.)

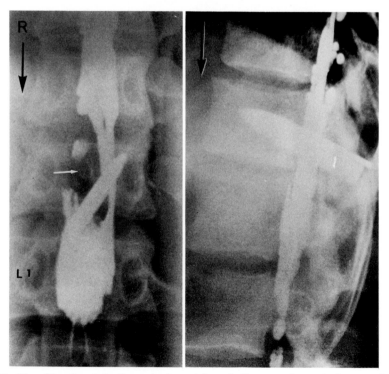

Fig 13–15.—Bleeding into the spinal cord from knife wound, producing arachnoiditis. The patient had a complete block at the lower border of L-1. Note sharply defined defect on the right at the level of the knife blade *(white arrow).* (Reprinted, with permission, from Hinkel C.L., Nichols R.L.: *Am. J. Roentgenol.* 55:689, 1946.)

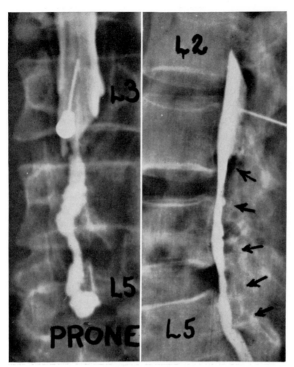
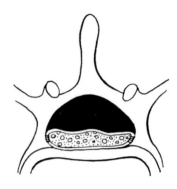

Fig 13–16.—Abscess resulting from penetrating injury. **Left,** anteroposterior and lateral myelographic spot films show a complete block due to an extradural abscess on the dorsal aspect of the cauda *(arrows),* producing a high-grade obstruction. **Right,** cross-sectional diagram demonstrating an almost complete block, with compression of the dura and the cauda equina filaments. (Reprinted, with permission, from Hinkel C.L., Nichols R.L.: *Am. J. Roentgenol.* 55:689, 1946.)

and the tear beyond the block cannot be seen. Compression of the thecal sac and intraspinal contents by bone can further increase the difficulty of demonstrating a tear (Fig 13–12). If the spinal canal is completely obliterated by a fracture-dislocation, a tear is very likely (Fig 13–11).

Penetrating injuries can also produce a meningeal tear (Fig 13–27). In either case, CSF leakage (which can be substantial) occurs into the surrounding soft tissues. The exposed neural tissues are susceptible to infection, thus necessitating immediate surgery. Extensive CSF extravasation may cause the spinal subarachnoid space to collapse due to decreased CSF pressure, thus making successful puncture difficult.

Pantopaque is the best contrast agent to demonstrate meningeal tears, which are frequently multiple. Large collections of Pantopaque are commonly found outside the canal. With metrizamide, the leakage site is difficult to identify, since this agent disperses within the extraspinal soft tissues. When it is not surgically important to identify the meningeal tear, metrizamide should be used because it is readily absorbed from the soft tissues (Mikhael and Hemmati).

Spinal-pleural and spinal-mediastinal fistulae have also been reported (Wilson and Jumer, Zilkha and Nicoletti, Compos et al., Overton et al.). These rare lesions are secondary to missile wounds or blunt trauma. While the formation of a sub-

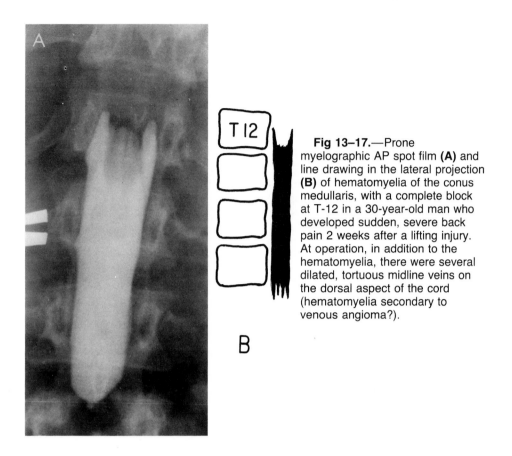

Fig 13–17.—Prone myelographic AP spot film **(A)** and line drawing in the lateral projection **(B)** of hematomyelia of the conus medullaris, with a complete block at T-12 in a 30-year-old man who developed sudden, severe back pain 2 weeks after a lifting injury. At operation, in addition to the hematomyelia, there were several dilated, tortuous midline veins on the dorsal aspect of the cord (hematomyelia secondary to venous angioma?).

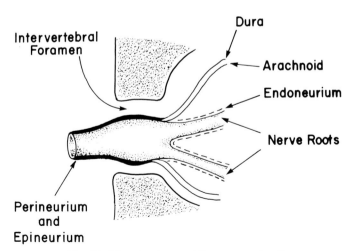

Fig 13–18.—Anatomy of the nerve sheath.

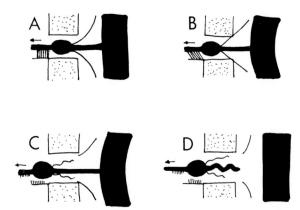

Fig 13–19.—Diagram of mechanism of brachial plexus avulsion injury (modified from Sunderland). **A,** normal anatomical arrangement of nerve root and nerve root sheath. **B,** with traction on the nerve root, the sheath is pulled into the intervertebral foramen. At the same time, the fibrous attachment of the nerve root to the transverse process is stretched. The spinal cord is also drawn in the direction of the pull. **C,** with increasing traction, the protective structures (meninges and ligaments) give way. **D,** finally, the elastic strength of the nerve root is exceeded, and it tears at its junction with the spinal cord. The spinal cord is now freed.

arachnoid-pleural fistula in penetrating injuries can be easily understood, its pathogenesis in blunt trauma is unclear. Compos et al. believe that a sudden deceleration of the body accompanied by extreme dorsiflexion of the spine causes the osseous prominences of the vertebral body to perforate the pleura. This, along with tearing of the neighboring root sleeves from the compressive effect of the dorsiflexion, produces a fistula. At Pantopaque myelography, the oil can be seen leaving the confines of the spinal canal and passing into the pleural space.

Penetrating Injury

The first detailed account of myelography in trauma was given by Hinkel and Nichols, based on their experience with penetrating injuries to the spinal cord in patients during World War II. Currently, such injuries are uncommon, accounting for less than 5% of all trauma to the spinal cord. They are caused by either gunshot or knife wounds (Fig 13–15), the latter rarely penetrating beyond the bony confines of the vertebral column. A gunshot wound, on the other hand, may shatter the vertebra, forcing numerous bone and bullet fragments into the spinal canal (Figs 13–13 and 13–14). Cord and nerve root injuries are frequently associated with meningeal tears and hematomas because of the severe disruptive effects of the bullet. Fistulae between the subarachnoid space and the mediastinum or pleura have also been reported.

POSTTRAUMATIC SYRINX

A posttraumatic syrinx was described by Holmes in 1915. Since then, this lesion has been variously referred to as ascending spinal paralysis, progressive myelopathy, or cystic degeneration of the spinal cord (Laha et al.). It occurs in 2% of all cord injuries and is most common in the thoracic region (Barnett and Jousse).

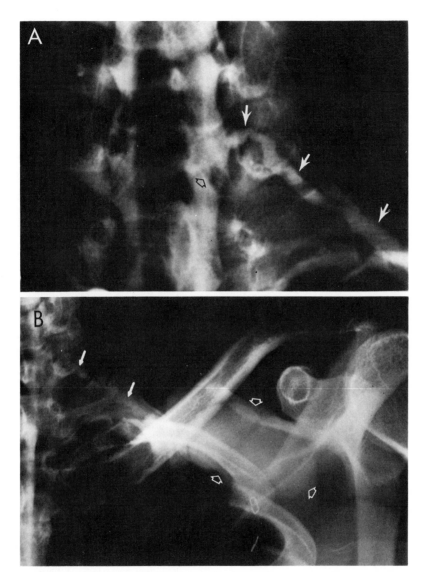

Fig 13–20.—Brachial plexus avulsion injury. Cervical metrizamide myelogram in a middle-aged male with a C-8 deficit after his arm was pulled into a baling machine. **A,** lateral tracking of contrast *(closed arrows)* indicates meningeal tear above the pedicle of C-7. Note that the C-8 root differs from its companion, being somewhat swollen *(open arrow).* **B,** contrast *(closed arrows)* extends along the axillary sheath and pools in the axilla *(open arrows),* indicating a probable tear of the sheath at this site in addition to the more proximal tear. Prior to the myelogram (which was performed several hours after injury), a laceration in the axilla was sutured. The patient was treated conservatively.

Symptoms may appear immediately after trauma (Williams and Turner) or be delayed. The latter is more common. Oakley et al. described a patient who presented 16 years after initial trauma. Patients usually experience pain on coughing and sneezing or an ascending sensory loss followed by motor changes.

The pathogenesis of posttraumatic syrinx is controversial. According to Gardner, this pathogenesis is similar to that of the congenital variety. Although there are

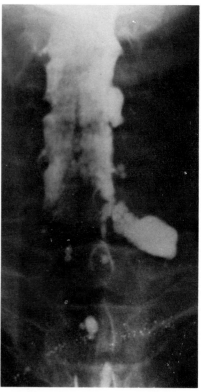

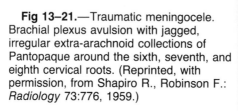

Fig 13–21.—Traumatic meningocele. Brachial plexus avulsion with jagged, irregular extra-arachnoid collections of Pantopaque around the sixth, seventh, and eighth cervical roots. (Reprinted, with permission, from Shapiro R., Robinson F.: *Radiology* 73:776, 1959.)

cases of posttraumatic syrinx communicating with the central canal and fourth ventricle (Oakley et al.), in most instances there is no communication. Williams believes that posttraumatic adhesions and scar tissue cause the pulsating CSF to dissect gradually into the substance of the spinal cord. Such cysts do not commonly communicate with the subarachnoid space. McLean et al. suggested that myelomalacia at the site of trauma is transformed over time into a cystic, glia-lined cavity

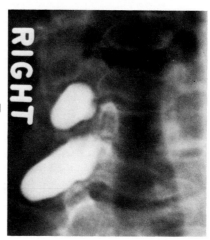

Fig 13–22.—Traumatic pseudomeningoceles of two lower cervical roots on the right in an elderly male who had suffered a severe avulsion of the brachial plexus some 20 years earlier.

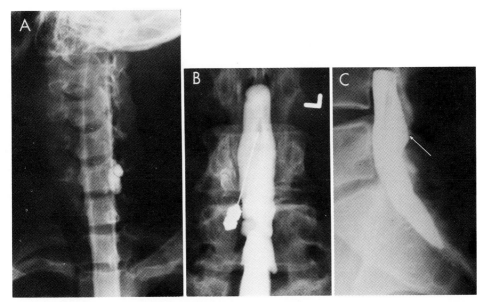

Fig 13–23.—Traumatic "meningocele" with avulsion of the left C-7 root. **A,** metrizamide myelogram in a 19-year-old man involved in an auto accident. The patient was unable to use his left arm. **B** and **C,** pseudomeningocele at L-4 and L-5 following lumbar
laminectomy *(arrow).*

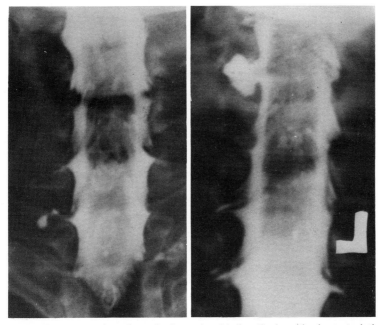

Fig 13–24.—Two examples of cervical arachnoid diverticula with characteristic smooth,
well-defined margins.

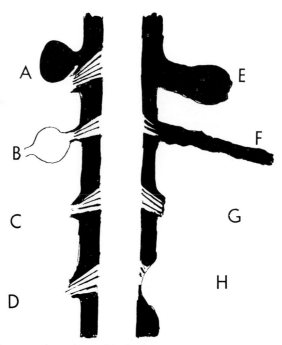

Fig 13–25.—Diagram of myelographic findings in brachial plexus avulsion. **A,** diverticulum. Note that it has a neck and is well rounded. **B,** perineural cyst, which may not fill with contrast. **C** and **D,** normal axillary sheaths. **E,** traumatic meningocele. Note long, irregular protuberance and the absence of normal nerve root shadow (as in Figs 13–21, 13–22). **F,** tracking of contrast down the axillary sheath (as in Fig 13–20). Note the paucity of nerve roots. **G,** amputated axillary sheath from marked meningeal and fibroblastic proliferation. **H,** a focal cystic collection within the subdural space that does not fill with contrast, secondary to a meningeal tear.

much like posttraumatic cystic CSF collections in the brain. DuBoulay et al. believe these cystic cavities enlarge with sudden changes in spinal venous pressure, as in sneezing and coughing.

At myelography, the cord is often enlarged (Figs 13–27 and 13–28). However, in many patients, it is normal in caliber. Seibert et al. found 14 of 25 (56%) patients with large cords, while 11 patients (44%) had normal or slightly enlarged cords. These statistics are similar to those found in nontraumatic syrinx. Also noteworthy is the fact that all Seibert's patients had associated cord adhesions, a finding that lends some support to Williams' hypothesis. Eleven patients in Seibert's series had a partial block, while 14 had a complete block. In eight patients, cyst punctures were attempted; six were successful. Seibert also reported the first cases of metrizamide uptake in a posttraumatic cyst on CT. A significant number of patients demonstrated this finding. In 1975, DiChiro et al. were the first to report metrizamide collection in a *non*traumatic cyst. Such contrast accumulation within a cyst is thought to be related to cord penetration, a finding which Dubois has verified experimentally. Hence, it can be assumed that the traumatic spinal cord cyst allows metrizamide to penetrate in a manner similar to that of the nontraumatic cyst. Metrizamide CT has obvious advantages over cyst puncture and is currently the best technique for demonstrating the syrinx cavity.

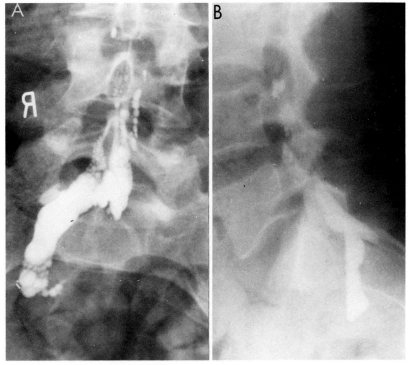

Fig 13–26.—Lumbar plexus injury. Frontal **(A)** and lateral **(B)** roentgenograms of a patient with traumatic avulsion of the right S-1 root. Note the jagged, irregular outline of the extra-arachnoid oil. (Reprinted, with permission, from Payne R.F., Thomson J.L.G.: *Br. J. Radiol.* 42:840, 1969.)

IATROGENIC TRAUMA

Extradural Hematoma

The first report of spinal epidural hematoma was published by Jackson in 1869. Since then, over 100 cases have been reported (Edelson et al., Brandt, Vinters et al.). Unlike intracranial extradural hematomas, spinal extradural hematomas are venous in origin, arising from the rich venous plexus surrounding the dura (Fig 13–29). Symptoms may be acute or chronic, depending on the level of the hemorrhage. Lumbar hematomas may be chronic because the nerve roots in that region can tolerate more compression than the spinal cord. In the cervical region, rapid progression of symptoms is the rule, since the spinal cord occupies a larger portion of the bony canal here than it does elsewhere (Boyd and Pear). The thoracic region is the most common site for hematomas, possibly because the posterior extradural space is larger here than elsewhere in the spine. Acute back pain, frequently interscapular, associated with radicular radiation, is the most common symptom. The pain is followed by paraplegia and poor sphincter control. Causes include anticoagulant therapy, arteriovenous malformation, rupture of vertebral hemangioma, trauma, penetrating and nonpenetrating injuries, lumbar puncture, arteriosclerosis, pregnancy and labor, infection, hemophilia, chronic alcoholism, and whooping

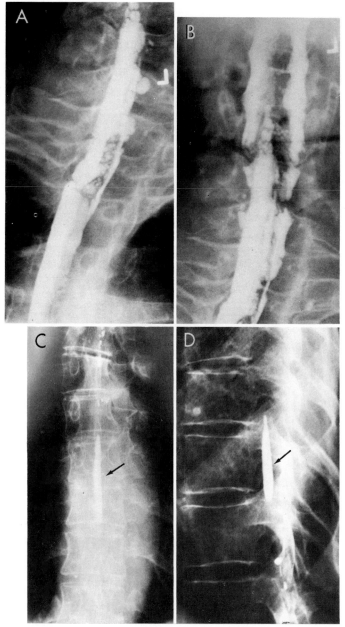

Fig 13–27.—Posttraumatic hydromyelia due to a fistula between the subarachnoid space and the central canal. A stab wound at T-2 17 years previously produced Brown-Séquard syndrome. The patient got along fairly well until a few years prior to admission, when she noted weakness in the arms and legs. One year before admission, she began to lose function in her right hand and arm. At admission, there was spasticity of the legs with dissociation of pain and temperature in both arms, more marked on the left. The oblique and frontal myelographic spot films, **A** and **B,** demonstrate displacement of the spinal cord to the left and irregularity of the Pantopaque column due to arachnoiditis. In **C** and **D,** an elongated collection of oil remained in the midline *(arrow)* and did not change its shape or position. At operation, the oil collection was found to be due to the fistula.

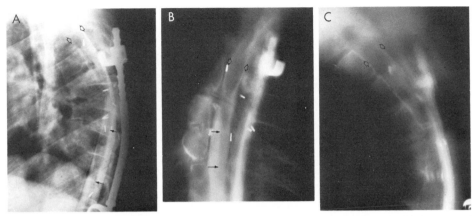

Fig 13–28.—Posttraumatic syrinx in a 29-year-old male who presented with increased difficulty in walking, and decreased sweating and numbness over the midthoracic region. As a child, he had had a neurofibroma removed from the thoracic region and several years later had a bicycle accident with compression fractures of the midthoracic vertebrae requiring Harrington rods. **A,** metrizamide myelogram in the lateral projection demonstrating a severe bone deformity secondary to blunt trauma and surgery. The cord shadow, widened *(open arrows)* above the apex of the scoliosis, almost completely fills the canal, while more caudad it is small *(closed arrows)*. **B,** and **C,** laminagrams show the widened cord better *(open arrows),* suggesting syringomyelia, and also cord narrowing, suggestive of associated cord atrophy *(closed arrows).*

cough. According to Pear, 45% of hematomas are spontaneous (no history of trauma or anticoagulation therapy) in patients under 50 years of age. The free reversal of blood flow within the vertebral venous plexus is thought to make it vulnerable to local pooling and rupture when subjected to a sudden increase in pressure, as in coughing and straining. This may account for the so-called spontaneous hemorrhage (Kaplan and Denker, Ventureyra et al.). Some unknown mechanisms must protect against mishap, because spontaneous hematomas are rare.

Myelographically, the spinal defect closely resembles its intracranial counterpart, with a convex inward configuration extending over several vertebrae (Figs 11–2, 13–29, 13–30). Anatomically, however, the relationship between the intracranial and the spinal dura and the periosteum is quite dissimilar. The intracranial dura lies close to the endocranium, making blood flow between the two surfaces difficult, while the spinal dura is widely separated from bone by loose areolar tissue, fat, and blood vessels. A possible explanation for the configuration in the spinal region is the resistance provided by the thick dura itself. Because the hematoma is commonly located on the posterior aspect of the cord, a supine lateral cross-table film is advisable when Pantopaque is used. Since the lesion does not usually extend circumferentially, the spinal cord is displaced ventrally and may be flattened. This results in spurious cord widening on the frontal view, which simulates an intramedullary lesion. The hematoma may cause a complete obstruction if it is sufficiently large. When situated posteriorly, it can be readily differentiated from a disk herniation by its location. When it occurs anteriorly, it can be differentiated by its length and its lack of relationship to the disk space. The rare chronic extradural hematoma involving the cauda equina may simulate an extradural tumor or granuloma.

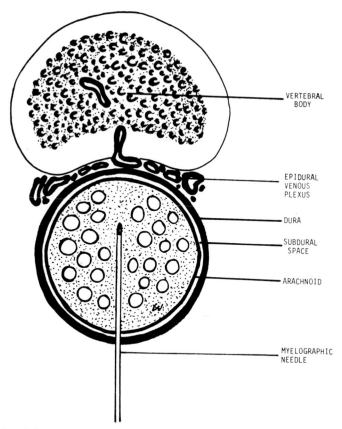

VERTEBRAL
BODY

EPIDURAL
VENOUS
PLEXUS

DURA

SUBDURAL
SPACE

ARACHNOID

MYELOGRAPHIC
NEEDLE

Fig 13–29.—Schematic drawing showing the rich extradural venous plexus and the absence of vessels in the subdural space, which accounts for the higher prevalence of traumatic extradural hematomas.

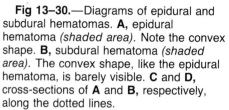

Fig 13–30.—Diagrams of epidural and subdural hematomas. **A,** epidural hematoma (shaded area). Note the convex shape. **B,** subdural hematoma (shaded area). The convex shape, like the epidural hematoma, is barely visible. **C** and **D,** cross-sections of **A** and **B,** respectively, along the dotted lines.

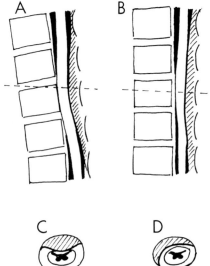

Subdural Hematoma

The first case report of a spinal subdural hematoma was published by Schiller et al. in 1948. Only about 35 cases have since been reported. The rarity of spinal subdural hematomas contrasts with their frequency in the intracranial cavity. In the skull, subdural hematomas can occur after minor trauma, while extradural hematomas are usually secondary to major trauma. This is due to the numerous anastomotic veins traversing the subdural space which are poorly supported by stromal tissue (Fig 13–29). Hence, any violent movement of the brain away from the inner table will result in tearing. The subdural space in the spine, on the other hand, is relatively avascular. Nonetheless, Manelfe found a longitudinal network of anastomotic veins along the inner lateral aspect of the dura, which is probably the source of bleeding. The causes of subdural hematomas are similar to those of extradural hematomas, with a large proportion occurring in patients on anticoagulant therapy (Paredes et al.). Edelson et al. reported eight patients with thrombocytopenia who developed subdural hematoma after lumbar puncture. Five patients had a platelet count below 20,000, and seven of the lumbar punctures were considered to be traumatic. Edelson and his co-workers cautioned against lumbar puncture in thrombocytopenic patients; the lower the platelet count, the more likely the chances of subdural hematoma development.

The most common site for a subdural hematoma is the thoracolumbar area. The symptoms and signs are similar to those of extradural hematoma. On myelography, the abnormality is reminiscent of the defects seen after inadvertent injection of contrast into the subdural space. Both blood and contrast spread circumferentially, conform to the contour of the spinal canal, and narrow the intraspinal cavity by displacing the arachnoid inward (Fig 13–30). The long, inward convex-inward configuration of the epidural hematoma may be absent with subdural hematoma, since the arachnoid is displaced uniformly inward (Fig 13–13). A subdural hematoma is also longer than an epidural hematoma. Only at its extremity will the defect form an obtuse angle with the opacified normal spinal canal (Fig 13–31). In this respect, spinal epidural and subdural hematomas are similar to their counterparts above the foramen magnum, where the former tend to be focal while the latter are more diffuse. This tendency to spread makes subdural collections of blood difficult to differentiate from neoplasms such as lymphomas, which frequently spread circumferentially. According to Zilkha, displacement of the spinal theca to one side in the presence of a normal ipsilateral axillary sleeve is indicative of spinal subdural hematoma.

Subarachnoid Hematoma

This unusual complication is even rarer than spinal subdural hematoma. It has appeared: (1) in patients with an underlying bleeding diathesis or previous spinal cord disease, (2) following lumbar puncture in normal patients or in those with bleeding tendencies, (3) spontaneously, with no obvious cause. Apparently the hematoma forms after massive bleeding, which prevents dilution of the blood by CSF. Normally, blood in the subarachnoid space disperses and becomes diluted by CSF so that it is not visible at myelography. In group 1, the underlying lesion may be a

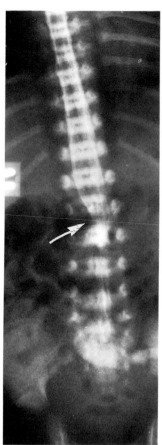

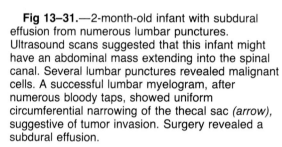

Fig 13–31.—2-month-old infant with subdural effusion from numerous lumbar punctures. Ultrasound scans suggested that this infant might have an abdominal mass extending into the spinal canal. Several lumbar punctures revealed malignant cells. A successful lumbar myelogram, after numerous bloody taps, showed uniform circumferential narrowing of the thecal sac *(arrow),* suggestive of tumor invasion. Surgery revealed a subdural effusion.

congenital vascular abnormality (e.g., aneurysm or angioma), an acquired disease that compromises the integrity of blood vessel walls (e.g., polyarteritis nodosa), or an abnormality in the bleeding or clotting mechanism. In the traumatic group, lumbar puncture may have lacerated a radicular vessel.

Clinically, these patients present with a sudden, dramatic onset of symptoms like those of acute epidural hematoma (severe back pain, sensory level, rapidly progressive paraparesis). However, unlike acute epidural hematoma, which is more common in the cervical region, acute subarachnoid hematoma occurs more frequently in the thoracolumbar area.

The myelographic findings depend on the size of the hematoma. A small hematoma is difficult to differentiate from other intradural, extramedullary lesions; but with increasing size, it envelops or displaces the cord. In the frontal projection, this can give a spurious appearance of cord enlargement, incorrectly suggesting an intramedullary lesion. Ultimately, a complete block may be found. Frager et al. point out that capping of the contrast column in the frontal and lateral projections indicates not only the superior margin of the clot but its subarachnoid location as well. These authors also point out that a C1-2 tap is usually necessary, since lumbar puncture may result in a dry tap. Spinal CT elegantly demonstrates the high-attenuation envelope of blood encasing or displacing the spinal cord.

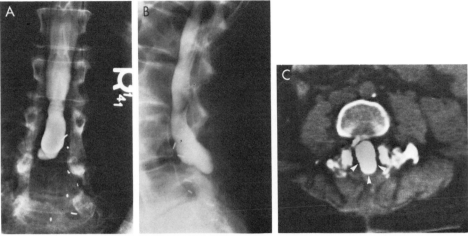

Fig 13–32.—Postlaminectomy pseudomeningocele. AP **(A)** and lateral **(B)** roentgeno-grams from a metrizamide lumbar myelogram demonstrating evidence of laminectomy at L-4 and L-5. The complete block at L-5 is due to adhesions associated with posterior herniation of the thecal sac through the laminectomy defect, simulating a meningocele. Note the irregular contour of the pseudomeningocele, which is similar to the traumatic meningocele in root avulsion. **C,** axial CT showing the pseudomeningocele *(arrowheads).*

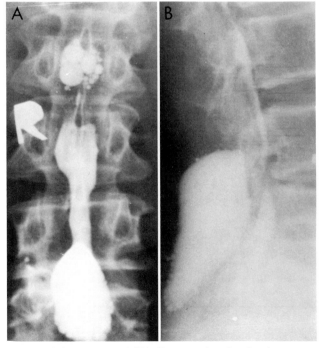

Fig 13–33.—Prone **(A)** and lateral **(B)** films made after laminectomy, demonstrating Pantopaque in a pseudomeningocele.

Pseudomeningocele

Pseudomeningoceles (Figs 13–32 and 13–33) occur most frequently along the dorsal aspect in the lumbar region at the site of previous surgery, usually a laminectomy. During such a procedure, the integrity of the thecal sac may be violated, causing CSF extravasation into the soft tissues behind the spine. These pockets of fluid may be large enough to produce a visible bulge below the incision scar. On myelography, a small posterior protuberance may indicate a pseudomeningocele, or a large cavity below the skin may communicate via a small tract with an otherwise normal thecal sac. In such circumstances, metrizamide should be used to locate the tract because Pantopaque is too viscous. Myelography can be supplemented by CT, which more precisely defines the extension of the tract beyond the confines of the vertebrae.

Postoperative Deformity

Localized arachnoiditis may occur at the site of previous surgery for tumor or herniated disk (Figs 13–34 and 13–35). When symptoms recur postoperatively, myelographic defects at the operative site must be interpreted with considerable

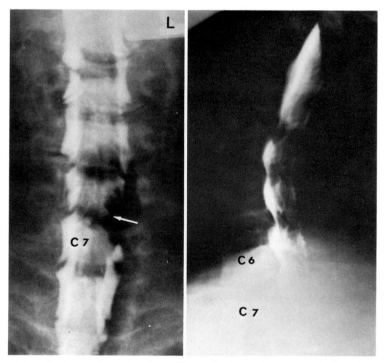

Fig 13–34.—Postoperative adhesions. The patient had been operated on 10 years earlier for removal of a neurilemoma of the left sixth cervical root. His complaint at admission was left radicular pain pointing to the same root. The question of recurrent tumor versus arachnoiditis arose. Myelography demonstrated generalized spondylosis of the cervical spine, with a prominent lateral defect localized at C6-7 on the left *(arrow)*. At operation, only arachnoiditis, with thickening of the meninges between the cord and dura, was found.

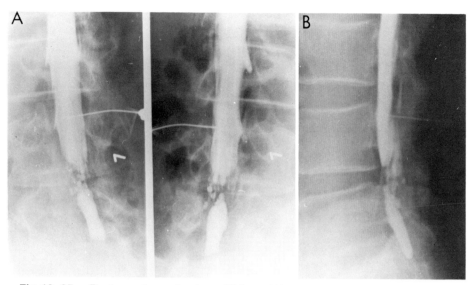

Fig 13–35.—Postoperative adhesions. Oblique **(A)** and lateral **(B)** roentgenograms in a 51-year-old man with a dense dural scar and adhesions at L4-5 consequent to a laminectomy 13 years earlier.

caution. They may be transient, due to edema in the immediate postoperative period, or they may persist indefinitely, due to fibrous adhesions. A postoperative scar presenting as an irregular, elongated, sharply defined defect between two nerve roots does not pose a great problem in differential diagnosis. However, a defect at the vertebral interspace may be indistinguishable from a herniated disk.

Acquired Spinal Cyst

Intradural and extradural spinal cysts may be found after traumatic or surgical spinal injury. Contrast entering the lesion at myelography can be considered pathognomonic of spinal cyst. However, the cyst may occasionally be closed off, producing a defect that mimics other lesions (Fig 13–36).

Acquired Epidermoid Sequestration Cyst

This rare lesion results from traumatic or iatrogenic inclusion of epidermal elements in the intradural or extradural space. Most of these cysts are lumbar in location, secondary to the implantation of skin fragments during spinal puncture (Fig 13–37). According to Pear, myelography demonstrates one or more posterior tumors adhering to the arachnoid and nerve roots. Unlike the congenital variety, no bone changes are visualized on the plain roentgenogram.

THE ROLE OF CT

The advantages of CT over conventional tomography in demonstrating fractures of the vertebral column are well documented (Mikhael and Hemmati, Coin et al.,

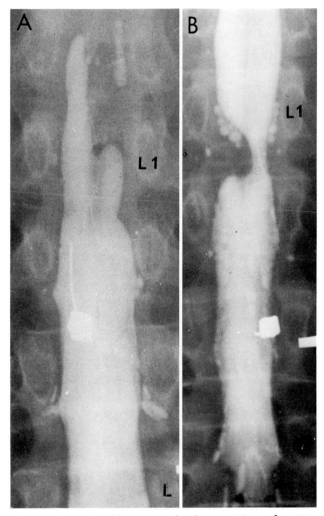

Fig 13–36.—Acquired arachnoid cyst postlumbar puncture. **A,** prone myelographic spot film (Nov. 1, 1968) in a 51-year-old man. Note the tip of the needle at L1-2 on the right. **B,** repeat myelogram (Apr. 1, 1970) because of persistent severe pain in the right thigh showed a constant defect at L1–2 on the right, at the site of the old lumbar puncture. At surgery, an acquired arachnoidal cyst was found.

Post et al.). Fractures of the vertebral body and neural arch not seen on tomography can be shown on CT. Moreover, CT offers a cross-sectional view of the spinal canal so that stenosis or bone fragments within the canal can be easily assessed. Ability to reformat these images in the sagittal and coronal planes provides another advantage. However, little is known of the role of CT in evaluating the spinal cord in trauma. Although Post et al. state that CT should be the prime imaging modality for studying the traumatized spinal cord followed by myelography, we believe the opposite to be true. Even though CT is an excellent modality for visualizing bone injuries, it cannot as yet be relied upon to reveal small soft tissue impingements on the cord. When used as an adjunct to metrizamide myelography, it can help in

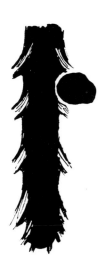
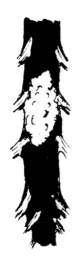

Fig 13–37.—Diagrams of a traumatic cyst filling with contrast *(left)* and an epidermoid cyst. Note the irregular surface. *Right,* postoperative adhesions.

assessing the amount of spinal cord compression by an osseous or soft tissue mass. Its role in visualizing the posttraumatic syrinx has already been mentioned.

BIBLIOGRAPHY

Allen W.E., D'Angelo C.M., Kier E.L.: Correlation of microangiographic and electrophysiologic changes in experimental spinal cord trauma. *Radiology* 110:107, 1974.

Barnes R.: Paraplegia in cervical spine injuries. *J. Bone Joint Surg.* 30B:234, 1948.

Barnett H.J., Jousse A.T.: Syringomyelia as a late sequel to traumatic paraplegia and quadriplegia—clinical features. *Major Probl. Neurol.* 1:129, 1973.

Beutel E.W., Roberts J.D., Langston H.T., Baker W.L.: Subarachnoid-pleural fistula. *J. Thorac. Cardiovasc. Surg.* 80:21, 1980.

Boyd H.R., Pear B.L.: Chronic spontaneous spinal epidural hematoma. *J. Neurosurg.* 36:239, 1972.

Brandt R.A.: Chronic spinal subdural hematoma. *Surg. Neurol.* 13:121, 1980.

Carter E.R., Jr.: Etiology of traumatic spinal cord injury: Statistics of more than 1100 cases. *Texas Med.* 73:61, 1977.

Cherazi B., Wagner F.C., Collins W.F., Freeman D.H.: A scale for evaluation of spinal cord injury. *J. Neurosurg.* 54:310, 1981.

Cloward R.: Acute cervical spine injuries. *Clinical Symposium CIBA*, vol. 32, no. 1, 1980.

Coin L.G., Pennick M., Ahmad W.D., Keranten V.J.: Diving-type injury of the cervical spine: Contribution of computed tomography to management. *J. Comput. Assist. Tomogr.* 3:362, 1979.

Collins W.F., Cherazi B.: Concepts of acute management of spinal cord injury, in Matthew, Glaser.: *Recent Advances in Neurology.* London, Churchill & Livingstone, 1980.

Compos B.A.R., Silva L.B., Ballaca N., Negrao M.M.: Traumatic subarachnoid-pleural fistula. *J. Neurol., Neurosurg. Psychiatr.* 37:269, 1974.

DeVanney J.W., Osher D.: Neurological clinical pathological conferences at Cincinnati General Hospital. *Dis. Nerv. Syst.* 13:53, 1952.

DiChiro G., Axelbaum S.P., Schellinger D., et al.: Computerized axial tomography in syringomyelia. *N. Engl. J. Med.* 292:13, 1975.

Dohrmann G.J., Allen W.E.: Microcirculation of traumatized spinal cord. *Trauma* 15:1003, 1975.

Dubois P.J., Drayer B.P., Sage M., et al.: Intramedullary penetrance of metrizamide in the dog spinal cord. *A.J.N.R.* 2:313, 1981.

duBoulay G., Shah S.H., Currie J.C., Logue V.: The mechanisms of hydromyelia in Chiari Type I malformations. *Br. J. Radiol.* 47:579, 1974.

Edelson R.N., Chernick N.L., Posner J.B.: Spinal subdural hematomas complicating lumbar puncture. *Arch. Neurol.* 31:134, 1974.

Fody E.P., Netsky M.G., Mrak R.E.: Subarachnoid spinal hemorrhage in a case of systemic lupus erythematosus. *Arch. Neurol.* 37:173, 1980.

Frager D., Zimmerman R.D., Wisoff H.S., Leeds N.E.: Spinal subarachnoid hematoma. *A.J.N.R.* 3:77, 1982.

Frantz P., Battaglini J.: Subarachnoid-pleural fistula: Unusual complication of thoracotomy. *J. Thorac. Cardiovasc. Surg.* 79:873, 1980.

Gardner W.J.: Hydrodynamic mechanism of syringomyelia: Its relationship to myelocele. *J. Neurol. Neurosurg. Psychiatr.* 28:247, 1965.

Goodman J.M.: Myelography in acute cervical injuries. *A.J.R.* 107:491, 1969.

Heiden J.S., Weiss M.H., Rosenberg A.W., et al.: Penetrating gunshot wounds of the cervical spine in civilians. *J. Neurosurg.* 42:575, 1975.

Henson R.A., Croft P.B.: Spontaneous spinal subarachnoid hemorrhage. *Q. J. Med.* 25:53, 1956.

Hinkel C.L., Nichols R.L.: Opaque myelography in penetrating wounds of the spinal canal. *A.J.R.* 55:689, 1946.

Hofstetter K.R., Bjelland J.C., Patton D.D., et al.: Detection of bronchopleural-subarachnoid fistula by radionuclide myelography: Case report. *J. Nuclear Med.* 18:981, 1977.

Holmes G.: The Goalstonian lectures on spinal injuries of warfare. *Br. Med. J.* 2:767, 1915.

Jackson R.: Case of spinal apoplexy. *Lancet* 2:5, 1869.

Kaplan L.I., Denker P.G.: Acute non-traumatic spinal epidural hemorrhage. *Am. J. Surg.* 78:356, 1949.

King O.J., Glas W.W.: Spinal subarachnoid hemorrhage following lumbar puncture. *Arch. Surg.* 80:574, 1960.

Krause J.F., Franti C.E., Riggins R.S.: Incidence of traumatic spinal cord lesions. *J. Chronic Dis.* 28:471, 1975.

Laha R.K., Malik H.G., Langill R.A.: Post-traumatic syringomyelia. *Surg. Neurol.* 4:519, 1975.

Lee B.C., Kazam E., Newman A.D.: Computed tomography of the spine and spinal cord. *Radiology* 128:95, 1978.

Leo J.S., Bergeron R.T., Ksischeff I.I., Benjamin M.V.: Metrizamide myelography for cervical cord injuries. *Radiology* 129:707, 1978.

Lippitt A.B.: Fracture of a vertebral body end plate and disk protrusion causing subarachnoid block in an adolescent. *Clin. Orthop.* 116:112, 1976.

McLean D.R., Miller J.D., Allen P.B., Ezzeddin S.A.: Post-traumatic syringomyelia. *J. Neurosurg.* 39:485, 1973.

Manelfe C.: Contribution a l'etude de la vascularisation arterielle de la dure-mere rachidienne chez l'homme: Etude anatomo-radiologique et histologique considerations pathologiques. Toulouse, France, Imprimerie Fourhie, 1969.

Masdeu J.C., Breuer A.C., Schoene W.C.: Spinal subarachnoid hematomas due to a source of bleeding in traumatic lumbar puncture. *Neurology* 29:872, 1979.

Mikhael M.A., Hemmati M.: Neuroradiologic assessment of the spinal cord injuries. In Calenoff L. (ed.): *Radiology of Spinal Cord Injury.* St. Louis, C.V. Mosby Co., 1981.

Murphy F., Hartung W., Kirklin J.W.: Myelographic demonstration of avulsion injury of the brachial plexus. *A.J.R.* 58:102, 1947.

Oakley J.C., Ojemann G.A., Alvord E.C.: Post-traumatic syringomyelia. *J. Neurosurg.* 55:276, 1981.

Overton M.C., III, Hood R.M., Farris R.G.: Traumatic subarachnoid-pleural fistula. Case report. *J. Thoracic Cardiovasc. Surg.* 51:729, 1966.

Paredes E.S.D., Kishmore P.R.S., Ward J.D.: Cervical spinal subdural hematoma. *Surg. Neurol.* 15:477, 1981.

Pay N.T.: Positive and negative contrast myelography in spinal trauma. *Radiology* 123:103, 1977.

Pear B.L.: Iatrogenic intraspinal epidermoid sequestration cysts. *Radiology* 92:251, 1969.

Pear B.L.: Spinal epidural hematoma. *A.J.R.* 115:155, 1972.

Plotkin R., Ronthal M., Froman C.: Spontaneous spinal subarachnoid hemorrhage. Report of three cases. *J. Neurosurg.* 25:443, 1966.

Post M.J.D., Green B.A., Quencer R.M., Stokes N.A.: The importance of computed tomography in spinal trauma. Presented at the 19th annual meeting of the American Society of Neuroradiology, 1981.

Quiles M., Marchisello P.J., Tsairis P.: Lumbar adhesive arachnoiditis: Etiologic and pathologic aspects. *Spine* 3:45, 1978.

Rice J.F., Shields C.B., Morris C.T., Neely B.D.: Spinal subarachnoid hemorrhage during myelography. *J. Neurosurg.* 48:645, 1978.

Roberson F.C., et al.: Myelopathy presenting as an intrinsic spinal cord tumor. *Surg. Neurol.* 9:317, 1978.

Scher A., Vambeck V.: An approach to the radiological examination of the cervico-dorsal junction following injury. *Clin. Radiol.* 28:243, 1977.

Schiller F., Neligan G., Budtz-Olsen O.: Surgery in hemophilia: A case of spinal subdural hematoma. *Lancet* 2:842, 1948.

Schneider R.C., Kahn E.A.: Chronic neurological sequelae of acute trauma to the spine and spinal cord: Problems pertaining to the treatment of retained foreign bodies. *J. Bone Joint Surg.* 41A:457, 1959.

Seibert C.E., Dresibach J.N., Swanson W.B., et al.: Progressive post-traumatic optic myelopathy: Neuroradiologic evaluation. *A.J.R.* 136:1161, 1981.

Ventureyra E.C.G., Ghanem W.M., Ivan L.P.: Spontaneous spinal epidural hematoma in a youngster. *Child's Brain* 5:103, 1979.

Vinters H.V., Barnett H.J.M., Kaufmann J.L.E.: Subdural hematoma of the spinal cord and widespread subarachnoid hemorrhage complicating anticoagulant therapy. *Stroke* 11:459, 1980.

Wagner F.L., Cherazi B.: Spinal cord injury: Indications for operative intervention. *Surg. Clin. North Am.* 60:1049, 1980.

Wagner F.L., Cherazi B.: Early decompression and neurological outcome in acute spinal cord injuries. *J. Neurosurg.* 56:699, 1982.

Webb B.J., Berzins E., Wingardner T.S., Lorenzi E.: Spinal cord injury: Epidemiologic implications, costs and patterns of care in 85 patients. *Arch. Phys. Med. Rehab.* 60:335, 1979.

Williams B.: The distending force in the production of communicating syringomyelia. *Lancet* 2:41, 1970.

Williams B., Turner E.: Communicating syringomyelia presenting immediately after trauma. *Acta Neurochirurg.* 24:97, 1971.

Wilson C., Jumer M.: Traumatic spinal-pleural fistula. *J.A.M.A.* 179, 1962.

Yashon D., Jane J.A., White R.J.: Prognosis and management of spinal cord and cauda equina bullet injuries in sixty-five civilians. *J. Neurosurg.* 32:163, 1970.

Zilkha A., Nicoletti J.M.: Acute spinal subdural hematoma. *J. Neurosurg.* 41:627, 1974.

14

Inflammatory Lesions

ARACHNOIDITIS

CHRONIC ARACHNOIDITIS may be caused by a variety of factors which can be grouped into six major categories: (1) agents injected into the subarachnoid space—therapeutic drugs, anesthetic agents, contrast media, (2) infection, (3) intrathecal hemorrhage, (4) trauma—iatrogenic and external, (5) space-occupying lesions, (6) idiopathic. Duke and Hashimoto reported a series of six members of a Japanese family who developed chronic adhesive spinal arachnoiditis. In these patients, the disease seemed to be a genetically determined (autosomal dominant) process producing marked fibrotic thickening of the arachnoid with secondary ischemic radiculomyopathy.

Lombardi and his co-workers were unable to pinpoint a specific etiology in over 50% of 41 patients with spinal arachnoiditis. It has long been my clinical impression that blood potentiates the minor irritative effects of Pantopaque. The experimental findings of Howland, Curry, and Butler support this opinion. This is apparently not true of metrizamide. Therefore, it is not advisable to perform elective Pantopaque myelography in the face of a bloody spinal tap. Clark questions a possible relationship between the development of postmyelographic arachnoiditis and disk surgery in the presence of a narrow spinal canal. Perhaps subarachnoid bleeding is enhanced in this setting, in light of the fact that atraumatic lumbar puncture is more difficult to achieve.

Because leptomeningeal adhesions often develop slowly, signs and symptoms of arachnoiditis may not manifest themselves for months or years after the original insult. The clinical picture is frequently obscure because of the protracted development of the disease process, the overlapping of cord and root signs, and the variability of localization. Although arachnoiditis has a predilection for the thoracic region, it may occur in any area. The patient usually complains of pain involving one or more roots, and paresthesias in an irregular distribution.

Quiles et al. reviewed the pathologic changes in chronic lumbar arachnoiditis. The initial acute response consists of a fibrinous exudate with minimal cellular infiltration and vascular response. As the process goes on, there is agglutination of the fibrin-covered nerve roots and meninges. Eventually fibrosis occurs, with involvement of the dura, leptomeninges, and nerve roots. In the lumbar region, the cauda equina may be matted together over several vertebral segments. The adhesions may produce multiple loculations of cerebrospinal fluid with intradural cyst formation, compression of the cord or cauda equina, and intramedullary cavitation of the cord. Wolfgang described the unique development of a neurotrophic shoulder joint secondary to adhesive arachnoiditis of the upper thoracic cord following saddle block anesthesia in childbirth.

Fisher's experimental studies in animals indicate that Pantopaque always produces some meningeal inflammatory reaction. The amount of residual Pantopaque seems to be less important with respect to clinical symptoms than individual sensitivity to the oil. This has been confirmed by Bergeron et al., who demonstrated that the histologic changes of arachnoiditis invariably produced by intrathecal Pantopaque in monkeys do not correlate well with the presence of clinical findings. This is also true of man, in whom clinically significant arachnoiditis due to Pantopaque is unusual, i.e., a fraction of 1%, according to Peterson.

Repeat myelography with metrizamide in a small group of patients who had undergone previous Conray and Dimer-X myelography revealed radiographic evidence of arachnoiditis in all, although neurologic findings were uncommon. It is too early to draw a final conclusion about metrizamide because the number of patients who have been restudied after previous metrizamide myelography is relatively small. In the latter group, it is interesting that patients who had not undergone laminectomy demonstrated no evidence of arachnoiditis on the repeat metrizamide myelogram.

Because the clinical pattern is often confusing, myelography is an important diagnostic aid. In these circumstances, metrizamide is the contrast medium of choice. Unfortunately, there is no single, clear-cut myelographic pattern characteristic of arachnoiditis (Figs 14–1 to 14–4). The myelographic appearance depends upon the

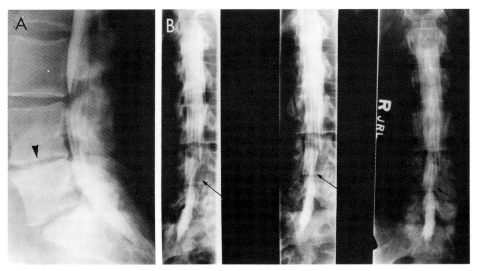

Fig 14–1.—Metrizamide myelogram in a 51-year-old female who had undergone a previous laminectomy at L4-5. Note the narrowing of the L4-5 disk space *(arrowhead)* on the lateral shoot-through film **(A)**. Note also at the same interspace the left-sided elongated defect that extends well above the disk space level *(arrow)* and the absence of focal nerve root swelling **(B)**.

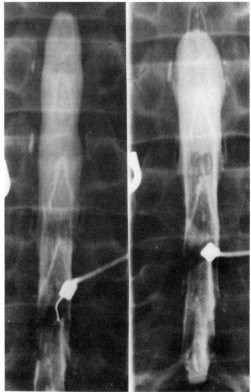

Fig 14–2.—Pantopaque myelogram in a 48-year-old man with diffuse matting together of the lumbar and sacral nerve roots due to arachnoiditis. The patient had undergone a cervical and lumbar Pantopaque myelogram one year previously. His current complaint was pain in the midback and both buttocks, but there were no objective neurologic findings.

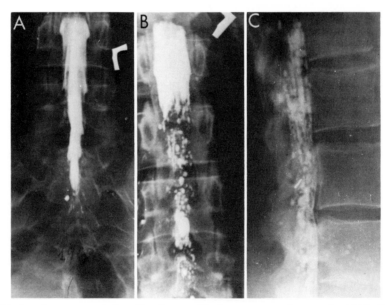

Fig 14–3.—**A,** representative film from a Pantopaque myelogram in 1962. **B** and **C,** upright frontal and lateral views of postlaminectomy myelogram 4 years later demonstrating a partial obstruction as well as irregular localized collections of oil due to arachnoiditis.

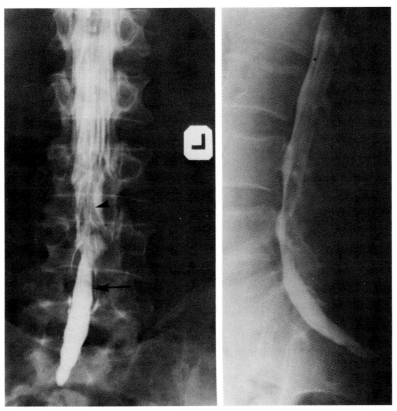

Fig 14–4.—Frontal and lateral radiographs of a metrizamide myelogram demonstrating arachnoiditis at L4-5 and L5-S1 in a patient who had a previous Pantopaque myelogram. Note the thickened, matted roots *(arrowhead)* and the constriction of the theca in the lower lumbar region *(arrow)* with absence of nerve root filling at the latter level.

nature and severity of the pathologic changes. The mildest radiographic findings include varying degrees of fusion of the nerve roots, blunting or absence of filling of one or more root sleeves, and small irregular defects on the lateral aspect of the contrast column. In patients with previous disk surgery, the deformity may extend above and below the disk space explored. More dorsal localization of the scar in patients with arachnoiditis helps to differentiate the deformity from recurrent disk herniation. Smith and Loeser described three patients with extensive lumbar and lumbosacral arachnoiditis after multiple fusions or diskectomies who exhibited a myelographic picture characterized by absence of root-sleeve filling. At operation, there was marked localized extradural scarring, with encasement of the involved nerve roots by thickened arachnoid. Because each root was densely adherent to the inner surface of the dura, the pattern was that of a Pantopaque-filled subarachnoid space devoid of nerve roots (Figs 14–5, 14–6).

Most patients with relatively severe arachnoiditis exhibit some obstruction (Figs 14–7 to 14–9). Conversely, patients with a high-grade or total obstruction due to tumor may also have arachnoiditis. In the latter patients, the arachnoiditis may possibly be related to the markedly elevated CSF protein levels. In Lombardi's

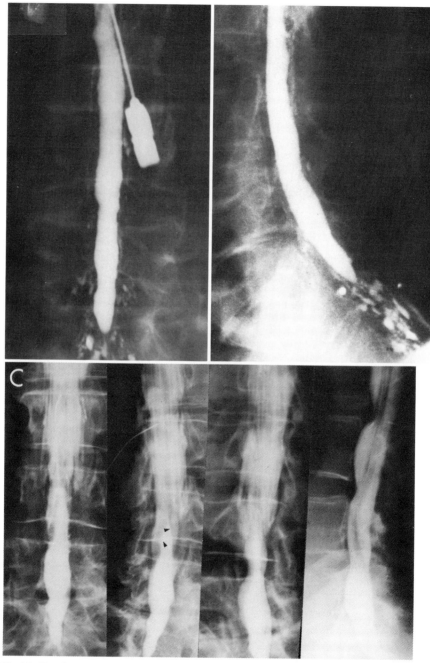

Fig 14–5.—Anteroposterior **(Top Left)** and lateral **(Top Right)** radiographs during myelography in a patient with severe arachnoiditis of the cauda equina. There is complete absence of filling of the axillary sleeves as well as irregular constriction of the oil column. The resected cauda (inset) clearly illustrates the spotty fixation of the oil. **C,** postoperative arachnoiditis shown on a metrizamide myelogram in a 60-year-old woman who had undergone a previous laminectomy. Note the denuded, irregular appearance of the margins of the thecal sac below the level of the upper third of the body of L-4. No nerve root sleeves are seen in this area. Note also the matted nerve roots *(arrowheads).*

study of arachnoiditis, approximately two thirds of the patients had a complete block. Many of the cases of severe arachnoiditis exhibit one or more of the following myelographic findings—localized clumping of the contrast medium, irregular streaks or droplets, angular defects, adhesive bands or webs. In a word, the myelographic picture in these patients is bizarre. If Pantopaque is used, one may see the oil column break up into a number of irregular, loculated, slowly moving droplets or streaks that may be separate or communicating. Occasionally, the multiple adhesions produce localized obliteration of the subarachnoid space, with a series of scalloped defects that can mimic an arteriovenous malformation of the cord (Figs 14–10, 14–11). Elkington likened the peripheral disposition of the arachnoidal adhesions to the guttering of a candle. At times, the contrast medium may pass with difficulty in a narrow, tortuous path that terminates in a cul-de-sac or reenters a normal subarachnoid segment. It is important to remember that the deformities of the contrast column are constant and reproducible. Because of its decreased viscosity and lesser tendency to irritate the arachnoid, metrizamide is vastly preferable to Pantopaque if arachnoiditis is suspected.

At times, differentiation between arachnoiditis and tumor may present a problem, particularly in the presence of a complete obstruction. The oval or circular defect in these patients differs from extramedullary, intradural tumor because it is less well defined, the ipsilateral subarachnoid space is not expanded, and the spinal cord is not displaced. The "paint-brush" effect seen in other cases of arachnoiditis with complete obstruction may mimic that produced by extradural tumor. The important differential criterion is absence of displacement of the cord in arachnoiditis (Fig 14–12). This finding holds up when the loculated CSF cyst is small. If, however, the cyst is large enough and under tension, the spinal cord may be displaced or invaginated. In the latter instance, differentiation from tumor can only be made if the cyst fills spontaneously with contrast medium or if the cyst is injected. Leptomeningeal infiltration by systemic carcinoma or lymphoma, producing longitudinal striations and irregularity of the contrast column, may be difficult to differentiate from arachnoiditis.

A number of cases of intramedullary cavities, i.e., syringomyelia, have been reported in association with chronic adhesive arachnoiditis. Presumably the arachnoiditis produces focal obliteration of the vascular supply to the cord with secondary necrosis and cavitation. These cavities are not lined by ependyma. The diagnosis of syringomyelia should be seriously considered in patients with arachnoiditis who exhibit evidence of an intramedullary mass. This diagnosis should also be entertained when there is obstruction or severe distortion in patients with clinical findings at a higher level than the site of the obstruction. Under these circumstances, the obstruction prevents visualization of a concomitant enlarged cord. In patients like this, an attempt should be made to visualize the cord from above, following a C1-2 puncture.

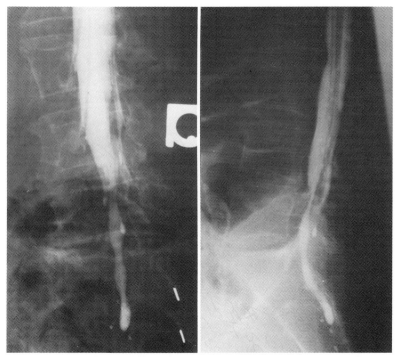

Fig 14–6.—Anteroposterior and lateral films of a metrizamide myelogram in a 76-year-old woman with extensive postoperative arachnoiditis below the level of the L4-5 interspace. Note the marked circumferential constriction of the theca below this level. The patient had a previous Pantopaque myelogram and laminectomy for disk herniation 2 years before the present study.

HYPERTROPHIC PACHYMENINGITIS

This entity, first described by Charcot in 1869, is characterized clinically by radicular pain in the neck and arms, with subsequent weakness and atrophy, spastic paralysis of the legs, and loss of sphincter control. Pathologically, there is compression of the nerve roots and cord by marked nonspecific, inflammatory hypertrophy of the dura mater. The inflammatory process of unknown etiology may spread to the leptomeninges and produce softening of the cord due to compression. The lesion has been found in all segments of the spinal cord.

Guidetti and LaTorre described myelographic findings in five patients, all of whom exhibited a partial or complete block. The lateral projection is helpful in diagnosis. In each instance, the spinal cord was displaced ventrally by the posterior inflammatory mass, producing a "beak-shaped" filling defect, with the apex at the anterior subarachnoid space (Fig 14–13). Wirth and Gado also described a case in the cervical region in which the thickened dura produced a symmetric increased distance bilaterally between the pedicles and the lateral margins of the contrast column in the frontal projection. I would think this would be difficult to differentiate from sheet-like infiltration of the dura by tumor. I have seen only a single case of hypertrophic pachymeningitis in the thoracic region—in a middle-aged man with extensive Paget's disease.

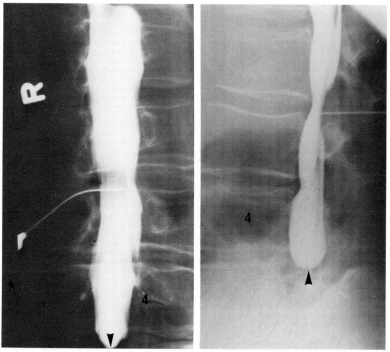

Fig 14–7.—Postoperative arachnoiditis in a 76-year-old woman who had a previous Pantopaque myelogram and a laminectomy at L4-5 2 years previously for a herniated disk. The present study was carried out because of persistent pain and weakness in the right leg. Note the total circumferential obstruction in the upright position at L4-5 *(arrowhead)* without evidence of a mass effect or displacement of the theca.

MYELITIS

Occasionally, myelitis may be associated with severe edema sufficient to produce a complete obstruction. Under these circumstances, it may not be possible to differentiate clinically among myelitis, extradural abscess, or cord tumor. Myelography merely demonstrates a complete block and suggests evidence of cord enlargement indistinguishable from that seen with intramedullary tumors (Fig 14–14).

RADIATION MYELITIS

Radiation myelopathy is a rare sequel of irradiation of a lesion within, or close to, the spinal cord. The radiation is usually given to treat a tumor of the pharynx, neck, upper esophagus, mediastinum, or lungs. Symptoms of radiation myelitis tend to develop slowly. Although the time interval from the completion of radiation therapy to the onset of symptoms may rarely be a few months, the average is well over 2 years. The early symptoms, which can appear acutely or gradually, consist of paresthesias in one or both upper or lower extremities and, less commonly, pain. The typical patient develops weakness and, sometimes, spasticity in one or both lower extremities along with subjective sensory alteration, which is ultimately as-

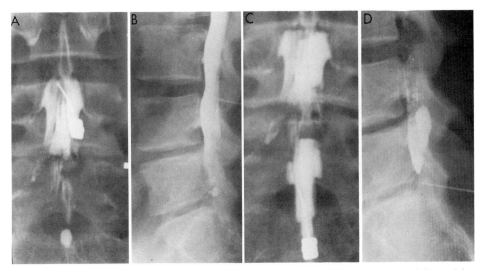

Fig 14–8.—The patient was a 30-year-old male who had a myelogram followed by removal of a herniated disk fragment at L4-5 on the left 8 years previously. Because of recurrent back pain with radiation down the left leg, he had another myelogram (lumbar puncture at L3-4). Frontal and lateral cross-table erect films from the latter study (**A** and **B**) demonstrate a high-grade obstruction at L4-5. A second puncture was performed at L5-S1, using 2 ml of Pantopaque to define the inferior margin of the defect (**C** and **D**). The irregular character of the defect with complete obstruction in a postlaminectomy patient is highly suggestive of arachnoiditis.

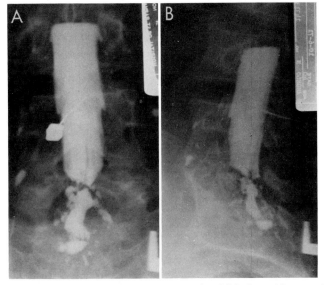

Fig 14–9.—Partial obstruction at L-5 due to arachnoiditis in a 40-year-old female who had had two previous myelograms a year before (one was unsuccessful because of an extra-arachnoid injection). Upright prone (**A**) and oblique (**B**) films from the present study demonstrate the ragged, irregular collection of oil at L-5 and S-1.

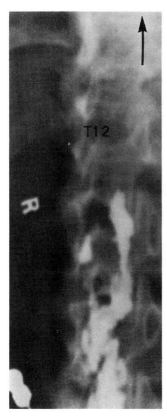

Fig 14–10.—Pantopaque myelogram in a patient with arachnoiditis, demonstrating irregular pocketing of the oil due to localized obliteration of the subarachnoid space. Note the resemblance to a vascular malformation. (Reprinted, with permission, from Sheinmel A., Glasser S.M., *Am. J. Roentgenol.* 67:415, 1952.)

sociated with a sensory level. There is also evidence of sensory and motor involvement of the long tracts and, in some cases, of the posterior columns as well. A partial Brown-Séquard syndrome is a common finding, with motor weakness and pyramidal tract signs in one lower extremity and alteration of pain and temperature in the opposite extremity. In many cases, the patient becomes paraplegic or quadriplegic and has bowel and bladder incontinence. Radiation myelitis should be suspected when motor and sensory signs occur in the segment of irradiated cord in a patient with normal CSF (except for a possible increase in protein) and no evidence of generalized metastases. According to Boden, relatively long lengths of cervical spinal cord should not receive more than 3,500 rad in 17 days.

Worthington and others have reported myelographic evidence of diffuse enlargement of the spinal cord in patients with radiation myelitis. The enlargement is nonspecific and cannot be differentiated from the enlargement produced by an intramedullary tumor. There may or may not be an associated complete block. The correct diagnosis can be established if the myelographic findings are present in a patient who received a cancericidal dose of radiation to the cervical or thoracic cord. The cord swelling, which invariably occurs after sharp clinical deterioration, is limited to the radiation field and adjacent segments. Histologic study demonstrates edema of the irradiated segment of cord, necrosis of gray matter, demyelination of white matter, and severe vascular damage. There are also changes above and below the margins of the irradiated segment due to edema fluid that passes

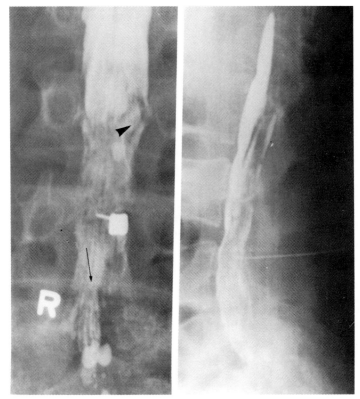

Fig 14–11.—Pantopaque myelogram in a 53-year-old man with extensive arachnoiditis after two previous myelograms and laminectomies. The entering complaint was low back pain radiating into the left lower extremity. Note the dilated vessels *(arrowhead),* which may superficially suggest a vascular malformation. The matted nerve roots *(arrow)* and the clinical history indicate the correct diagnosis of arachnoiditis.

through the injured vessel walls in the field of irradiation and diffuses throughout the white matter.

Mikhael reported a unique case of radiation necrosis of a cervical root which presented both an intradural and an extradural mass at myelography. The patient also had a focal, well-defined area of destruction of the left lateral mass of C-2 and C-3 due to radiation necrosis.

INTRAMEDULLARY ABSCESS AND GRANULOMA

Rarely, an intramedullary abscess (Fig 14–15) or chronic granuloma (Fig 14–16) may produce a myelographic picture indistinguishable from that of an intramedullary neoplasm. There may or may not be a complete obstruction present.

Subdural Granuloma

Reddy et al. reported a unique case of a radiopaque granuloma in the spinal subdural space, with a myelographic block at T-6. The granuloma followed the use

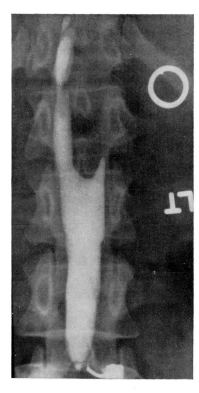

Fig 14–12.—Smooth filling defect at L1-2 due to arachnoiditis, obliterating the subarachnoid space on the left side. The absence of displacement of the cauda by the apparent mass should serve to differentiate arachnoiditis from tumor. (Reprinted, with permission, from Seaman W.B., et al., *J. Neurosurg.* 10:145, 1953.)

of sterile micropulverized BaSO₄ to outline a cerebellar abscess complicated by a subdural empyema. At operation, the granulation tissue in the subdural space extended from C-1 to T-8, particularly posteriorly on the left side.

Subdural Abscess

Patronas et al. reported a rare case of subdural abscess in the spinal canal. At myelography, performed through a C1-2 puncture, there was a complete block at T-8 with a defect on the dorsal aspect of the Pantopaque column. The interface of the block showed a gradual transitional zone with irregularities of the oil column due to thick pus projecting into it. A laminectomy from T-6 to L-5 demonstrated a subdural abscess extending the length of the laminectomy. In the 12 cases of subdural abscess reported in the literature, there was an antecedent distant focus of infection in 10 patients. The subdural space can become infected by (1) direct extension, (2) spinal puncture, or, more commonly, (3) hematogenous spread from a distant focus. *Staphylococcus aureus* was the offending organism in seven cases, *Streptococcus hemolyticus* in two cases, and *Pneumococcus* in one case. Unlike extradural abscess, spinal subdural abscess is not associated with vertebral osteomyelitis.

Extradural Abscess

Inflammatory lesions of the spinal extradural space arise either by direct extension from a contiguous infected area or as a blood-borne metastatic focus from a

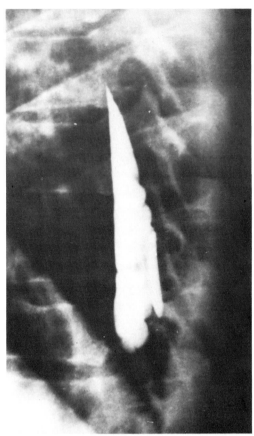

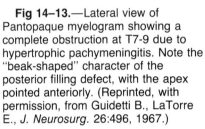

Fig 14–13.—Lateral view of Pantopaque myelogram showing a complete obstruction at T7-9 due to hypertrophic pachymeningitis. Note the "beak-shaped" character of the posterior filling defect, with the apex pointed anteriorly. (Reprinted, with permission, from Guidetti B., LaTorre E., *J. Neurosurg.* 26:496, 1967.)

primary infection elsewhere in the body (frequently staphylococcic) (Figs 14–17 to 14–21). In many instances, however, no definite source for the extradural infection is found. Some investigators believe that such cases are secondary to an occult focus of osteomyelitis in the bony spine. It is important to remember that infection in the urinary tract is a common source for metastatic osteomyelitis of the vertebral column. Vertebral osteomyelitis and diskitis have also been reported in heroin addicts.

The lesion may present as a diffuse suppurative process of the entire extradural space or as a localized abscess. Extradural infections in the cervical and thoracic regions usually occur on the dorsal aspect of the spinal cord below the level of the fourth thoracic vertebra. This is due to the fact that there is only a potential extradural space anteriorly and a relatively wide space posteriorly containing fat and many veins. The extradural space is potential in the cervical region and widest in the thoracolumbar area.

The clinical picture is one of fulminating cord compression. Routine spine radiographs may or may not demonstrate a focus of vertebral osteomyelitis. Myelography usually discloses either a complete block or an extradural defect. When the clinical findings suggest involvement at multiple cord segments, it may be advisable to introduce the contrast medium by lateral C1-2 puncture as well as via the lumbar route to outline the full extent of the disease.

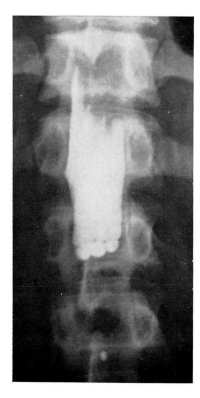

Fig 14–14.—Myelitis with pronounced edema of the conus medullaris, resulting in a complete block at T-11 and T-12. (Reprinted, with permission, from Sheinmel A., Glasser S.M., *Am. J. Roentgenol.* 67:415, 1952.)

Chronic Nonspecific Extradural Granuloma

The syndrome of chronic nonspecific spinal extradural granuloma is essentially that of back and nerve root pain followed by symptoms of compression of the spinal cord or cauda equina. There are a number of striking differences between the clinical manifestations of acute extradural infection and those of the chronic inflammatory mass. The former is usually accompanied by a definite history of an antecedent infection (e.g., furuncle, tonsillitis, or osteomyelitis) 2–3 weeks prior to the abrupt onset of severe, relentless back pain, with or without radicular extension. This is frequently followed, within approximately 1 week, by the appearance and rapid progression of motor and sensory deficits and sphincter disturbance often culminating in signs of a transverse spinal lesion. The clinical picture is one of acute fulminating sepsis. In contrast, a history of infection is not usually elicited from the patient with a chronic extradural granuloma. The pain is more insidious in onset and may be attributed to a specific episode of trauma. Localized tenderness over the spine may be present or absent. The onset of pain may precede the neurologic findings by a variable but significantly prolonged interval and be disproportionately severe, compared with the paucity of motor or sensory changes.

Although there is little difficulty in distinguishing the acute from the chronic spinal extradural inflammatory process, it may not be possible on clinical grounds alone to differentiate chronic extradural granuloma from neoplasm or intervertebral disk herniation. Examination of the cerebrospinal fluid is, in many instances, of little help, since all three lesions may produce spinal block with CSF protein elevation or xanthochromia.

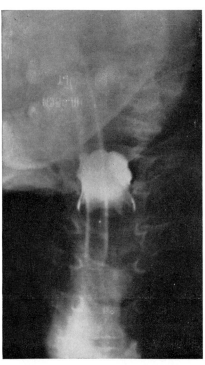

Fig 14–15.—Cisternal Pantopaque myelogram in a 4½-year-old boy demonstrating widening of the cord and a complete block at the lower border of T-1 owing to an abscess within the cord itself. (Reprinted, with permission, from Dutton J.E.M., Alexander G.J., *J. Neurol., Neurosurg. Psychiatr.* 17:303, 1954.)

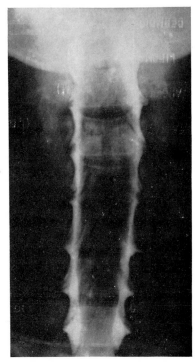

Fig 14–16.—Intramedullary granuloma in a 37-year-old man, with myelographic findings indistinguishable from those of intramedullary neoplasm.

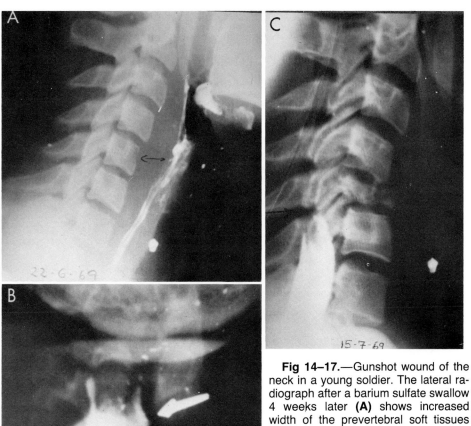

Fig 14–17.—Gunshot wound of the neck in a young soldier. The lateral radiograph after a barium sulfate swallow 4 weeks later **(A)** shows increased width of the prevertebral soft tissues anterior to C-5 and destruction of the anterior margin of this vertebra. Note the metallic foreign body fragments in the neck. Myelography 3 weeks later, following the development of neurologic signs, shows progressive destruction of C-5, with a pathologic compression fracture. There is a complete block at C5-6, with displacement of the spinal cord posteriorly and to the right by an extradural abscess on the left anterior aspect of the cord **(B** and **C)**. (Courtesy of A. Bartal.)

The granuloma can originate either as a direct extension from a contiguous vertebral infection or as a hematogenous metastasis from a remote focus. Although early reports in the literature mention the possibility of a primary extradural space infection, this seems unlikely. The failure to detect a primary source of infection elsewhere in the body does not exclude the presence of occult focal vertebral osteomyelitis. The extensive venous anastomoses within the extradural space demonstrated by Batson may explain the route of infection in some cases. Ordinarily, no specific organism can be cultured from either the bloodstream or the extradural space and tissue. Occasionally, however, staphylococcus, brucella, pneumococcus, and other organisms have been recovered.

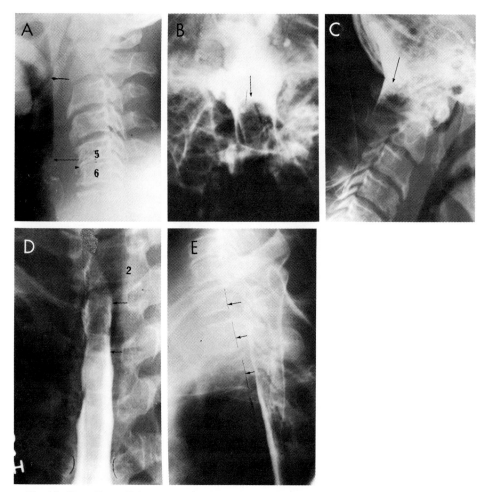

Fig 14–18.—C5-6 disk space infection with extension into the prevertebral soft tissues and formation of an extensive ventral granuloma from C-2 to T-4. The patient was a 50-year-old male who had a 2-week history of meningitis-like symptoms and a gram-positive septicemia. He suddenly developed loss of strength in both upper extremities without a definite sensory level. A C1-2 puncture failed. Cisternal puncture was successfully performed and showed a complete obstruction at C1-2. An L2-3 puncture was then performed to outline the lower level of the obstruction. **A,** lateral cervical spine, showing narrowing of the C5-6 space *(arrowhead)* and widening of the prevertebral soft tissues at C-5 *(arrow)* compared with the normal width at C-2 *(arrow)*. **B,** frontal, and, **C,** lateral myelographic films after cisternal puncture indicating a complete block *(arrow)*. **D,** frontal myelographic films following L5-S1 puncture, showing a block at T-2 with displacement of the contrast column away from the left pedicles *(arrow)*. **E,** lateral shoot-through radiograph made at the same time showing a ventral epidural mass. At operation, a dense thick mass of epidural granulation tissue was found ventrally extending from C-2 to T-4.

At operation, the lesion presents as a firm, well-localized, extradural mass variably adherent to the adjacent dura. The most common location is the posterior thoracic or lumbar region, although it may extend laterally or, less frequently, anteriorly. It may not be possible to differentiate granuloma from benign or malignant neoplasm grossly at surgery, and frozen section may be extremely helpful. Micro-

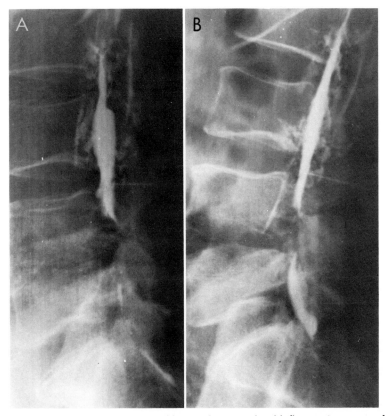

Fig 14–19.—Osteomyelitis at L4-5 with anterior extradural inflammatory mass following diskectomy in a 67-year-old man. Note the destructive changes at the L4-5 interspace and the apparent complete obstruction and posterior displacement of the theca from the body of L-4 **(A)**. The patient was placed in the upright position for 15 minutes and a repeat film made **(B)**. Some of the oil has passed caudally, demonstrating the entire extent of the lesion.

scopically, the picture is that of a nonspecific chronic inflammatory process in which a dense fibrous stroma is infiltrated by lymphocytes, plasma cells, and polymorphonuclear leukocytes.

Dandy's dissections in cadavers readily explain the anatomical basis for preferential localization of extradural infections in the posterior thoracic and lumbar areas. Dandy points out that the spinal extradural space containing fat, loose areolar tissue, and veins is present as an actual space posterior only to the spinal nerve attachments. Anteriorly, except the lumbosacral area, the extradural space is a potential one throughout the spinal axis, with the dura in close apposition to the posterior longitudinal ligament and the vertebral body. In the cervical region, the spinal extradural space begins posteriorly at the level of C-7 and gradually increases to a depth of 0.5–0.75 cm in the midthoracic region (T4-8). Below this level, it tapers somewhat to the level of T11-L2 and ultimately attains its greatest depth at L3-S2.

Since establishment of the diagnosis of chronic extradural granuloma on clinical grounds is, at best, difficult or impossible, the radiologic findings assume particular importance. The preliminary study should consist of conventional radiography of

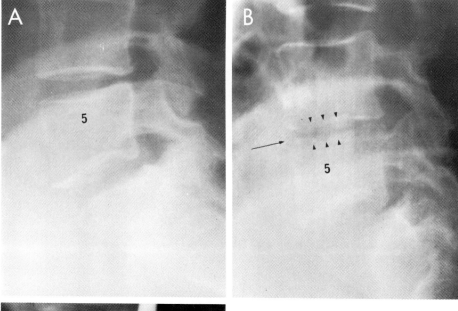

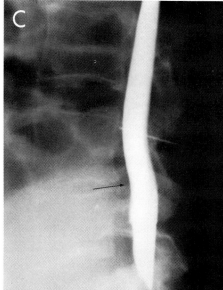

Fig 14–20.—Epidural abscess secondary to osteomyelitis at L4-5 in a 50-year-old man. **A,** lateral radiograph on October 30, 1975, showing a normal L4-5 disk space. **B,** repeat film 19 days later (November 18), showing loss of sharpness of opposing cortical margins of L-4 and L-5 (arrowheads), narrowing of the interspace, and early destruction of the anterosuperior aspect of L-5 (arrow). The lateral shoot-through film **(C)** shows definite posterior displacement of the theca with an anterior concavity of the oil column (arrow) indicative of a ventral epidural mass. At operation, pus was drained from this site.

the spine supplemented by tomography. These films may either be entirely negative or demonstrate one or more of the following changes: (1) narrowing of the intervertebral disk space; (2) changes in vertebral body or bodies contiguous to the intervertebral disk space (early, this may consist of loss of sharpness of outline of the bone immediately adjacent to the articular plate. As the lesion progresses, there may be actual bone destruction and eventual wedging and collapse of the involved vertebra). Similar changes may involve the bony neural arch or the vertebral end of the rib; (3) there also may be localized paravertebral soft tissue mass (Fig 14–22).

The plain roentgenograms should be succeeded by myelography. It is important

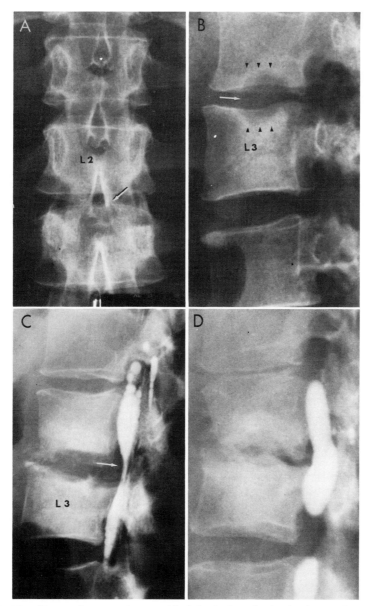

Fig 14–21.—The patient, a 50-year-old diabetic female, had a large abscess on the back of her neck from which *Staphylococcus aureus* was cultured in October 1962. Early in April 1963, she complained of lumbar pain of several weeks' duration. On April 13, 1963, a diagnosis of osteomyelitis at L2-3 was made *(arrow)*, **A** and **B.** Note the narrowing of the involved intervertebral disk space and the subchondral destruction on either side of the joint *(arrowheads)*. At this time, the L2-3 interspace was curetted and approximately 500 ml of pus (positive for *S. aureus*) aspirated from the left psoas region. Although the patient received antibiotic therapy for 3 months, the lesion progressed. **C,** on October 9, 1963, myelography revealed a partial block, an elongated defect on the anterior aspect of the oil column at L2-3 *(arrow)* and further narrowing of the disk space, destruction, and sclerosis. Operation at that time disclosed an extradural abscess, which was drained. Further curettage and anterior fusion of the involved vertebral bodies were carried out. **D,** a repeat study on September 1, 1964 showed reparative changes in the vertebrae with no evidence of extradural abscess. The defect on the anterior aspect of the Pantopaque column at L2-3 is probably due to chronic granulation tissue plus spurring from the posterior margins of the vertebral bodies.

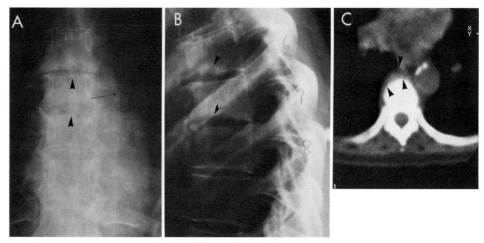

Fig 14–22.—A and **B,** extradural granuloma and abscess in a 70-year-old male secondary to disk space infection at T6-7 and T7-8 *(arrowheads).* Note the localized paraspinal mass *(arrow).* CT **(C)** confirms the presence of the paraspinal soft tissue mass *(arrowheads).*

that the lumbar puncture not be made in an area of demonstrable bone involvement. Myelography reveals a prominent extradural defect with or without incomplete or complete block (Fig 14–23). The lateral decubitus film with a horizontal beam is important in demonstrating the anterior or posterior localization of the lesion. Early in the course of the disease, there may be only unilateral impingement on the contrast column extending over one or more vertebral segments. This may progress to a more prominent defect with partial obstruction. Large granulomas may compress the theca and produce complete obstruction, with tapering of the head of the column of contrast medium. Hassin has demonstrated that the extradural inflammatory process may also extend into the subarachnoid space and produce an intense arachnoiditis. Both of these abnormalities may contribute to the partial block at myelography. The myelographic findings per se are not sufficiently specific to be diagnostic. However, the presence of a prominent myelographic defect, particularly if it extends over one or more vertebral bodies, in association with erosion of the articular margins of one or more vertebrae and narrowing of the intervertebral disk space, should suggest the diagnosis of chronic extradural granuloma.

Chronic Tuberculous Extradural Granuloma

A tuberculous extradural granuloma cannot be distinguished from its nonspecific counterpart at myelography. However, plain radiographs of the spine may be helpful in differential diagnosis. Tuberculosis usually produces less bone reaction on either side of the involved intervertebral disk space. An associated paraspinal soft tissue mass is more common in tuberculosis, whereas pyogenic infections tend to progress more rapidly and respond more promptly to appropriate antibiotic therapy (Fig 14–24). Tuberculous spondylitis must be differentiated from a low-grade, nonspecific, self-limited inflammation of the intervertebral disk in children, termed

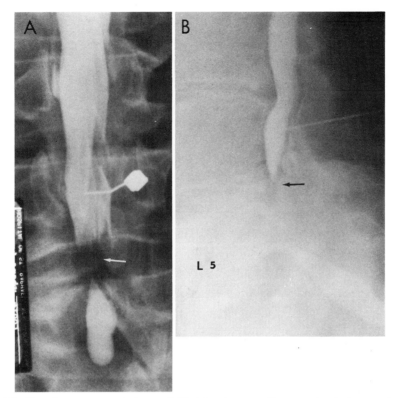

Fig 14–23.—A, anteroposterior and, **B,** lateral prone films made during myelography in a 55-year-old man complaining of low back pain of 2 years' duration. Note the prominent extradural defect at L4-5 *(arrow).* At laminectomy, an extradural granuloma was found.

spondylarthritis by Saenger. Although the radiologic findings in the two entities may be similar, the negative tuberculin reaction and the spontaneous regression with no specific therapy eventually rule out tuberculosis (Fig 14–25).

Bell has described a series of 10 patients with tuberculosis of the vertebral pedicles in the thoracolumbar region without involvement of the intervertebral disks. As the lesion progresses, it may involve the adjacent transverse process and medial end of the rib. It may also involve the posterior portion of the vertebral body. A characteristic feature of this type of spinal tuberculosis is the presence of a large paraspinal abscess. Four of the patients presented with paraplegia. Myelography was carried out in only one patient because the level of the bone lesion usually was obvious by conventional roentgenography. The films in this case demonstrated a left-sided extradural lesion at T-12. At operation, an extradural granuloma was found, which proved to be tuberculosis by histologic examination.

SCHISTOSOMIASIS

Schistosomes are bisexual trematodes of the family Bilharziadae whose primary host is man; snails serve as the intermediate host. Schistosomiasis of the spinal cord is a rare lesion, indeed. According to Herskowitz, there are only 30 reported cases

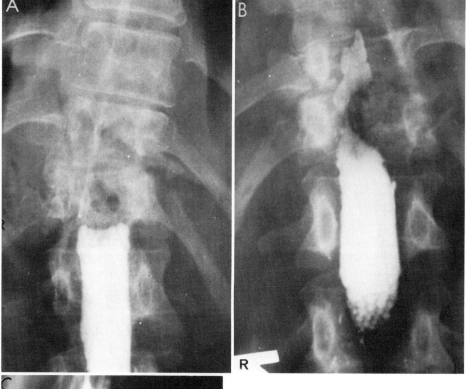

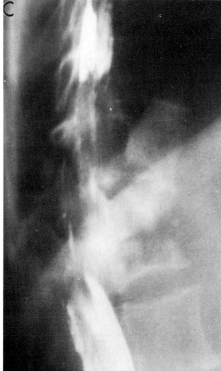

Fig 14–24.—Frontal film **(A)** during myelography in a patient with Pott's disease with a complete block at T12-L1. Note the prominent paraspinal mass and the destructive changes at T11-12. The Pantopaque was left in place. Re-examination 1 month later **(B** and **C)** demonstrates some oil above the lesion, with displacement of the Pantopaque posteriorly and to the right by the tuberculous extradural mass.

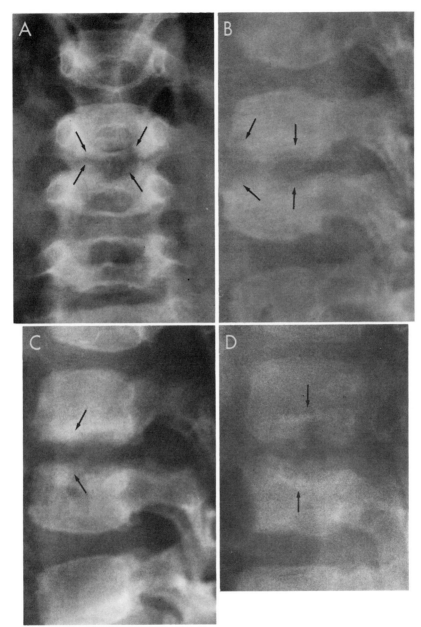

Fig 14–25.—The patient, a 2-year-old girl, complained of backache and limp. The PPD was negative. Skin tests for fungi, agglutinins for undulant fever, and various enteric pathogens, as well as blood cultures were also negative. The sedimentation rate was elevated, and the patient's temperature spiked up to 105 F. Roentgenograms, **A** and **B,** of the lumbar spine on February 13, 1958, showed narrowing of the disk space at L3-4, with subchondral erosive changes anteriorly involving L-3 and L-4 *(arrows).* **C,** repeat examination on September 22, 1958, showed some healing, which is still more pronounced on the final film, **D,** made on May 16, 1961. The last film demonstrates residual narrowing of the involved disk space. This is a typical example of so-called spondylarthritis.

in the world's literature. The most common sites of involvement are the lower thoracic or lumbar cord and the cauda equina. This anatomical predilection may be due to the rich anastomoses between the pelvic veins and the vertebral venous plexus and between the hemorrhoidal and systemic veins. Thus, parasites in the bladder or bowel can readily find their way into the vertebral venous plexus. Schistosomiasis may produce radiculitis, acute hemorrhagic necrotic myelitis and leptomeningitis, chronic granuloma of the spinal cord, or cauda equina. According to Hutton and Holland, and Maciel et al., myelitis is the most common manifestation of this disease when it involves the spinal axis. The responsible organisms are S. *mansoni* and S. *hematobium*; S. *japonicum* rarely involves the spinal cord.

The myelographic findings depend on the pathologic lesion and the degree of involvement and are indistinguishable from similar inflammatory lesions produced by other organisms.

CYSTICERCOSIS

Cysticercosis is acquired by eating inadequately cooked pork containing ova of the pig tapeworm, *Taenia solium*. The emerging embryos penetrate the human intestinal wall and become widely disseminated throughout the body. Ultimately they die, become encysted, and often calcified. Cysticercosis of the central nervous system is usually confined to the brain and its meninges; intraspinal cysticercosis is extremely rare. Bärtschi-Rochaix and Cuadra reported a case of extensive arachnoiditis in the upper thoracic region demonstrated at myelography and confirmed by operation.

ECHINOCOCCOSIS

Man acquires hydatid disease by the inadvertent ingestion of echinococcus ova in the feces of carnivores harboring the worm. The ingested ova hatch in the human gut; the larvae migrate through the mucosa into the bloodstream and are disseminated throughout the body. Hydatid disease is most common in the liver (75%) and lungs (15%), but cysts also occur in many other organs. According to Rayport et al., the skeleton is involved in 0.3%–3% of human echinococcosis and the spine in one third to one half of the latter group of patients.

Primary intramedullary, intradural and extradural cysts are extremely rare. Spinal echinococcosis usually is a compressive extradural inflammatory process secondary to hydatid disease of the vertebrae (Fig 14–26). The disease is most common in the thoracic region (50% of cases) and less frequent in the lumbar (20%), sacral (20%), and cervical (10%) areas. According to Dévé, 84% of patients with vertebral echinococcosis develop a myelopathy due to extradural compression.

Plain films of the spine demonstrate bubble-like radiolucencies in a vertebral body or its appendages that may show peripheral sclerosis with the passage of time. Often there is similar involvement of the head and neck of the contiguous rib. Initially, the intervertebral disk is spared, but later it may also become involved and show narrowing. A paravertebral soft tissue mass is present in patients with neurologic findings. Myelography is nonspecific and merely demonstrates extradural displacement of the spinal cord or cauda equina, with varying degrees of obstruction.

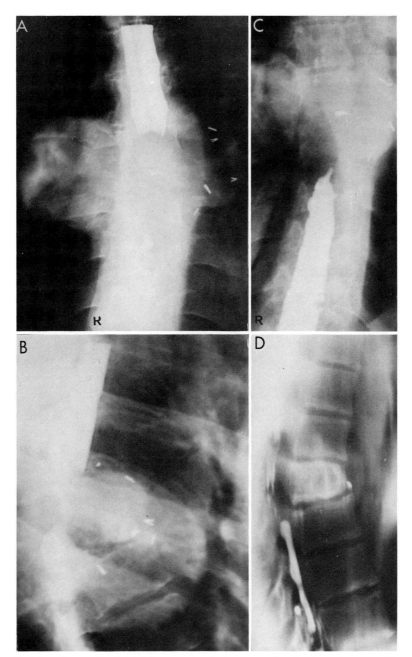

Fig 14–26.—The patient had been operated on previously for a large echinococcal granuloma in the lower midthoracic spine. Pantopaque introduced via cisternal puncture demonstrates complete extradural obstruction at T-7 **(A** and **B)**. Additional oil was introduced via lumbar puncture to outline the inferior extent of the lesion **(C** and **D)**. Note the sclerosis and cystic changes at T-7 as well as involvement of the T-7 and T-8 disk space. (Courtesy of S. Schorr.)

CRYPTOCOCCOSIS (TORULOSIS)

Cryptococcus neoformans is a small, yeastlike spherule that reproduces by budding and has no mycelia. It is widespread in nature and, at times, produces infection in man by inhalation of the spherules. The organism is disseminated from the lungs via the bloodstream to all organs, including the central nervous system, which appears to be particularly susceptible. There are several types of reaction in the spinal region: (1) a granulomatous leptomeningitis diffusely involving the subarachnoid space of the cord or cauda equina, (2) a granulomatous extradural mass that may be necrotic, (3) an intramedullary granuloma of the spinal cord, (4) acute myelitis. Needless to say, the myelographic findings are not specific; the correct diagnosis can be made only by identifying the organism.

BLASTOMYCOSIS

North American blastomycosis is caused by *Blastomyces dermatitidis* and the South American variety by *Blastomyces brasiliensis*. *Blastomyces dermatitidis* is a double-walled, single, budding yeast cell that grows as a yeast at body temperature and in the mycelial form at room temperature. Because the organism occurs in the soil, the disease is generally acquired by farmers as a chronic granulomatous infection of the skin and subcutaneous tissues. Less often, the lungs are involved, and rarely there is systemic dissemination via the bloodstream to other viscera, including the skeleton and the central nervous system. Under these circumstances, the spinal cord may be involved in a generalized leptomeningitis. More commonly, there is an extradural abscess secondary to vertebral osteomyelitis.

COCCIDIOIDOMYCOSIS

The causative organism, *Coccidioides immitis,* is a filamentous fungus commonly found in the soil of the arid southwestern United States. The organism is usually inhaled and produces a mild, self-limited, febrile disease. Rarely, it may take the form of a progressive infection, with visceral and skeletal lesions. The literature contains many reports of involvement of the brain and spinal cord in a granulomatous leptomeningitis, in some cases associated with parenchymal granulomas. There also may be a compressive myelopathy due to an extradural granuloma secondary to vertebral osteomyelitis. The destruction of the vertebral body and disk associated with a paraspinal soft tissue mass makes differential diagnosis difficult on the basis of the roentgenographic findings alone.

ASPERGILLOSIS

Involvement of the spinal cord by aspergillosis occurs almost exclusively as a terminal manifestation of an opportunistic infection in an immunocompromised host. Kingsley et al. reported a case of intradural extramedullary aspergillosis complicating chronic lymphatic leukemia. At myelography, there was irregularity of the theca anteriorly between T-7 and T-9, with a number of separate intradural extramedullary defects at that level. At operation, in addition to the intradural lesion at T-7, there were also three focal deposits on nerve roots somewhat more proximally.

ACTINOMYCOSIS

This infection is caused by a fungus of the actinomyces group, most often *Actinomyces bovis*. The mouth is the common portal of entry, and the lesion usually presents as a chronic, discharging osteomyelitis of the mandible. When the infection spreads to other organs via the bloodstream, it may produce vertebral osteo-

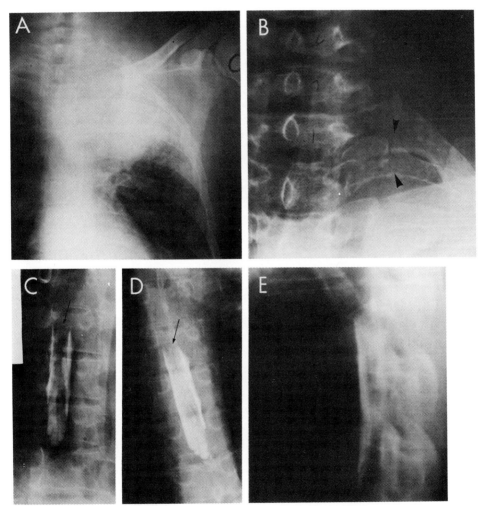

Fig 14–27.—Actinomycosis of the left lung and chest wall in a 45-year-old man which spread by contiguity into the paraspinal region. **A,** PA chest film demonstrating extensive density in region of left upper lobe. **B,** overpenetrated film showing destruction of the left second and third ribs *(arrowheads)*. **C,** oblique and, **D,** frontal films from a Pantopaque myelogram showing an obstruction at T-7 and displacement of the oil column away from the left pedicle *(arrowhead)*. **E,** lateral myelographic film demonstrating a complete extradural obstruction on the body of T-7 *(arrow)*. Involvement of the chest wall should always raise the question of actinomycosis.

myelitis with a paraspinal inflammatory mass. It may also spread by contiguity to the paraspinal region from the chest wall (Fig 14–27). The extradural abscess or granuloma may compress the spinal cord. Again, the findings are nonspecific; the correct diagnosis can be made only by isolating the organism.

IDIOPATHIC RETROPERITONEAL FIBROSIS

Warkentin reported a case of idiopathic retroperitoneal fibrosis in a 59-year-old female with unusual extension to the right thoracolumbar extradural space. Panto-

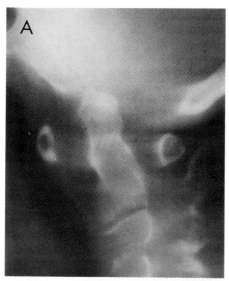

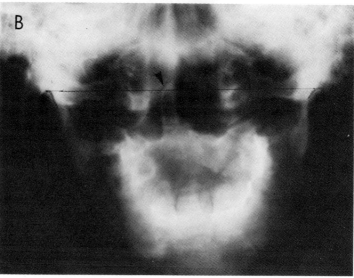

Fig 14–28.—Dislocation of the dens in a 55-year-old female with rheumatoid arthritis. The lateral tomogram **(A)** clearly demonstrates the posterior displacement of the dens, while the AP film **(B)** shows craniad displacement of the dens above the digastric line *(arrowhead)*. The patient had minimal neurologic findings.

paque myelography showed a complete extradural block at T12-L1, with displacement of the oil column to the left by an extradural mass. The cross-table lateral film demonstrated posterior encroachment on the Pantopaque column. Laminectomy revealed an extradural inflammatory mass compressing the cord from the level of T-10 to the lower border of L-1. The inflammatory tissue, which encased the right T-12 nerve root, extended into the intervertebral foramen and retroperitoneal space. Histologically, the mature hyalinized fibrous tissue with round cell infiltrate was identical to specimens removed during two previous ureterolyses.

Retroperitoneal fibrosis also occurs in association with various lymphomas.

ANKYLOSING SPONDYLITIS

In 1961, Bowie and Glasgow described three cases of chronic ankylosing spondylitis with axial and vesical sphincter disturbance, sensory loss in the sacral der-

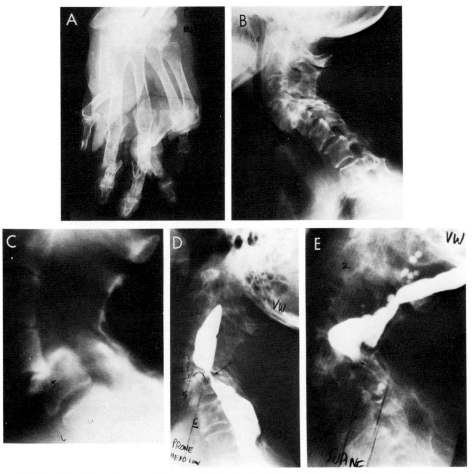

Fig 14–29.—Far advanced rheumatoid arthritis **(A)** in a 45-year-old female with involvement of the cervical spine and a pseudoarthrosis at C4-5. Note the marked dislocation of C-4 upon C-5 **(B and C).** The patient presented with quadriparesis. The lateral shootthrough Pantopaque myelogram in the prone **(D)** and supine **(E)** positions demonstrates the marked impingement on the cord at the site of dislocation *(arrow).*

matomes, and myelographic abnormalities. Rosenkranz, in a review of the literature, found eight more cases with a cauda equina syndrome and added one of his own. In addition to the classic findings of chronic ankylosing spondylitis, plain roentgenograms of the lumbar spine reveal multiple, well-defined, cystic erosions of the laminae and spinous processes. These changes are produced by varying-sized, cyst-like arachnoidal protrusions from the posterolateral aspects of a dilated lumbar thecal sac. Arachnoid cyst formation apparently is fairly common in patients with long-standing ankylosing spondylitis and a cauda equina syndrome. Matthews made an important contribution to the pathology of the arachnoidal cysts. In a postmortem report, he described diverticulae lined by a membrane composed of periosteum, dura, and arachnoid, without associated inflammatory changes in the meninges. Some of the nerve roots exhibited demyelinization and fibrosis. Matthews suggested that the arachnoid cysts might be the end result of preexisting arachnoiditis early in the disease. Presumably, CSF-filled blind pouches between adhesions produced pressure on adjacent neural structures and bone.

RHEUMATOID ARTHRITIS

An isolated, nontraumatic dislocation of the dens in a patient without a congenital anomaly is secondary to inflammation, i.e., pharyngitis, tonsillitis, rheumatoid arthritis (Fig 14–28). There may or may not be associated neurologic findings. Far advanced rheumatoid arthritis of the spine may result in a pseudoarthrosis with secondary dislocation and marked impingement upon the spinal cord or medulla (Fig 14–29).

BIBLIOGRAPHY

Aicardi J., Lapintre J.: Spinal epidural abscess in a one month old child. *Am. J. Dis. Child.* 114:666, 1967.

Alajovanine T., Houdart R., Drouhet E.: Les formes chirurgicales spinales de la torulosa; toruloma de la quene de cheval, *Rev. Neurol.* 88:153, 1953.

Ard R.W.: Paraplegia caused by unusual extradural granuloma simulating neoplasm: Presentation of case with complete recovery following surgical removal. *Arch Intern. Med.* 46:808, 1957.

Arseni C., Horvath L., Sander G.: Compression of the spinal cord due to hydatid disease. *Acta Psychiatr.* 35:1, 1960.

Autio E., Suolanen J., Norrbäck S., Slätis P.: Adhesive arachnoiditis after lumbar myelography with meglumine iothalamate (Conray). *Acta Radiol. (Diagn.)* 12:17, 1972.

Barnett H.J.M., Foster J.B., Hudgson P.: Syringomyelia associated with spinal arachnoiditis (chap. 15) in *Major Problems in Neurology: Syringomyelia*. London, W.B. Saunders Co., 1973, p. 220.

Barnett H.J.M., Foster J.B., Hudgson P.: The pathogenesis of syringomyelia cavitation associated with arachnoiditis localized to the spinal cord (chap. 16) in *Major Problems in Neurology: Syringomyelia*. London, W.B. Saunders Co., 1973, p. 245.

Bärtschi-Rochaix W., De La Cuadra, Jr.: Spinal cysticercosis. *Helvet. Med. Acta* 13:192, 1946.

Batson O.V.: The vertebral vein system. *A.J.R.* 78:195, 1957.

Bell D.: Tuberculosis of the vertebral pedicles. Personal communication.

Bergeron R.T., Rumbaugh C.L., Fan H., Cravioto H.: Experimental Pantopaque arachnoiditis in the monkey. *Radiology* 99:95, 1971.

Betty M., Lorber J.: Intramedullary abscess of spinal cord. *J. Neurol., Neurosurg. Psychiatr.* 26:236, 1963.

Boden G.: Radiation myelitis of the cervical spinal cord. *Br. J. Radiol.* 21:464, 1948.

Boharas S., Koskoff Y.D.: Early diagnosis of acute epidural abscess. *J.A.M.A.* 117:1085, 1941.

Bowie E.A., Glasgow G.: Cauda equina lesions associated with ankylosing spondylitis: Report of three cases. *Br. Med. J.* 2:24, 1961.

Brett J., Himmelfarb E., Gerald B.: Myelographic appearance of meningo-vascular lymphoma involving cauda equina. *J. Can. Assoc. Radiol.* 26:88, 1975.

Browder J., Meyers R.: Infections of spinal epidural space. Aspect of vertebral osteomyelitis. *Am. J. Surg.* 37:1, 1937.

Browder J., Meyers R.: Pyogenic infections of spinal epidural space. *Surgery* 10:296, 1941.

Budzilovich G.N., Most N., Feigen I.: Pathogenesis and latency of spinal cord schistosomiasis. *Arch Pathol.* 77:383, 1964.

Cabieses F., Vallenas M., Landa R.: Cysticercosis of the spinal cord. *J. Neurosurg.* 16:337, 1959.

Campbell J.A., Silver R.A.: Roentgen manifestations of epidural granulomas of the spine with report of 10 cases. *Am. J. Roentgenol.* 72:229, 1954.

Campbell M.M.: Pyogenic infections within the vertebral canal. *Bull. Neurol. Inst. New York* 6:574, 1937.

Carton C.A., Mount L.A.: Neurosurgical aspects of cryptococcosis. *J. Neurosurg.* 8:143, 1951.

Chait A., Gannon W.E.: Schistosomiasis of the spinal cord. *Am. J. Roentgenol.* 105:400, 1969.

Charcot J.M., Joffroy A.: Deux cas d'atrophie musculaire progressive avec lésions de la substance grise et des faisceaux antérolateraux de la moelle épinière. *Arch. Physiol. Norm. Pathol.* 2:354, 1869.

Christensen E.: Chronic adhesive spinal arachnoiditis. *Acta Psychiatr. Scandinav.* 17:23, 1942.

Clark K.: Significance of the small lumbar spinal canal: Cauda equina compression syndromes due to spondylosis. Clinical and surgical significance. *J. Neurosurg.* 31:495, 1969.

Cohen I.: Epidural spinal infections. *Ann. Surg.* 108:992, 1938.

Craig W.M., Dockerty M.B., Harrington S.W.: Intravertebral and intrathoracic blastomycoma simulating dumb-bell tumors. *South. Surg.* 9:759, 1940.

Dandy W.E.: Abscesses and inflammatory tumors in spinal epidural space (so-called pachymeningitis externa). *Arch Surg.* 13:477, 1926.

Davidoff L.M., Gass H., Grossman J.: Postoperative spinal arachnoiditis and recurrent spinal cord tumor. *J. Neurosurg.* 4:451, 1947.

Dazzi A., Verga P.: Di uno raro caso di cisticerco racemoso a localizzazione spinale. *Policlinico (Sez. Med.)* 33:65, 1926.

Decker H.G., Shapiro S.W., Porter H.R.: Epidural tuberculous abscess simulating herniated lumbar intervertebral disk. A case report. *Ann. Surg.* 149:294, 1959.

Dévé F.: L'echinococcose vertébrale. Son processus páthogénique et ses lesions. *Ann. Anat. Pathol.* 5:841, 1928.

Dew H.R.: *Hydatid Disease. Its Pathology, Diagnosis and Treatment.* Sydney, Australasian Medical Publishing Company, Ltd., 1928.

Diabal P.W., Mullins J.D., Coltman C.A., Jr.: An unusual manifestation of non-Hodgkin's lymphoma. Fibrosis masquerading as Ormond's disease. *J.A.M.A.* 243:1161, 1980.

DiTullio M.V., Jr.: Intramedullary spinal abscess: A case report with a review of 53 previously described cases. *Surg. Neurol.* 7:351, 1977.

Duke R.J., Hashimoto S.A.: Familial spinal arachnoiditis. *Arch. Neurol.* 30:300, 1974.

Durity F., Thompson G.B.: Localized cervical extradural abscess. Case report. *J. Neurosurg.* 28:387, 1968.

Dyke C.G.: The roentgen ray diagnosis of diseases of the spinal cord, meninges, and vertebrae, in Elsberg, C.A. (ed.), *Surgical Diseases of the Spinal Cord, Membranes, and Nerve Roots: Symptoms, Diagnosis and Treatment.* New York, Paul B. Hoeber, Inc., 1941.

Dynes J.B., Smedal M.J.: Radiation myelitis. *A.J.R.* 83:78, 1960.

Echols D.H.: Emergency laminectomy for acute epidural abscess: 4 cases with recovery in 3. *Surgery* 10:287, 1941.

Elkington J. St. C.: Meningitis serosa circumscripta spinalis (spinal arachnoiditis). *Brain* 59:181, 1936.

Elkington J. St. C.: Arachnoiditis, in Feiling, E. (ed.), *Modern Trends in Neurology*. New York: Paul B. Hoeber, Inc., 1941, p. 42.

Fisher R.L.: An experimental evaluation of Pantopaque and other recently developed myelographic contrast media. *Radiology* 85:537, 1965.

Fitchett M.S., Weidman F.D.: Generalized torulosis associated with Hodgkin's disease. *Arch. Pathol.* 18:225, 1934.

Fogeholm R., Halta M., Anderrson L.C.: Radiation myelopathy of the cervical spinal cord simulating intramedullary neoplasm. *J. Neurol., Neurosurg. Psychiatr.* 37:1177, 1974.

Freedman H., Alpers B.: Spinal subdural abscess. *Arch. Neurol. Psychiatr.* 60:49, 1948.

French J.D.: Clinical manifestations of lumbar spinal arachnoiditis. *Surgery* 20:718, 1946.

French J.D.: Recurrent arachnoiditis in the dorsal spinal region. *Arch. Neurol. Psychiatr.* 58:200, 1947.

Frey E., Zimmerli B.: Pantopaque myelography in tuberculous arachnoiditis. *Radiol. Clin.* 31:178, 1962.

Gasul B.M., Jaffe R.H.: Acute epidural spinal abscess—a clinical entity. *Arch. Pediatr.* 52:361, 1935.

Godwin-Austen R.B., Howell D.S., Worthington B.: Observations in radiation myelopathy. *Brain* 98:557, 1975.

Gordon A.L., Yudell A.: Cauda equina lesion associated with rheumatoid spondylitis. *Ann. Intern. Med.* 78:555, 1973.

Grant F.C.: Epidural spinal abscess. *J.A.M.A.* 128:509, 1945.

Greenfield J.G.: *Textbook of Neuropathology*, ed. 2. Baltimore, Williams & Wilkins Co., 1967, p. 224.

Greenwood R.C., Voris A.C.: Systemic blastomycosis with spinal cord involvement. *J. Neurosurg.* 7:450, 1950.

Guidetti B., LaTorre E.: Hypertrophic spinal pachymeningitis. *J. Neurosurg.* 26:496, 1967.

Hart G.M.: Circumscribed serous spinal arachnoiditis simulating protruded lumbar intervertebral disk. *Ann. Surg.* 148:266, 1958.

Hauge T.: Chronic rheumatoid polyarthritis and spondylarthritis associated with neurological symptoms and signs and occasionally simulating an intraspinal expansive process. *Acta Chir. Scandinav.* 120:395, 1961.

Herskowitz A.: Spinal cord involvement with Schistosoma mansoni. Case report. *J. Neurosurg.* 36:494, 1972.

Howland W.J., Curry J.L.: Experimental studies of Pantopaque arachnoiditis. *Radiology* 87:253, 1966.

Howland W.J., Curry J.L., Butler A.K.: Pantopaque arachnoiditis. Experimental study of blood as a potentiating agent. *Radiology* 80:489, 1963.

Hunt J.R.: Acute infectious osteomyelitis of spine and acute suppurative perimeningitis. *Med. Rec.* 65:641, 1904.

Hurteau E., Baird W.C., Sinclair E.: Arachnoiditis following the use of iodized oil. *J. Bone Joint Surg.* 36A:393, 1954.

Hutton P.W., Holland H.J.: Schistosomiasis of the spinal cord. *Br. Med. J.* 2:1931, 1960.

Hyndman O.R., Gerber W.F.: Spinal extradural cysts, congenital and acquired. Report of cases. *J. Neurosurg.* 3:474, 1946.

Jackson F.E., Kent D., Clarke F.: Quadriplegia caused by involvement of cervical spine with *Coccidioides immitis*. *J. Neurosurg.* 21:512, 1964.

Jakobson J.K.: Clinical evaluation of a histologic examination of the side effects of myelographic contrast media. *Acta Radiol. (Diagn.)* 14:638, 1973.

Jakoby R.K., Koos W.T.: Intradural extramedullary tuberculoma of the spinal cord. *J. Neurosurg.* 18:557, 1961.

Janz H.: Zur differential Diagnose zwischen Arachnoiditis spinalis und Tumor spinalis im Myelogramm. *Nervenarzt* 18:175, 1947.

Jones A.: Transient radiation myelopathy. *Br. J. Radiol.* 37:727, 1964.

Jorgensen J., Hansen P.H., Steenskov V., Ovesen N.: A clinical and radiological study of chronic lower arachnoiditis. *Neuroradiology* 9:139, 1975.

Joseph S.I., Denson J.S.: Spinal anesthesia, arachnoiditis, and paraplegia. *J.A.M.A.* 168:1333, 1958.

Kamman G.R., Baker A.B.: Syphilitic pan-meningitis (so-called chronic hypertrophic spinal pachymeningitis). *Ann. Intern. Med.* 15:748, 1941.

Kingsley D.P.E., White E., Marks A., Coxon, A.: Intradural extramedullary aspergilloma complicating chronic lymphatic leukemia. *Br. J. Radiol.* 52:916, 1979.

Knutsson F.: The myelogram following operation for herniated disc. *Acta Radiol.* 32:60, 1949.

Korbsch H.: Über Rückenmarksysticerkose. *Deutsche Ztschr. Chir.* 237:779, 1932.

Kozlowski K.: Late spinal blocks after tuberculous meningitis. *Am. J. Roentgenol.* 90:1220, 1963.

Lee M.L.H., Waters D.J.: Neurological complications of ankylosing spondylitis. *Br. Med. J.* 1:798, 1962.

Lerner M.A.: Progression and regression of myelographic block in acute transverse myelopathy. *Clin. Radiol.* 19:337, 1968.

Lewtas N.A., Dimant S.: The diagnosis of hypertrophic interstitial polyneuritis by myelography. *J. Fac. Radiologists* 8:276, 1957.

Ley A., Jacas R., Oliveras C.: Torula granuloma of the cervical spinal cord. *J. Neurosurg.* 8:327, 1951.

Lichtenstein R.S.: Arachnoiditis following myelography (letter). *Spine* 4:93, 1979.

Lindquist P.R., McDonald E.: Rheumatoid cyst causing extradural compression. *J. Bone Joint Surg.* 52A:1235, 1970.

Lombardi G., Passerini A.: Myelographic aspects of spinal arachnoiditis. *Radiol. Med.* 41:654, 1955.

Lombardi G., Passerini A., Migliavacca F.: Spinal arachnoiditis. *Br. J. Radiol.* 35:314, 1962.

Long R., Rachmaninoff N.: Spinal adhesive arachnoiditis with cyst formation. Injection of cyst during myelography. Case report. *J. Neurosurg.* 27:73, 1967.

Maciel A., Coelho B., Abath G.: Myelite schistosomique due au S. mansoni: Étude anatomico-clinique. *Rev. Neurol.* 91:241, 1963.

Marty R., Minkler D.S.: Radiation myelitis simulating tumours. *Arch. Neurol.* 29:352, 1973.

Mason M.S., Raaf J.: Complication of Pantopaque myelography. Case report and review. *J. Neurosurg.* 19:302, 1962.

Matheis H.: Die cryptococcose (torulose) des nervensystems. *Deutsche Ztschr. Nervenh.* 180:595, 1960.

Matthews W.B.: The neurological complications of ankylosing spondylitis. *J. Neurol. Sci.* 6:561, 1968.

Mayher W.E., Daniel E.F., Allen M.B.: Acute meningeal reaction following Pantopaque myelography. *J. Neurosurg.* 34:396, 1971.

McGill I.G.: An unusual neurological syndrome associated with ankylosing spondylitis. *Guy's Hosp. Rep.* 115:33, 1966.

Mikhael M.A.: Delayed radiation necrosis of a spinal nerve root presenting as an intra-spinal mass. *Br. J. Radiol.* 52:905, 1979.

Miller P.R., Elder W.: Meningeal pseudocysts (meningocele spurius) following laminectomy. *J. Bone Joint Surg.* 50A:268, 1968.

Mixtér W.J., Smithwick R.H.: Acute intraspinal epidural abscess. *N. Engl. J. Med.* 207:127, 1932.

Moniz E.: La pachyméningite spinale hypertrophique et les cavités médullaires. *Rev. Neurol.* 2:433, 1925.

Mulvey R.B.: Unusual myelographic patterns of arachnoiditis. *Radiology* 75:778, 1960.

Naffziger H.C., Stern W.E.: Chronic pachymeningitis: Report of case and review of literature. *Arch. Neurol. & Psychiatr.* 62:38, 1949.

Nelson J.: Intramedullary cavitation resulting from adhesive spinal arachnoiditis. *Arch. Neurol. Psychiatr.* 50:1, 1943.

Odeku E.L., Lucas A.O., Richard D.R.: Intramedullary spinal cord schistosomiasis. *J. Neurosurg.* 29:417, 1968.

Odin M., Runstrom G., Lindblom A.: Iodized oils as an aid to the diagnosis of lesions of the spinal cord and a contribution to the knowledge of adhesive circumscribed meningitis. *Acta Radiol.* (Suppl.) 7, 1928.

Pagni C.A., Cassinari V., Bernasconi V.: Meningocele spurius following hemilaminectomy in a case of lumbar discal hernia. *J. Neurosurg.* 18:709, 1961.

Pallis C.A., Louis S., Morgan R.L.: Radiation myelopathy. *Brain* 84:460, 1961.

Palmer J.J.: Radiation myelopathy. *Brain* 95:109, 1972.

Patronas N.J., Marx W.J., Duda E.E.: Radiographic presentation of spinal abscess in the subdural space. *A.J.R.* 132:138, 1979.

Peterson H.O.: The hazards of myelography. *Radiology* 115:237, 1975.

Praestholm J., Olgard K.: Comparative histological investigation of the sequelae of experimental myelography using sodium methiodal and meglumine iothalamate. *Neuroradiology* 14:14, 1972.

Quencer R.M., Tenver M., Rothman L.: The postoperative myelogram. Radiographic evaluation of arachnoiditis and dural/arachnoid tears. *Radiology* 123:667, 1977.

Quiles M., Marchisello P.J., Tsairis P.: Lumbar adhesive arachnoiditis: Etiologic and pathologic aspects. *Spine* 3:45, 1978.

Radberg C., Werrnberg E.: Late sequelae following lumbar myelography with water soluble contrast media. *Acta Radiol. (Diagn.)* 14:507, 1973.

Ramamurthi B., Anguli, V.C.: Intramedullary cryptococcic granuloma of the spinal cord. *J. Neurosurg.* 11:622, 1954.

Rand C.W.: Coccidioidal granuloma. Report of two cases simulating tumour of spinal cord. *Arch. Neurol. Psychiatr.* 23:502, 1930.

Ransford A.O., Harries B.J.: Localized arachnoiditis complicating lumbar disc lesions. *J. Bone Joint Surg.* 54B:656, 1972.

Rayport M., Wisoff H.S., Zaiman H.: Vertebral echinococcosis. Report of case of surgical and biological therapy with review of the literature. *J. Neurosurg.* 21:647, 1964.

Reddy G.N.N., Harris P., Gordon A.: Spinal subdural granuloma caused by micropulverized barium sulfate. Case report. *J. Neurosurg.* 26:425, 1967.

Reeves D.L., Butt E.M., Hammock R.W.: Torula infection of the lungs and central nervous system. *Arch. Intern. Med.* 68:57, 1941.

Richter J.A., Danziger A., Price H.I.: The postoperative myelogram. *S. Afr. Med. J.* 55:409, 1979.

Robinson R.G.: Hydatid disease of the spine and its neurological complications. *Br. J. Surg.* 47:301, 1959.

Rosenblath: Ein Fall von Cysticerkenmeningitis mit vorwiegender Beteilung des Rückenmarks. *Deutsche Ztschr. Nervenh.* 46:113, 1913.

Rosenkranz W.: Ankylosing spondylitis: Cauda equina syndrome with multiple spinal arachnoid cysts. *J. Neurosurg.* 34:241, 1971.

Russell M.L., Gordon D.A., Ogryzlo M.A., McPhedran R.S.: The cauda equina syndrome of ankylosing spondylitis. *Ann. Intern. Med.* 78:551, 1973.

Saenger E.L.: Spondylarthritis in children. *A.J.R.* 64:20, 1950.

Seaman W.B., Marder S.N., Rosenbaum H.E.: The myelographic appearance of adhesive spinal arachnoiditis. *J. Neurosurg.* 10:145, 1953.

Sehgal A.D., Gardner W.J., Dohn D.F.: Pantopaque arachnoiditis. Treatment with subarachnoid injection of corticosteroids. *Cleveland Clin. Quart.* 29:177, 1962.

Selby R.C., Pillay K.V.: Osteomyelitis and disc infection secondary to pseudomonas aeruginosa in heroin addiction. Case report. *J. Neurosurg.* 37:463, 1972.

Sheinmel A., Glasser S.M.: Uncommon compressing lesions of the spinal cord and its membranes. *Am. J. Roentgenol.* 67:415, 1952.

Shenkin H.A., Horn R.C., Jr., Grant, F.C.: Lesions of spinal epidural space producing cord compression. *Arch. Surg.* 51:125, 1945.

Skalpe I.O.: Adhesive arachnoiditis following lumbar radiculography with water-soluble contrast agents. A clinical report with special reference to metrizamide. *Radiology* 12:647, 1976.

Skalpe I.O., Amundsen P.: Lumbar radiculography with metrizamide. A non-ionic water soluble contrast medium. *Radiology* 115:91, 1975.

Skalpe I.O., Amundsen P.: Thoracic and cervical myelography with metrizamide. Clinical experiences with a water-soluble, non-ionic contrast medium. *Radiology* 116:101, 1975.

Skalpe I.O., Sortland O.: Adhesive arachnoiditis in patients with spinal block. *Neuroradiology* 22:243, 1982.

Skultety F.M.: Cryptococcic granuloma of the dorsal spinal cord. *Neurology* 2:1066, 1961.

Smith F.B., Crawford J.S.: Fatal granulomatosis of the central nervous system due to a yeast (torula). *J. Path. Bact.* 33:291, 1930.

Smith R.W., Loeser J.D.: A myelographic variant in lumbar arachnoiditis. *J. Neurosurg.* 36:441, 1972.

Smolik E.A., Nash F.P.: Lumbar spinal arachnoiditis. A complication of the intervertebral disc operation. *Ann Surg.* 133:490, 1951.

Spiegel P.G., Kengla K.W., Isaacson A.S., Wilson J.C., Jr.: Intervertebral disc-space inflammation in children. *J. Bone Joint Surg.* 54A:284, 1972.

Stevenson L.D., Eckhardt R.E.: Myelomalacia of cervical portion of spinal cord, probably the result of roentgen therapy. *Arch. Pathol.* 39:109, 1945.

Sullivan C.R.: Diagnosis and treatment of pyogenic infections of intervertebral disc. *Surg. Clin. North Am.* 41:1077, 1961.

Sullivan C.R., Bickel W.H., Svien H.J.: Infections of vertebral interspaces after operations on intervertebral discs. *J.A.M.A.* 166:1973, 1958.

Suolanen J.: Adhesive arachnoiditis following myelography with various water soluble contrast media. *Neuroradiology* 9:83, 1975.

Teng P., Papatheodorou C.: Myelographic findings in adhesive spinal arachnoiditis. *Br. J. Radiol.* 40:201, 1967.

Vogel P.J.: Circumscribed spinal arachnoiditis with cavitations of the spinal cord. *Bull. L.A. Neurol. Soc.* 11:48, 1946.

Wakefield G.S., Carroll J.D., Speed D.E.: Schistosomiasis of the spinal cord. *Brain* 85:535, 1962.

Warkentin J.H.: An unusual manifestation of idiopathic retroperitoneal fibrosis. *Radiology* 93:1313, 1969.

Wilson G., Bartle H.D., Jr., Dean J.S.: Chronic hypertrophic spinal pachymeningitis. *Am. J. Med. Sci.* 198:616, 1939.

Winkelman N.W., Gotten N., Schiebert D.: Localized adhesive spinal arachnoiditis. A study of 25 cases with reference to etiology. *Trans. Am. Neurol. Assoc.* 78:15, 1953.

Wirth F.P., Jr., Gado M.: Incomplete myelographic block with hypertrophic spinal pachymeningitis. Case report. *J. Neurosurg.* 38:368, 1973.

Wolfgang G.L.: Neurotrophic arthropathy of the shoulder—a complication of progressive adhesive arachnoiditis. A case report. *Clin. Orthop.* 87:217, 1972.

Worthington B.S.: Diffuse cord enlargement in radiation myelopathy. *Clin. Radiol.* 30:117, 1979.

Zilka A., Reiss J., Shulman K., Schechter M.M.: Traumatic subarachnoid-mediastinal fistula. A case report. *J. Neurosurg.* 32:473, 1970.

15

Vascular Malformations

RENE DJINDJIAN, M.D.

THIS CHAPTER will consider the vascular anatomy of the normal spinal cord, the technique of selective spinal arteriography, and the angiographic findings in various pathologic states.

ANATOMY

Traditional anatomy texts describe the arterial supply of the spinal cord as the anterior and posterior spinal branches of the vertebral artery. According to this description, the paired anterior spinal arteries unite between the pyramids of the medulla to form a single channel coursing down the anterior median fissure to the filum terminale. The smaller posterior spinal arteries run down either side of the posterior aspect of the cord medial to the posterior nerve roots. The inaccuracy of this simplistic account has been apparent since Adamkiewicz's demonstration of segmental anastomotic branches in 1882. In 1889, Kadyi's classic monograph confirmed and extended these observations. More recently, studies by Tanon, Suh and Alexander, Bolton, Tureen, Adams, Gillilan, Lazorthes et al., Corbin, Doppman and DiChiro, and Djindjian and his co-workers have further clarified the blood supply of the cord.

In fact, the spinal cord is asymmetrically supplied at a few levels in each region by arterial branches accompanying the anterior and posterior spinal nerve roots (Figs 15–1 to 15–3). These anterior and posterior radiculomedullary arteries reinforce the anterior and posterior spinal arteries, resulting in two relatively independent arterial networks—a larger anterior and a smaller posterior system. The branches of the radiculomedullary arteries that supply the spinal cord may penetrate into the depths of the cord or encircle the cord as part of the pial arterial plexus (Fig 15–4).

In the cervical region, the cord is supplied by the vertebral, thyrocervical and costocervical branches of the subclavian artery (Figs 15–5, 15–6), in the thoracic region by the paired supreme intercostal branches of the subclavian artery and the aortic intercostals, and in the lumbar region by the lumbar arteries. The sacral nerves and roots are supplied by the lumbar branches of the iliolumbar division of the hypogastric artery or by the sacral arteries. According to Lazorthes, these ana-

318

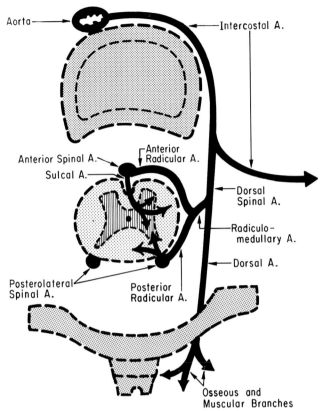

Fig 15–1.—Schematic cross-section showing the extra- and intraspinal (extramedullary) branches of an intercostal artery.

tomical divisions, i.e., cervical, thoracic, and lumbar, do not have exact functional counterparts. Lazorthes suggests that it is more appropriate to consider the functional circulation of the cord as: (1) cervico-upper thoracic, corresponding to the cervical cord and the first two thoracic segments; (2) midthoracic (consisting of the first seven thoracic segments), representing a watershed with a marginal blood supply, since it receives only a few, sparse radiculomedullary branches from the proximal thoracic supply and some craniad flow from the lumbar area; (3) thoracolumbar, extending from T-8 to the filum terminale.

Usually, there are three anterior radiculomedullary arteries in the cervico-upper thoracic region that anastomose with the anterior spinal artery. The most proximal vessel arises from the vertebral artery and accompanies the C-3 nerve root. A second larger vessel, commonly originating from the deep cervical artery, accompanies the C-6 nerve root (artery of the cervical enlargement). The third artery, arising from the costocervical trunk or the supreme intercostal artery, accompanies the C-8 nerve root. Although the level of entry of the artery of the cervical enlargement usually is at C6-7, it may occur at C5-6 or, rarely, at C4-5.

In the anteroposterior projection, the anterior spinal artery to the upper cord can be visualized as a thin linear vessel arising from the vertebral artery, coursing downward and medially to reach the midline at C-1. The most proximal arterial

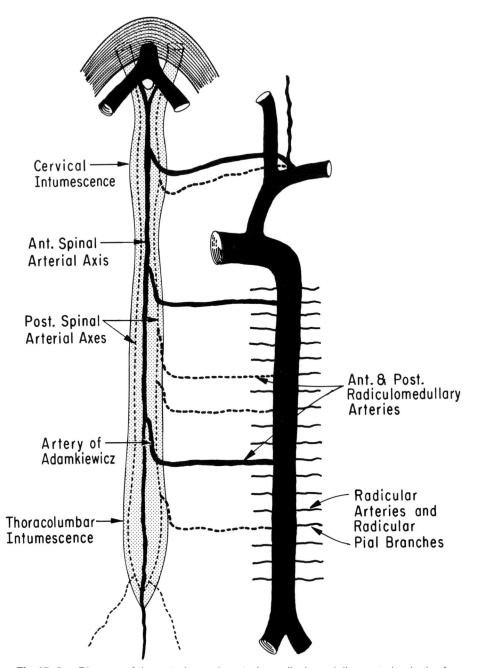

Fig 15–2.—Diagram of the anterior and posterior radiculomedullary arteries in the frontal projection.

feeder accompanying the C-3 root rarely is visualized in the normal patient. However, the artery of cervical enlargement often is seen as a hairpin-like vessel with ascending and descending limbs connecting the cervical and the superior thoracic segments of the anterior spinal artery. A break in continuity between the latter areas is not unusual. The artery of the cervical enlargement commonly arises from

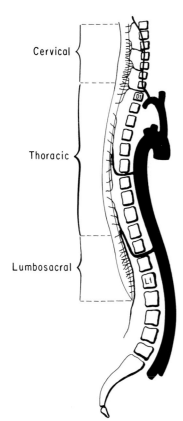

Cervical

Ant. Spinal A.

Radicular arteries
to the cervical cord
and intumescence

Thoracic

Dorsal radicular A.

Fig 15–3.—Schematic lateral
view of the segmental functional
blood supply of the spinal cord.

Lumbosacral

Radicular arteries
to the lumbar cord
and intumescence

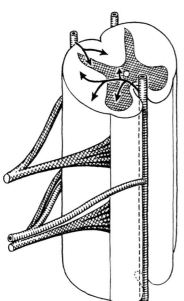

Fig 15–4.—Diagram of the
intramedullary arterial distribution.

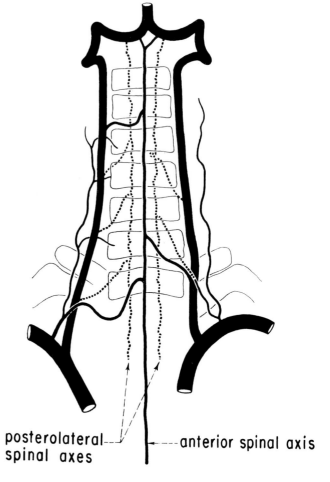

Fig 15–5.—Diagram of the anterior and posterior radiculomedullary arteries in the cervical region (frontal projection).

posterolateral spinal axes · · · · anterior spinal axis

either deep cervical artery to enter the spinal canal at C6-7. However, it may arise from the supreme intercostal artery on either side to enter the spinal canal at C7-T1, from either vertebral artery to enter the spinal canal at C5-6 (Fig 15–7) or, rarely, from the subclavian artery, describing a wide curve parallel to the deep cervical artery before it enters the spinal canal at C5-6. The artery of the cervical enlargement is often reinforced by an anterior radiculomedullary artery arising from the deep cervical artery or from the contralateral supreme intercostal artery. All of these branches participate in the formation of the anterior spinal arterial trunk. In the lateral projection, the anterior spinal artery is visualized just posterior and parallel to the vertebral bodies, in front of the spinal cord.

The anterior meningeal branch of the vertebral artery may be opacified at the level of the axis, coursing superiorly to the region of the foramen magnum, anterior to the anterior spinal artery. The muscular branches of the deep cervical arteries supplying the neck muscles are opacified also. In the lower cervical spine, these vessels anastomose with their analogues of the opposite side and with the muscular branches of the vertebral artery to produce a "stepladder" appearance in the region of the spinous processes. This should not be confused with the anterior radiculomedullary arteries.

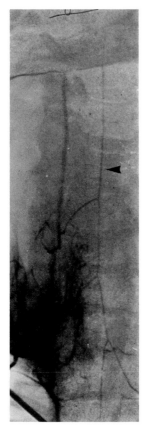

Fig 15–6.—Selective opacification of the right deep cervical artery filling the anterior spinal artery *(arrowhead)* in the cervico-upper thoracic region.

In the midthoracic region, the anterior spinal artery usually is reinforced by a narrow anterior radiculomedullary artery from the third, fourth, or fifth intercostal artery, commonly on the left side. This vessel also has a hairpin configuration with a narrow ascending branch that sometimes can be followed up to the cervical anterior spinal artery and a slightly larger descending branch that may anastomose with the ascending branch of the arteria radicularis magna.

The well-developed muscular branches make it possible at times to opacify the deep cervical artery and a segment of the subclavian artery from a selective injection of the third or fourth intercostal artery. Occasionally, an area of hypervascularization can be seen at the lateral border of T-3 and T-4, which should not be mistaken for a tumor. The muscular branches at or near the midline can be differentiated from the radiculomedullary arteries by their anastomoses with the adjacent segments.

The principal arterial supply of the thoracolumbar cord is the arteria radicularis magna (great anterior medullary artery, artery of Adamkiewicz, artery of the lumbar enlargement [Lazorthes]) (Figs 15–8, 15–9). This vessel usually arises on the left side (75%)—between T-9 and L-2 (85%), between T-5 and T-8 (15%). The arteria radicularis magna enters the spinal canal through the corresponding intervertebral foramen and ascends obliquely for a variable distance to reach the midline (usually at T-10). Here, it divides into a small, narrow ascending branch to the midthoracic segment and a larger descending branch. At the site of bifurcation in the anterior

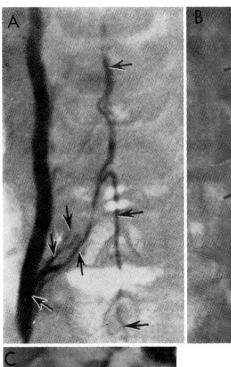
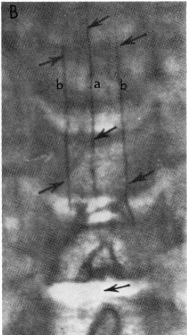
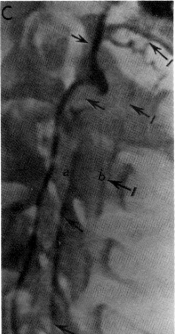

Fig 15–7.—Selective injection of the right vertebral artery demonstrating the artery to the cervical enlargement entering the spinal canal at the C6-7 interspace. The posterior spinal artery *(twin arrows)* arises from the same trunk close to the origin of the radiculomedullary artery **(A).** A later film at 11.5 sec shows the anterior spinal artery *(a)* and both posterior spinal arteries *(b)* in the anteroposterior **(B)** and lateral **(C)** projections.

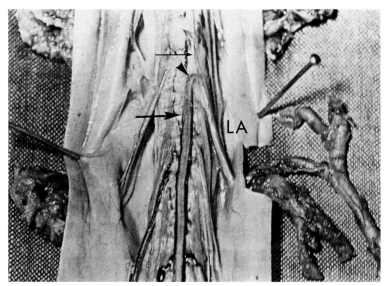

Fig 15–8.—Photograph of an anatomical preparation demonstrating the arteria radicularis magna. *LA* = lumbar artery; *arrowhead* = hairpin turn; *thin arrow* = thin ascending branch; *thick arrow* = large descending branch.

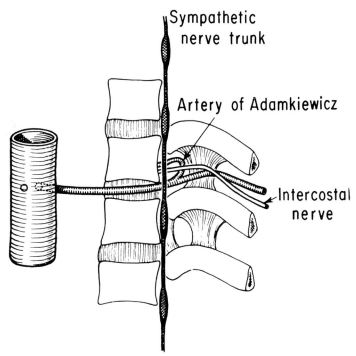

Fig 15–9.—Lateral diagram illustrating the origin of the arteria radicularis magna *(upper arrow)* from an intercostal artery.

median fissure, it makes a hairpin bend to descend as the anterior spinal trunk to the lumbar intumescence. The latter branch usually is straight at its origin but soon becomes undulating or tortuous. This is particularly true in younger children, in whom the tortuosity should not be mistaken for a vascular malformation at contrast myelography (see Fig 9–11,*B*). In the anteroposterior angiogram, the arteria radicularis magna can be readily identified by its characteristic hairpin bend (Figs 15–10, 15–11). In the lateral projection, this vessel can be seen arising from an intercostal or upper lumbar artery, entering the spinal canal through the intervertebral foramen, coursing craniad and slightly anteriorly, and bending sharply caudad in a straight line close to the posterior surface of the vertebral bodies (Fig 15–12).

At the level of the distal conus, the arteria radicularis magna anastomoses with both posterior spinal arteries (anastomotic loop of Lazorthes). It also anastomoses with the sacral radicular arteries, which normally supply the cauda equina and the filum terminale. The anastomotic arch and the lumbosacral radicular arteries are never opacified in normal patients. In severe occlusive disease, however, where the vessels can also supply the lower thoracic cord, they may be visualized.

The rich muscular arteries in the thoracolumbar region frequently produce homogeneous opacification of the hemivertebra on the side of injection. This should not be confused with the posterior spinal arteries, the arteries to the dura or vertebral angiomas that contain vascular lakes.

The anterior spinal artery supplies the anterior two thirds to four fifths of the spinal cord. In general, it tends to be fairly well defined and sometimes paired in the cervical region, tapering in a somewhat undulating course to the upper thoracic

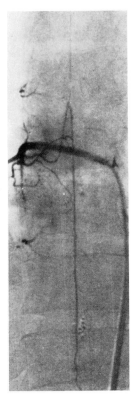

Fig 15–10.—Selective injection of the eighth right intercostal artery filling the arteria radicularis magna. Note the characteristic hairpin bend, the small ascending and the larger descending branch (frontal projection).

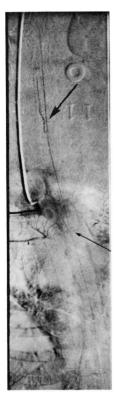

Fig 15–11.—Opacification of the anterior spinal artery in the midthoracic region, the arteria radicularis magna *(thick arrow)* and a supplementary artery of Adamkiewicz *(thin arrow)* in an infant by selective injection of the left ninth intercostal artery.

area. It varies considerably, depending on its proximity to, and the size of, reinforcing arterial feeders from segmental radiculomedullary vessels. Usually a small vessel just above its junction with the arteria radicularis magna, it attains its maximal caliber at or below this site, where it anastomoses with the posterior spinal arteries.

The posterior spinal arteries represent two freely anastomosing, plexiform channels that course longitudinally on a line with the entrance of the posterior nerve rootlets (see Fig 15–7,*B*). Shortly after their origin from the vertebral arteries, they form an irregular anastomotic plexus and, at intervals, are joined on each side by small posterior radiculomedullary arteries. Usually the anterior and posterior radiculomedullary arteries do not anastomose with their respective spinal arteries at the same level. However, the anterior spinal artery and the posterior spinal plexus encircle the spinal cord and freely anastomose to form the pial arteriolar plexus.

In the anteroposterior projection, the posterior spinal artery rarely is visualized at angiography in the cervical region. In the lateral view, the posterior spinal artery is visualized as a thin linear vessel coursing longitudinally anterior to the base of the spinal processes parallel to the anterior spinal artery (see Fig 15–7,*C*). The distance between the anterior and posterior spinal arteries in the lateral view represents the sagittal diameter of the spinal cord. In the thoracic region, the posterior spinal arteries are slender vessels that usually are not visualized. In the thoracolumbar area, the posterior spinal arteries usually can be identified as narrow vessels in the frontal and lateral projections, particularly at T-11, T-12, and L-1. In the frontal view, they are always lateral to the midline arteria radicularis magna, with ascend-

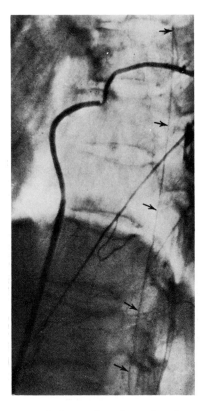

Fig 15–12.—Lateral arteriogram of the arteria radicularis magna, which is visualized *(arrows)* posterior to the vertebral bodies and anterior to the spinal cord.

ing and descending branches forming a tight network of vessels. In the lateral view, the posterior spinal arteries are seen well behind the posterior border of the vertebral bodies, lying on the dorsal surface of the distal spinal cord.

The venous drainage of the spinal cord is similar to, but not an exact replica of, the arterial supply (Figs 15–13, 15–14). The principal venous chain is the posterior spinal vein, a somewhat tortuous, longitudinal trunk running in the posterior median sulcus. It receives posterolateral venous channels and drains the posterior two thirds of the cord. The anterior spinal vein (or veins) is a smaller vessel that parallels the anterior spinal artery. In addition, there are numerous anterior and posterior radiculomedullary veins that drain into the anterior and posterior spinal veins. The radiculomedullary veins are irregular in distribution and do not necessarily course with the corresponding radiculomedullary arteries. The radiculomedullary veins accompany the corresponding nerve roots to the intervertebral foramina and pierce the dura to empty into the segmental intervertebral veins and ultimately into the venous plexus draining the vertebrae. The latter (external vertebral) along with the extradural (internal vertebral) veins drain via the intervertebral veins into the azygos system. There is no direct transdural communication between the intradural and extradural veins.

TECHNIQUE

A thorough medical evaluation is a necessary prerequisite for patients undergoing selective arteriography of the spinal cord. Since many of the patients are paraplegic,

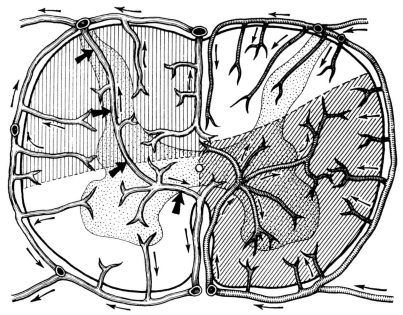

Fig 15–13.—Cross-sectional diagram of the intramedullary veins. (From Suh and Alexander.)

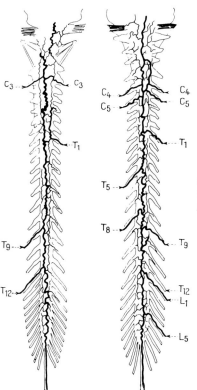

Fig 15–14.—Diagram of the anterior and posterior spinal and radicular veins. (From Suh and Alexander.)

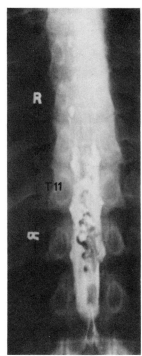

Fig 15–15.—Arteriovenous malformation at T11-12 in a 26-year-old white male who presented with a 2-year history of a Brown-Séquard syndrome at T-11. Note the characteristic coiled, serpentine appearance of the abnormal vessels. (Reprinted, with permission, from Sheinmel A., Glasser S. M., *Am. J. Roentgenol.* 67:415, 1952.)

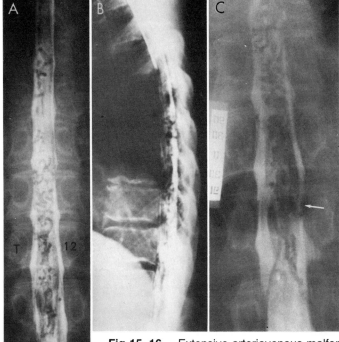

Fig 15–16.—Extensive arteriovenous malformation involving the thoracic cord and conus in a 45-year-old dentist with characteristic serpentine filling defects in the Pantopaque column produced by the tortuous pathologic vessels **(A** and **B).** In **C,** note the widening of the cord in the region of the conus medullaris (proved by arteriography and surgery).

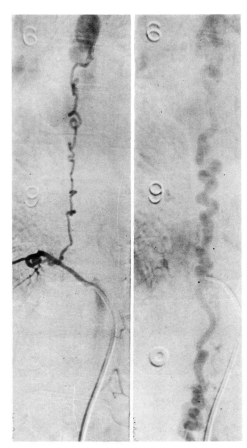

Fig 15–17.—Arteriovenous malformation in the midthoracic region in a patient with Rendu-Osler-Weber syndrome. The lesion is fed by a dilated posterior spinal artery arising from the right ninth intercostal artery; **(left)** arterial and **(right)** venous phases. Note the voluminous venous drainage.

Fig 15–18.—Dilated, tortuous arterial collaterals of the cervical and upper thoracic cord in a patient with coarctation of the aorta. (Reprinted, with permission, from Lombardi G., Migliavacca F., *Br. J. Radiol.* 32:810, 1959.)

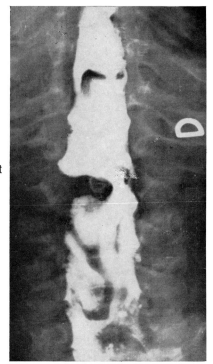

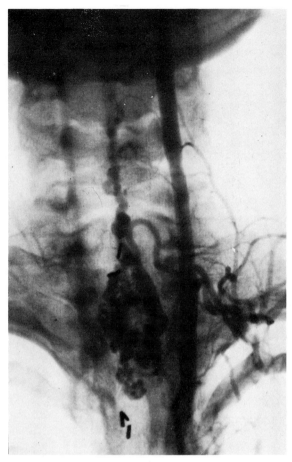

Fig 15–19.—Left subclavian arteriogram in the late phase showing a cervicothoracic arteriovenous malformation fed by the left deep cervical artery. Note the prominent venous drainage.

particular attention should be given to the treatment of existing urinary tract infections and bedsores. An intravenous sensitivity test, although notoriously unreliable, should be carried out for medicolegal purposes. Although some investigators successfully use local anesthesia, I prefer general anesthesia with intratracheal intubation after appropriate premedication. Apnea is produced during the period of rapid serial filming to eliminate the blurring effect of respiratory motion. The blood pressure is monitored carefully throughout the examination. Diazepam (Valium) is used intravenously in the event of chronic contractions of the lower extremities.

Subtraction is a vitally important part of the technique; the first film devoid of contrast material is used for the subtraction mask. Percutaneous catheterization of the femoral artery is carried out with a Seldinger PE 160 needle and a suitable guidewire. A green, end-hole Odman catheter with an S-shaped curve is used. The curvature is adapted to the size of the aorta, i.e., a wide curve of the proximal part of the S for a wide aorta and a more acutely angled curve for a narrow aorta. The outer segment of the curve should rest against the aortic wall, permitting the tip of the catheter to be guided into the intercostal or lumbar ostium respectively in the

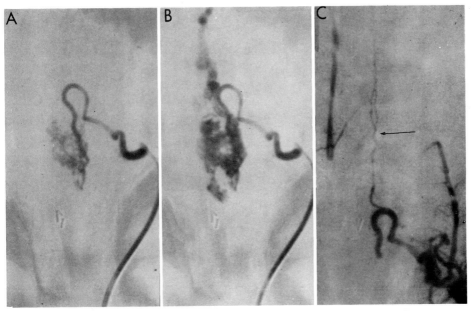

Fig 15–20.—Same case as Figure 15–19 after selective catheterization of the left deep cervical artery prior to embolization **(A** and **B)** and after embolization **(C).** Note filling of the anterior spinal artery *(arrow)* and absence of filling of the malformation after embolization (subtraction).

thoracic and lumbar regions. For the cervical region, the catheter should have less of a terminal curve to facilitate its introduction into the branches of the subclavian artery. Methylglucamine iothalamate (Conray 60) is the contrast medium of choice; a maximum of 250 ml of contrast medium should not be exceeded during an examination.

Because the various functional segments of the spinal cord present different problems, they will be discussed separately.

Cervicothoracic Region

A detailed study of the arterial supply of the cervical spinal cord requires bilateral catheterization of the subclavian artery. At present, I selectively catheterize and opacify the vertebral artery, the costocervical and the thyrocervical trunks. To avoid complications, I perform the examination in two stages, each side being catheterized separately, with a few days separating the two studies. Coned-down serial films are made in both the anteroposterior and lateral projections, with manual injection of 5 ml of contrast material.

Midthoracic and Thoracolumbar Regions

In these areas, selective catheterization of the intercostal and/or lumbar arteries is imperative for adequate visualization of the radiculomedullary arteries. Arteriography of the thoracolumbar region in adults implicitly requires catheterization of the intercostal or upper lumbar artery, which gives rise to the arteria radicularis magna. However, in small children, in whom selective catheterization may be dif-

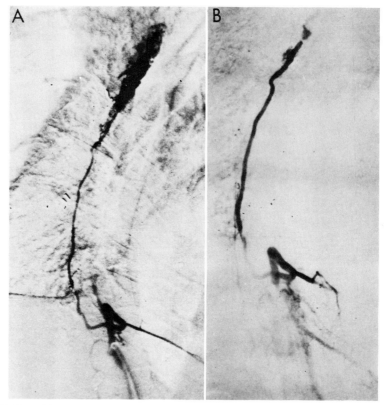

Fig 15–21.—Midthoracic arteriovenous malformation supplied by the left ninth intercostal artery before **(A)** and after **(B)** embolization (subtraction).

ficult or impossible, midstream aortography is a valid procedure, since it often opacifies the anterior spinal artery. A characteristic "jump" is felt as the catheter enters an intercostal or lumbar ostium. The position of the catheter in each vessel is verified on the television monitor by the manual injection of 2–3 ml of contrast material. Each injection is accompanied by a series of three rapid spot films at intervals of 1 second for survey purposes. If any pathologic process is demonstrated, serial anteroposterior and lateral films are made after the forceful manual injection of 5–8 ml of contrast material followed immediately by flushing of the catheter with physiologic saline (two films per second for 4 seconds followed by 1 film per second for 10 seconds). If there is delayed venous drainage, the series is prolonged, i.e., one film every 2 seconds for 30 seconds. Since the arteria radicularis magna arises on the left side from T-9 to L-2 in 75% of patients, these vessels are catheterized initially. The number and the location of the vessels injected vary with the individual program. If the principal arteries feeding the cord are not opacified from these injections, additional vessels are catheterized as necessary. The maximal volume of 250 ml of contrast medium should not be exceeded in order to minimize complications. It is wise to terminate the examination, even though incomplete, and finish it a few days later rather than risk harming the patient.

At the end of the examination, firm compression is applied to the femoral puncture site as long as necessary to prevent a local hematoma. The pulses in the corre-

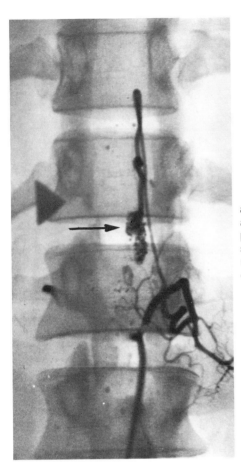

Fig 15–22.—Selective arteriography of the left first lumbar artery, with opacification of the left posterior spinal artery supplying a small thoracolumbar vascular malformation on the dorsal aspect of the spinal cord.

sponding limb are checked carefully and the patient's blood pressure, urinary output, and neurologic status monitored for several hours after the examination. In general, repeated, protracted selective injections of small volumes of contrast medium are better tolerated by the spinal cord than is a single, large intra-aortic bolus.

SELECTED PATHOLOGIC STATES

Vascular Malformations

Pantopaque myelography is a useful screening procedure in the diagnosis of vascular malformations of the spinal cord because of the frequent atypical clinical and neurologic findings. In our series, specific myelographic evidence of a vascular malformation occurred in 48% of the cases. The characteristic appearance is that of multiple, serpiginous filling defects in the oil column (Fig 15–15). Abnormalities not considered to be characteristic occurred in 42% of the cases, whereas 10% of the patients had a normal myelogram. The quality of the study in the latter group of patients was not always satisfactory. The myelographic findings depend on the size, number, and configuration of the abnormal vessels, as well as the patency of

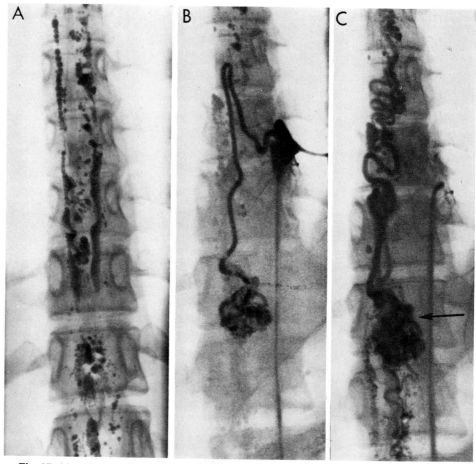

Fig 15–23.—A, myelogram in a patient with a thoracolumbar arteriovenous malformation. **B,** angiogram in the same case demonstrating the upper role of the vascular malformation supplied by the dilated arteria radicularis magna. The film was taken 4.2 sec following selective injection of the left ninth intercostal artery. **C,** later film at 8 sec showing the round angioma at T11-12 *(arrow)* as well as the prominent superior and inferior draining veins.

the subarachnoid space. In the presence of a freely communicating subarachnoid space and an extensive anomaly, the lesion commonly presents as coiled, curvilinear defects in the contrast column (Fig 15–16). However, in the presence of arachnoiditis, often secondary to bleeding, the myelogram may exhibit various atypical filling defects. Under these circumstances, the irregular spotty defects may not suggest a vascular lesion. Moreover, the so-called characteristic appearance of enlarged tortuous vessels may also be associated with some tumors, i.e., hemangioblastoma. In the latter situation, there usually is also evidence of a block suggestive of an intramedullary or an intradural extramedullary mass. Occasionally a vascular malformation alone may produce obstruction to the flow of contrast. It is important to examine the entire spinal canal in the supine as well as in the prone position. This is necessary because many vascular malformations have a predilection for the posterior surface of the cord. In addition, pulsations or changes in the size and

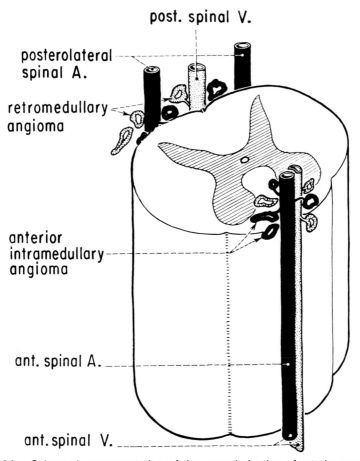

Fig 15–24.—Schematic representation of the vascularization of arteriovenous malformation of the cord, depending on their location. The anterior spinal artery supplies the anterior intramedullary or anterior juxtaspinal malformations; the two posterior spinal arteries supply the posterior intramedullary or posterior juxtaspinal malformations.

shape of a defect at fluoroscopy following the Valsalva maneuver are helpful diagnostic signs.

In summary, positive contrast myelography is useful in a significant number of cases in suggesting the possibility of a vascular abnormality. However, it does not provide an accurate anatomical or dynamic evaluation of the lesion, nor is it helpful in planning therapy. Finally, a negative myelogram does not exclude an angioma.

Vascular malformations occur much more commonly in the brain than in the cord. In most patients, symptoms first appear in childhood or early adult life. In our series, 80% of patients were under 45 years of age and half of them under 14 years at the onset of symptoms; males predominated (70%). The clinical presentation is one of variable progression of radiculomedullary involvement. Subarachnoid hemorrhage is the first sign in approximately one third of the patients. The classic picture consists of spinal subarachnoid hemorrhage with severe radicular pain and corresponding neurologic signs of spinal cord or root involvement. Associated cutaneous angiomas may be present (14% in our series), sometimes at the same seg-

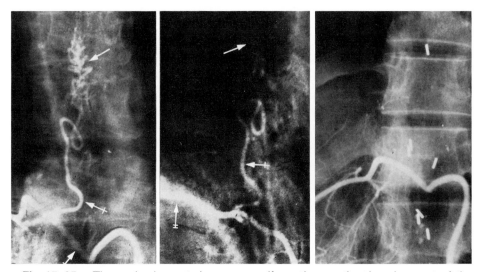

Fig 15–25.—Thoracolumbar arteriovenous malformation on the dorsal aspect of the spinal cord fed by the right twelfth intercostal artery. Preoperative frontal and lateral projections and postoperative frontal arteriogram, respectively, from left to right. Note absence of filling of the malformation in the postoperative selective arteriogram.

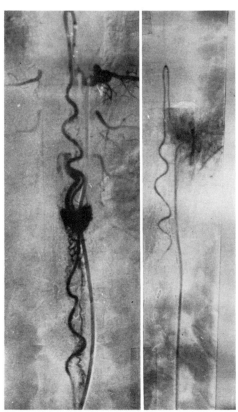

Fig 15–26.—Thoracolumbar arteriovenous malformation supplied by the left tenth intercostal artery. Pretreatment **(left)** and postembolization **(right).** Note the opacification of the osseous and muscular branches and absence of filling of the malformation on the postembolization film.

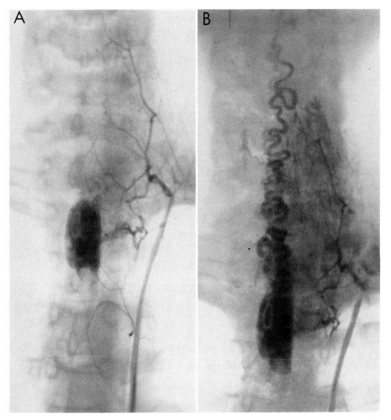

Fig 15–27.—Hemangioblastoma of the upper thoracic spinal cord supplied by the left supreme intercostal artery. The early arterial film is not reproduced. Later films show homogeneous uniform opacification of the tumor **(A)** and late filling of draining veins **(B)**.

mental dermatome. Other abnormal associations may include vertebral abnormalities, i.e., scoliosis and kyphoscoliosis, segmental vertebral hemangioma, vertebral erosions due to large arteriovenous channels, Rendu-Osler-Weber syndrome (Fig 15–17), venous and lymphatic dysplasia, combined cutaneous-vertebral-cord angiomas (Louis-Bar).

The pathology of spinal cord vascular malformations is relatively simple. Apart from the arterial dilatations associated with coarctation of the aorta (Fig 15–18), pure arterial aneurysms of the spinal cord are extremely rare. Indeed, some authorities doubt their existence. Capillary malformations such as telangiectasis and cavernous hemangioma also constitute a rare entity. These anomalies usually occur in the posterior columns and frequently are associated with similar lesions in the brain, notably the pons. I have never demonstrated such a lesion by selective arteriography. The most common abnormality is the arteriovenous malformation. In my experience (105 vascular malformations of the cord studied angiographically), every case proved to be an arteriovenous aneurysm.

Spinal arteriovenous malformations have an unequal regional distribution—12% cervical, 28% upper thoracic, 60% thoracolumbosacral, i.e., below T-8. The cervical malformations usually are medium sized, with numerous bilateral arterial feed-

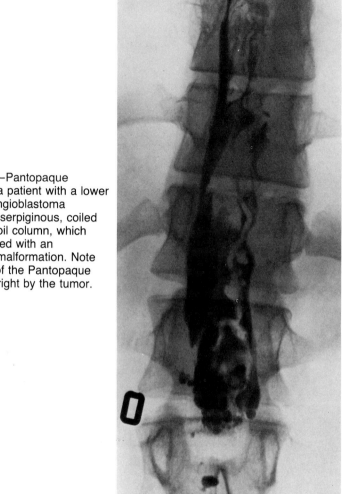

Fig 15–28.—Pantopaque myelogram in a patient with a lower thoracic hemangioblastoma demonstrating serpiginous, coiled defects in the oil column, which may be confused with an arteriovenous malformation. Note displacement of the Pantopaque column to the right by the tumor.

ers from branches of the subclavian artery, i.e., vertebral, costocervical and thyrocervical trunks (Figs 15–19, 15–20). The upper thoracic lesions tend to be large, extending over three or more vertebral segments with afferent arteries, often unilateral, arising from the aortic intercostals (Fig 15–21). The thoracolumbar malformations generally are small and tend to have a single arterial feeder like a simple arteriovenous fistula (Figs 15–22, 15–23). From a surgical point of view, the important feature is the presence or absence of intramedullary penetration of the abnormal vessels. The relatively uncommon intramedullary angiomas (18%) are nourished by an anterior blood supply and are inoperable. The mixed malformations, supplied by both anterior and posterior arterial feeders, constitute 32% of the cases. Fortunately, half of the vascular malformations lie on the dorsal aspect of the cord and are perfused solely by posterior vessels (Fig 15–24). Surgical treat-

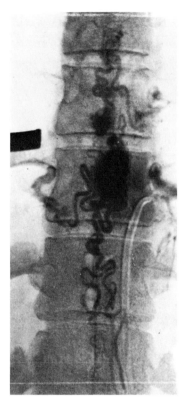

Fig 15–29.—Late film during myelography in the patient shown in Figure 15–28 after selective catheterization of the feeding intercostal artery on the left side. Note the homogeneous tumor blush and the extensive persisting venous drainage.

ment of the latter group consists of intradural ligation of the feeding vessel or vessels followed by extirpation of the malformation when feasible (Fig 15–25). Embolization by the injection of Gelfoam or clot into the catheter is an alternative method of treatment (Fig 15–26).

Hemangioblastoma

The association of spinal cord and cerebellar hemangioblastomas is a common one, especially in von Hippel-Lindau disease. If a lesion is found in either of these sites, the other should be investigated by appropriate radiologic studies, as clinically indicated. Since multiple hemangioblastomas of the cord may occur, control angiography of the entire cord is indicated.

As of January 1972, our experience consisted of angiography of 85 spinal cord tumors, including 20 cases of hemangioblastoma. The latter is a highly vascular tumor with a characteristic angiographic appearance similar to that seen in cerebellar hemangioblastoma. Although the findings may superficially resemble those of an arteriovenous malformation, they can readily be differentiated from the latter (Figs 15–27 to 15–29). Hemangioblastoma is characterized by (1) relatively early opacification of the tumor blood supply in the form of a fine network of vessels with later filling of vascular lakes within the tumor, (2) a sharply defined, persistent tumor blush, (3) late filling of draining veins. The last occasionally may be large enough to produce a block of the contrast column at a distance from the tumor, thereby resulting in false localization. These signs are in contrast to the rapid succession of the arterial, arteriovenous, and venous phases, and the absence of a tumor blush in vascular malformations. In addition, most arteriovenous malformations have an accelerated blood flow with early venous filling. Also, the malformation has an irregular areolar appearance suggestive of the superimposition of the malformed arteries and veins that constitute the lesion.

BIBLIOGRAPHY

Adamkiewicz A.: Die Blutgefässe des menschlichen Rückenmarkes. *S.B. Heidelberg Akad. Wiss.* 84:469, 1883; 85:101, 1882.

Adams H.D., van Geertruyden H.H.: Neurologic complications of aortic surgery. *Ann. Surg.* 144:574, 1956.

Ainslie J.P.: Paraplegia due to spontaneous extradural or subdural haemorrhage. *Br. J. Surg.* 45:565, 1958.

Antoni N.: Spinal vascular malformations (angiomas) and myelomalacia. *Neurology* 12:795, 1962.

Bar G.F.J.M., Hesslinga E.M.: Extradural varix resembling protrusion of nucleus pulposus; case. *Nederl. Tijdschr. Geneesk.* 85:3897, 1941.

Bassett R.C., Peet M.M., Holt J.F.: Pial medullary angiomas. Clinicopathologic features and treatment. *Arch. Neurol. Psychiatr.* 61:558, 1949.

Bergstrand A., Höök O., Lidvall H.: Vascular malformations of the spinal cord. *Acta Neurol. Scandinav.* 40:169, 1964.

Black W.C., Faber H.K.: Blood vessel tumor of spinal cord in a boy aged 9 years, with special reference to a new diagnostic syndrome. *J.A.M.A.* 104:1889, 1935.

Bolton B.: The blood supply of the human spinal cord. *J. Neurol., Neurosurg. Psychiatr.* 2: 137, 1939.

Brion S., Netsky M.G., Zimmerman H.M.: Vascular malformations of the spinal cord. *A.M.A. Arch. Neurol. Psychiatr.* 68:339, 1952.

Buchanan D.N., Walker A.E.: Vascular anomalies of spinal cord in children. *Am. J. Dis. Child.* 61:928, 1941.

Buckley A.C.: Hematomyelia secondary to hemangioma. *J. Nerv. Ment. Dis.* 83:422, 1936.

Bucy P.C.: Blood vessel tumors of the spinal canal. *Surg. Clin. North Am.* 12:1323, 1932.

Cobb S.: Haemangioma of the spinal cord, associated with skin naevi of the same metamere. *Ann. Surg.* 62:641, 1915.

Cohen I.: Extradural varix simulating herniated nucleus pulposus. *J. Mt. Sinai Hosp.* 8:136, 1941.

Corbin J.L.: *Rechesches anatomiques sur la vascularisation artérielle de la moelle; leur contribution à l'étude de l'ischémie médullaire d'origine artérielle.* Paris, Masson et Cie, 1961.

Cross G.O.: Subarachnoid cervical angioma with cutaneous hemangioma of a corresponding metamere. Report of a case and review of the literature. *Arch. Neurol. Psychiatr.* 58:359, 1947.

DiChiro G.: Combined retino-cerebellar angiomatosis and deep cervical angiomas. *J. Neurosurg.* 14:685, 1957.

DiChiro G., Doppman J., Ommaya A.S.: Selective arteriography of arteriovenous aneurysms of the spinal cord. *Radiology* 88:1065, 1967.

Djindjian R.: L'angiographié en couleurs en neuro-radiologie. Une methóde nouvelle de soustraction en couleurs. *Atlas Radiol. Clin.* 72:1, 1964.

Djindjian R., Cophignon J., Theron J., et al.: Embolization in vascular neuroradiology (technique and indications in connection with 30 cases). *Nouv. Presse Méd.* 1:2153, 1972.

Djindjian R., Dumesnil M., Fauré C., et al.: Étude angiographique d'un angioma intrarachidien. *Rev. Neurol.* 106:278, 1962.

Djindjian R., Dumesnil M., Fauré C., Tavernier J.B.: Angiome medullaire dorsal (étude clinique et arteriographique). *Rev. Neurol.* 108:432, 1963.

Djindjian R., Fauré C.: Investigations neuroradiologiques (arteriographie et phlebographie) dans les malformations vasculaires medullaires. *Roentgen-Europ.* 6–7:171, 1963.

Djindjian R., Fauré C.: Die neuroradiologischen Untersuchungsmethoden bei den Gefassmissbildungen im Rückenmark (Arteriographie and Phlebographie). *Roentgen-Europ.* 6–7:184, 1963.

Djindjian R., Fauré C., Houdart R., Lefebvre J.: *Arteriographie des Angiomes Medullaires. La Radiographie des Formations Intra-Rachidiennes.* Paris, Masson, 1965.

Djindjian R., Fauré C., Hurth M., et al.: Exploration angiographique des malformations vasculaires de la moelle épinière. *Acta Radiol.* 5(n.s.):142, 1966.

Djindjian R., Fauré C., Hurth M.: *Explorations Arteriographiques des Aneurysmes Arterioveineux de la Moelle Epiniere.* Paris, Expansion Scientifique, 1966.

Djindjian R., Hurth M., Houdart R.: *L'angiographie de la Möelle Épinière (Angiography of the Spinal Cord).* Paris, Masson, 1970.

Djindjian R., Hurth M., Houdart R.: Medullary angiomas, segmental or generalized vascular dysplasias and phacomatoses. *Rev. Neurol.* 124:121, 1971.

Djindjian R., Hurth M., Houdart R.: Medullary hemangioblastomas and von Hippel-Lindau disease. *Rev. Neurol.* 124:495, 1971.

Doppman J., DiChiro G.: The arteria radicularis magna: Radiographic anatomy in the adult. *Br. J. Radiol.* 41:40, 1968.

Epstein B.S.: Low back pain associated with varices of the epidural veins simulating herniation of the nucleus pulposus. *Am. J. Roentgenol.* 57:736, 1947.

Epstein B.S., Davidoff L.: The roentgenological diagnosis of dilatation of the spinal cord veins. *Am. J. Roentgenol.* 49:476, 1943.

Ernst E.C., Jr., Heilbrun N.: Diagnosis of intraspinal hemangiomas by myelography. *Radiology* 54:417, 1950.

Fine R.D.: Angioma racemosum venosum of spinal cord with segmentally related angiomatous lesions of skin and forearm. *J. Neurosurg.* 18:546, 1961.

Gilbert I.: Angioma venosum racemosum with angiomatous lesions of skin and omentum. *Br. Med. J.* 1:468, 1952.

Gillilan L.A.: The arterial blood supply of the human spinal cord. *J. Comp. Neurol.* 110:75, 1958.

Globus J.H., Doshay L.J.: Venous dilatations and other intraspinal vessel alterations, including true angiomata with signs and symptoms of cord compression. *Surg., Gynecol. Obstet.* 48:345, 1929.

Gold M.E.: Spontaneous spinal epidural hematoma. *Radiology* 80:823, 1963.

Gross S.W., Ralston B.L.: Vascular malformations of the spinal cord. *Surg., Gynecol. Obstet.* 108:673, 1959.

Hare C.C., Everts W.H.: Calcified subpial lesions of the spinal cord with associated varicose veins. *Bull. Neurol. Inst., New York* 6:295, 1937.

Henson R.A., Croft P.B.: Spontaneous subarachnoid hemorrhage. *Quart. J. Med.* 25:53, 1956.

Hieke I.: Über Hämatomyelie bei intramedullären Telangiektasien. *Beitr. Path. Anat.* 110:433, 1949.

Höök O., Lidvall H.: Arteriovenous aneurysms of the spinal cord. A report of 2 cases investigated by vertebral angiography. *J. Neurosurg.* 15:84, 1958.

Houdart R., Djindjian R., Hurth M.: Vascular malformations of the spinal cord. *J. Neurosurg.* 24:583, 1966.

Jackson F.E.: Spontaneous spinal epidural hematoma coincident with whooping cough. Case report. *J. Neurosurg.* 20:715, 1963.

Kadyi H.: Quoted by Wyburn-Mason, R.: *Vascular Abnormalities and Tumours of the Spinal Cord and Its Membranes.* London, H. Kimpton, 1943.

Kortzeborn A.: Laminektomie bei angioma racemosum des Rückenmarks. *Zentralbl. Chir.* 56:868, 1929.

Lazorthes G., Gouaze A., Zadeh J.O., et al.: Arterial vascularisation of the spinal cord. Recent studies of the anastomotic substitution pathways. *J. Neurosurg.* 35:253, 1971.

Levy A., Klinger M.: Spontaneous spinal epidural hematoma. *Acta Neurochir.* 11:530, 1964.

Lombardi G., Migliavacca F.: Angiomas of the spinal cord. *Br. J. Radiol.* 32:810, 1959.

Longheed W.M., Hoffman H.J.: Spontaneous spinal extradural hematoma. *Neurology* 10:1058, 1960.

Louis-Bar D.: Report of angiomatoses of the Sturge-Weber type and other dysplasias. Jubilee vol., *J. Belge Neurol. et Psychiatr.*, 1951, pp. 287–317.

Lowrey J.J.: Spinal epidural hematomas. Experiences with three patients. *J. Neurosurg.* 16:508, 1959.

Manelfe C., Gouaze A., Djindjian R.: *Vascularization and Circulation of the Spinal Cord.* Paris, Masson, 1973.

Margolis G., Odom G.L., Woodhall B., Bloor B.M.: Role of small angiomatous malformations in production of intracerebral hematomas. *J. Neurosurg.* 8:564, 1951.

Morris L.: Angioma of cervical spinal cord. Case report. *Radiology* 75:785, 1960.

Newman M.J.: Racemose angioma of the spinal cord. *Quart. J. Med.* 28:97, 1959.

Nichols P., Jr., Manganiello L.O.J.: Extradural hematoma of the spinal canal. Report of a case. *J. Neurosurg.* 13:638, 1956.

Odom G.L., Woodhall B., Margolis G.: Spontaneous hematomyelia and angiomas of the spinal cord. *J. Neurosurg.* 14:192, 1957.

Pia H.N., Vogelsang H.: Diagnosis and treatment of spinal angiomas. *Ztschr. Nervenheilk.* 187:74, 1965.

Piatt A.D.: Varicosities of spinal canal veins in lumbar region simulating disk herniations. *Ohio Med. J.* 45:979, 1949.

Richardson J.C.: Spontaneous haematomyelia: A short review and a report of cases illustrating intramedullary angioma and syphilis of the spinal cord as possible causes. *Brain* 61:17, 1938.

Schultz E.C., et al.: Paraplegia caused by spontaneous spinal epidural hemorrhage. *J. Neurosurg.* 10:608, 1953.

Suh T.H., Alexander L.: Vascular system of the human spinal cord. *Arch. Neurol. Psychiatr.* 41:659, 1939.

Svien H.J., Baker H.L.: Roentgenographic and surgical aspects of vascular anomalies of spinal cord. *Surg., Gynecol. Obstet.* 112:729, 1961.

Svien H.J., Peserico L.: Spontaneous epidural hematoma of the cervical region; report of case. *Proc. Staff Meet. Mayo Clin.* 34:309, 1959.

Tanon L.: Les artéres de la moelle dorso-lumbaire. Thesis. Paris, Vigo, 1908.

Taylor A.R.: Surgical treatment of spinal arterio-malformations. *J. Neurol., Neurosurg. Psychiatr.* 4:578, 1964.

Teng P., Papatheodoru C.: Myelographic appearance of vascular anomalies of the spinal cord. *Br. J. Radiol.* 37:358, 1964.

Teng P., Shapiro M.J.: Arterial anomalies of spinal cord. Myelographic diagnosis and treatment by section of dentate ligaments. *A.M.A. Arch. Neurol. Psychiatr.* 80:577, 1958.

Therkelsen J.: Angioma racemosum venosum medullae spinalis. *Acta Psychiatr. et Neurol. Scandinav.* 33:219, 1958.

Tureen L.L.: Circulation of the spinal cord and the effect of vascular occlusion. *Res. Publ. Ass. Res. Nerv. Ment. Dis.* 18:394, 1938.

Turner O.A., Kernohan J.W.: Vascular malformations and vascular tumors involving the spinal cord: Pathologic study of 46 cases. *Arch. Neurol. Psychiatr.* 46:444, 1941.

Van Bogaert L.: Pathology of the angiomatoses. Jubilee vol., *J. Belge Neurol. et Psychiatr.*, 1951, pp. 393–516.

Verbiest H., Calliauw L.: Les angiomes racemeux intraduraux de la moelle épinière. *Rev. Neurol.* 102:230, 1960.

Vraa-Jensen G.: Angioma of the spinal cord. *Acta Psychiatr. et Neurol. Scandinav.* 24:709, 1949.

Wende S.: Neuroradiological diagnosis of spinal vascular malformations. *Radiologe* 2:227, 1962.

Wyburn-Mason R.: *Vascular Abnormalities and Tumors of the Spinal Cord and Its Membranes.* London, H. Kimpton, 1943.

16

Tumors

TUMORS OF THE SPINAL CORD are pathologically similar, although less common than brain tumors (1:6). They may arise from the neural tissue, from the meninges, from the surrounding bone and soft tissues, from embryonal rests, or as metastases from neoplasms in the cranial cavity or elsewhere in the body.

For purposes of discussion, spinal cord tumors may be classified as intramedullary, extramedullary intradural, and extramedullary extradural. In the adult, the incidence of intramedullary tumors has been variously estimated to be 7–22% (15% probably is a fair average), extramedullary intradural tumors 53–65%, and extramedullary extradural tumors 28–30%. Some extramedullary tumors may penetrate through openings in the dura to involve the subdural and extradural spaces. In a series of 317 spinal tumors reported by Lombardi and Passerini, 11% of the lesions were both intradural and extradural. Most of the latter tumors were dumbbell neurilemomas, although there also were a few meningiomas. In a series of 557 intraspinal tumors from the Mayo Clinic, Rasmussen, Kernohan, and Adson reported the following incidence of location:

Cervical	18%
Thoracic	54%
Lumbar	21%
Sacral	7%
Multiple levels	1%

Although spinal cord tumors may occur at any age, they are more common between the third and sixth decades, with no apparent sex preponderance.

There are a number of significant differences between spinal tumors in childhood and in adults. First, the anatomical distribution differs, with a greater concentration in the cervical, lumbar, and sacral regions in childhood, largely due to the increased frequency of congenital lesions in these areas. In a series of 61 intraspinal tumors in children reported by Ingraham and Matson, 17 were cervical and cervicothoracic, 22 thoracic and thoracolumbar, and 22 lumbar and sacral in location. Second, intramedullary and extradural tumors occur with greater frequency and extramedullary intradural tumors with considerably less frequency in childhood. Finally, the relative incidence of the various pathologic types of spinal cord tumor differs considerably (Fig 16–1). Gliomas and congenital tumors are more common

345

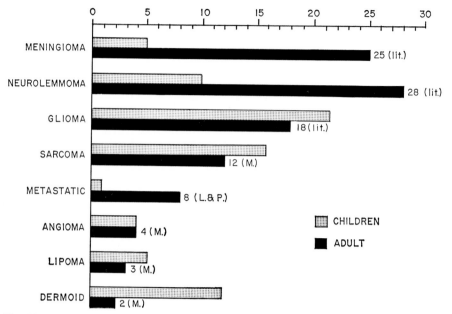

Fig 16–1.—Graph showing comparison of tumor types in children and adults (modified from Haft, Ransohoff and Carter). Abbr.: *lit.,* literature; *M,* Merritt, H. H., *Textbook of Neurology.* Philadelphia, Lea & Febiger, 1955; *L. & P.,* Lombardi G., Passerini A.: *Spinal Cord Diseases.* Baltimore, Williams & Wilkins Co., 1965.

in children, whereas meningiomas and neurilemomas are much more frequent in the adult (meningioma: 6 to 1; neurilemoma: 3 to 1). Ependymomas and astrocytomas constitute approximately one third of the acquired tumors in children. Occasionally they are quite bulky and may extend from the foramen magnum to the lumbar area. These so-called giant tumors of the spinal cord are often associated with scoliosis.

In addition to the local bone changes due to expanding intraspinal lesions described in Chapter 6, metastatic tumors may produce osteoblastic or osteolytic lesions in the spine with or without an associated paraspinal mass.

INTRAMEDULLARY TUMORS

These neoplasms are predominantly gliomas (Figs 16–2 to 16–9). Subgroups in this category include ependymoma, astrocytoma, oligodendroglioma, glioblastoma multiforme, and medulloblastoma.

By far the most common glioma of the spinal cord is the ependymoma (65% of all intraspinal gliomas), which may involve the cord or the conus and filum terminale. In the filum terminale, it may appear as a fusiform swelling or as one or more fairly well-encapsulated nodules. The latter type of tumor lends itself to almost complete surgical removal, since it presents more or less as an extramedullary lesion. Rarely, the tumor may be confined to the extradural portion of the filum terminale or have both an intradural and an extradural localization. Ependymomas of the conus and filum are frequently large, bulky lesions extending over a consid-

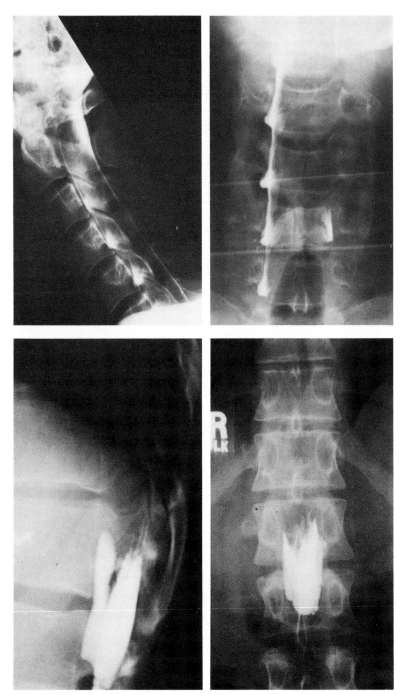

Fig 16–2.—Metrizamide myelogram of the cervical cord performed via C1-2 puncture **(top)** and Pantopaque study carried out by lumbar puncture **(bottom)** in a 30-year-old man with a cystic astrocytoma involving the entire cord down to the conus.

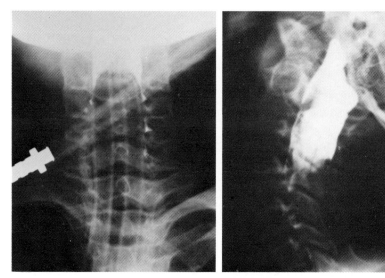

Fig 16–3.—Metrizamide cervical myelogram performed via C1-2 puncture in a 13-year-old girl with an ependymoma involving the cervical cord from C-3 to C-7. Note the almost total obstruction at C3-4.

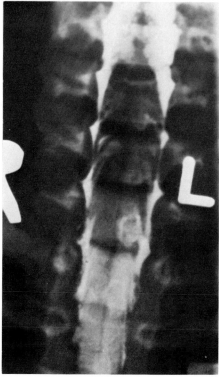

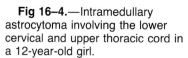

Fig 16–4.—Intramedullary astrocytoma involving the lower cervical and upper thoracic cord in a 12-year-old girl.

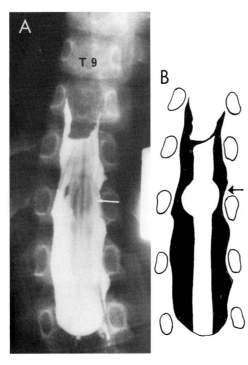

Fig 16–5.—Intramedullary glioblastoma multiforme of the lower thoracic cord. The patient was a 6½-year-old boy with paresis of the right lower extremity of 6 months' duration, without pain or bladder dysfunction. Physical examination revealed moderate weakness of the right leg, more marked in the proximal half, but no sensory level. Note the complete block and splaying of the oil column due to enlargement of the cord. Note also the separate tumor nodule at T-12 *(arrow)*. At surgery, the tumor, which extended from T-7 to L-1, presented anterolaterally with a well-delineated firm capsule within the substance of the cord.

erable distance, filling the entire circumference of the spinal canal. Under these circumstances, they may produce thinning and erosion of the pedicles, with enlargement and scalloping of the bony canal over several vertebral segments (see Fig 16–7). However, the small encapsulated ependymoma may not give rise to any detectable bone changes. Woltman has recorded an unusually mobile, 7-cm-long ependymoma of the filum terminale that moved freely in an axial direction during myelography and at surgery because of unusual laxity of the filum terminale. Rarely, ependymomas of the cauda equina may mimic intracranial lesions by presenting with increased intracranial pressure due to subarachnoid hemorrhage or the secretion of abnormal proteins.

The second most common glioma is the astrocytoma, which constitutes approximately 30% of intraspinal gliomas. Less common gliomas include glioblastoma multiforme, oligodendroglioma, and medulloblastoma. The remaining uncommon intramedullary tumors are made up of a miscellaneous group including dermoid cyst, melanoma, sarcoma, and hemangioblastoma.

Hemangioblastoma may be found as an isolated intramedullary lesion throughout the spinal axis with some predilection for the cervicothoracic and thoracolumbar regions. Rarely, hemangioblastoma may occur as a purely extradural tumor. The tumors may be multiple or part of von Hippel-Lindau disease, a congenital complex consisting of hemangioblastomas (often cystic) of the cerebellum, medulla, or cord; angiomatosis of the retina; and cysts or benign tumors of the pancreas, adrenals, kidneys, or ovaries. When the tumor extends out to the pia mater, it is often associated with marked pial varicosities that may resemble a vascular malformation (Fig 16–10). The syndrome also may be associated with vascular nevi and dilated pial veins above and below the spinal cord tumor. The disease has been reported oc-

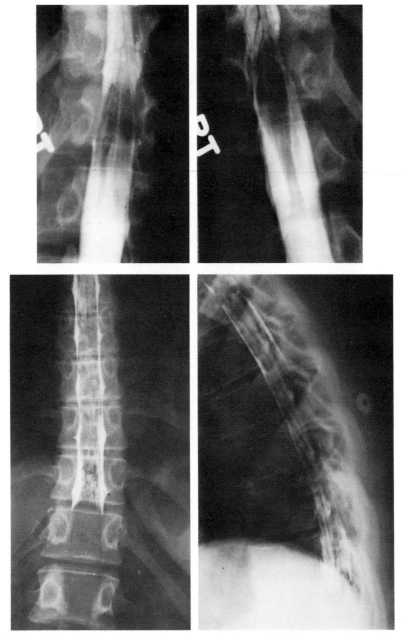

Fig 16–6.—Oligodendroglioma (a rare tumor in the cord) of the conus in a 20-year-old female who presented with a foot drop on July 26, 1971 **(top).** The patient had a surgical decompression followed by radiation therapy. Because of progression of symptoms, repeat metrizamide myelography was done via C1-2 puncture on November 26, 1971 **(bottom).** This demonstrates a complete block at T11-12.

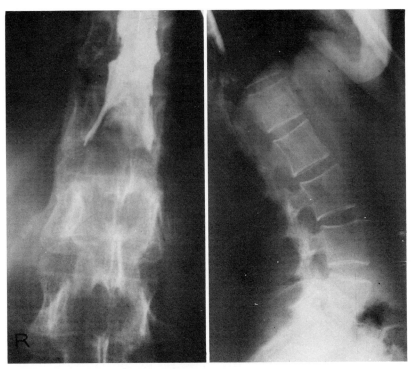

Fig 16–7.—Large ependymoma involving the conus medullaris and cauda equina and extending from T-11 to L-5. The anteroposterior view demonstrates erosion of the pedicles and widening of the interpediculate distance, whereas the lateral projection shows enlargement of the vertebral canal and excavation of the posterior surface of several lumbar vertebrae. The marked splaying and widening of the conus medullaris indicates the intramedullary location of the lesion.

casionally in families with transmission as a simple, nonsex-linked dominant. When multiple tumors are present, one or more lesions may be found along the nerve roots or cauda equina in addition to the underlying intramedullary tumor. Both cerebellar and spinal hemangioblastomas frequently have a cystic component containing fluid with a high protein content.

The diagnosis of hemangioblastoma should be considered in (1) patients with a spinal tumor who have an associated retinal angioma and/or cerebellar lesion, (2) patients who present with a spinal cord lesion after surgical excision of a cerebellar hemangioblastoma, and (3) patients with serpiginous, worm-like defects at myelography and intramedullary expansion of the cord (although similar findings may occur in other intramedullary gliomas). Confusion of the myelographic findings with arteriovenous malformation of the cord may present a problem that can be resolved by selective arteriography with subtraction. Hemangioblastoma is characterized by diffuse, uniform staining of the tumor nodule, whereas AV malformations show congeries of individual, separate vessels. In addition, there is no evidence of rapid shunting from arteries to veins in hemangioblastoma.

Primary neuroblastoma of the spinal axis is extremely rare. When it occurs, it presents either as (1) an intramedullary tumor of the spinal cord similar to its coun-

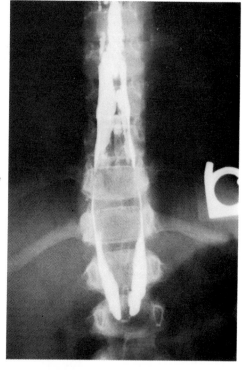

Fig 16–8.—Astrocytoma of conus in a 10-year-old boy first diagnosed 8 years previously. Note the cord expansion extending from T-10 to the conus at L1-2.

terpart in the brain, or (2) a lesion arising from ganglion cells, e.g., in the dorsal ganglion.

Myelography plays a vital role in the diagnosis of all intramedullary tumors (Figs 16–2 to 16–14). When the tumor produces complete obstruction, correct differential diagnosis from various extramedullary tumors may not always be possible. In this situation, contrast medium injected below the level of the tumor may delineate a well-defined, smooth, lower border of the lesion. More frequently, however, the tumor produces a partial block. Under such circumstances, the diffusely infiltrated swollen cord usually displaces the subarachnoid contrast on either side. This produces a wide, central radiolucency representing the dilated cord, with a linear, streak-like density to one or both sides corresponding to the narrowed subarachnoid space. In addition, there may be a beaded appearance on either side of the cord for several segments when the nerve root sheaths are filled with contrast. It is important to remember that this appearance merely represents enlargement of the spinal cord and is not necessarily pathognomonic of neoplasm. It may also be seen in myelitis, intramedullary granuloma or abscess, intramedullary hematoma, and syringomyelia (see Figs 16–11 to 16–14).

Syringohydromyelia

Syringomyelia and hydromyelia may manifest themselves as a relatively localized lesion involving a segment of the cord, or they may involve the entire length of the cord. In the former instance, the lesion is usually localized to the cervical cord but

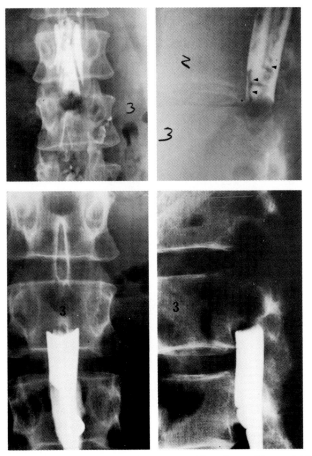

Fig 16–9.—Ependymoma of conus in a 51-year-old patient with a total block extending from the L2-3 interspace to the inferior aspect of L-3. The Pantopaque was introduced both via C1-2 puncture **(top)** and via lumbar puncture **(bottom).** Note the dilated veins *(arrowheads).*

may also extend into the thoracic region. Positive-contrast myelography in the frontal projection demonstrates symmetric narrowing of the subarachnoid space associated with an enlarged cord, an appearance identical to that produced by intramedullary tumors. The enlarged cord may be fairly round because of increased transverse and sagittal diameters (Figs 16–22, 16–23), or it may be flattened in the sagittal diameter. In patients with an abnormally small cord due to atrophy or a normal-sized cord, there is no problem in differential diagnosis from an intramedullary tumor. Air myelography demonstrates a collapsing cord in the semierect position, thereby indicating a cystic process and excluding a solid tumor. Uncommonly, the upper cervical cord will collapse, but the enlarged lower cord will remain distended because of adhesions. Collapse of the cervical cord presumes a communication with the fourth ventricle. In patients with collapsed syringohydromyelia, a metrizamide myelogram commonly shows narrowing of the sagittal diameter of the spinal cord in the lateral projection. The concomitant widening of the transverse

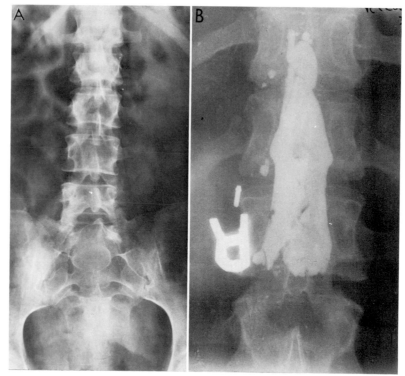

Fig 16–10.—Anteroposterior radiograph of the lumber spine **(A)** in a young woman with a large hemangioblastoma extending from L-1 to S-3. Note the erosion of the pedicles and the lumbosacral vertebral bodies. The prone myelographic spot film **(B)** shows a complete block at the lower border of L-1 as well as dilated serpiginous pial vessels.

diameter of the flattened cord may be difficult to assess on the routine frontal film. If laminography does not resolve the problem, CT is most helpful.

Kendall and Symon recommend cyst puncture and endomyelography to facilitate the specific diagnosis of elongated expanding cord lesions. This technique was originally described in 1928 by Vitek, who used Lipiodol as the contrast medium. In 1966, Westburg reported nine patients with intramedullary cystic lesions of the cervical cord diagnosed by pneumomyelography in whom he aspirated the cysts. Kendall and Symon indicate that puncture should be performed on patients with extensive expansion of the spinal cord to determine whether a cyst is present. They introduce a fine spinal needle as low as possible into the lesion and aspirate the cyst fluid. Complete aspiration is preferable if the cyst puncture is meant to be therapeutic. For diagnostic purposes, however, only enough fluid is aspirated for chemical and cytologic analysis, to avoid collapse of the cyst. This is followed by the injection of 1–2 ml of Pantopaque or metrizamide to outline the entire cyst and to demonstrate the presence or absence of a mural tumor nodule.

The introduction of Pantopaque into the cystic cavity by direct puncture may demonstrate a unique pattern, i.e., a series of constrictions of the dilated oil column resembling a stack of coins or a string of sausages. Harwood-Nash and Fitz suggest that the constrictions are due to irregular collections of glial fibers arranged in a circumferential fashion. This appearance, which is strongly suggestive of syringo-

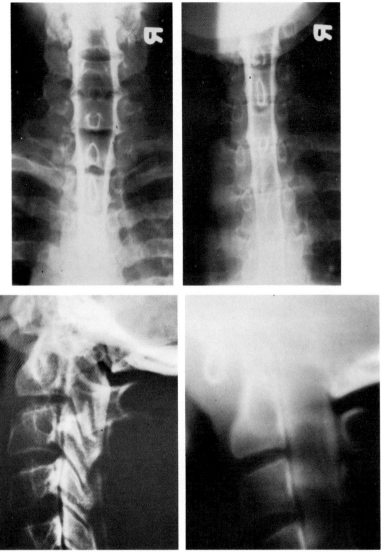

Fig 16–11.—Metrizamide myelogram in a 30-year-old woman with syringomyelia (surgically proved). The frontal films **(top)** demonstrate the extent of the lesion down to T-1. The lateral films **(bottom)** demonstrate the associated assimilation of the posterior arch of C-1 into the basiocciput, subluxation of a hypoplastic dens, and basilar invagination.

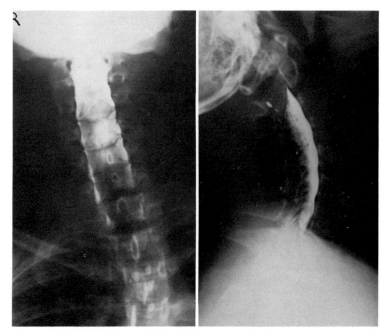

Fig 16–12.—Anteroposterior and lateral myelographic films in a patient with syringo-myelia of the lower cervical and upper thoracic cord.

myelia, is helpful in arriving at the correct diagnosis in patients without cord collapse because of absence of communication with the fourth ventricle. The presence of a smooth-walled cyst, cerebellar tonsillar herniation, and a collapsing cord favor the diagnosis of hydromyelia.

CT has greatly facilitated the diagnosis of syringohydromyelia. The characteristic appearance is a well-defined, low-attenuation intramedullary cyst in an enlarged cord (see Fig 16–14). Following injection of metrizamide into the subarachnoid space, the contrast medium slowly enters the cystic cavity and opacifies it after several hours (see Fig 16–14,C). However, the hydrodynamic aspects of the lesion, i.e., whether there is free communication of fluid within the cystic cavity, are best studied by myelography with air and metrizamide.

Primary Melanoma

Primary melanoma of the spinal cord is extremely rare, with only 27 cases reported in the literature. To qualify for this category, the cord tumor should be the only lesion in the central nervous system, with no history or evidence of a melanoma elsewhere. According to Hirano and Carton, their patient is the only recorded case of primary intramedullary melanoma established by operation and biopsy in which subsequent complete postmortem examination failed to reveal any other central nervous system lesion. Since melanin-containing cells are normally found in the meninges, it is presumed that primary spinal melanomas are meningeal in origin. The tumor may be intramedullary with minimal local meningeal involvement, intra- and extramedullary, or extramedullary-intradural (see Fig 16–15). In a review of 25 cases reported in the literature by Hirano and Carton, mye-

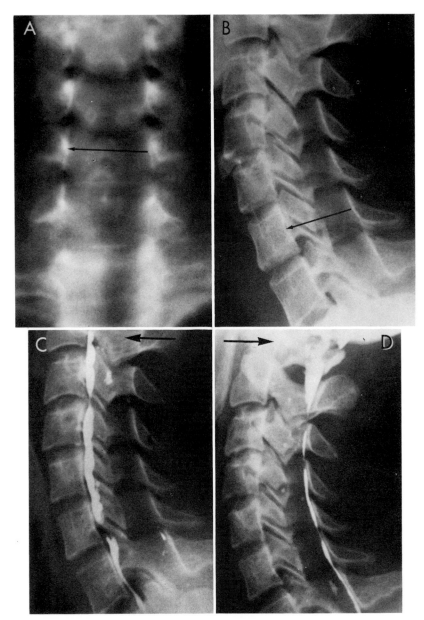

Fig 16–13.—Syringomyelia with diffuse symmetric expansion of the entire cervical cord. Note the thinning of the pedicles in the anteroposterior tomogram *(arrow)* in **A,** as well as the wide sagittal diameter of the bony cervical canal *(arrow)* in **B.** Lateral radiographs with the horizontal beam in **C,** the prone, and **D,** the supine positions provide an accurate index of the anteroposterior diameter of the spinal cord.

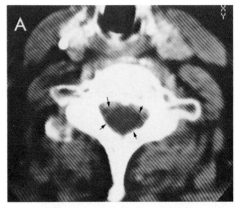
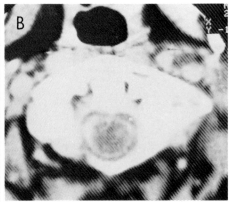
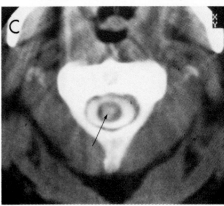

Fig 16–14.—A, axial CT of the cervical spine at level of T-4 in a patient with syringomyelia. Note the widened cord *(arrows)*. **B,** axial CT study at level of C-1 after lumbar injection of 5 ml of metrizamide (170 mg I/ml). Note the marked asymmetric narrowing of the subarachnoid space due to the enlarged cord. **C,** delayed metrizamide myelogram in a 32-year-old man with syringomyelia extending from C5-7. Axial scan at C-6 demonstrating penetration of the contrast into the cystic cavity *(arrow)*.

lography had been performed in 10 patients. There were abnormalities in nine patients, seven of whom had a complete block. Total surgical extirpation was accomplished in three cases of extramedullary intradural tumor and in one case of extradural tumor. In only one case was the correct preoperative diagnosis made because of "coal-black" cerebrospinal fluid at myelography. At the time of operation, the diagnosis may not be obvious if there is a pigmented mass associated with a vascular lesion, for melanoma often is hemorrhagic and difficult to distinguish grossly from a hematoma. Although these tumors tend to recur and seed throughout the cerebrospinal axis, they do not usually metastasize outside the central nervous system.

EXTRAMEDULLARY INTRADURAL TUMORS

This group represents the largest number of spinal cord tumors, mostly benign, and is composed principally of meningiomas and nerve sheath tumors, which occur with equal frequency in several series.

Meningiomas

According to Wolf, spinal meningiomas originate from cells covering the arachnoidal villi. They have a definite predilection for females (80–85% are found in

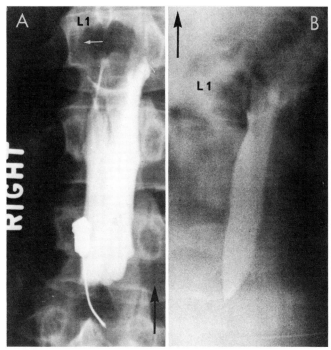

Fig 16–15.—Melanoma of the conus medullaris. The patient, a 17-year-old girl, was seen originally because of low back pain and left-sided sciatica. She had a hemilaminectomy by an orthopedic surgeon for a bulging disk at L5-S1 without previous myelography. She was readmitted 10 months later because her pain had not improved postoperatively. At the time of readmission, there was evidence of thinning of the right pedicle at L-1 *(arrow),* **A.** Lumbar puncture performed at myelography revealed a spinal fluid protein level of 920 mg/100 ml. Myelography, **A** and **B,** demonstrated a complete block at L-1, with a sharply defined cap defect anterior to the conus characteristic of an extradural tumor. At operation, an elongated extramedullary intradural tumor was found anterior to the conus. The tumor was firm, jet black in color, and extended from T-12 to the lower border of L-1. Excision was incomplete because of recurrent brisk hemorrhage. A near total removal of the tumor was accomplished at a second-stage procedure. At this time, a few fragments of tumor capsule intimately associated with the conus were left behind. The patient received a course of postoperative radiation.

women), tend to occur later in life than neurilemomas (average age at diagnosis was 50 years in Bull's series), and favor the thoracic segment of the spine. Thus, in the Mayo Clinic series of 140 spinal meningiomas, Rasmussen and his colleagues reported the following distribution:

Cervical	16.5%
Thoracic	82%
Lumbar	1.5%

These tumors vary in size from a small nodule to a large, lobulated mass. The usual spinal meningioma is a fairly small, single, discrete, round or oval, intradural tumor (Figs 16–16 to 16–26). Occasionally it may be multiple; at times, it may be both intradural and extradural (7%). Extradural meningiomas are rare, representing less than 77% of all spinal meningiomas. They tend to occur in younger patients, particularly in males. The correct preoperative diagnosis can be established by an-

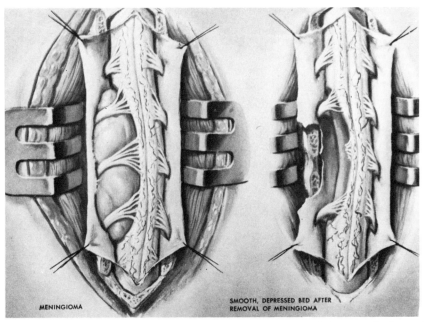

Fig 16–16.—Artist's drawing of lateral-lying intradural extramedullary meningioma demonstrating narrowing of the cord with displacement to the contralateral side at the site of the tumor. (From the Ciba Collection of Medical Illustrations by Frank H. Netter, M.D. Copyright Ciba.)

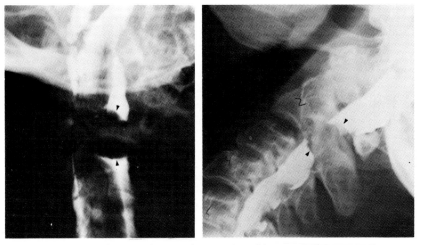

Fig 16–17.—Metrizamide myelogram in 52-year-old woman demonstrating a meningioma on the left posterolateral aspect of the cord at C-2 *(arrowheads).*

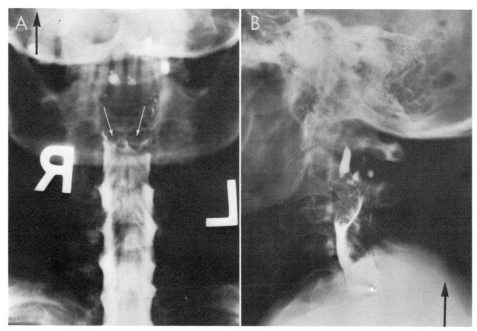

Fig 16–18.—Meningioma at C2-3 in a middle-aged woman. Note the bilobate appearance of the defect *(arrows)* in the frontal projection, **A,** and the anterior location with respect to the cord, in the lateral view, **B.**

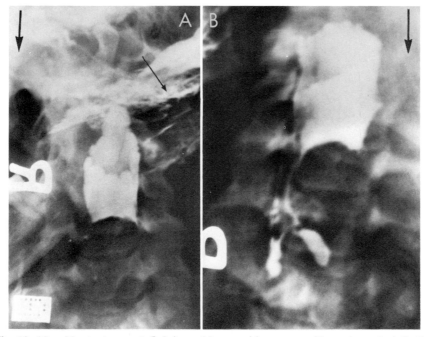

Fig 16–19.—Meningioma at C-3 in a 44-year-old woman with a characteristic "cap" defect. The contrast medium, Lipiodol, was introduced by cisternal puncture and is partially extra-arachnoid at the site of injection *(thin arrow).*

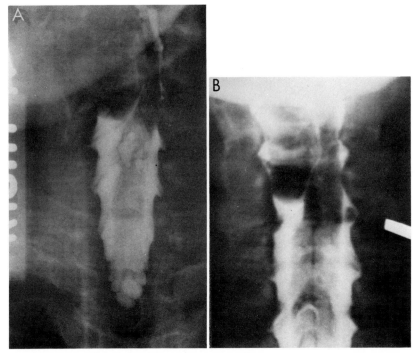

Fig 16–20.—A, intradural extramedullary meningioma of the right anterolateral aspect of the upper cervical cord, displacing the latter to the left. Note the dilated ipsilateral subarachnoid space and the similarity to the artist's drawing in Figure 16–16. **B,** intradural extramedullary neurilemoma on the right side of the cord, extending from C-2 to C-5. Obviously it would be impossible to differentiate between spinal meningiomas and neurilemomas by myelography alone.

giography, since myelography demonstrates only a nonspecific extradural mass lesion.

Meningiomas commonly exhibit microscopic calcification. Unfortunately, gross calcification recognizable on the plain roentgenogram is infrequent. When present, however, it is helpful in differential diagnosis because nerve sheath tumors do not, as a rule, calcify (see Fig 16–25). It may be difficult to differentiate calcification in a meningioma from a calcified herniated thoracic intervertebral disk. However, the disk usually lies in juxtaposition to a narrowed intervertebral disk space. Although bony changes (thinning or erosion of the pedicle in contact with the tumor, widening of the interpediculate distance) can be produced by both meningioma and neurilemoma, they are four times as common in the latter lesion. Lombardi and Passerini reported widening of an intervertebral foramen in one case of a malignant extradural meningioma.

Meningioma is the most common extramedullary intradural tumor in the region of the foramen magnum (see Fig 16–26). Although these tumors usually arise high in the cervical cord, they may have a small extension into the posterior fossa. As they compress the cord, they produce cervico-occipital pain and paresthesia, disturbed position sense (more marked in the upper extremity), weakness of the ipsilateral arm, atrophy of the small muscles of the hand, and spastic paraparesis. The

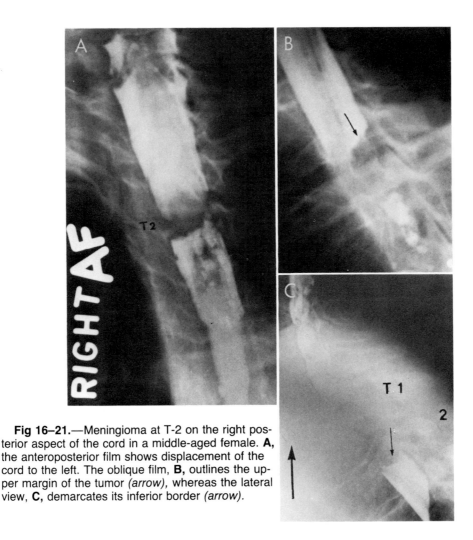

Fig 16–21.—Meningioma at T-2 on the right posterior aspect of the cord in a middle-aged female. **A,** the anteroposterior film shows displacement of the cord to the left. The oblique film, **B,** outlines the upper margin of the tumor *(arrow)*, whereas the lateral view, **C,** demarcates its inferior border *(arrow)*.

spinal accessory nerve also may be involved. Foramen magnum meningiomas are more common on the anterior surface of the cord. At myelography, the anteriorly situated tumors displace the cord posteriorly, thereby increasing the normal distance (2 mm in adults, 3 mm in children) between the dens and the anterior margin of the oil-filled subarachnoid space. These changes are best demonstrated with the patient in the prone lateral projection using the horizontal beam. Tumors on the posterior aspect of the cord produce a filling defect on the posterior margin of the contrast column, best shown in the supine lateral projection with the horizontal beam. The frontal views demonstrate displacement of the cord away from a laterally-lying tumor. Foramen magnum meningiomas commonly produce some degree of obstruction and may cause a complete block. These lesions must be distinguished from the Arnold-Chiari malformation and from chordomas of the clivus. There are some findings that may be helpful in differential diagnosis when the obstruction is incomplete. Most meningiomas are located anterolaterally, whereas the displaced cerebellar tonsils in the Arnold-Chiari malformation produce a defect on the pos-

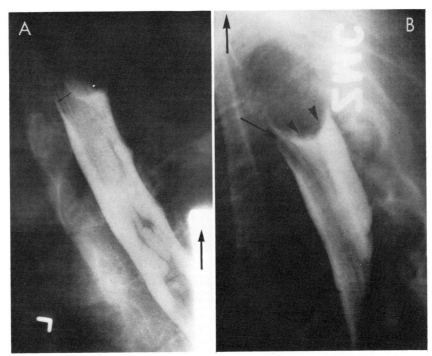

Fig 16–22.—Upper thoracic meningioma in a 60-year-old female. The cord *(arrow)* is displaced anteriorly and to the left by the tumor *(arrowheads)* lying on its right posterior aspect.

terior and lateral aspects of the contrast column. In the absence of adhesions, the Arnold-Chiari defect tends to be bilaterally symmetric. Chordomas can be suspected if they produce demonstrable bone destruction and an extradural defect at myelography (Fig 16–27).

Nerve Sheath Tumors

Unfortunately, these tumors (Figs 16–28 to 16–47) have been designated by a variety of names: neurofibroma, neurinoma, perineurial fibroblastoma, neurilemoma, schwannoma. At present, it is generally thought that these tumors arise from the cells of Schwann in the nerve sheath. Consequently, they are more properly termed neurilemomas or schwannomas. In contrast to meningiomas, neurilemomas tend to occur somewhat earlier in life (average age at diagnosis was 38 years in Bull's series) and have no predilection for sex or location. The last is illustrated by the following distribution pattern in the Mayo Clinic series of 163 neurilemomas:

Cervical	22%
Thoracic	43%
Lumbar	33.5%
Sacral	1%
Multiple levels	0.5%

Although quite variable in size and shape, these tumors tend to be larger than

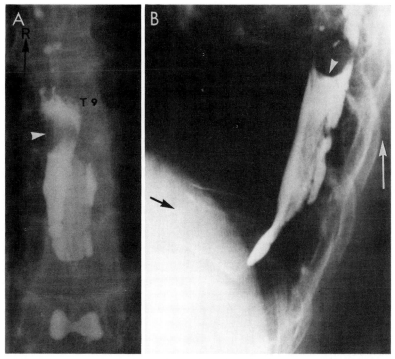

Fig 16–23.—Meningioma at T9-10 *(arrowhead)* on the right posterior aspect of the cord **(A)** in a 59-year-old woman complaining of back pain. Note the compression fracture of T-12 in **B** *(arrow)*. Conventional radiography showed a generalized decreased density of the spine as well as the fracture. The clinical impression prior to myelography was extradural cord compression at T-12 due to either osteoporosis or multiple myeloma.

meningiomas. The average neurilemoma is a smooth, soft, often cystic lesion attached to a posterior root. Unlike meningioma, it is rarely adherent to the dura. Although most neurilemomas are intradural (67%), some 16% extend from the nerve root through a dural opening to occupy both an intradural and an extradural position. An additional 16% are entirely extradural in location. These tumors usually are single but on occasion may be multiple (Fig 16–39). Rarely, meningioma and neurilemoma have been reported in the same patient. Grossly recognizable calcification in neurilemomas is extremely rare (I have seen only one case). However, calcification in extradural neuroblastoma and ganglioneuroma does occur more commonly. It is also interesting that Bull, Tönnis and associates, and Lombardi and Passerini report no neurilemomas involving the first cervical nerve at the occipitoatlantal junction. Although bone changes are four times as frequent in neurilemoma compared with meningioma, the small, purely intradural neurilemoma does not usually produce recognizable bone erosion. However, large tumors frequently are responsible for erosion of the pedicles, an increased interpediculate distance, scalloping of the posterior margins of vertebral bodies, and thinning of the laminae. Unlike the usual meningioma, which tends to produce a localized bony change, the large neurilemoma often involves two or more vertebrae. In addition, the dumbbell type of neurilemoma, which extends out of the vertebral canal along the spinal nerve root into the paraspinal region, usually enlarges the intervertebral

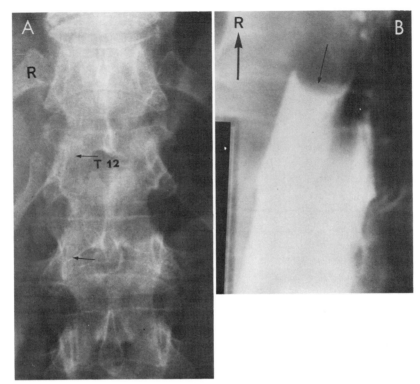

Fig 16–24.—Meningioma at T11-12 in a 49-year-old female complaining of back pain and right-sided sciatica for 10 months. The plain film of the spine, **A,** shows erosion of the right pedicles of T-12 and L-1. **B,** the oblique spot film at myelography, demonstrates the tumor *(arrow)* on the right anterolateral aspect of the cord.

foramen (Fig 16–40). It also frequently erodes adjacent ribs and produces a variable-sized soft tissue mass.

Schubiger and Yasargil reported a case of neurofibromatosis associated with a large saccular aneurysm of the vertebral artery at the level of C-4 and C-5. The conventional roentgenograms of the cervical spine and the Pantopaque myelogram were compatible with a preoperative diagnosis of neurinoma, i.e., intradural extramedullary lesion with widening of the intervertebral foramina and thinning of the pedicles at the level of the lesion. Deans et al. also described three female patients with neurofibromatosis who had arteriovenous fistulas that became symptomatic during the fifth or sixth decade. Two of the lesions involved the cervical spine and demonstrated bony erosion; one lesion involved the face. Deans suggested two possible mechanisms: (1) dysplastic smooth wall or neural proliferation in the arterial wall with secondary formation of an arteriovenous fistula, and (2) congenital AV fistula as a manifestation of the widespread mesodermal dysplasia.

Multiple neurilemomas occur occasionally, as do multiple meningiomas. Although the former may be found as isolated tumors, they are more likely to be part of generalized neurofibromatosis. In Lombardi and Passerini's series of 317 spinal tumors in 312 patients, there were 12 cases of multiple tumors, i.e., one patient with ependymomas, two with meningiomas, two with isolated neurilemomas, and

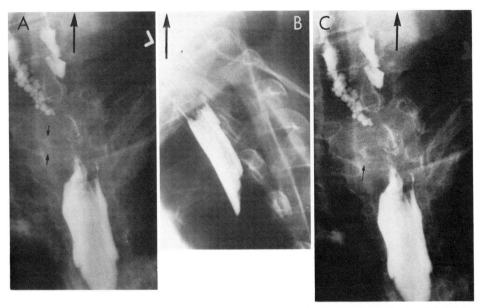

Fig 16–25.—The patient, a female in her late sixties, had old tuberculosis of the right upper lobe. She was seen because of the sudden onset of paraplegia. Anteroposterior **(A)** and lateral **(B)** myelographic films demonstrated an intradural extramedullary tumor on the right side of the cord at T1-2. The Pantopaque coats the left lateral margin of the tumor. Although a preoperative diagnosis of meningioma was made because of the patient's age and sex, the location of the tumor, and the myelographic findings, the calcification *(arrow),* in **C,** was not originally appreciated. This clinches the diagnosis of meningioma.

seven with neurofibromatosis. The patients with neurofibromatosis often exhibit characteristic bone changes as well as multiple scattered intradural and extradural myelographic defects. Myers et al. have recorded the unusual occurrence of solitary spinal neurolemmoma in three members of the same family who had no evidence of von Recklinghausen's disease. These authors also mention other similar examples of solitary neurilemoma in multiple members of the same family without neurofibromatosis reported by Elsberg and by Romeo Orbegozo and Ortega Nuñez.

Myelography in extramedullary intradural tumors may demonstrate either complete obstruction or an intraspinal mass without a block. In the former instance, the contrast medium outlines the upper or lower margin of the tumor as a sharply defined, concave filling defect. When the tumor is lateral in position, the contrast medium may outline more than one side of the lesion, with contralateral displacement of the spinal cord (above the level of the conus medullaris). Wood has pointed out that neurilemomas, because of their sharp encapsulation, tend to be more completely outlined by contrast than meningiomas, which have a broad dural attachment and a somewhat irregular surface. In my experience, these criteria alone have not been helpful in differentiating meningioma from neurilemoma. However, when sex, age, location, bony changes, and calcification are considered together with the myelographic findings, a correct preoperative diagnosis often is possible.

Rarely, a neurilemoma of the cauda may present with an abrupt onset of intractable sciatica, violent headache, and bloody CSF due to acute subarachnoid hem-

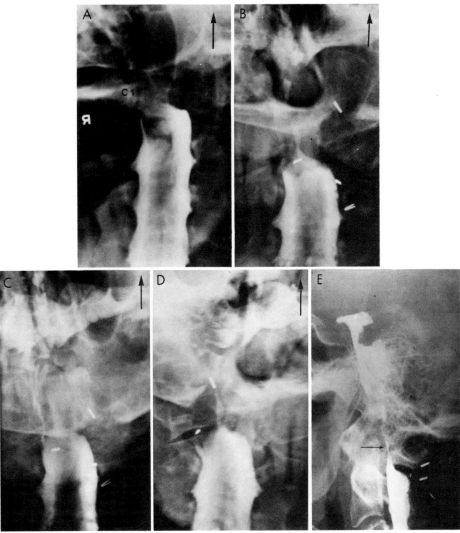

Fig 16–26.—Foramen magnum meningioma incompletely removed from a middle-aged female in 1960. **A,** the original myelogram demonstrates a complete block at C1-2. The patient was reoperated on 2 years later, when the tumor was thought to have extended into the region of the foramen of Magendie. The anteroposterior, **B,** oblique, **C** and **D,** and lateral, **E,** films demonstrate the posterior location of the tumor, with resultant anterior displacement of the cord. Note the thin midline streak of Pantopaque in the anterior subarachnoid space at C-1 *(arrow).*

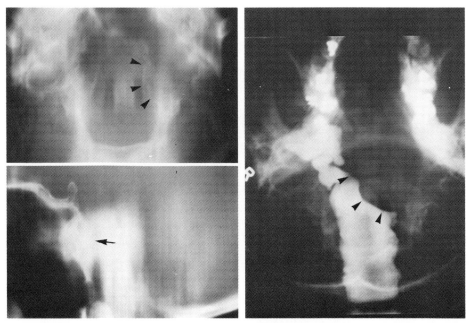

Fig 16–27.—Recurrent clivus chordoma in an 18-year-old girl who presented with diplopia, difficulty in swallowing, and paresis of cranial nerves IV, IX, X, and XII on the right side. The tumor was originally discovered 6 years previously during a transpalatal adenoidectomy and was partially resected. Two additional subtotal resections were done. The myelogram demonstrates a large left-sided extra-axial mass at C1-2 *(arrowheads)*. Note the extensive destruction of the clivus and the left occipital bone on the tomograms *(arrow and arrowheads)*.

orrhage. The lumbar and root pain usually increases in severity whereas the headache recedes, thereby suggesting a spinal rather than an intracranial origin. Myelography clinches the diagnosis.

Intracanalicular Neurilemomas

The very small (0.25–0.5 mm) intracanalicular acoustic neurinoma does not usually produce localized bone erosion or widening of the internal auditory canal. However, it can be diagnosed by Pantopaque myelography because it presents as a round filling defect in the oil-filled canal (Figs 16–41, 16–42). This technique is now obsolete and has been replaced by CT pneumocisternomeatography (see Fig 4–26). The slightly larger intracanalicular tumor may produce a partial or complete cutoff of the oil column, with the lateral aspect of the tumor visualized as a cup-shaped filling defect (Figs 16–43 to 16–47). Valvassori has called attention to two filling defects in the lateral half of the canal caused by normal variants: (1) a fine, crescentic radiolucency between the fundus of the canal and the convex lateral margin of the oil column due to a short arachnoidal sac and (2) a small, round filling defect in the lower half of the canal about 3 mm from the fundus due to the forward bend of the cochlear nerve as it enters the modiolus (see Fig 9–31,*B*). Lin and Silverstein reported two cases of unilateral hearing loss, vertigo, and tinnitus, with

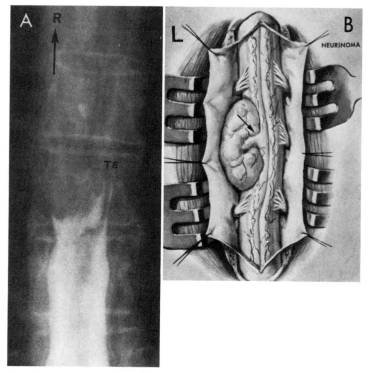

Fig 16–28.—Neurilemoma extending from T-6 to T-8 on the right posterolateral aspect of the cord in a 42-year-old female is shown in **A.** In **B**, the artist has depicted a similar (slightly smaller) neurilemoma producing narrowing and displacement of the cord to the right. Note the resemblance of this illustration to Figure 16–16. (**B** is from the Ciba Collection of Medical Illustrations by Frank H. Netter, M.D. Copyright Ciba.)

small defects in the lateral end of the internal auditory canal at tomomyelography. No tumor was found at operation in either case. In one patient, the defect was thought to be due to inflamed vestibular nerves or incomplete filling of the canal. In the second patient, the defect was caused by arachnoiditis, which produced adhesions between the dura and cranial nerves VII and VIII. As a result of their experience, the authors recommend diagnostic labyrinthotomy in similar cases prior to operation, i.e., in patients with severe hearing loss. Patients with intracanalicular neurilemomas have a markedly elevated perilymph protein level (>1000 mg/100 ml). On the other hand, patients with large cerebellopontine angle tumors not invading the internal auditory canal have a normal perilymph protein level. In Lin and Silverstein's experience with 50 acoustic neurilemoma suspects, there were no false positives or false negatives.

Bilateral acoustic neurinomas rarely occur in the absence of generalized neurofibromatosis. Occasionally, one sees bilateral symmetric enlargement of the internal auditory canals in patients who are totally asymptomatic, i.e., in the absence of tinnitus or a neurosensory hearing loss (see Fig 16–41). This represents either a normal variant or a forme fruste of neurofibromatosis. Prior to high-resolution CT scanning, we examined two such patients by pneumoencephalography and found no evidence of intracanalicular tumor.

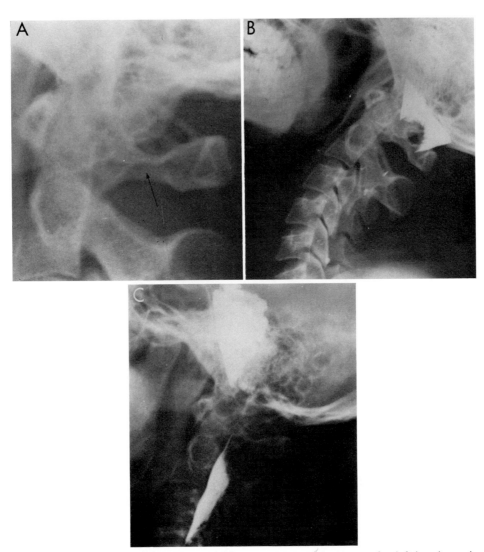

Fig 16–29.—The patient, a 28-year-old man, was seen because of a left hemiparesis and numbness of the left upper extremity of several months' duration. The lateral plain radiograph **(A)** shows a well-defined, localized erosion of the undersurface of one posterior arch of C-1 *(arrow)*. **A,** Pantopaque introduced via cisternal puncture. **B** demonstrates a "cap" defect at the upper border of C-1, marking the superior extent of the tumor. Additional oil introduced from below **(C)** defines the inferior margin of the tumor on C-2. At operation, a 3 × 5-cm neurilemoma was removed. The tumor was both intradural and extradural in location. (Courtesy of R. Cobb.)

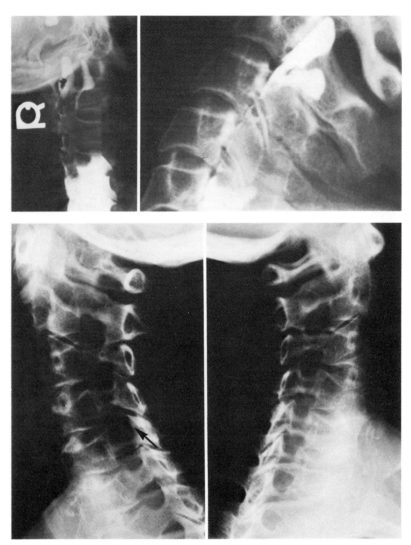

Fig 16–30.—Top, neurilemoma on the left posterolateral aspect of the upper cervical cord in a 65-year-old woman. The cord is displaced to the right and anteriorly by the tumor mass. At surgery, the lesion extended from the C2-3 to the C4-5 level. **Bottom,** preliminary films demonstrate erosion of the left intervertebral foramen at C4-5 *(arrow).* The contralateral normal foramina are shown for comparison.

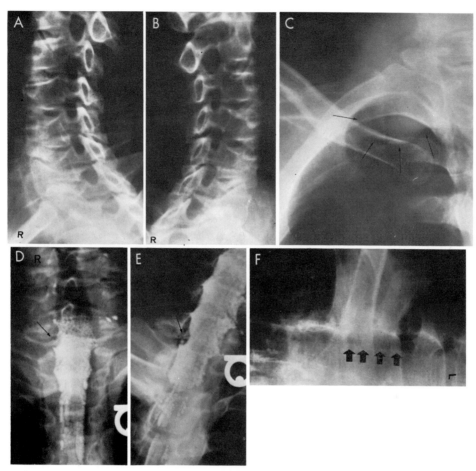

Fig 16–31.—Neurilemoma arising from the right eighth cervical nerve distal to its exit from the intervertebral foramen. **A** and **B,** plain films of the cervical spine, show no bony changes. The spot film, **C,** of the right apex demonstrates a sharply defined tumor in the pulmonary sulcus *(arrows),* with a suggestive pleural attachment. At myelography, **D** and **E,** a constant defect is noted along the right lateral aspect of the Pantopaque column *(arrow),* but no oil entered the apical mass. The differential diagnosis of lateral intrathoracic meningocele should be considered because the viscous oil does not always penetrate the narrow channel leading to a meningocele. Hence, pneumomyelography was carried out, **F.** A left lateral decubitus film made with the horizontal beam demonstrates a column of air along the right lateral margin of the subarachnoid space *(arrows),* with no air entering the apical mass. At operation, a neurilemoma was resected.

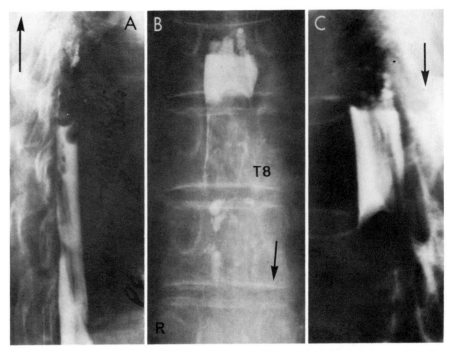

Fig 16–32.—Neurilemoma at T-8 in a 59-year-old man. Lumbar myelography shows the lobular character and the inferior margin of the tumor at T8-9. The head of the table was tilted approximately 80 degrees craniad in **A.** Cisternal puncture with the introduction of 2 ml of Pantopaque defines the upper margin of the lesion at T7-8, **B** and **C.**

Extrameatal Angle Tumors

The size of the defect in the Pantopaque-filled cerebellopontine (CP) cistern depends on the tumor size. The typical defect has a lobulated or crescentic border corresponding to the medial aspect of the tumor, which deforms the apex of the cerebellopontine cistern. Although the histologic nature of the angle tumor cannot be determined from the defect, the tomographic findings prior to myelography may be helpful in differential diagnosis. Smooth, uniform enlargement of the meatus is highly suggestive of acoustic neurinoma; localized sclerosis or hyperostosis of the petrous ridge is likely to be due to a meningioma; erosion of the petrous apex without enlargement of the internal auditory canal favors the diagnosis of epidermoid (Figs 16–48, 16–49). Rarely, a large aneurysm of the basilar artery may present as a CP angle mass (Fig 16–50).

Wilner and Kashef described a series of patients with clinical signs of an eighth-nerve tumor in whom an arachnoidal cyst or adhesions in the cerebellopontine angle were found at operation (Figs 16–51, 16–52). The cyst and adhesions, localized to the angle, probably were due to previous inflammation. Such cysts cannot be distinguished from angle tumors by the myelographic findings alone. However, none of the patients with arachnoiditis or cyst exhibited changes in the internal auditory canal. Also, the patients with adhesions tended to show tapering of the oil column in the region of the porus acusticus rather than the abrupt, cup-shaped cutoff characteristic of tumor.

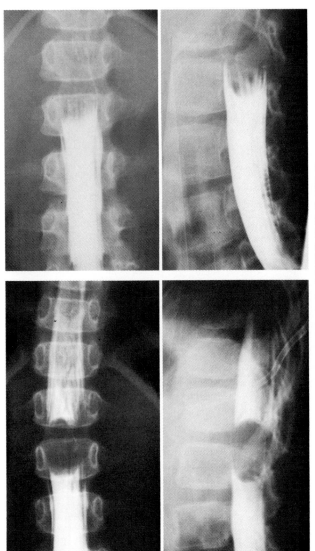

Fig 16–33.—Metrizamide myelography in a 5-year-old girl with a 6-week history of leg pain and a reluctance to walk. Metrizamide was originally introduced at L3-4 **(top),** and the lower border of an intradural obstructing lesion was encountered at the level of the body of L-2. The CSF protein level in the fluid removed from the lumbar puncture was 350 mg%. Metrizamide was also injected from above via C1-2 puncture to demarcate the superior margin of the neurilemoma **(bottom).** The protein level in the CSF obtained from the C1-2 puncture was 35 mg%.

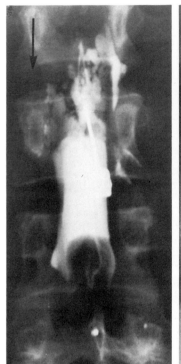 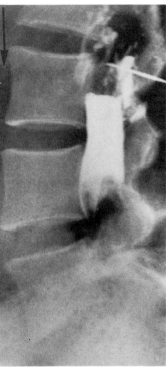

Fig 16–34.—Neurilemoma at L-4 producing a complete obstruction. Some of the Pantopaque at the site of injection is extra-arachnoid. The patient presented with clinical findings suggestive of a herniated lumbar disk. Note that the defect is at the level of the midbody of L-4 and not at the interspace.

There have been several case reports of elderly patients with tortuous basilar arteries looping laterally to indent the ipsilateral cerebellopontine cistern. These patients usually present with twitching of the eye, which ultimately spreads to the entire hemiface, facial weakness and paresis of the trigeminal nerve. The correct diagnosis can be established by vertebral arteriography or by contrast enhanced CT.

Intraspinal Metastatic Implants

Metastases to the spinal cord and cauda equina are usually secondary to primary brain tumors (Fig 16–53). Uncommonly, tumors outside the central nervous system, particularly melanoma, bronchogenic carcinoma and carcinoma of the breast, may metastasize via the bloodstream to the spinal cord and cauda. Since the latter structures are not routinely examined at necropsy, the exact incidence of such metastases is not known. Metastatic implants from primary brain tumors may be secondary not only to cerebellar medulloblastomas and ependymomas but also to other types of supra- and infratentorial gliomas (Figs 16–53, 16–54). Cairns and Russell reported spinal metastases in more than one third of a series of 22 cerebral gliomas, with a fairly equal distribution above and below the tentorium. Brain tumors spread into the spinal subarachnoid space by seeding into the cerebrospinal fluid. Metastatic implants may either be asymptomatic or produce symptoms of spinal cord or

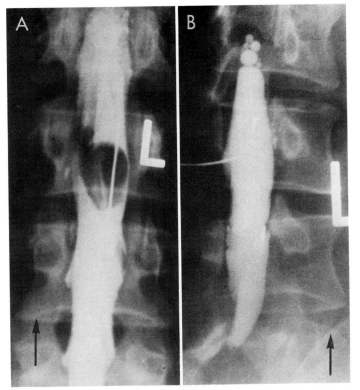

Fig 16–35.—**A,** lobulated neurilemoma arising from the left fourth lumbar root. **B,** reexamination at a later date shows complete excision of the tumor, with no evidence of recurrence. The tumor represented an incidental finding during cervical myelography in a 29-year-old man who sustained a whiplash injury in an auto accident. The patient's complaints consisted of pain in the neck radiating to the left hand and some weakness of this hand.

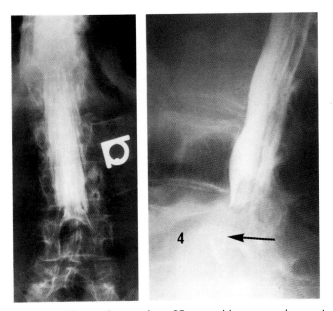

Fig 16–36.—Metrizamide myelogram in a 65-year-old woman, demonstrating a neurilemoma at the level of the body of L-4. Note the excavation of the posterior aspect of this vertebral body *(arrow)*.

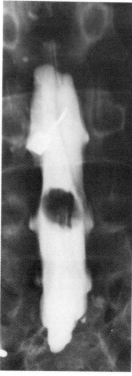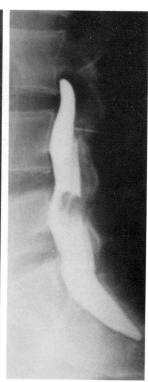

Fig 16–37.—Neurilemoma in a 32-year-old man arising from the left L-5 nerve root. The posterior location of the tumor on the body of L-4 and the sharply defined margins of the lesion differentiate it from the herniated intervertebral disk.

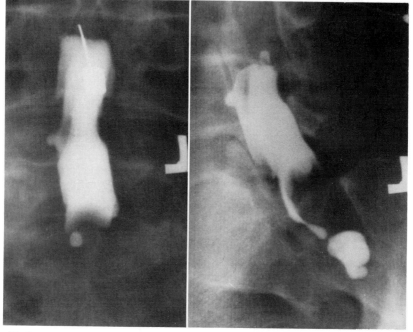

Fig 16–38.—Intradural neurilemoma arising from the first sacral nerve root, presenting as a sharply defined cap defect.

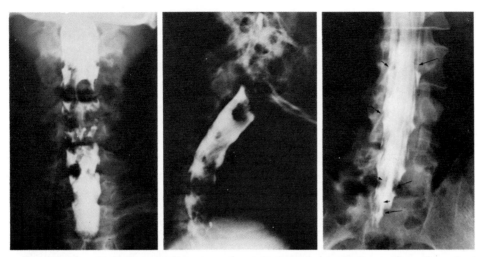

Fig 16–39.—Multiple neurofibromas of cervical cord (surgically confirmed) and of cauda equina *(arrows)* (unconfirmed) in a 65-year-old man who was admitted with a 6-month history of quadriparesis. The cervical portion of the myelogram suggested an AV malformation. The thoracic cord was normal. Selective injection showed both vertebral and costocervical arteries to be normal. At operation, multiple neurofibromas were found studding the cervical cord. (Courtesy of H. Hawkins.)

cauda equina compression, i.e., weakness in both lower extremities, with impairment of bowel and bladder control. The implants may occur at any level of the cord or cauda equina as a single discrete nodule or multiple nodules; less commonly, they take the form of diffuse gliomatosis of the meninges. The nodular implants vary from a pinhead to several centimeters in size, are grayish white, firm, and adherent to the cord and meninges. They are more common on the dorsal aspect of the spinal cord. Not infrequently, they invade the cord itself. The more diffuse type of metastasis usually infiltrates the arachnoid extensively for a considerable distance. Rarely, diffuse meningeal gliomatosis or reticulum cell sarcoma of the meninges has been reported as a primary lesion. Metastatic gliomas usually do not produce any recognizable changes on plain radiographs. However, Black and Keats have reported osteoblastic metastases to the spine in association with metastatic seeding of the spinal axis by cerebellar medulloblastoma.

Myelographically, the nodular type of metastasis presents as multiple round or oval constant filling defects of varying size in the contrast column (Figs 16–53 to 16–56). Because these metastases frequently involve the entire circumference of the cord, they do not usually displace the cord as extramedullary lesions characteristically do. They may further be differentiated from extramedullary intradural tumors in that they usually do not have as sharply defined margins because of their more intimate fusion with the cord. Occasionally, however, they may be sharply outlined. Although the smaller lesions do not cause any obstruction to the flow of contrast medium, larger metastases may produce a partial or complete obstruction. When the cauda equina is involved by medium-sized or large tumor masses, the affected roots may be displaced and irregularly thickened by the tumor nodule. Less commonly, there may be an irregular streaky appearance of the contrast medium due to diffuse infiltration of the nerve roots, which can be confused with

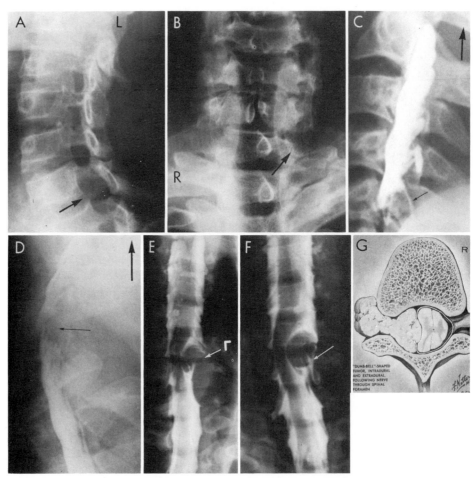

Fig 16–40.—Dumbbell neurilemoma in a young male. Note the enlargement of the intervertebral foramen at C6-7 on the left, **A,** and the change in the corresponding pedicle, **B.** Incidentally, there is failure of bony fusion of the posterior neural arch of C-6. **C** and **D,** lateral radiographs made at myelography demonstrate the posterior location of the tumor *(arrows),* whereas **E** and **F,** the frontal films, show the tumor to lie on the left side *(arrows).* In **E,** the bilobate character of the tumor is readily appreciated, with the extradural component inferior. In **F,** the arrow points to the cervical nerve root intimately related to the tumor. In **G,** an artist's drawing of a typical "dumbbell" tumor is shown. (From the Ciba Collection of Medical Illustrations by Frank H. Netter, M.D. Copyright Ciba.)

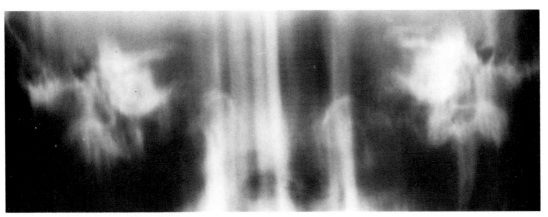

Fig 16–41.—AP tomogram demonstrating bilateral symmetric enlargement of the internal auditory canals in an asymptomatic patient.

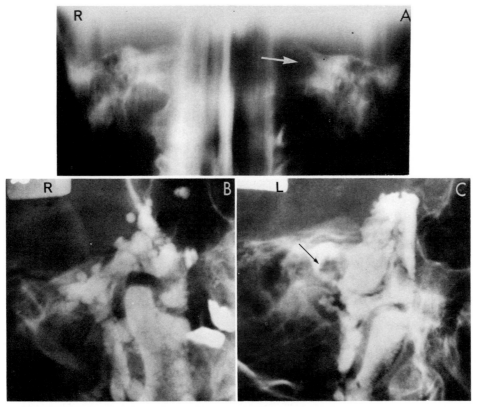

Fig 16–42.—Intracanalicular eighth-nerve neurilemoma in a 60-year-old man with old bilateral hearing deficit due to otitis media. There was a recent sudden complete loss of hearing on the left side. Note the widening of the left internal auditory canal and flaring of the porus acusticus *(arrow)* on the AP tomogram **(A)**. **B** and **C**, posterior fossa myelography showed a normal right side and a rounded filling defect produced by the tumor in the left canal *(arrow)*.

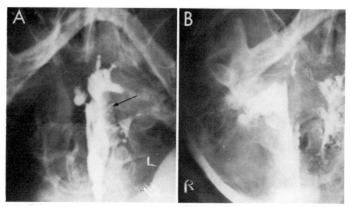

Fig 16–43.—Large eighth-nerve neurilemoma bulging out of the left porus acusticus producing a prominent filling defect in the oil column as well as preventing filling of the canal itself *(arrow)* **(A).** The right canal fills normally **(B).**

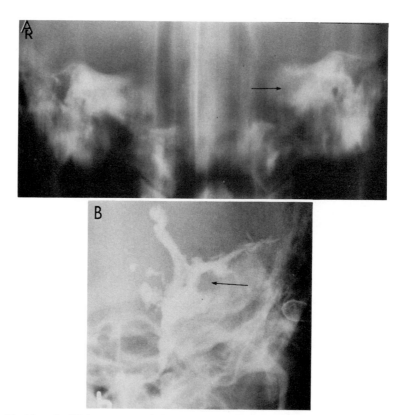

Fig 16–44.—**A,** AP tomogram of the petrous bones in a young woman showing widening of the left internal auditory canal and flaring of the porus acusticus. The Towne projection of the posterior fossa myelogram **(B)** demonstrates failure of the Pantopaque to enter the left canal because of an intracanalicular neurilemoma projecting out from the porus acusticus.

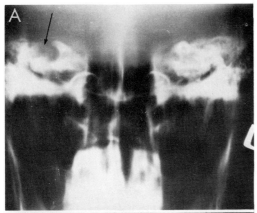

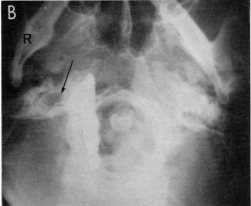

Fig 16–45.—Large dumbbell neurilemoma of the right eighth nerve in a middle-aged woman. The sharply defined bone defect in the right petrous ridge *(arrow)* was produced by the tumor growing out of the internal auditory canal **(A).** The Pantopaque does not enter the right internal auditory canal because of tumor occluding the porus acusticus *(arrow)* **(B).** The canal on the left side fills normally **(C).**

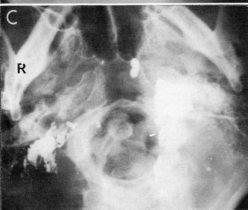

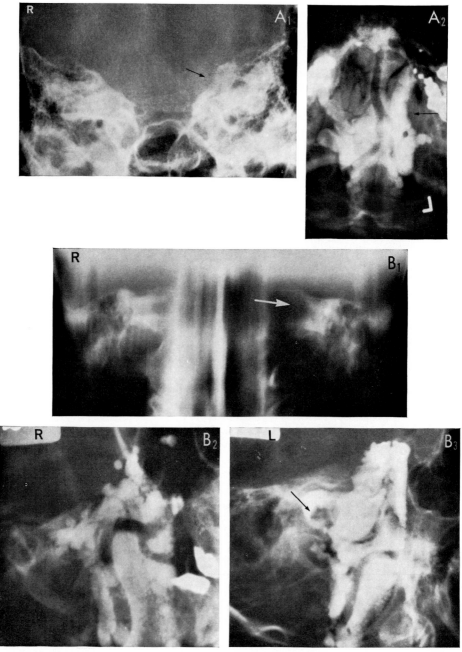

Fig 16–46.—Neurilemoma of the left eighth nerve in a young man with a nerve conduction deficit in the left ear. The Towne view **(A₁)** shows erosion of the left porus acusticus *(arrow)* and widening of the canal. Posterior fossa myelography **(A₂)** demonstrates a prominent filling defect *(arrow)* in the left cerebellopontine angle produced by the tumor. Compare this with the findings in **(B)**, a 60-year-old man in whom the tumor is confined to the bony canal. The AP tumorgram **(B₁)** shows widening of the left internal auditory meatus with flaring of the porus acusticus. Posterior fossa myelography demonstrates a normal right side **(B₂)**, and the intracanalicular tumor on the left *(arrow)* surrounded by Pantopaque **(B₃)**.

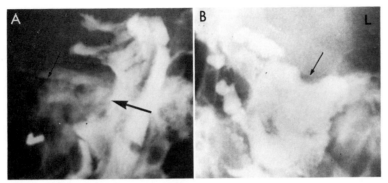

Fig 16–47.—Large eighth-nerve tumor on the right in a 45-year-old woman with an ipsilateral nerve conduction deficit. The AP Towne view showed enlargement of the right internal auditory meatus. The posterior fossa myelogram on the right **(A)** shows the dilated canal with trumpeting of the porus acusticus *(thin arrow),* failure of filling of the canal, and a large defect in the oil column produced by the tumor in the right cerebellopontine angle *(thick arrow).* The left side is normal **(B).** Note the defect produced by the trigeminal nerve as it crosses the tentorium *(arrow).*

hypertrophic interstitial polyneuritis or chronic arachnoiditis. The presence of nodular masses on the nerve roots and extradural tumor, as well as the clinical setting, are helpful in differential diagnosis (Figs 16–57 to 16–59).

If intraspinal metastases are suspected and myelography in the usual prone position is uninformative, the patient should be examined in the supine position. This maneuver may demonstrate metastases on the dorsal aspect of the cord, a common site for these lesions. When I use Pantopaque, I frequently leave the oil in the spinal canal in cases of metastatic medulloblastoma and occasionally of other lesions characterized by multiple metastatic intraspinal deposits. This facilitates re-examination after radiation therapy to evaluate the efficacy of the treatment and to detect new or recurrent metastases.

PACHYMENINGEAL CARCINOMATOSIS OR LYMPHOMATOSIS (FIG 16–60)

Diffuse sheetlike infiltration of the dura by metastatic carcinoma is extremely rare. Kim et al. reported such a case in a 66-year-old man with a primary adenocarcinoma of the colon. Pantopaque myelography demonstrated uniform concentric narrowing of the subarachnoid space from C-2 to C-6 with an increased distance between the medial margins of the pedicles and the lateral aspects of the subarachnoid space. At laminectomy, the dura was markedly thickened and whitish in appearance due to infiltration by tumor. The subarachnoid space was normal.

The myelographic findings are identical to those produced by hypertrophic pachymeningitis and the mucopolysaccharidoses, since all of these processes produce diffuse thickening of the dura. Differentiation from arachnoiditis associated with marked narrowing of the subarachnoid space can usually be made because of the irregularity of the contrast column and the presence of varying degrees of obstruction in the latter entity.

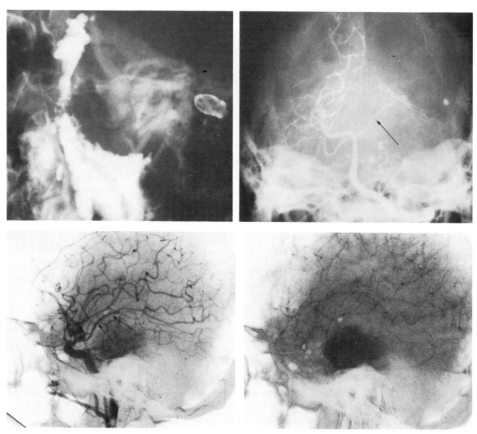

Fig 16–48.—Middle-aged woman admitted with a 6-month history of tinnitus, decreased hearing, and "wax" in her left ear. **Top,** the myelogram demonstrates a large mass in the left cerebellopontine angle. A barium-coated cotton applicator is in the external auditory canal. The vertebral arteriogram shows marked elevation and narrowing of the left posterior cerebral artery *(arrow)*. **Bottom,** subtraction films of early *(left)* and late *(right)* arterial phase of a left carotid arteriogram show elevation of the left posterior cerebral artery *(arrows)* and an intense tumor stain. The stain and the supratentorial extension favor the diagnosis of meningioma (confirmed at surgery).

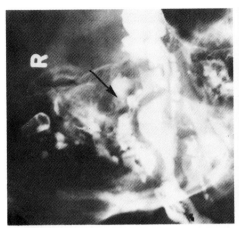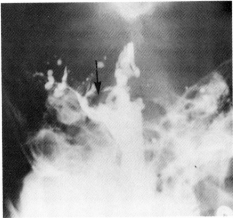

Fig 16–49.—Large cholesteatoma (epidermoid) of the left cerebellopontine (CP) angle in a 32-year-old man. The oblique spot film and the Towne view demonstrate a large mass in the CP angle with irregular margins *(arrows)*. There is a barium-coated cotton applicator in the external auditory canal. The correct diagnosis was suggested because of the irregularity of the tumor mass at myelography and pneumoencephalography (not shown).

Lymphoma

Hunt and his associates reported a case of primary reticulum cell sarcoma of the nervous system with extensive involvement of the leptomeninges, the frontal-lobe white matter, the subependymal regions of the ventricles, and multiple areas of the spinal cord at various levels. There also was widespread involvement of nearly all the nerve roots and spinal ganglia but no evidence of lymphoma outside the nervous system. The patient, a 75-year-old woman, originally presented with a left foot drop and severe pain in the left hip and leg. Myelography showed pronounced enlargement of the right fifth lumbar nerve root (Fig 16–61). At operation and necropsy, both the sensory and motor roots of the fifth lumbar nerve were irregularly enlarged and purplish brown in color. Frozen and permanent sections, as well as necropsy findings, established the diagnosis of malignant lymphoma of the reticulum cell sarcoma type (histiocytic lymphoma).

Rarely, lymphosarcoma may occur as a primary solitary extradural lesion. Bucy and Jerva reported a series of eight patients with this lesion, five of whom made gratifying recoveries after surgical extirpation. The tumor is as common in males as in females and may occur at any age, although it is more common after age 40. It usually involves the thoracic segment of the spinal cord. Plain films of the spine are of little diagnostic aid. Myelography demonstrates evidence of an extradural lesion with varying degrees of obstruction.

The usual type of cord involvement in lymphoma is extradural, indistinguishable myelographically from metastatic carcinoma or sarcoma (Figs 16–62, 16–63). Van Allen and Rahme reported a case of diffuse lymphosarcoma in a 31-year-old man with extensive invasion of the leptomeninges and massive involvement of the cauda equina, producing gross enlargement of the roots. The myelographic picture clearly revealed the marked swelling of the roots of the cauda equina, not unlike the appearance in hypertrophic interstitial polyneuritis (Figs 16–64, 16–65). Britt et al.

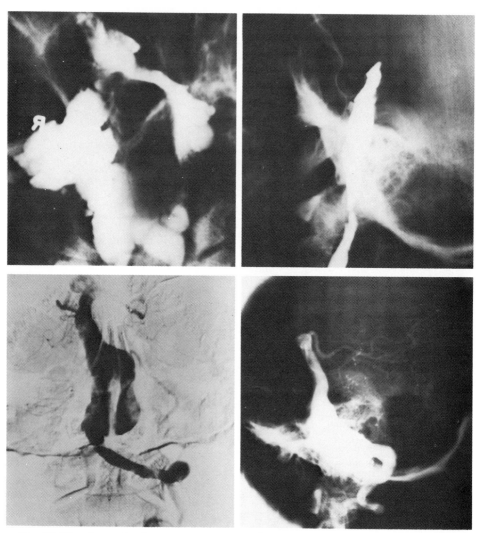

Fig 16–50.—Large basilar artery aneurysm in a 50-year-old man which presented as an extrameatal angle mass at myelography. Note that the aneurysm conforms to the defect in the myelogram.

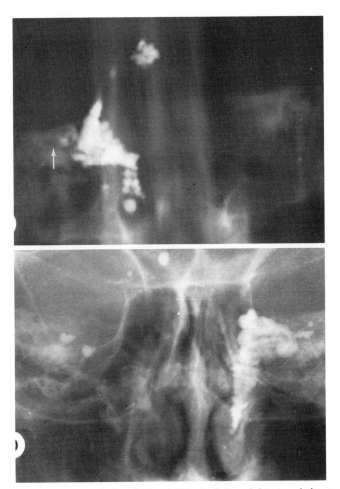

Fig 16–51.—Tomography shows lack of filling of the right canal *(arrow)*, proved at operation to be caused by arachnoidal adhesions with cyst formation **(top).** Posterior fossa myelogram demonstrating normal filling of the left internal auditory canal **(bottom).** (Reprinted, with permission, from Wilner H.I., Kashef R., *Am. J. Roentgenol.* 115:126, 1972.)

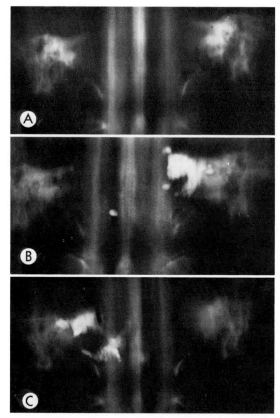

Fig 16–52.—AP tomogram reveals a localized erosion of the right petrous bone inferior to the internal auditory canal; the left canal is normal **(A).** The normal left canal fills with Pantopaque **(B).** The right internal auditory canal also fills with oil, but there is a defect in the oil column below and medial to the meatus, corresponding to the bone defect **(C).** At operation, an arachnoidal cyst was found with no evidence of tumor. (Reprinted, with permission, from Wilner H.I., Kashef R., *Am. J. Roentgenol.* 115:126, 1972.)

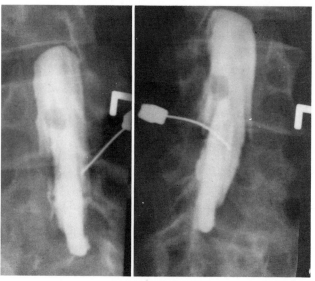

Fig 16–53.—Intraspinal metastases in a patient with a cerebellar astrocytoma. Note the round filling defect produced by a nodular gravitational implant.

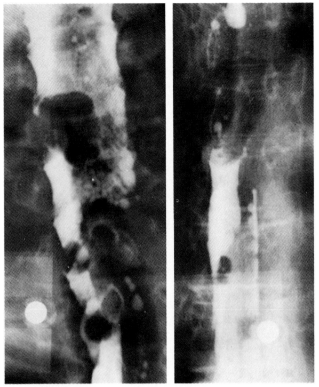

Fig 16–54.—Multiple subarachnoid metastases to the cervical and thoracic cord in a patient with an ependymoma of the fourth ventricle.

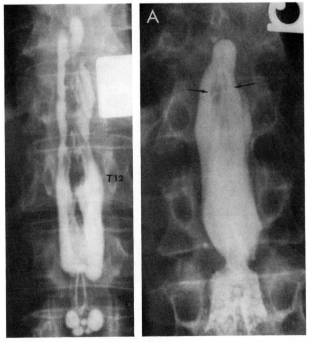

Fig 16–55.—Myelogram in a patient with bronchogenic carcinoma of the right upper lobe with extensive intramedullary metastasis in the region of the conus medullaris (confirmed at necropsy).

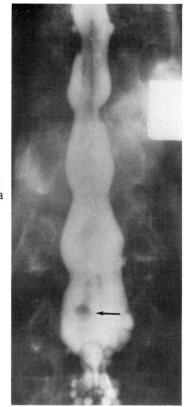

Fig 16–56.—Nodular metastasis *(arrow)* to the conus medullaris in a patient with carcinoma of the pancreas (confirmed at necropsy).

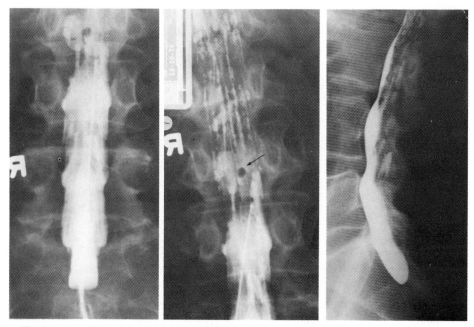

Fig 16–57.—The patient was a middle-aged man with bronchogenic carcinoma. The myelogram shows nodular implants *(arrow)* as well as diffuse infiltration of the nerve roots resembling hypertrophic interstitial polyneuritis.

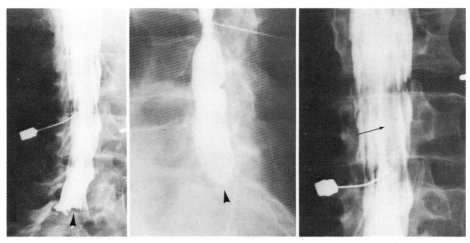

Fig 16–58.—Metrizamide myelogram in a 60-year-old man with bronchogenic carcinoma showing a cutoff of the caudal sac *(arrowheads)* in addition to diffuse infiltration of the nerve roots *(arrow)*.

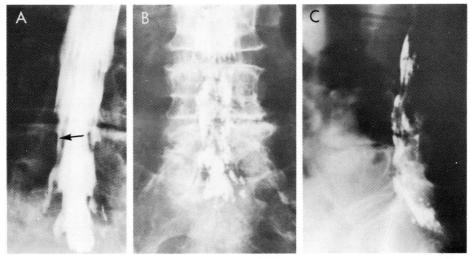

Fig 16–59.—The patient was a 63-year-old woman with breast carcinoma. The original Pantopaque myelogram **(A)** shows an extradural defect *(arrow)* and some irregularity of the nerve roots. Some of the Pantopaque was removed, and the patient was restudied 3 days later **(B** and **C)**. The delayed study demonstrates nodular defects as well as irregular coating of thickened nerve roots. At necropsy, there was diffuse neoplastic infiltration of the nerve roots of the cauda as well as extradural tumor.

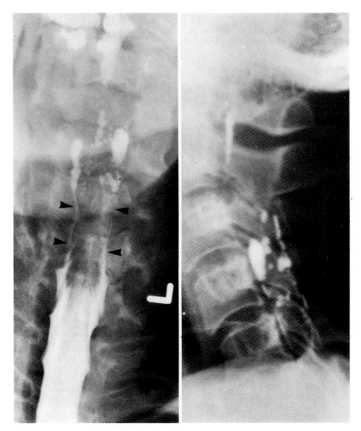

Fig 16–60.—Lymphosarcoma in a 51-year-old woman infiltrating and thickening the dura bilaterally at C-5 and C-6. Note the resemblance to chronic hypertrophic pachymeningitis with displacement of the symmetrically thinned lateral margins of the subarachnoid space away from the pedicles *(arrowheads).*

reported a similar case in a patient with diffuse involvement of the subarachnoid and perineural spaces of the cauda equina by lymphoma cells. The resulting myelographic appearance was one of diffuse symmetric swelling of the nerve roots resembling a mass of spaghetti. The differential diagnosis should include arteriovenous malformation, adhesive arachnoiditis, hypertrophic interstitial polyneuritis, Guillain-Barré syndrome, and subarachnoid metastases.

EXTRADURAL TUMORS

Approximately 25–30% of all spinal tumors are extradural in location. By and large, the greatest number of these tumors, particularly in the older age group, are malignant. The high incidence of malignant tumors and the low incidence of benign tumors in the extradural space contrast sharply with the situation in the subdural space, where most of extramedullary tumors are benign. The benign extradural tumors include neurilemoma (most common), meningioma (often malignant in the extradural space), lipoma, dermoid, and epidermoid. Extradural tumors may origi-

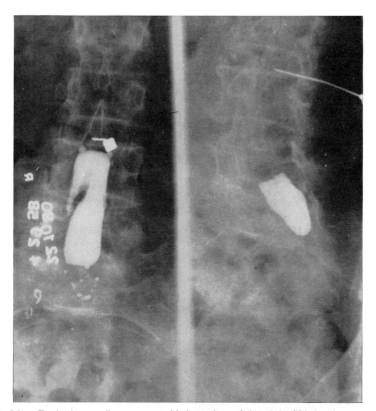

Fig 16–61.—Reticulum cell sarcoma with invasion of the right fifth lumbar root resulting in marked enlargement of this root. (Reprinted, with permission, from Hunt T.R. Jr., et al., *J. Neurosurg.* 17:342, 1960.)

nate as primary benign or malignant tumors of the dura, extradural or soft tissues, or nerve roots, as primary or metastatic tumors of the vertebrae and contiguous structures, with secondary extension into the extradural space (Fig 16–66), or as extradural metastases from tumors elsewhere in the body. The largest group of extradural tumors is composed of metastatic lesions of the vertebrae with extension into the spinal canal. Although this type of metastasis may be secondary to almost any malignant tumor, it is particularly common with carcinoma of the breast and lung. Osteolytic or osteoblastic changes are often demonstrable on plain films; pathologic fractures of one or more vertebrae are common as well. Spinal cord compression is not uncommon in various lymphomas and multiple myeloma.

The lymphomas (particularly Hodgkin's disease) may produce localized osteoblastic involvement of one or more vertebrae with or without a recognizable paraspinal soft tissue mass. Cockshott and Evans reported a series of 18 Nigerian children with Burkitt's tumor (lymphosarcoma) who presented with paraplegia. Plain films of the spine demonstrated vertebral destruction or a paraspinal mass in 14 patients. The intervertebral disks were spared, unlike the usual case of Pott's disease. The paraspinal masses sometimes were quite large, extending over several segments, frequently bilateral and asymmetric. Erosion of a pedicle and widening of the interpediculate distance were noted in only four children, presumably because of the

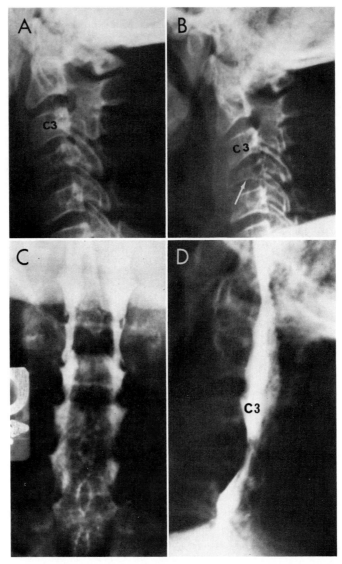

Fig 16–62.—Extradural deposits in a patient with chronic lymphatic leukemia. **A,** the original lateral radiograph of the cervical spine on August 25, 1964, showed a slight loss of the normal bone density of C-4, which was not appreciated. **B,** repeat examination on October 4, 1965 revealed a pathologic fracture of C-4 *(arrow).* **C** and **D,** myelography demonstrated an elongated anterior defect of the Pantopaque column extending from C-3 to C-5 due to extradural leukemic infiltration.

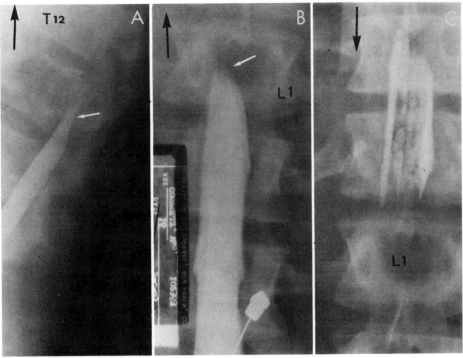

Fig 16–63.—Extradural deposit at L-1 in a 17-year-old boy with diffuse reticulum cell sarcoma. Note, in **A,** the destructive changes involving the body of L-1 and, in **A** and **B,** the block defining the lower limit of the lesion at lumbar myelography *(white arrow)*. Cisternal injection of Pantopaque defined the upper limit of the lesion at the T12-L1 interspace in **C.**

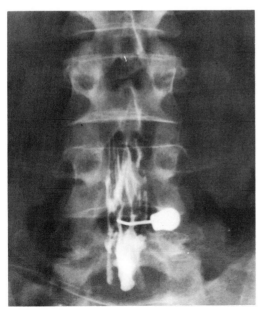

Fig 16–64.—Myelogram in a patient with diffuse lymphosarcoma of the cauda equina and leptomeninges. The neoplastic infiltration has produced enlargement of the roots of the cauda, resulting in an appearance similar to that seen in hypertrophic interstitial polyneuritis. (Reprinted, with permission, from Van Allen M.W., Rahme E.S., *Arch. Neurol.* 7:476, 1962.)

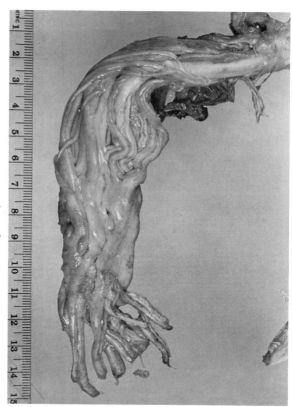

Fig 16–65.—Photograph of the lumbosacral cord and the cauda equina of the patient whose myelogram is shown in Figure 16–64. (Reprinted, with permission, from Van Allen M.W., Rahme E.S., *Arch. Neurol.* 7:476, 1962.)

rapid growth of the tumor. Myelography demonstrated either complete obstruction or displacement of the theca away from the tumor. Rarely, lymphoma may arise in, and be limited to, the extradural space.

In the McKissock et al. series of 22 patients with spinal cord compression due to myeloma, only two patients had evidence of generalized myelomatosis prior to surgery. Plain films of the spine demonstrated bone destruction at the site of the lesion in 19 patients (Fig 16–67); half of the patients had destruction of one or more pedicles. All of the patients exhibited some degree of obstruction at myelography; 19 had a complete block and four a partial block. The anatomical distribution is of interest; 16 were in the thoracic region, three in the cervical region, and three in the lumbar region. In my experience, spinal myelomas seem to have a predilection for the thoracic segment of the spine. Sod and Wiener reported a rare case of extramedullary intradural plasmocytoma, apparently the only such example in the literature.

Chordomas are rare. In a 35-year study at Memorial Hospital, Higinbotham et al. found 46 cases with an age span of 2.5 to 71 years. Seventy per cent of the patients were male, and only 10 cases occurred in the cervical, thoracic and lumbar areas. Myelography reveals evidence of nonspecific extradural compression when present (Fig 16–68).

Although extradural tumors secondary to malignant disease of the vertebral column often produce osteolytic or osteoblastic bone changes on the plain film (50–

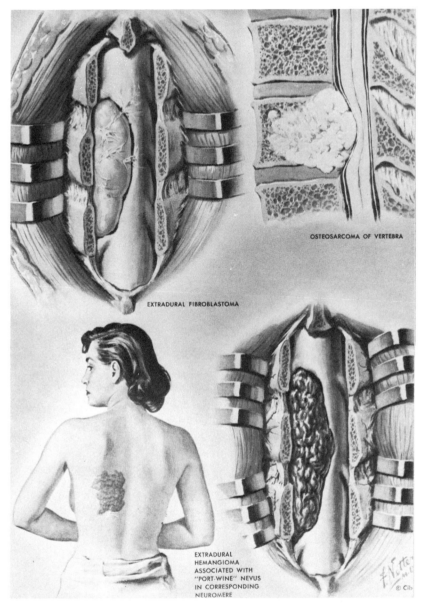

OSTEOSARCOMA OF VERTEBRA

EXTRADURAL FIBROBLASTOMA

EXTRADURAL
HEMANGIOMA
ASSOCIATED WITH
"PORT-WINE" NEVUS
IN CORRESPONDING
NEUROMERE

Fig 16–66.—Artist's representation of a variety of extradural tumors. (From the Ciba Collection of Medical Illustrations by Frank H. Netter, M.D. Copyright Ciba.)

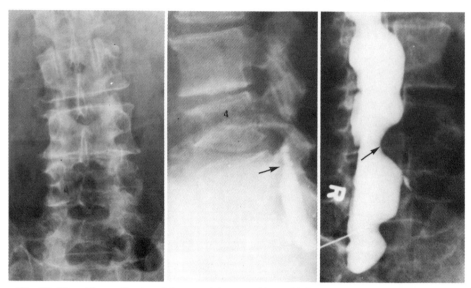

Fig 16–67.—The patient, a 66-year-old man with multiple myeloma, complained of diffuse bone pain. The plain films showed multiple osteolytic lesions of the ribs and a pathologic fracture of L-4 with a localized extradural mass *(arrow)*.

60%) (Figs 16–69, 16–70), extensive neoplastic disease of the spine may exist without recognizable changes on the roentgenogram. Consequently, myelography is often of considerable help in elucidating the cause of backache or radicular pain in these patients. The myelographic findings vary, depending on the location of the tumor and the degree of obstruction. The basic characteristic of an extradural mass is displacement of the entire thecal sac to the contralateral side (Fig 16–71).

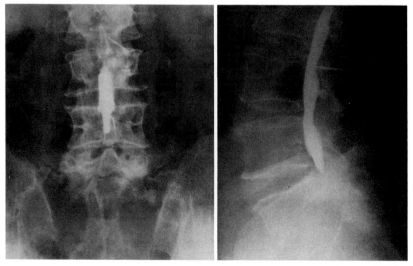

Fig 16–68.—Lumbosacral chordoma with extensive destruction of the sacrum and a complete block at L4-5 due to extradural tumor.

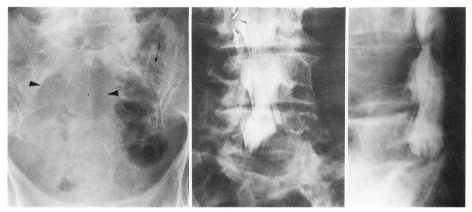

Fig 16–69.—Osteogenic sarcoma secondary to Paget's disease of the sacrum in a 76-year-old man. Note the Pagetoid changes in the wings of the sacrum *(arrow)* and the large osteolytic lesion in the midsacrum *(arrowheads).* Both of these findings were confirmed by CT. Metrizamide myelography shows a sharp cutoff of the left inferior aspect of the caudal sac at the lower end of L-5 secondary to involvement by tumor.

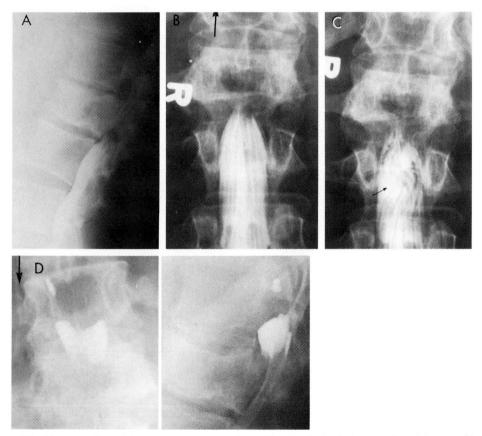

Fig 16–70.—Osteoblastic metastases to L-1 with a pathologic fracture in a 36-year-old man with a malignant bronchial carcinoid. **A,** metrizamide injected at L3-4 outlines the lower end of the block. **B** and **C,** note the redundant nerve roots secondary to the neoplastic spinal stenosis *(arrow).* **D,** 1.5 ml of Pantopaque was introduced via a C1-2 tap outline the upper margin of the lesion.

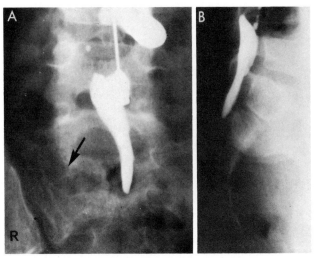

Fig 16–71.—The patient, a 9-year-old boy, had pain in the back radiating down the right lower extremity due to a Ewing's sarcoma of the sacrum. Note the destructive lesion of the right sacral wing *(arrow)* and the associated extradural mass indenting and distorting the right anterolateral aspect of the Pantopaque column **(A** and **B).**

Partial Obstruction

When the extradural tumors lie above the lumbosacral level, the defects they produce may be indistinguishable from those due to herniated intervertebral disks (that is, localized, unilateral indentations of the Pantopaque column). Localization of the defect at the level of the vertebral body instead of the interspace, extent of the defect over several vertebral segments, and marked scalloping of the defect

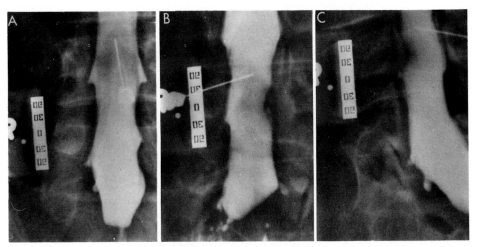

Fig 16–72.—Metastatic extradural carcinoma from a primary oat cell bronchogenic carcinoma in a 45-year-old male with low back and sciatic pain. The patient's pulmonary lesion was minute and not seen on the original chest roentgenogram. Note the irregularity of the oil column on the left at the level of the body of L-5 and the asymmetry at S-1 **(A)** and the multiple bilateral defects **(B** and **C).**

favor a diagnosis of extradural metastasis (Figs 16–72 to 16–76). At the lumbosacral level, a more characteristic appearance frequently is seen—an asymmetric tapering of the Pantopaque column in the form of an inverted cone or triangle with distortion of the ipsilateral axillary pouch (see Fig 16–73). The very caudal end of the subarachnoid space may be smoothly cut off due to circumferential encasement of the distal cauda equina by the tumor (see Figs 16–75, 16–76).

Complete Obstruction

In the presence of a complete block, a smooth, concave margin usually marks the contrast column. If there is uniform infiltration of the tumor around the cord or cauda equina, the contrast column is narrowed to a point of complete obstruction, but the cord or cauda remains in the midline. This is in contrast to the intramedullary tumor with complete obstruction, in which enlargement of the cord frequently can be recognized at the head of the contrast column. Usually, the margin of the defect is not as sharply defined as that seen with an intradural extramedullary lesion (Figs 16–77 to 16–81). This diagnostic criterion, however, does not always hold true, and correct differentiation between extramedullary intradural lesions and extradural tumors may not always be possible. In general, the presence of a complete block makes consistently accurate differential diagnosis difficult. In this regard, the injection of a small amount of additional Pantopaque, saline, or metrizamide, as the case may be, with the head of the table tilted down will frequently succeed in getting some contrast above the "complete block" and define the upper end of the lesion. If this fails, a C1-2 puncture can be done to achieve the same goal.

Benign tumors of the spine, such as hemangioma, aneurysmal bone cyst, and giant cell tumor, rarely have neurologic complications. Cavernous hemangioma of the spine, most common in the lower thoracic or upper lumbar region, is usually an asymptomatic lesion incidentally discovered on either a chest or an abdominal film (Fig 16–82). Neurologic complications are the result of bleeding or pathologic fracture (Figs 16–83, 16–84). Similar rare complications in giant cell tumor or aneurysmal bone cyst are caused either by a pathologic fracture or by extension of the lesion beyond the vertebra with extradural compression of the cord or cauda (Fig 16–85). The myelographic findings are those found with any extradural lesion.

LESS COMMON TUMORS

Lipoma

Lipomas in adults are rare lesions which constitute less than 1% of all spinal tumors. These tumors are probably mesenchymal rather than neural in origin, although their exact origin is not definitely known. They may arise from fat cells normally found in the pia mater or by metaplasia of pluripotential connective tissue cells. These tumors tend to occur on the posterior aspect of the cord. Although they are more commonly extramedullary intradural in location, they may be intramedullary, intra-extramedullary (Figs 16–86, 16–87), or even extradural. The larger, more extensive tumors have a tendency to split the posterior columns as they grow, thus giving the impression that they arose within the cord. This impres-

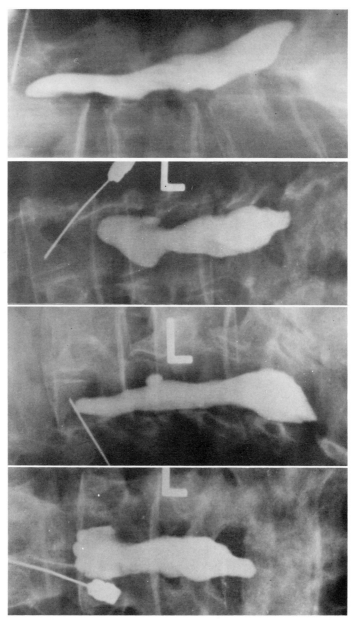

Fig 16–73.—Anteroposterior and oblique spot myelographic films, **left,** and lateral decubitus film, **right,** in a patient with extensive extradural metastases from a primary bronchogenic carcinoma. Note the irregular scalloping of the Pantopaque column, with elongated defects at the level of the vertebral bodies.

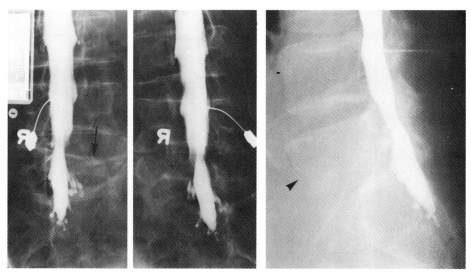

Fig 16–74.—Myelogram in a 70-year-old man with an extradural defect on the left posterolateral aspect of the thecal sac. Note the pathologic fracture of the left half of the L-5 vertebral body *(large arrow)*, with destruction anteriorly as well *(arrowhead)*. Pathologic diagnosis—fibrosarcoma.

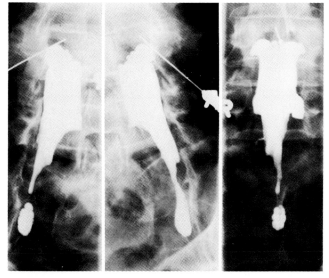

Fig 16–75.—Extradural metastases to the distal cauda equina from an oat cell carcinoma of the lung. Note that the lesion which begins at the level of the distal body of L-5 has the appearance of an asymmetric inverted cone. As it proceeds distally, the tumor encases and markedly narrows the distal caudal sac.

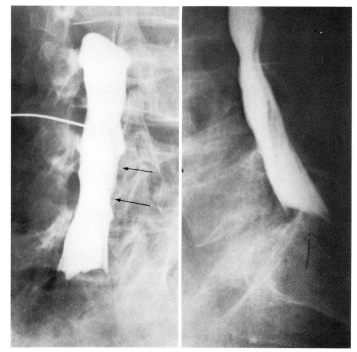

Fig 16–76.—Encasement of the distal caudal sac by tumor. Note also the irregularity of the left side of the contrast column on the body of L-5 due to extradural tumor *(arrows).*

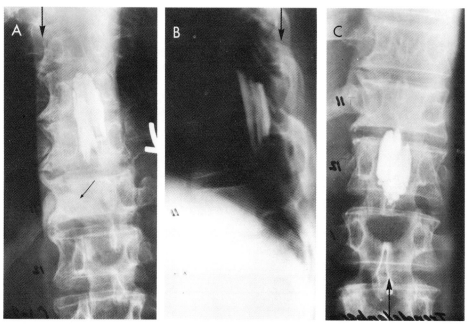

Fig 16–77.—Metastatic carcinoma of the prostate in a 60-year-old man with osteoblastic metastases to the body of T-11 *(small arrow)* and a complete obstruction. **A** and **B,** Pantopaque was introduced via C1-2 puncture to define the upper margin of the block. **C,** the oil was introduced by lumbar puncture to determine the lower extent of the lesion. At laminectomy, there was a tumor mass extending out from the body of T-12 into the spinal canal.

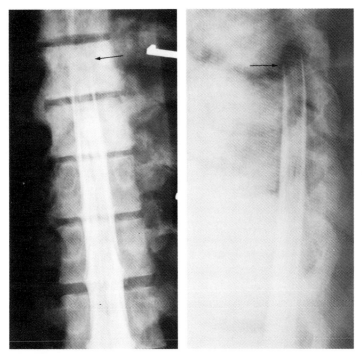

Fig 16–78.—Metrizamide myelogram in a 68-year-old man with extensive osteoblastic metastases from a prostatic carcinoma. Note the complete extradural obstruction at the level of T-8 *(arrow).*

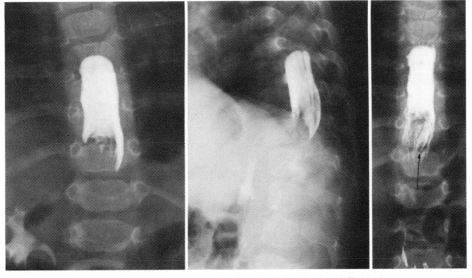

Fig 16–79.—Complete obstruction at the level of the body of T-11 due to metastatic neuroblastoma in a 5-month-old boy. There was a progressive loss of function of both lower extremities and a sensory loss at T-10. Note the redundant nerve roots due to the obstruction *(arrow).*

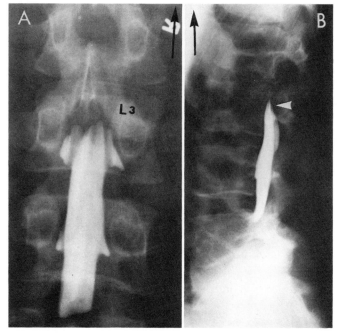

Fig 16–80.—Extradural metastasis at the level of L-3 10 years after removal of a cerebellar sarcoma and postoperative irradiation of the cerebrospinal axis. The posterior location of the defect and its position on the body of the vertebra *(arrowhead)* exclude a herniated intervertebral disk.

Fig 16–81.—Myelogram in a 6-year-old boy with metastatic extradural neuroblastoma at the level of L-3. The tumor displaces the cauda equina anteriorly and to the right *(arrows)*.

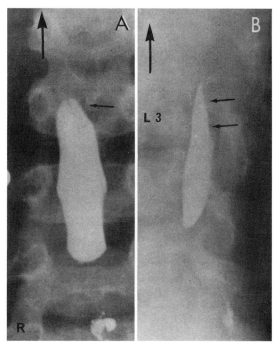

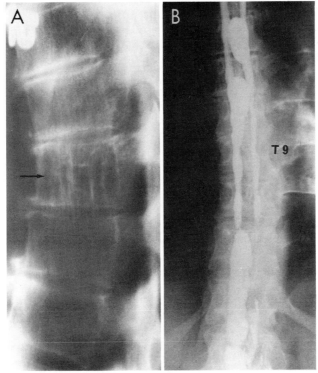

Fig 16–82.—Lateral radiograph in a middle-aged female with midthoracic backache. The hemangioma of the body of T-9 is well demonstrated in **A** *(arrow)*. **B,** myelography in the supine as well as the prone position was negative. The clinical complaint probably was unrelated to the hemangioma.

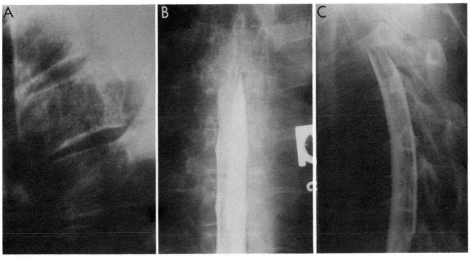

Fig 16–83.—Hemangioma of T-4 in a 43-year-old man with a long history of pain in the upper back complicated by the onset of bilateral lower-extremity weakness and a sensory level at T-5 of 3 weeks' duration. The lateral radiograph demonstrates the characteristic parallel vertical trabeculation of a vertebral hemangioma **(A).** The frontal **(B)** and lateral **(C)** myelographic films show displacement of the spinal cord anteriorly and to the right by extradural extension of the hemangioma. (Courtesy of D. Bloom.)

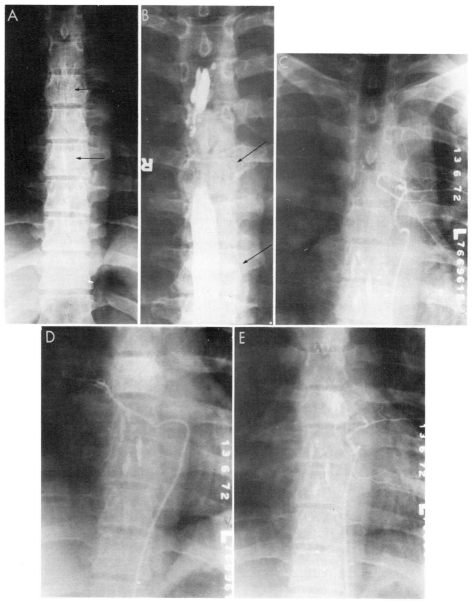

Fig 16–84.—The patient was a 23-year-old man with a 2-year history of paraparesis and a sensory level at T-8. The AP radiograph of the thoracic spine **(A)** demonstrates two vertebral hemangiomas at T-5 and T-7 *(arrows)*. The frontal myelogram shows displacement of the spinal cord to the right at T6-7 by an extradural hematoma, confirmed at operation **(B)**. Bilateral selective arteriography was carried out at multiple levels. Selective injection of the left fourth intercostal artery is negative **(C)**. Selective injection of the left fifth intercostal artery shows slight opacification of the left superior portion of the body of T-5 **(D)**. Selective injection of the right fifth intercostal artery shows further opacification of the hemangioma **(E)**. (Courtesy of M. Hirsch.)

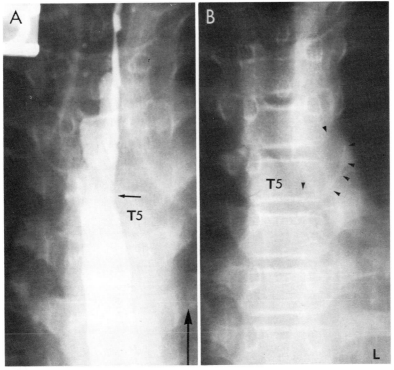

Fig 16–85.—Shallow extradural defect on the left side of the Pantopaque column at the level of T4-5 *(arrow),* with displacement of the spinal cord to the right, **A.** The patient, a 10-year-old boy, complained of sharp pain in the left posterior thoracic region, which radiated anteriorly. The anteroposterior roentgenogram of the thoracic spine, **B,** demonstrates erosion of the left lamina, pedicle and costal process of T-5 *(arrowheads)* and normal intervertebral disk spaces. At operation, an aneurysmal bone cyst was found extending out from T-5 into the extradural space.

sion may be enhanced by the presence of adhesions between these structures. Probably, however, even when these lesions appear to be intramedullary at operation, they actually originate outside the cord itself. Lipomas have a distinct tendency to occur at three distinct age periods—during infancy, at puberty, and during the third to fifth decades of life. There is no predilection for either sex. Because these tumors are slow-growing, they frequently are associated with bony changes on the roentgenogram, e.g., widening of the vertebral canal, erosion of the pedicles and vertebral bodies. The syndrome of lipoma of the cauda equina in childhood has been discussed in Chapter 12 and will not be considered further here. Intradural lipoma of the lower spinal cord may produce symptoms identical to those seen in patients with spinal dysraphism. Lipomas have a unique predilection for the cervical, midthoracic, and lumbosacral regions, where there may be delayed closure of the neural tube, according to Stookey. In a review of 51 spinal cord lipomas, Caram and his associates found the following distribution:

Cervical	6
Cervicothoracic	11
Thoracic	20

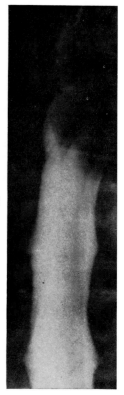

Fig 16–86.—Myelographic spot film in a 51-year-old female, demonstrating a complete block at T-8 produced by a large intradural lipoma. The tumor also infiltrated widely into the substance of the spinal cord and could not be completely removed. (Reprinted, with permission, from Caram P.C., et al., *J. Neurosurg.* 14:28, 1957.)

Conus and cauda equina	5
Thoracolumbar	1
Thoracic to sacral	1
Lumbosacral	1
Entire cord	5
Unlocalized	1

Although myelography is not diagnostic of the histologic nature of the tumor, it may help in establishing a diagnosis preoperatively. For example, a tumor extending over several segments in a young patient with myelographic findings suggestive of both an intramedullary and an extramedullary mass should arouse the strong suspicion of lipoma or congenital cyst. Localization to the cervical or thoracic segments should strengthen this suspicion. CT scanning can provide the specific diagnosis, obviating the need for biopsy.

Dermoids and Epidermoids

These uncommon (less than 1%) benign tumors are grossly similar in appearance, with a smooth, glistening white capsule enclosing a cystic structure filled with epithelial debris, cholesterol, and other lipoids. In the case of the dermoid, the tumor not only contains epithelial elements but also derivatives of the dermis, such as hair and sebaceous glands. Because of their shiny capsule, they commonly are referred to as "pearly tumors." Both the dermoid and the epidermoid are encapsulated,

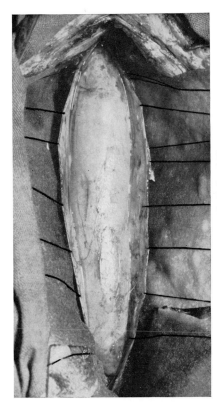

Fig 16–87.—Operative photograph of a large intradural lipoma in a 15-year-old girl. The tumor extended from C-5 to T-3 and diffusely infiltrated the cord, making removal impossible. Conventional radiographs of the cervical spine demonstrated widening of the neural canal, erosion of the pedicles and the posterior surface of the vertebral bodies. (Reprinted, with permission, from Caram, P.C., et al., *J. Neurosurg.* 14:28, 1957.)

slow-growing intradural neoplasms. Although most of these tumors are extramedullary, occasionally they may have an intramedullary site. When the tumor is extramedullary intradural in position, it cannot be distinguished from a neurilemoma. Both lesions are well defined and sharply delineated by the contrast column, tend to produce some degree of obstruction, and displace the cord or the cauda equina to the opposite side.

Dermoids and epidermoids arise from epithelial rests that become sequestered during closure of the neural tube between the third and fifth fetal weeks. Consequently, they occupy a midline or near-midline position characteristically. If the cleavage of the cutaneous and neural ectoderm persists locally anywhere along the neuraxis, a dermal sinus is formed connecting the skin with the neuraxis. Such sinuses, although rare, have also been reported in the cervical and thoracic regions; however, they are more common in the lumbosacral area. Indeed, dermoids and epidermoids both are, in general, more common in the lower spine. List, in a review of the literature in 1941, found that 65% of these lesions were located below the twelfth thoracic vertebra.

According to Sachs and Horrax, dermoids are slightly more common than epidermoids. Of the 61 cases of dermoids and epidermoids they collected from the literature, at least 36 were dermoids; of the 14 cases associated with dermal sinuses, all but one were dermoids.

Dermoids and epidermoids may be associated with varying degrees of spina bifida and may present as cauda equina tumors. The latter lesions are prone to be quite large and extensive, often filling the spinal canal over several lumbosacral segments. Myelography is not diagnostic in itself, merely demonstrating an intradural tumor, intramedullary or extramedullary in position as the case may be, often with a complete block (Fig 16–88). These lesions have been previously discussed in Chapter 12 in association with spinal dysraphism. They are probably hamartomas rather than true neoplasms.

Acquired epidermoids following lumbar puncture or laminectomy are discussed in Chapter 20.

Teratoma

Teratoma represents a relatively rare type of spinal cord tumor, occurring only once in Rasmussen's group of 557 spinal neoplasms and not at all in Elsberg's series of 253 cord tumors. These lesions contain derivatives of all three germ layers and probably constitute the most complex type of congenital spinal cord tumor histologically, with the more simple dermoid at the opposite end of the scale. Although there is not absolute proof, teratomas are thought to arise from multipotential germinal cells early in embryonic development. They may be intradural or extradural in location. Some teratomas are well encapsulated, whereas others are so intimately

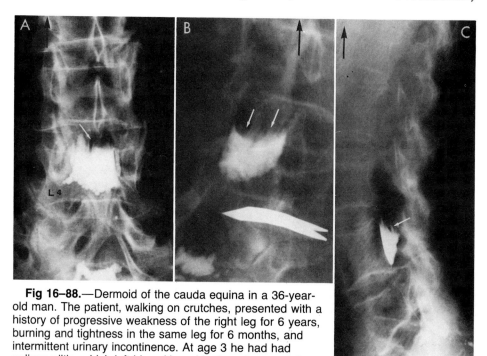

Fig 16–88.—Dermoid of the cauda equina in a 36-year-old man. The patient, walking on crutches, presented with a history of progressive weakness of the right leg for 6 years, burning and tightness in the same leg for 6 months, and intermittent urinary incontinence. At age 3 he had had poliomyelitis, which left him with residual weakness of the right foot. Neurologic examination disclosed weakness and atrophy of the right thigh and calf, loss of sensation below the level of L-4, and an absent right ankle jerk. At operation, he had a cystic intradural tumor that extended from the tip of the conus to L-4. Note the enlargement of the lumbar intervertebral canal, the scalloping of the posterior border of the vertebral bodies, and the defect at the upper border of L-4 *(white arrow)* outlining the inferior margin of the tumor. In **B** and **C,** the white arrows point to the inferior margin of the tumor.

attached to the spinal cord and cauda equina that no satisfactory cleavage plane can be established at operation. Characteristically, a varying-sized portion of the tumor is cystic. In addition, the tumor may extend over several segments and produce bony changes detectable on plain roentgenograms, such as fusiform enlargement of the spinal canal, thinning of the pedicles, with an increase in the interpediculate distance, erosion of the laminae and posterior aspects of several vertebrae. Occasionally, these patients may exhibit a pigmented nevus on the skin at the site of the lesion.

Myelography demonstrates the location of the lesion with or without an associated block. The diagnosis of teratoma should be suspected when a child or young adult presents the clinical picture of a slowly growing spinal cord tumor associated with a pigmented nevus of the skin at the site of the lesion, and the bone changes mentioned above.

Hoefnagel and his colleagues reported an extramedullary intradural cyst in the cervical region in a 6-year-old girl, with observations on the occurrence of sex chromatin in such cysts. The authors indicate that the absence of nuclear chromatin in the cells of the fibrous capsule along with chromatin-positive cells in the epithelial lining suggest a teratomatous origin. Cyst puncture and endomyelography may be quite helpful in the preoperative diagnosis of these and other cystic tumors of the spinal cord. Cytology of the contents of a cyst or histology of a tumor nodule can give a preoperative cellular diagnosis in addition to differentiating tumor from syringomyelia and demonstrating the precise localization of tumor nodules in a cystic neoplasm.

BIBLIOGRAPHY

Adson A.W.: Tumours of the spinal cord; diagnosis and treatment. *Can. Med. Assoc. J.* 40:448, 1939.

Adson A.W.: Diagnosis and treatment of tumors of the spinal cord. *Northwest Med.* 24:309, 1925.

Appleby A., Batson G.A., Lassman L.P., Simpson C.A.: Spinal cord compression by extramedullary haematopoiesis in myelosclerosis. *J. Neurol., Neurosurg. Psychiatr.* 27:313, 1964.

Bailey P., Bucy P.C.: Tumors of the spinal canal. *Surg. Clin. North Am.* 10:233, 1930.

Barron K.D., Hirano A., Araki S., Terry R.D.: Experiences with metastatic neoplasms involving spinal cord. *Neurology* 9:91, 1959.

Bassett R.C.: The neurologic deficit associated with lipomas of the cauda equina. *Ann. Surg.* 131:109, 1950.

Beehler E.: Metastases to spinal subdural space: Report of case. *Bull. Los Angeles Neurol. Soc.* 25:44, 1960.

Benson D.F.: Intramedullary spinal cord metastases. *Neurology* 10:281, 1960.

Black S.P.W., German W.J.: Four congenital tumors found at operation within the vertebral canal, with observations on their incidence. *J. Neurosurg.* 7:49, 1950.

Black S.P.W., Keats T.F.: Generalized osteosclerosis secondary to metastatic medulloblastoma of the cerebellum. *Radiology* 82:395, 1964.

Bobroff L.M., Leeds N.E.: Minimal terminal irregularities of the distal subarachnoid space as a sign of epidural seeding. *Am. J. Roentgenol.* 118:601, 1973.

Bonafé A., Ethier R., Melancon D., et al.: High resolution computed tomography in cervical syringomyelia. *J. Comput. Assist. Tomogr.* 4:42, 1980.

Bonafé A., Manelfe C., Espagno J., et al.: Evaluation of syringomyelia with metrizamide computed tomographic myelography. *J. Comput. Assist. Tomogr.* 4:797, 1980.

Bonstelle C.T., Vines F.S.: Calcification in a cervical intraspinal neurolemmoma. *Neuroradiology* 10:231, 1976.

Botterell E.H., Fitzgerald G.W.: Spinal cord compression produced by extradural malignant tumors: Early recognition, treatment and results. *Can. Med Assoc. J.* 80:791, 1959.

Britt J., Himmelfarb E., Gerald B.: Myelographic appearance of meningo-vascular lymphoma involving cauda equina. *J. Can. Assoc. Radiol.* 26:88, 1975.

Bucy P.C., Jerva M.J.: Primary epidural spinal lymphosarcoma. *J. Neurosurg.* 19:142, 1962.

Bucy P.C., Ritchey H.: Klippel-Feil syndrome associated with compression of the spinal cord by an extradural hemangiolipoma. *J. Neurosurg.* 4:476, 1947.

Bull J.W.D.: Spinal meningiomas and neurofibromas. *Acta Radiol.* 40:283, 1953.

Cabot Case 44401: *N. Engl. J. Med.* 259:688, 1958.

Cairns H., Russell D.S.: Intracranial and spinal metastases in gliomas of the brain. *Brain* 54:377, 1931.

Càlogero J.A., Moossy J.: Extradural spinal meningiomas. Report of four cases. *J. Neurosurg.* 37:442, 1972.

Camp J.D.: Multiple tumors within the spinal canal; diagnosis by means of Lipiodol injected into the subarachnoid space (myelography). *Am. J. Roentgenol.* 36:775, 1936.

Camp J.D.: The roentgenologic localization of tumors affecting the spinal cord. *Am. J. Roentgenol.* 40:540, 1938.

Camp J.D., Adson A.W., Shugrue J.J.: Roentgenographic findings associated with tumors of the spinal column, spinal cord and associated tissues. *Am. J. Cancer* 17:348, 1933.

Caram P.C., Scarcella G., Carton C.A.: Intradural lipomas of the spinal cord, with particular emphasis on the "intramedullary" lipomas. *J. Neurosurg.* 14:28, 1957.

Clarke E.: Spinal cord involvement in multiple myelomatosis. *Brain* 79:332, 1956.

Clifford J.H., McClintock H.G., Lubchenko A.E.: Primary spinal cord malignant melanoma. Case report. *J. Neurosurg.* 29:410, 1968.

Cloward R.B., Bucy P.C.: Spinal extradural cyst and kyphosis dorsalis juvenilis. *Am. J. Roentgenol.* 38:681, 1937.

Cockshott W.P., Evans K.T.: Childhood paraplegia in lymphosarcoma (Burkitt's tumor). *Br. J. Radiol.* 36:914, 1963.

Conway L.W.: Hydrodynamic studies in syringomyelia. *J. Neurosurg.* 27:501, 1967.

Cooper I.S., Craig W. McK., Kernohan J.W.: Tumors of the spinal cord; primary extramedullary gliomas. *Surg., Gynecol. Obstet.* 92:183, 1951.

Critchley M., Greenfield J.G.: Spinal symptoms in chloroma and leukemia. *Brain* 53:11, 1930.

Crosby R.M.N., Wagner J.A., Nicholas P., Jr.: Intradural lipoma. *J. Neurosurg.* 10:81, 1953.

Crowell R.M., Wepsic J.G.: Thoracic cord compression due to chondrosarcoma in two cousins with hereditary multiple exostoses. Report of two cases. *J. Neurosurg.* 36:86, 1972.

da Roza A.C.: Primary intraspinal tumors: Their clinical presentation and diagnosis. *J. Bone Joint Surg.* 46B:8, 1964.

Deans W.R., Block S., Leibrock L., et al.: Arteriovenous fistula in patients with neurofibromatosis. *Radiology* 144:103, 1982.

Decker R.E., Gross S.W.: Intraspinal dermoid tumor presenting as chemical meningitis. Report of a case without dermal sinus. *J. Neurosurg.* 27:60, 1971.

deLorimier A.A., Bragg K.V., Lindern G.: Neuroblastoma in childhood. *Am. J. Dis. Child.* 118:441, 1969.

Desorgher G., Cécile J.P., Bonte G., et al.: Scoliosis revealing a spinal cord mass. *J. Radiol. et Électrol.* 50:695, 1969.

Deutsch M., Scotti L.N., Hardman D.R., et al.: Myelography in patients with medulloblastoma. *Radiology* 117:467, 1975.

Dodge H.W., Jr., Love J.G., Gottlieb C.M.: Benign tumors at the foramen magnum; surgical considerations. *J. Neurosurg.* 13:603, 1956.

Dolan K.D.: Expanding lesions of the cervical spinal canal. *Radiol. Clin. North Am.* 15:203, 1977.

Dorwart R.H., Wara W.M., Norman D., Levin V.A.: Complete myelographic evaluation of spinal metastases from medulloblastoma. *Radiology* 139:403, 1981.

du Boulay G.H., Macdonald J.S.: Elusive tumors in the cervical spinal canal. *Br. J. Radiol.* 37:465, 1964.

Dubowitz V., Lorber J., Zachary R.B.: Lipoma of the cauda equina. *Arch. Dis. Child.* 40:207, 1965.

Ehni G., Love J.G.: Intraspinal lipomas. Report of case; review of the literature and clinical and pathologic study. *Arch. Neurol. Psychiatr.* 53:1, 1945.

Ellertsson A.B.: Semiologic diagnosis of syringomyelia related to roentgenologic findings. *Acta Neurol. Scandinav.* 45:385, 1969.

Elsberg C.A.: *Tumors of the Spinal Cord.* New York, Paul B. Hoeber, Inc., 1925.

Elsberg C.A.: *Surgical Diseases of the Spinal Cord, Membranes and Nerve Roots.* New York, Paul B. Hoeber, Inc., 1941.

Epstein B.S.: Myelographic diagnosis of epidural metastases in lumbosacral spinal canal. *Am. J. Roentgenol.* 68:730, 1952.

Epstein B.S.: Spinal canal mass lesions. *Radiol. Clin. North Am.* 4:185, 1961.

Epstein B.S., Davidoff L.M.: The myelographic diagnosis of extramedullary cervical spinal cord tumors. *Am. J. Roentgenol.* 55:413, 1946.

Epstein B.S., Epstein J.A., Carras R.: Extension of posterior fossa tumors particularly intraventricular fourth ventricle tumors into the upper cervical spinal canal. *Am. J. Roentgenol.* 110:31, 1970.

Fagan C.J., Swischuk L.E.: Dumbbell neuroblastoma or ganglioneuroma of the spinal canal. *A.J.R.* 120:453, 1974.

Feiring E.H., Hubbard J.H.: Spinal cord compression from intradural carcinoma. *J. Neurosurg.* 23:635, 1965.

Garrett M.J.: Spinal myeloma and cord compression in diagnosis and management. *Clin. Radiol.* 21:42, 1970.

Gass H.: Unilateral numbness of the face and the basal cisterns. *Neurology* 19:66, 1970.

Gautier-Smith P.C.: Clinical aspects of spinal neurofibromas. *Brain* 90:359, 1967.

Gibberd F.B., Ngan H., Swann G.F.: Hydrocephalus, subarachnoid haemorrhage and ependymomas of the cauda equina. *Clin. Radiol.* 23:422, 1972.

Goldenberg D.B., Rienhoff W.F., III, Rao P.S.: Osteochondroma with spinal cord compression. *J. Can. Assoc. Radiol.* 19:192, 1968.

Graham D.I., Bondi M.R.: Intradural spinal ossifying schwannoma. Case report. *J. Neurosurg.* 36:487, 1972.

Grant F.C., Austin G.M.: The diagnosis, treatment and prognosis of tumors affecting the spinal cord in childhood. *J. Neurosurg.* 13:355, 1956.

Greenberg A.D., Scatliff J.H., Selker R.G., Marshall M.D.: Spinal cord metastases from bronchogenic carcinoma: Case report. *J. Neurosurg.* 23:72, 1965.

Greenwald C.M., Eugenio M., Hughes C.R., Gardner W.J.: The importance of the air shadow of the cisterna magna in encephalographic diagnosis. *Radiology* 71:695, 1958.

Griffin J.W., Thompson R.W., Mitchison M.J., et al.: Lymphomatous leptomeningitis. *Am. J. Med.* 52:200, 1971.

Gupta S.K., Bhandari Y.P.: Intraspinal dermoids and epidermoids. *Am. J. Roentgenol.* 105:386, 1969.

Guyer P.B., Cook P.L.: The myelographic appearance of spinal cord metastases. *Br. J. Radiol.* 41:615, 1968.

Haft H., Ransohof J., Carter S.: Spinal cord tumors in children. *Pediatrics* 23:1152, 1959.

Haft H., Shenkin H.A.: Spinal epidural meningioma. Case report. *J. Neurosurg.* 20:801, 1963.

Halaby F.A., Peterson R.B., Leaver R.C.: Spinal lipoma. *Am. J. Roentgenol.* 92:1292, 1964.

Hall J.H., Fleming J.F.: Lumbar disc syndrome produced by sacral canal metastases. *Can. J. Surg.* 13:146, 1970.

Hallpike J.F., Stanley P.: A case of extradural spinal meningioma. *J. Neurol., Neurosurg. Psychiatr.* 31:195, 1968.

Hamby W.B.: Tumors in the spinal canal in childhood. An analysis of the literature with report of a case. *J. Nerv. Ment. Dis.* 81:24, 1935.

Hannan J.R., Geist R.M., Jr.: Teratomatous tumors of spinal canal: 2 cases. *Am. J. Roentgenol.* 63:875, 1950.

Hannan J.R., Hughes C.R., Mulvey B.E.: Spinal cord tumors. *Radiology* 53:711, 1949.

Harwood-Nash D.C., Fitz C.R.: Myelography and syringohydromyelia in infancy and childhood. *Radiology* 113:661, 1974.

Hatam A., et al.: Myelography in metastatic lesions. *Acta Radiol. (Diagn.)* 16:321, 1975.

Häussler G.: Indication for contrast roentgenography of tumors in spinal canal. *Fortschr. Geb. Röntgenstrahlen* 74:525, 1951.

Heiser S., Swyer A.J.: Myelography in spinal metastases. *Radiology* 62:695, 1954.

Higinbotham N.L., Phillips R.F., Farr H.W., Hustu H.O.: Chordoma. Thirty-five-year study at Memorial Hospital. *Cancer* 20:1841, 1967.

Hirano A., Carton C.A.: Primary malignant melanoma of the spinal cord. *J. Neurosurg.* 17:935, 1960.

Hoefnagel D., Benirschke K., Duarte J.: Teratomatous cysts within the vertebral canal. Observations on the occurrence of sex chromatin. *J. Neurol., Neurosurg. Psychiatr.* 25:159, 1962.

Holaday W.J., Evans E.B.: Spinal (meningeal) melanoma. A case report. *J. Bone Joint Surg.* 50A:738, 1968.

Horrax G.: Extramedullary spinal cord tumors. *Surg. Clin. North Am.* 27:535, 1947.

Hunt T.R., Jr., Poser C.M., Williamson W.P.: Lymphoma of spinal nerve root. *J. Neurosurg.* 17:342, 1960.

Ingraham F.D.: Intraspinal tumors in childhood. *Am. J. Surg.* 39:342, 1938.

Ingraham F.D., Bailey O.T.: Cystic teratomas and teratoid tumors of the central nervous system in infancy and childhood. *J. Neurosurg.* 3:511, 1946.

Ingraham F.D., Matson D.D.: *Neurosurgery of Infancy and Childhood.* Springfield, Ill., Charles C Thomas, Publisher, 1954.

Jacobson H.H., Lester J.: Myelographic manifestation of diffuse leptomeningeal melanomatosis. *Neuroradiology* 1:30, 1970.

Johnson D.F.: Intramedullary lipomas of the spinal cord. Review of literature and report of case. *Bull. Los Angeles Neurol. Soc.* 15:37, 1950.

Jorgensen J., Ovesen N., Poulsen J.O.: Intraspinal tumours in the first two decades of life. Clinical and radiological features. *Acta Orthop. Scand.* 47:391, 1976.

Kane C.A., Foley J.M.: Primary reticulum cell sarcoma of leptomeninges. *A.M.A. Arch. Intern. Med.* 101:333, 1958.

Katz P.B., Lee Y., Wallace S., Ray R.D.: Myelography of spinal block from epidural tumor: A new approach. *A.J.R.* 136:945, 1981.

Kendall B.: Application of angiography to tumours affecting the spinal cord. *Proc. Roy. Soc. Med.* 63:185, 1970.

Kendall B., Russell J.: Haemangioblastomas of the spinal cord. *Clin. Radiol.* 39:817, 1966.

Kendall B., Symon L.: Cyst puncture and endomyelography in cystic tumours of the spinal cord. *Br. J. Radiol.* 46:198, 1973.

Kenefick J.S.: Hereditary sacral agenesis associated with presacral tumours. *Br. J. Surg.* 60:271, 1973.

Kerber C.W., Margolis M.T., Newton T.H.: Tortuous vertebrobasilar system: A cause of cranial nerve signs. *Neuroradiology* 4:74, 1972.

Kernohan J.W., Woltman H.W., Adson A.W.: Gliomas arising from the region of the cauda equina: Clinical, surgical and histologic considerations. *Arch. Neurol. Psychiatr.* 29:287, 1933.

Kiel F.W., Starr L.B., Hansen J.L.: Primary melanoma of the spinal cord. *J. Neurosurg.* 18:616, 1961.

Kim K.S., Ho S.U., Weinberg P.E., Lee C.: Spinal leptomeningeal infiltration by systemic cancer: Myelographic features. *A.J.N.R.* 3:233, 1982.

Kim S.W., Jeon C.S.: Spinocranial neurofibroma. Case report. *J. Neurosurg.* 27:565, 1971.

Kinney T.D., Fitzgerald P.J.: Lindau-von Hippel disease with haemangioblastoma of the spinal cord and syringomyelia. *Arch. Pathol.* 43:439, 1947.

Klefenberg G., Saltzman G.: Gas myelographic studies in syringomyelia. *Acta Radiol.* 52:129, 1959.

Krishnan K.R., Smith W.T.: Intramedullary hemangioblastoma of the spinal cord associated with pial varicosities simulating intradural angioma. *J. Neurol., Neurosurg. Psychiatr.* 24:350, 1961.

Lerman R.I., Kaplan E.S., Daman L.: Ganglioneuroma-paraganglioma of the intradural filum terminale. *J. Neurosurg.* 36:652, 1972.

Lin S., Silverstein H.: False positive roentgenologic diagnosis of small intracanalicular acoustic neurinoma. *Am. J. Roentgenol.* 118:511, 1973.

List C.F.: Intraspinal epidermoids, dermoids and dermal sinuses. *Surg., Gynecol. Obstet.* 73:525, 1941.

Lombardi G., Passerini A.: Spinal cord tumors. *Radiology* 76:381, 1961.

Lombardi G., Passerini A.: Multiple lesions of the spinal cord. *Am. J. Roentgenol.* 92:1298, 1964.

Love J.G., Miller R.H., Kernohan J.W.: Lymphomas of the spinal epidural space. *A.M.A. Arch. Surg.* 69:66, 1954.

Love J.G., Thelen E.P., Dodge H.W., Jr.: Tumors of the foramen magnum. *J. Internat. Coll. Surgeons* 22:1, 1954.

MacCarty C.S., et al.: Dermoid and epidermoid tumors in the central nervous system of adults. *Surg., Gynecol. Obstet.* 108:191, 1959.

Manno N.J., Uihlein A., Kernohan J.W.: Intraspinal epidermoids. *J. Neurosurg.* 19:754, 1962.

Martin C.F., Jr., Gedgaudas E., D'Angio G.J.: Residual radiopaque bolus in managing intraspinal neoplasms. *Am. J. Roentgenol.* 97:980, 1966.

McCrae D.L., Standen J.: Roentgenologic findings in syringomyelia and hydromyelia. *Am. J. Roentgenol.* 98:695, 1966.

McKissock W., Bloom W.H., Chynn K.Y.: Spinal cord compression caused by plasma cell tumors. *J. Neurosurg.* 18:68, 1961.

Melot C.J., Potvliege R., Martin P., Brihaye J.: Myélographie dans les infiltrations néoplastiques de l'espace épidural. *Acta Radiol. (Diagn.)* 1:736, 1963.

Meyer J.D., Latchaw R.E., Roppolo H.M., et al.: Computed tomography and myelography of the postoperative lumbar spine. *A.J.N.R.* 3:223, 1982.

Moes C.A.F., Hendrick E.B.: Diastematomyelia. *J. Pediatr.* 63:238, 1963.

Murphy W.T., Bilge N.: Compression of the spinal cord in patients with malignant lymphomas. *Radiology* 82:495, 1964.

Myers R.N., Austin G.M., Walker A.E., Gallagher J.P.: Solitary spinal cord tumors occurring in multiple members of a family. *J. Neurosurg.* 17:783, 1960.

Nassar S.I., Correll J.W.: Subarachnoid hemorrhage due to spinal cord tumors. *Neurology* 18:87, 1968.

Nassar S.I., Correll J.W., Housepian E.M.: Intramedullary cystic lesions of the conus medullaris. *J. Neurol., Neurosurg. Psychiatr.* 31:106, 1968.

Otenasek F.J., Silver M.L.: Spinal hemangioma (hemangioblastoma) in Lindau's disease. Report of 6 cases in a single family. *J. Neurosurg.* 18:295, 1961.

Parsms M.: The spinal form of carcinomatous meningitis. *Q. J. Med.* 41:509, 1972.

Perlmutter I., Horrax G., Poppen J.I.: Cystic hemangioblastomas of the cerebellum. End results in 25 verified cases. *Surg., Gynecol. Obstet.* 91:89, 1950.

Piehl M.R., Reese H.H., Steelman H.F.: The diagnostic problem of tumors at foramen magnum. *Dis. Nerv. System* 11:67, 1950.

Pinto R.S., Lin J.P., Firooznia H., Lefleur R.S.: The osseous and angiographic features of vertebral chordomas. *Neuroradiology* 9:231, 1975.

Porro N.: L'esplorazione radiologica dello spazio sotto aracnoideo (miklografia). *Radiol. Med.* 22:475, 1935.

Prentice W.B., Kieffer S.A., Gold L.H.A., Bjornson R.G.: Myelographic characteristics of metastasis to the spinal cord and cauda equina. *Am. J. Roentgenol.* 118:682, 1973.

Prieto A., Jr., Cantu R.C.: Spinal subarachnoid hemorrhage associated with neurofibroma of the cauda equina. Case report. *J. Neurosurg.* 27:63, 1967.

Punt J., Pritchard J., Pincott J.R., Till K.: Neuroblastoma: A review of 21 cases presenting with spinal cord compression. *Cancer* 45:3095, 1980.

Quencer R.M., Tenner M.S., Rothman L.M.: Percutaneous spinal cord puncture and myelocystography. Its role in the diagnosis and treatment of intramedullary neoplasms. *Radiology* 118:637, 1976.

Rasmussen T.B., Kernohan J.W., Adson A.W.: Pathologic classification, with surgical considerations, of intraspinal tumors. *Ann. Surg.* 111:513, 1940.

Rath S., Mathai K.V., Chandy J.: Multiple meningiomas of the spinal canal. Case report. *J. Neurosurg.* 26:639, 1967.

Raynor R.B.: Spinal cord compression in Gaucher's disease. *J. Neurosurg.* 19:902, 1962.

Reiser E.: Die Myelographie, ihre Technik und ihre Ergebnisse. *Roentgenpraxis* 10:217, 1938.

Reyes M.G., Fresco R., Bruetman M.E.: Mediastinal paraganglioma causing spinal cord compression. *J. Neurol., Neurosurg. Psychiatr.* 40:276, 1977.

Rhea A.H., Jensen L.B.: Spinal leptomeningeal carcinomatosis visualized by Amipaque myelography. *Neuroradiology* 17:283, 1979.

Rogers L., Heard G.: Intrathecal spinal metastases (rare tumors). *Br. J. Surg.* 45:317, 1958.

Roller G.J., Pribram H.F.W.: Lumbosacral intradural lipoma and sacral agenesis. *Radiology* 84:507, 1965.

Romeo Orbegozo J.M., Ortega Nuñez A.: Compression medulas por neurofibroma de presentacion familiar. *Rev. Clin. Españ.* 46:315, 1952.

Ross A.T., Bailey O.T.: Tumors arising within spinal canal in children. *Neurology* 3:922, 1953.

Roth M., Gotfryd O., Moravek V.: Intraspinal dermoid and spinal extradural cyst: Pneumomyelographic findings. *Neuroradiology* 5:127, 1973.

Sachs E., Horrax G.: Cervical and lumbar pilonidal sinus communicating with intraspinal dermoids. *J. Neurosurg.* 6:97, 1949.

Schubiger O., Yasargil M.G.: Extracranial vertebral aneurysm with neurofibromatosis. *Neuroradiology* 15:171, 1978.

Schuster J., Markovitz E.: Die Darstellung der Vena longitudinalis posterior cerebrospinalis bei intramedullarem Tumor. *Fortschr. Geb. Röntgenstrahlen* 38:675, 1928.

Shahinfar A.H., Schechter M.M.: Traumatic extradural cysts of the spine. *Am. J. Roentgenol.* 98:713, 1966.

Shapiro J.H., Och M., Jacobson H.G.: Differential diagnosis of intradural (extramedullary) and extradural spinal canal tumors. *Radiology* 76:718, 1961.

Shenkin H., Alpers B.: Gliomas of the spinal cord. *Arch. Neurol. Psychiatr.* 52:87, 1944.

Shephard R.H., Sutton D.: Dumb-bell ganglioneuromata of spine: 4 cases. *Br. J. Surg.* 45:305, 1958.

Sloof J.L., Kernohan J.W., MacCarty C.S.: *Primary Intramedullary Tumors of the Spinal Cord and Filum Terminale.* Philadelphia, W.B. Saunders Co., 1964.

Smith M.J., Stenstrom K.W.: Compression of spinal cord caused by Hodgkin's disease. *Radiology* 51:77, 1948.

Smith W.T., Turner E.: Solitary intramedullary carcinomatous metastasis in spinal cord: Case report. *J. Neurosurg.* 29:648, 1968.

Smolik E.A., Sachs E.: Tumors of the foramen magnum of spinal origin. *J. Neurosurg.* 11:161, 1954.

Snyder L.J., Wilhelm S.K.: Multiple myeloma with spinal cord compression as initial finding. *Ann. Intern. Med.* 28:1169, 1948.

Sod L.M., Wiener L.M.: Intradural extramedullary plasmocytoma. Case report. *J. Neurosurg.* 16:107, 1959.

Sparling H.J., Adams R.D., Parker F., Jr.: Involvement of nervous system by malignant lymphoma. *Medicine* 26:286, 1947.

Stanley P., Siegel S.E., Isaacs H.: Calcification in a paraspinal malignant melanoma in a child. *A.J.R.* 129:143, 1977.

Stein B.M., Leeds N.E., Taveras J., Pool J.L.: Meningiomas of the foramen magnum. *J. Neurosurg.* 20:740, 1963.

Stookey B.: Intradural lipoma. *Arch. Neurol. Psychiatr.* 18:16, 1927.

Strang R.R.: Metastatic tumor of the cervical spinal cord. *Med. J. Aust.* 1:205, 1962.

Svien H.J., Thelen E.P., Keith H.M.: Intraspinal tumors in children. *J.A.M.A.* 155:959, 1954.

Swanson H.S., Barnett J.C.: Intradural lipomas in children. *Pediatrics* 29:911, 1962.

Taniguchi T., Mufson J.A.: Intradural lipoma of the spinal cord, report of a case. *J. Neurosurg.* 7:584, 1950.

Tarlov I.M.: Extradural hemangioblastoma roentgenologically visualized with Diodrast at operation and successfully removed. *Radiology* 49:717, 1947.

Thomas M.L., Andress M.R.: Osteochondroma of the cervical spine causing cord compression. *Br. J. Radiol.* 44:549, 1971.

Till K.: Observations on spinal tumors in childhood. *Proc. Roy. Soc. Med.* 52:333, 1959.

Tönnis W., Friedmann G., Nittner K.: Zur röntgenologischen Diagnose und Differential-diagnose der intraspinalen Tumoren; unter Berücksichtigung der klinischen Symptomato-logie. *Fortschr. Geb. Röntgenstrahlen* 88:288, 1958.

Törmä T.: Malignant tumours of the spine and the spinal extradural space. A study based on 250 histologically verified cases. *Acta Chir. Scandinav.*, Suppl. 225, 1957.

Traub S.L.: Mass lesions in the spinal canal. *Semin. Radiol.* 7:240, 1972.

Tucker A.S., Aramsri B., Gardner W.J.: Primary spinal tumors: A seven year study. *Am. J. Roentgenol.* 87:371, 1962.

Tucker A.S., Aramsri B., Hughes C.R.: Roentgenographic diagnosis of spinal tumors. *Am. J. Roentgenol.* 78:54, 1957.

Valvassori G.E.: Myelography of the internal auditory canal. *Am. J. Roentgenol.* 115:578, 1972.

Van Allen M.W., Rahme E.S.: Lymphosarcomatous infiltration of the cauda equina. Mye-lography in an unusual case. *Arch. Neurol.* 7:476, 1962.

Verda D.J.: Malignant lymphomas of spinal epidural space. *Surg. Clin. North Am.* 24:1228, 1944.

Verity G.: The neurologic manifestations and complications of lymphoma. *Radiol. Clin. North Am.* 6:97, 1968.

Vinstein A.L., Franken E.A., Jr.: Hereditary multiple exostoses. Report of a case with spinal cord compression. *Am. J. Roentgenol.* 112:405, 1971.

Vitek J.: La ponction dorsale therapeutique et diagnostique des cavites syringomyeliques. *Bruxelles Med.* 91:311, 1928–29.

Vitek J.: Ponction bipolaire de la cavite syringomyelique. *Presse Méd.* 40:1507, 1932.

Von Pechy K.: Zur Kenntnis der gutartigen Wirbelsäulengeschwülste in Wirbelkanal. *Frank-furt. Ztschr. Path.* 37:562, 1929.

Walker A.E., Jessico C.M., Marcovich A.W.: Myelographic diagnosis of intramedullary spinal cord tumors. *Am. J. Roentgenol.* 45:321, 1941.

Walker H.R.: Extradural osseous lesions simulating the disc syndrome. *J.A.M.A.* 172:691, 1960.

Webb J.H., Craig W.M., Kernohan J.W.: Intraspinal neoplasms in the cervical region. *J. Neurosurg.* 10:360, 1953.

Westburg G.: Gas myelography and percutaneous puncture in the diagnosis of spinal cord cysts. *Acta Radiol.* Suppl. 252, 1966.

Whitehouse G.H., Griffiths G.J.: Roentgenologic aspects of spinal involvement by primary and metastatic Ewing's tumor. *J. Can. Assoc. Radiol.* 27:290, 1976.

Wickbom I., Hanafee W.: Soft tissue masses immediately below the foramen magnum. *Acta Radiol. (Diagn.)* 1:647, 1963.

Wilkinson A., Mark V.H.: Thoracic extramedullary astrocytoma. Case report. *J. Neurosurg.* 28:504, 1968.

Wilner H.I., Kashef R.: Unilateral arachnoidal cysts and adhesions involving the eighth nerve. *Am. J. Roentgenol.* 115:126, 1972.

Wolf A.: Tumors of the spinal cord, nerve roots and membranes. II. pathology, in Elsberg C.A.: *Surgical Diseases of the Spinal Cord, Membranes and Nerve Roots.* New York, Paul B. Hoeber, Inc., 1941.

Woltman H.W., et al.: Intramedullary tumors of spinal cord and gliomas of intradural por-tion of filum terminale. Fate of patients who have these tumors. *A.M.A. Arch. Neurol. & Psychiatr.* 65:378, 1951.

Wood E.H., Jr.: Diagnosis of spinal meningiomas and schwannomas by myelography. *Am. J. Roentgenol.* 61:683, 1949.

Wood E.H., Jr., Taveras J.M., Pool J.L.: Myelographic demonstration of spinal cord metas-tases from primary brain tumors. *Am. J. Roentgenol.* 69:221, 1953.

Wortzman G., Botterell E.H.: A mobile ependymoma of the filum terminale. *J. Neurosurg.* 20:164, 1963.

Zilkha A., Nicoletti J.M.: Direct visualization of spinal dermoid cyst by positive contrast study. *Br. J. Radiol.* 45:859, 1972.

17

The Herniated Intervertebral Disk

LUMBAR

History

THE INTERVERTEBRAL DISK was first described by Vesalius in 1555 in his classic monograph "De Humani Corporis Fabrica." In 1857, Virchow elaborated on the anatomy of the intervertebral disk. The following year, von Luschka published a more detailed description of the anatomy and embryology of this structure. Remak (1855), Kölliker (1860), Robin (1868), and Löwe (1879) made further contributions to the embryology of the intervertebral disk, pointing out the role of the notochord. Bardeen, Williams, and Compere and Keyes have added to this phase of the subject.

The earliest known report of traumatic rupture of an intervertebral disk was made by Kocher in 1896. The latter described a posterior L1-2 herniation at post mortem in a man who landed upright after a fall of 100 feet. In 1911, Middleton and Teacher reported on a young man who developed pain and flaccid paralysis of the lower extremities after lifting a heavy weight. Sixteen days after the injury, the patient died and necropsy disclosed a posterior disk herniation at T12-L1. The same year, Goldthwait discussed and diagrammatically illustrated the role of trauma in a typical posterior L5-S1 herniation of the nucleus pulposus. Two years later, Elsberg described the benign extradural spine "tumor," which he termed chondroma. Thereafter, an increasing number of intraspinal "chondromas" and "enchondromas" were reported by various surgeons, some of whom appreciated the diskogenic origin of these lesions. In 1918, Sicard pointed out the role of irritation of the intraspinal sciatic nerve roots in the production of sciatica. Interestingly enough, the clinical syndrome of sciatica had been described by an Italian, Dominico Cotunio (Cotugnio), approximately a century and a half before (1764).

The most exhaustive contribution to the anatomy and pathology of the intervertebral disk was made by Schmorl, whose incomparable postmortem studies of the spine appeared between 1927 and 1932. Beadle, working in Schmorl's laboratory in Dresden, added to these brilliant studies. In 1929, Dandy reported two cases of nerve root compression due to extruded cartilaginous fragments of the intervertebral disk. However, it remained for Mixter and Barr in 1934 to correlate the anatomical, pathologic and clinical features in a distinct syndrome. Their classic publication resulted in universal acceptance of the role of the intervertebral disk in the production of low back pain and sciatica, and its surgical treatment.

Embryology

The embryology of the vertebral column and the intervertebral disk has been reviewed thoroughly by Keyes and Compere. According to these authors, a ridge of entodermal cells known as the chordal plate develops in the midsagittal plane in the early embryo (3½ weeks). This ridge separates off as the notochord and is soon surrounded by mesenchymal cells from the sclerotomes to form a column. The latter becomes segmented by a series of parallel arterial branches from the aorta. In the 5-week-old embryo, each segment of the column consists of a light cephalic and a dark caudal mass. The cells closest to the vessels (the cephalic and caudal cells above and below each segmental artery) have the richest blood supply, grow more rapidly, and fuse to form the primordia of the vertebral bodies. The cells farther away from the blood vessels (the cranial portion of each dark caudal mass) remain relatively unchanged and give rise to a portion of the intervertebral disks. As the cells closest to the vessels increase in size, they encroach on the notochord and compress it toward the intervertebral spaces. Eventually, progressive ossification all but obliterates the notochord in the vertebral bodies, leaving only a vestigial mucoid streak (Fig 17–1).

In the development of the intervertebral disk from the two sites described above, the embryonic nucleus pulposus is originally formed from the notochordal cells, which are extruded from the primitive vertebral bodies. The annulus fibrosus is derived from cells in the cranial portion of the dark caudal masses. The latter cells

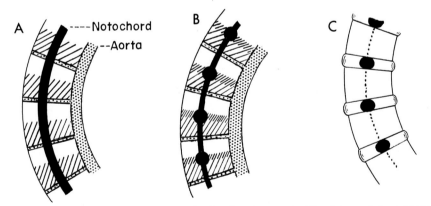

Fig 17–1.—Three successive stages in the development of the intervertebral disks (after Armstrong). **A,** in the 5-week embryo, the notochord is surrounded by mesenchymal cells to form a column that is segmented by parallel arterial branches from the aorta. Each segment consists of a lighter cephalic mass and a darker caudal mass. **B,** the cells closest to the vessels, i.e., the cephalic and caudal cells above and below each segmental artery, grow more rapidly and fuse to form the primitive vertebral bodies; the cells more remote from the blood vessels, i.e., the cranial portion of each darker caudal mass, form part of the intervertebral disks. **C,** as the cells close to the vessels grow, they compress the notochord into the intervertebral spaces and eventually obliterate all but a remnant, which persists as the nucleus pulposus.

differentiate into elongated fibroblasts, which envelop the nucleus and become centrally attached to the vertebral bodies above and below. Later, invaginations from the center of the annulus invade the nucleus so that the adult nucleus pulposus has a dual origin from the notochord and the annulus.

Anatomy

The adult intervertebral disk consists of three parts: (1) the articular plates, (2) the nucleus pulposus, and (3) the annulus fibrosus. The adult disk is thicker anteriorly throughout the spine, particularly in the lumbar region. The disks are adherent to the thin hyaline cartilaginous articular plates which cover the superior and inferior surfaces of the vertebral bodies. The intervertebral disks themselves lack blood vessels, lymphatics, and nerves. They are nourished by a diffusion process that provides a metabolic exchange via the vessels supplying the vertebral bodies. This is borne out by the fairly rapid disappearance of aqueous contrast material from the nucleus pulposus after disk puncture. The exchange takes place through the perforated cartilaginous end-plate between the disk and the adjacent vertebral spongiosa.

ARTICULAR PLATE.—In the growing spine, the cartilaginous articular plate overlaps the anterior and lateral margins of each vertebral body, forming the "epiphyseal ring" or "rim ledge" (Schmorl) (Fig 17–2). When full growth is attained, enchondral bone formation stops and fusion between the epiphyseal ring and vertebral body takes place. In the adult, the rim ledge measures approximately 2–3 mm in width and 1.5–2.0 mm in height, projecting above the articular surface of the vertebral body as an incomplete bony ring that encloses the disk anterolaterally but not posteriorly. The fibers of the annulus fibrosus (Sharpey fibers) are firmly attached to the compact bony ring. The residual central portion of the articular surface of the vertebral body consists of spongy bone, which abuts on the cartilaginous plate. This spongy surface is subject to erosion by nuclear tissue, which may prolapse into it (Schmorl's nodes).

NUCLEUS PULPOSUS.—The demarcation between the nucleus pulposus and the annulus fibrosus, although definite, is not sharply defined. The nucleus pulposus is variable in size but usually occupies a position posterior to the center of the verte-

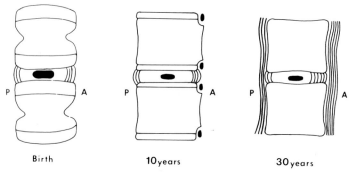

Birth   10 years   30 years

Fig 17–2.—The appearance of the vertebrae at birth, at 10 years of age, and in the adult. Note the progressive decrease in the height of the articular plate and the appearance and fusion of the epiphyseal rings.

bra. This position varies slightly in different segments of the spine, being somewhat more anterior in the upper thoracic region. Grossly, the fibrocartilaginous nucleus has a semigelatinous, white, glistening appearance. Microscopically, it consists of a loose network of fine fibrous strands coursing in irregular, wavy bundles. Within the meshes of the fibrous network are numerous spindle-shaped connective tissue and cartilage cells (Fig 17–3). The turgor of the nucleus depends on its water content, which diminishes with age. The decrease in fluid content of the nucleus normally begins in the third and fourth decades, and usually progresses slowly. It is accelerated by any condition that produces disk degeneration, i.e., trauma or inflammation. As degeneration occurs, some obliteration of the cellular elements takes place along with fibrous tissue infiltration, yellow-brown discoloration, cleft formation and thinning.

ANNULUS FIBROSUS.—The annulus, the strongest portion of the intervertebral disk, firmly binds the vertebrae together. It also determines the size and configuration of the disk. Basically, it consists of a variable number (6 in the lower thoracic, 10–12 in the lumbar region) of concentric lamellae, which encircle the nucleus and extend out over the entire disk surface. In the lumbar region, the lamellae are quite large and thick, especially at the lateral margins of the disk. At the anterior and lateral margins of the vertebral body, the annulus is firmly fused to the bony rim ledge. Anteriorly also, the annulus merges imperceptibly with the strong anterior longitudinal ligament, which is attached to the anterior surface of the vertebral bodies. Posteriorly, however, the attachment is much less secure because of the deficient bony rim ledge, the decrease in the number and thickness of the lamellae, and the relative weakness of the posterior longitudinal ligament (Fig 17–4).

Pathology

The intervertebral disk is subject to the following pathologic processes:

PROLAPSE OF THE NUCLEUS PULPOSUS INTO THE VERTEBRAL BODY (SCHMORL'S NODE).—Fissures and other hiati in the cartilaginous articular plates may permit the prolapse of nuclear tissue into the spongy portion of the vertebral body (Figs 17–5 to 17–8). This finding is relatively common, occurring in 38% of Schmorl's necropsy material. Only a small number of these protrusions are demonstrable by conventional radiography, depending on the size of the protrusion, the presence or absence of calcification, and the degree of reactive sclerosis in the surrounding bone. These intervertebral prolapses are probably not symptomatic per se, partic-

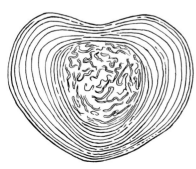

Fig 17–3.—Cross-section of an adult lumbar intervertebral disk, showing the loose mesh of connective tissue and cartilage cells in the central nucleus pulposus together with the concentric annular lamellae.

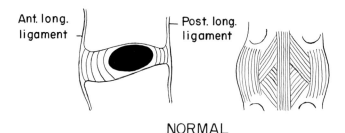

NORMAL

Fig 17–4.—Diagram of a normal intervertebral disk. **Left,** lateral view; **right,** posterior view.

ularly when they are small. However, they may lead to progressive disk degeneration which can cause symptoms.

BALLOONING OF THE INTACT INTERVERTEBRAL DISK INTO THE VERTEBRAL BODY.—This condition may occur in diseases characterized by profound weakening of the structure of the vertebral body; for instance, osteoporosis, osteomalacia, hyperparathyroidism. Presumably as a result of increased imbibition of water, the disk expands into a globular structure, which diffusely indents the articular surfaces of the softened vertebral bodies, thus producing a biconcave fish-type of vertebra (Fig 17–9).

CALCIFICATION.—Calcification may occur to a varying degree in the nucleus pulposus or the annulus fibrosus (Figs 17–10, 17–11). This calcification commonly is asymptomatic, although in children it may occasionally be associated with pain (Fig 17–12). In children, the calcification may be resorbed as the symptoms disappear. Diffuse calcification of the intervertebral disks occurs in ochronosis as part of the widespread degenerative changes in cartilage associated with this disease.

DIFFUSE DEGENERATION.—Diffuse degeneration of the intervertebral disk is associated with dehydration, fibrillation of the fibrocartilage, narrowing of the intervertebral disk space, reactive sclerosis of the subchondral bone, and spur formation

Fig 17–5.—Lateral tomogram showing a typical Schmorl's node protruding through the superior articular plate into the body of L-5. Note the peripheral sclerosis.

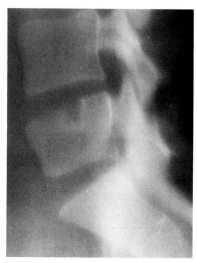

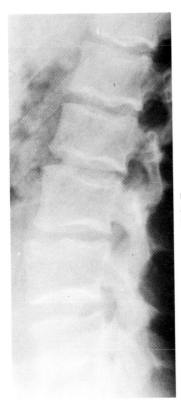

Fig 17–6.—Multiple Schmorl's nodes in a 26-year-old asymptomatic male without dorsal kyphosis.

(Fig 17–13). Gas may be seen in the degenerated disk, presumably due to diffusion from the interstitial fluid space into a partial vacuum within the pathologic disk (Fig 17–14). This is elegantly demonstrated by CT. These changes may be the result of aging, trauma or inflammation.

INFLAMMATION.—Inflammation of the intervertebral disk space may follow direct trauma by needle puncture or surgical removal of the nucleus pulposus (Fig 17–15), or via the bloodstream secondary to infection elsewhere in the body. The organisms vary in virulence. Although they are usually confined to the intervertebral disk, extradural abscess, paravertebral abscess, or sinus can occur as a complication. The patient usually complains of excruciating back pain. The pain, when a lumbar disk is involved, is centered in the low back but may be referred to the lower abdomen, groin, or testes. The pain may come on as early as a week, or as late as 10 weeks, following trauma. Fever and leukocytosis are not prominent, but an elevated sedimentation rate is almost invariably present.

The complications of extradural abscess and granuloma are discussed in Chapter 14. The present section is limited to infections confined to the disk space. Radiographs of the spine may fail to disclose a lesion until 4–6 weeks have elapsed. The earliest roentgen sign is a loss of the sharp detail of the dense white epiphyseal plates on either side of the involved interspace. Localized areas of erosion often can be seen at the anterior margins of the involved interspace, which gradually becomes narrower (see Fig 14–21). In the healing phase, proliferation of new bone

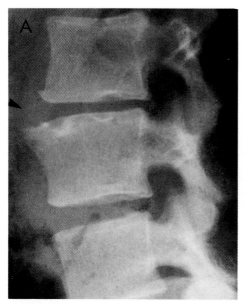

Fig 17–7.—A, multiple Schmorl's nodes at the L2-3 interspace in an asymptomatic young woman associated with narrowing of the interspace and an anterior disk herniation *(arrowhead)*. **B,** asymptomatic anterior disk herniation at L3-4 *(arrow)* in a 14-year-old boy with low back pain. Note the pronounced uptake of the radioisotope by the lesion *(arrow)*.

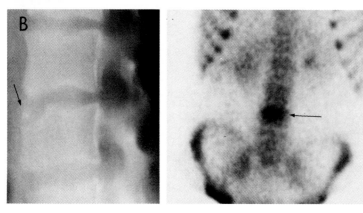

appears from the anterolateral margins of the two vertebrae bordering the pathologic interspace. Completely bony fusion eventually occurs within 6–24 months.

An interesting lesion involving the intervertebral disk in children has been described under the term of spondylarthritis. The lesion represents a low-grade inflammatory process affecting the disk and adjacent vertebral bodies. The patient presents with pain in the back, hip, or buttock, limitation of motion of the involved extremity, low-grade fever, mild leukocytosis, and elevated sedimentation rate. Blood cultures are negative, as are skin tests for tuberculosis, brucellosis, and other specific infections that can produce similar involvement of the spine. Approximately 2–4 weeks after the onset of clinical symptoms, roentgenograms of the spine reveal narrowing of the involved intervertebral disk space with some resorption or destruction of the adjacent vertebrae (see Fig 14–25). These changes persist for approximately 1–3 months. Thereafter, early sclerosis of the vertebral body may be seen, and healing progresses during the next 2–8 months with gradual widening of the intervertebral disk space and new bone formation in the areas of destruction.

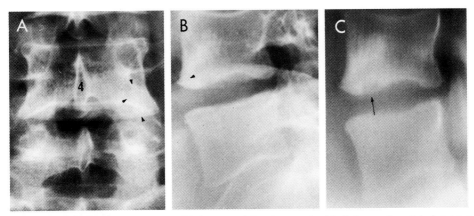

Fig 17–8.—Striking sclerosis of left anterolateral aspect of L-4 *(arrowheads)* due to a Schmorl's node on the inferior aspect of the vertebral body. Note that the node itself is not well visualized on the conventional AP and lateral films **(A and B)**. However, it is clearly seen *(arrow)* on the lateral tomogram **(C)**.

In young children, there is frequently a remarkable restitution to normalcy within a year. It is important to differentiate this lesion from tuberculosis. The correct diagnosis can be made by appropriate bacteriologic studies and skin tests, the clinical course, and serial roentgenograms of the spine.

HERNIATION OF THE NUCLEUS PULPOSUS THROUGH THE ANNULUS FIBROSUS.— Herniation of the nucleus through a tear in the annulus is an important entity. The earliest pathologic changes in this lesion are softening of the nucleus and mild fray-

Fig 17–9.—Tracing of a lateral radiograph of the lumbar spine in a 75-year-old female with severe senile osteoporosis, showing ballooning of the intervertebral disks into the vertebral bodies.

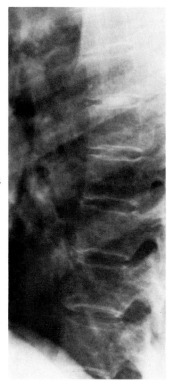

Fig 17–10.—Calcification of a single nucleus pulposus in the upper thoracic spine.

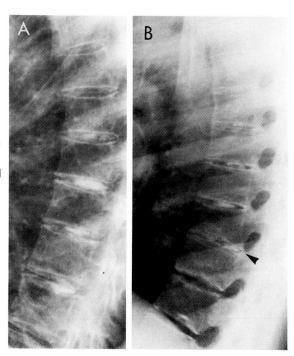

Fig 17–11.—Two examples of calcification of multiple disks in the thoracic spine in middle-aged asymptomatic females. Note the associated disk herniation *(arrowhead)* at T9-10 in **B.**

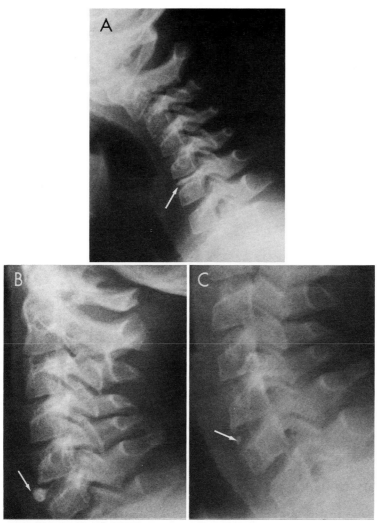

Fig 17–12.—Calcification of the intervertebral disk at C5-6 *(arrow)* in a 4-year-old boy. **A,** at the time of the original radiograph on February 18, 1963, the patient complained of pain in the neck. **B,** re-examination on August 2, 1965, showed anterior protrusion of the calcified disk *(arrow)*. However, the patient had no pain referable to the neck at that time. **C,** follow-up films on January 6, 1966, showed considerable reabsorption of the calcification with only a small residual fleck *(arrow)*.

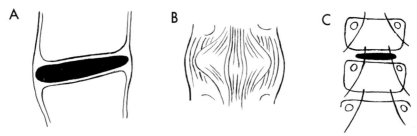

Fig 17–13.—Diffuse degeneration in a lumbar intervertebral disk with an intact annulus. **A,** lateral view of a degenerated lumbosacral disk; **B,** posterior view of a degenerated disk at L4-5 showing diffuse bulging of the disk and thinning of the annulus and posterior longitudinal ligament; **C,** frontal projection showing the relationship of the bulging disk to the nerve roots.

ing of the annulus, usually posteriorly at its weakest point (Fig 17–16). Progressive disintegration and fragmentation of the nucleus eventually occurs, along with actual rupture of the annulus. Extrusion of nuclear material through the defect in the annulus may be gradual or sudden, secondary to trauma of varying severity. The most common site of nuclear herniation is posterolateral, although posterior central and, less commonly, anterior protrusions also occur (Figs 17–17, 17–18). The herniated fragment may lie in the lateral recess or in the intervertebral foramen. The latter is clearly demonstrable by high-resolution CT but cannot be visualized by myelography because metrizamide does not extend out laterally in the nerve root sheath beyond the pedicle (Fig 17–19). The extruded fragment varies in size and is

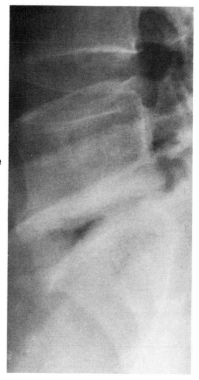

Fig 17–14.—Lateral view of the lumbosacral spine, demonstrating degeneration of the L5-S1 intervertebral disk with gas in the disk substance.

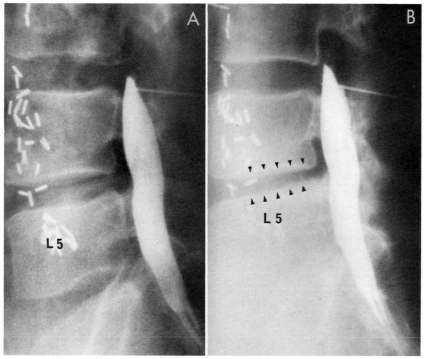

Fig 17–15.—Lateral radiographs made during myelography demonstrating progressive narrowing *(arrowheads)* of the L4-5 intervertebral disk space following laminectomy with removal of a disk fragment. **A,** radiograph made on March 26, 1963; **B,** radiograph made on November 21, 1963.

usually covered by the thinned-out, stretched, posterior longitudinal ligament. The protrusion may burst through the posterior longitudinal ligament to present as a free fragment in the spinal canal either at the level of the involved interspace or somewhat above or below it (Fig 17–20). Occasionally, the nuclear fragment may dissect the posterior longitudinal ligament away from its attachment and come to lie some distance away from its point of rupture (Figs 17–21, 17–22). Uncommonly, the completely extruded fragment is large enough to occlude the spinal canal, resulting in a complete block with paresis or paraplegia. Rarely, a herniated disk fragment may penetrate through the dura and arachnoid to present in the subarach-

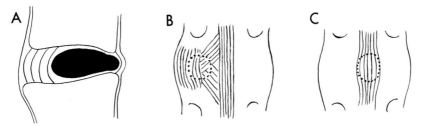

Fig 17–16.—A bulging disk with an intact annulus. **A,** lateral view of a central or a lateral bulge. **B,** posterior view of a posterolateral bulge. **C,** posterior view of a central bulge.

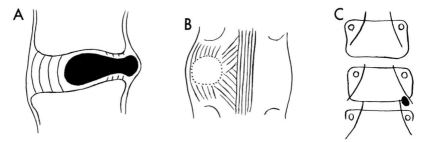

Fig 17–17.—Posterolateral disk herniation. **A,** lateral view showing the herniated fragment protruding through a tear in the annulus beneath the intact posterior longitudinal ligament. **B,** posterior view demonstrating the defect in the annulus. **C,** frontal view showing the disk fragment medial to the nerve root at the level of the interspace.

noid space. Slater and his co-workers reported two midline intradural disk extrusions in a series of 1,000 patients operated on for lumbar disk herniation. The authors emphasize the rarity of this occurrence and suggest intradural exploration when the extradural findings fail to account for the clinical findings. Bilateral protrusions may also occur, due either to extension of the original protrusion across the midline or to the development of a second protrusion on the opposite side (Fig 17–23). In diffuse degeneration of the disk, the entire posterior portion of the annulus is thinned out and lax in the absence of an actual tear. Under these circumstances, the nucleus bulges posteriorly to a varying degree (Fig 17–24).

Clinical Findings

A series of 1,000 herniated lumbar disks operated upon by Finneson disclosed the following localization:

L5-S1	516	(52%)
L4-L5	218	(22%)
L5-S1 and L4-L5	243	(24%)
		98.0%
L3-L4	16	1.5%
L2-L3	3	0.2%
L1-L2	2	0.15%
T12-L1	2	0.15%

In a composite series of approximately 3,000 cases of single lumbar disk herniations culled from the literature (Raaf, Lansche and Ford, Gurdjian et al., Lombardi

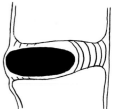

Fig 17–18.—Anterior disk herniation (lateral view).

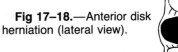

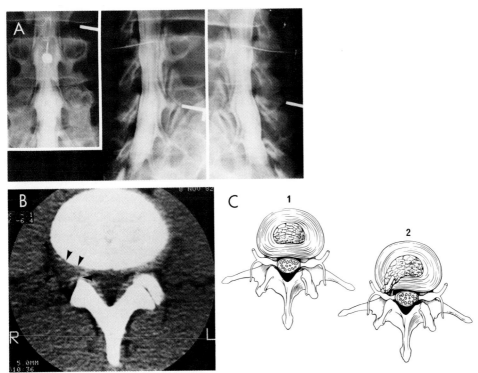

Fig 17–19.—Lateral disk herniation into the intervertebral foramen which cannot be visualized by myelography but is clearly demonstrable by CT. **A,** negative metrizamide myelogram. **B,** CT showing the large herniated fragment at L4-5 in the right intervertebral foramen obliterating the epidural fat in the foramen *(arrowheads)*. Note also minimal bulging of the disk on the left. **C,** artists's rendition of the CT findings in a normal patient *(1)* in the axial projection and of the disk herniation *(arrow)* into the intervertebral foramen *(2)*.

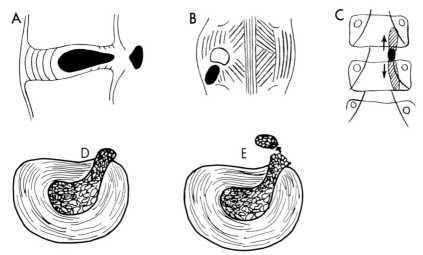

Fig 17–20.—Herniated disk presenting as a free fragment in the extradural space through a rent in the posterior longitudinal ligament. **A,** lateral view showing the fragment at the level of the interspace. **B,** posterior view showing migration of the free fragment inferiorly. **C,** frontal view showing the relationship of the fragment to nerve roots at the interspace and above and below it. **D,** axial projection of a posterolateral herniation. **E,** axial projection of a posterolateral herniation with a migratory free fragment.

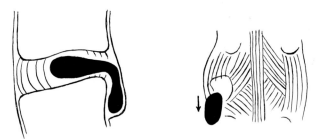

Fig 17–21.—Posterolateral herniation elevating the posterior longitudinal ligament and coming to rest at the level of the vertebral body below the interspace.

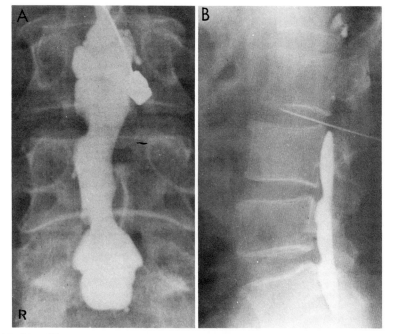

Fig 17–22.—The patient was a 51-year-old man with a large tear in the posterior longitudinal ligament through which a massive, irregularly shaped fragment of disk herniated. It came to lie as a free fragment anterior to the left fifth lumbar nerve, compressing the common dural sac **(A).** The large size and irregular shape of the fragment are unusual and make it difficult to distinguish from extradural metastases. The lateral position of the disk fragment accounts for the minimal defect in the lateral cross-table film **(B).**

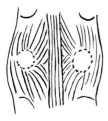 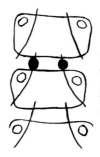

Fig 17–23.—Bilateral herniation. Posterior view, **left,** and frontal view, **right,** showing the relationship of the protruded fragments to the corresponding nerve roots.

and Passerini), 43% involved the L5-S1 disk, 47% involved the L4-5 disk, and 10% involved the remaining higher lumbar levels (Figs 17–25, 17–26). Multiple herniations occurred in 10.3% of the Lansche and Ford series and in 15% of Lombardi and Passerini's patients (Fig 17–27). The most frequent associations of multiple herniations in the latter series involved the L4-5 disk (69% of the multiple herniations), L3-4 disk (17%), and other sites (14%). It is important to remember that an obstructive disk herniation may mask a second more cephalad or caudal herniation, depending on the site of lumbar puncture (Fig 17–28).

A history of trauma is frequently elicited. Although unreliable in some patients, the traumatic history is unmistakable in many others. Thus, some patients with an acute onset of symptoms describe lifting a heavy object or twisting the back, accompanied by a snapping sensation and low back pain with or without sciatic radiation. The acute pain may disappear completely, or it may be followed by a dull backache. In contrast to the acute group, the chronic cases are more likely to present with a dull, low backache, often relieved by rest. This type of pain tends to be intermittent and not so definitely episodic as the acute type. At times, sciatic pain of acute or insidious onset may be the initial symptom. Frequently, the patient complains of both backache and sciatic pain. Aggravation of the pain by coughing, sneezing, or straining is a common symptom. Although the sciatic pain is usually confined to one leg, it may be bilateral when the disk fragment or fragments compress roots on both sides. Rarely, the patient presents with a compression syndrome, with a varying degree of paraplegia.

Physical examination during the acute attack demonstrates erector spini spasm in the lumbar region, straightening of the lumbar spine, and limitation of flexion and

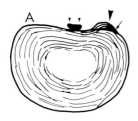 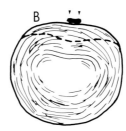

Fig 17–24.—Axial diagram of **(A)** posterolateral bulge *(arrowhead)* with an intact annulus *(arrow);* **B,** diffuse generalized bulge with an intact annulus. Dotted line represents the normal position of the annulus; double arrowhead points to the posterior longitudinal ligament.

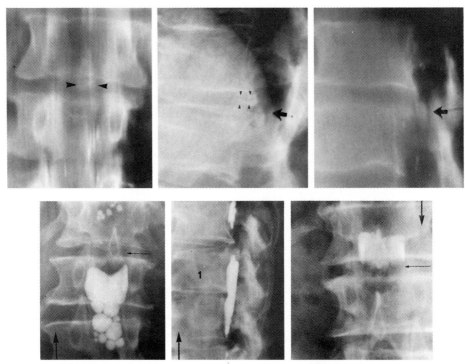

Fig 17–25.—**Top** *(left to right),* AP tomogram, lateral radiograph, and lateral tomogram demonstrating a calcified free disk fragment in the neural canal at T12-L1 which has migrated somewhat caudally. Note the residual disk calcification in the posterior portion of the T12-L1 interspace *(small arrowheads).* **Bottom** *(left to right),* frontal and lateral spot films demonstrating the lower limit of high-grade block after the introduction of 2 ml of Pantopaque from below (head down 90 degrees), and the upper limit of the block after the injection of 1 ml of oil via a C1-2 puncture.

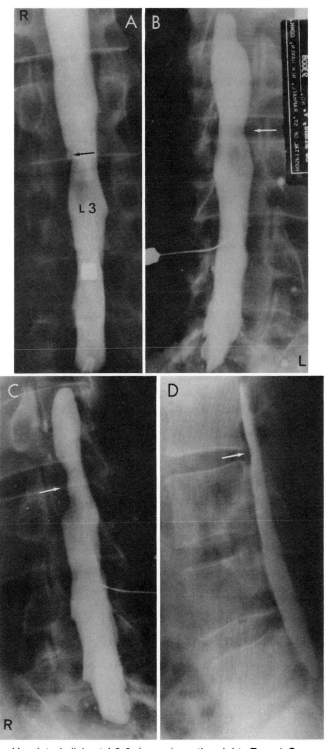

Fig 17–26.—Herniated disk at L2-3 *(arrow)* on the right; **B** and **C** represent oblique views. Note, in **C,** how much more prominent the defect is when the right side of the Pantopaque column is seen in profile *(arrow).*

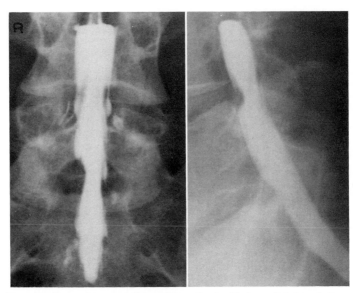

Fig 17–27.—Myelographic spot films of a patient with two disk herniations, i.e., a central herniation at L4-5 and a lateral herniation at the lumbosacral interspace on the right.

extension. About half of the patients exhibit scoliosis, most often with the convexity toward the side of the disk herniation. Production of pain in the leg, hip, or back by stretching the sciatic nerve is one of the most classic signs (positive straight leg raising test). Sensory changes such as hypalgesia may occur in the dermatome supplied by the involved root. Because of overlap between adjacent dermatomes and individual variations in dermatomal distribution, the sensory findings should be interpreted in the light of the pain distribution and the reflex changes. For instance, since the roots involved in the knee jerk are L-3 and L-4, impairment of either of these roots may result in a diminished tendon reflex at the knee; likewise, since the S-1 and S-2 roots are responsible for the ankle jerk, pressure on these

Fig 17–28.—Six months prior to admission, the patient, a 50-year-old male, experienced low back pain with radiation along the posterior aspect of both thighs. The pain disappeared only to recur 5 months later. Two weeks before admission, there was a sudden onset of numbness of the left leg below the knee and a left foot drop. In the hospital, the pain was somewhat less intense and confined entirely to the low back and right leg. There was no urinary or bowel difficulty. Physical examination showed marked impairment of pain sensation along the distribution of lumbar dermatomes 4 and 5 on the left. Both knee jerks were present, but the ankle jerks were absent. Radiographic examination of the thoracic and lumbar spines revealed 12 thoracic vertebrae with complete sacralization of L-5. Hence, the most caudal recognizable intervertebral disk space was L4-5. At the time of the initial myelogram, the needle was inserted at the upper margin of the body of L-2. Note the complete block of L2-3, with feathering of the distal end of the Pantopaque column in the frontal projection *(arrow),* **A.** The lateral decubitus film, **B,** made with the horizontal beam demonstrates elevation of the anterior aspect of the oil column from the posterior surface of L-2 adjacent to the L2-3 interspace *(arrows).* This type of extradural defect is highly suggestive of a herniated disk. The diagnosis of a large free fragment of disk in the spinal canal was considered. Because of the midline position of the defect and the previous history of left-sided symptoms and signs, the possibility of a second disk

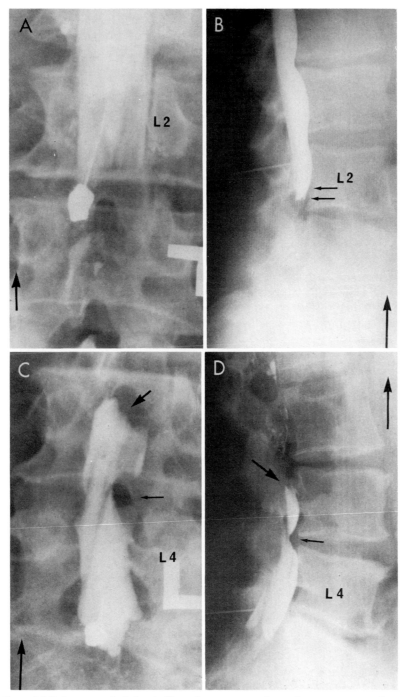

herniation at L3-4 was entertained. Therefore, a repeat myelogram was performed the following day with the needle at the L4-5 interspace. Note the prominent defect at L3-4 on the left side *(thin arrows)*, **C** and **D.** Note also the inferior margin of the obstructing lesion at L2-3 *(broad arrows)*. At operation, there was large nuclear fragment free in the spinal canal at L2-3 and a second disk herniation at L3-4 on the left side.

roots may produce a diminished or absent ankle jerk. An abnormal ankle jerk is helpful in differentiating between L-5 and S-1 root involvement, since this reflex usually is normal in L-5 root lesions and abnormal when the S-1 root is involved. Precise localization is not always possible from the clinical findings alone (Fig 17–29).

A herniated intervertebral disk may or may not be associated with some degree of elevation of the spinal fluid protein level. When disk herniation produces significant spinal block, the protein is considerably elevated.

Radiography

Routine radiography may demonstrate a normal spine or localized narrowing of the involved intervertebral disk space, with or without associated osteophyte formation and subchondral sclerosis. Occasionally, calcification of the herniated fragment in the spinal canal can be seen at the level of the involved interspace (Fig 17–30). There also may be some calcification in the residual disk within the intervertebral space. Calcification of an intervertebral disk (particularly of the nucleus pulposus) without herniation is common in the middle and lower thoracic regions and has no pathologic significance per se. At times, the soft tissue shadow of a protruded lumbar disk fragment can be recognized in the lateral projection, especially when the protrusion is anterior. In acute disk herniation, the normal lordosis may be lost due to erector spini spasm. Most important of all, radiographs of the lumbar spine help to exclude other pathologic processes, i.e., tumor (Fig 17–31)

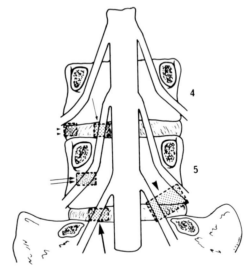

Fig 17–29.—Diagram illustrating how medial and lateral disk herniations at different lower lumbar levels produce variable neural compression. Thus, a lateral L4-5 herniation can compress the L-4 nerve *(small arrowheads)*, while a more medial herniation at the same interspace *(small arrow)*, as well as a lateral herniation of the lumbosacral disk at the foraminal level *(double arrow)* compress the L-5 root. The more common medial lumbosacral herniation compresses the S-1 root *(large arrow)*. However, a large lateral herniation of the lumbosacral disk can compress both the S-1 root as it crosses the interspace and the L-5 root as it exists through the lumbosacral neural foramen *(large arrowhead)*.

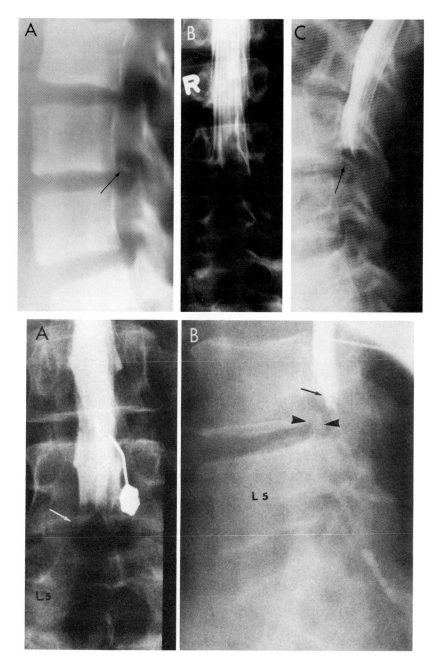

Fig 17–30.—**Top,** calcified free fragment in the neural foramen at L3-4 in a 15-year-old weight lifter. The lateral tomogram **(A)** clearly shows the calcification in the foramen *(arrow)*. The AP **(B)** and lateral **(C)** views of a metrizamide myelogram demonstrate a complete extradural obstruction. Note the "feathering" of the distal end of the contrast column, suggestive of an extradural defect. The CSF protein level was markedly elevated. At surgery, a large free fragment was found, only a portion of which was calcified. **Bottom: A,** herniated disk at L4-5 with a calcified disk fragment free in the spinal canal producing a complete block *(arrow)*. In **B,** note the calcified free fragment *(arrowheads),* which is responsible for the tent-like displacement of the Pantopaque column away from the posterior inferior margin of the L-4 vertebral body *(arrow)*. Because the herniated disk fragment is extradural, the dura is not stripped away from the cauda equina but is displaced with the cauda as a unit. In the presence of a complete obstruction, this finding is highly suggestive of a herniated disk.

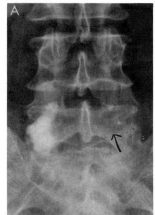

Fig 17–31.—A 64-year-old man with extradural metastatic tumor who presented with a typical story of a herniated disk involving the fifth left lumbar root. Note the destruction of the left pedicle and superior articular process of L-5, which led to the correct preoperative diagnosis (*arrows,* **A** and **B**). At laminectomy, a tongue of extradural tumor presented at the margin of the left L-5 lamina and encased the left L-5 root. The frontal myelogram **(C)** demonstrates a swollen left L-5 root. The lateral cross-table film was essentially negative.

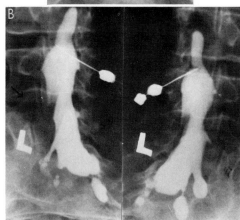

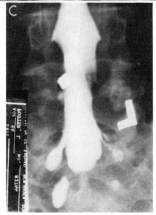

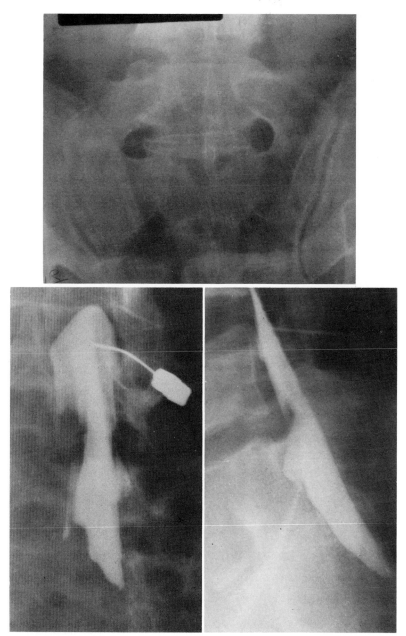

Fig 17–32.—**Top,** anteroposterior view of the lumbosacral region, demonstrating bilateral sacralization of the transverse processes of the last lumbar vertebra. **Bottom,** oblique and lateral myelographic spot films of the same patient, showing a right posterolateral disk herniation at the space above the transitional interspace.

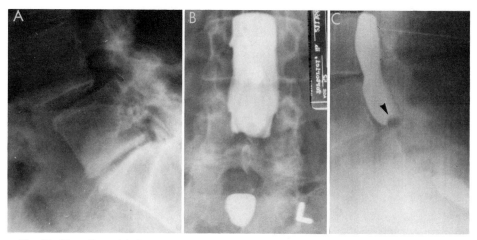

Fig 17–33.—Spondylolisthesis at L4-5 in a 52-year-old female who also had diskogenic disease at the lumbosacral interspace **(A).** The myelogram shows a high-grade obstruction at L4-5 **(B** and **C)** with a defect on the lateral film *(arrowhead)* due to a completely extruded disk fragment lying free in the canal.

and various congenital abnormalities, such as transitional vertebra, spondylolisthesis, achondroplasia, and lesions associated with a widened spinal canal.

Transitional vertebra is a term used to designate sacralization of the last lumbar vertebra or lumbarization of the first sacral vertebra. This process, which may be partial or complete, is characterized by a narrow joint space and a rudimentary intervertebral disk. When the sacralization or lumbarization is fairly complete, the intervertebral disk space above the transitional interspace becomes the physiologic lumbosacral joint. Consequently, degenerative changes, including herniation, are more likely to occur at that level (Fig 17–32). Similarly, patients with spondylolis-

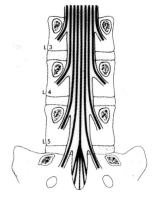

Fig 17–34.—Schematic diagram of normal lower lumbar metrizamide myelogram in AP projection *(above)* and axial projection *(below)* as seen in metrizamide CT.

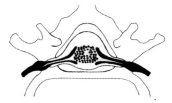

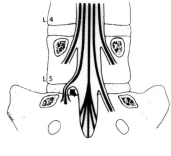

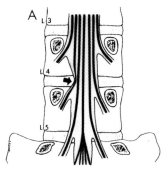

Fig 17–35.—Schematic diagram of a metrizamide myelogram in a patient with a lateral disk herniation at L5-S1 on the right, compressing and widening the corresponding S-1 root. There is no deformity of the thecal sac. AP projection *(above);* axial projection *(below)* as seen in metrizamide CT *(below).*

thesis at the L5-S1 level occasionally have a herniated disk at the L4-5 interspace (Fig 17–33). Marked narrowing of the spinal canal and a dorsolumbar gibbus are important findings in the achondroplastic dwarf, since they predispose to cauda equina compression in the presence of a herniated disk or spondylosis.

Myelography may be entirely normal (Fig 17–34) in the presence of disk hernia-

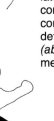

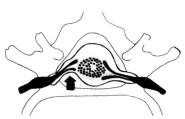

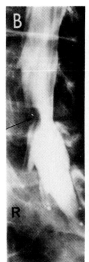

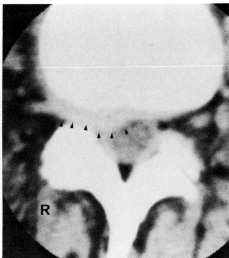

Fig 17–36.—**A,** schematic diagram in the AP and axial projections of a metrizamide myelogram in a patient with a large disk herniation at L4-5 on the right, compressing both the intradural segment of the L-5 nerve root and the adjacent thecal sac. **B,** oblique myelographic spot film *(left)* and axial CT scan *(right)* illustrating compression of the nerve root and thecal sac at L4-5 on the right.

tion, or it may reveal various abnormalities. A significant defect is constant and reproducible, regardless of the contrast medium used. With respect to contrast media, metrizamide has sounded the death knell to the use of Pantopaque for the diagnosis of lumbar disk herniation. CT has focused attention on the importance of minimal myelographic abnormalities in metrizamide myelography when the defects correspond to the patient's clinical findings (see Fig 17–45). Such defects cannot be accurately assessed with Pantopaque.

Most myelographic defects due to disk herniation can be classified into three major categories: (1) compression of the nerve root (Fig 17–35), (2) compression of the nerve root and thecal sac (Fig 17–36), (3) compression of the thecal sac (Fig 17–37).

1. COMPRESSION OF THE NERVE ROOT.—Kieffer has emphasized the significance of fusiform widening of the distal end of the involved nerve root due to compression by the herniated disk fragment. This abnormality was rarely demonstrated with Pantopaque because of its high viscosity and radiodensity. However, the widened nerve root is readily visible with metrizamide because the latter fills the subarachnoid space surrounding the nerve root sleeve. This type of defect is produced by a

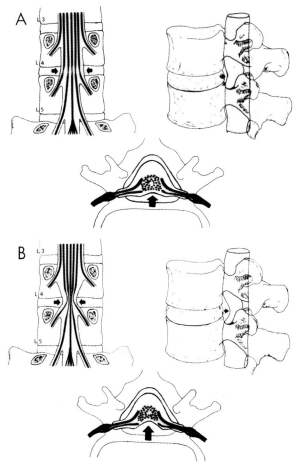

Fig 17–37.—Schematic diagram of a metrizamide myelogram in a patient with a small central bulge or herniation at L4-5 **(A)** in the frontal, lateral, and axial projections and in a second patient with a larger central bulge or herniation at the same level **(B)** in the frontal, lateral, and axial projections.

herniated disk fragment adjacent to the lateral margin of the dural sac, compressing the emerging nerve root (Fig 17–38).

2. COMPRESSION OF THE NERVE ROOT AND THECAL SAC.—This defect (Figs 17–39 to 17–47), the most common in frequency, is produced by a posterolateral disk herniation. It is characterized by a varying-sized indentation on the anterolateral aspect of the contrast column at the level of the interspace. The indentation is angular with a transverse or slightly sloping superior margin, which may extend above the level of the interspace, and a sharper oblique inferior margin, which may project below the level of the interspace. The defect tends to be more pronounced in the oblique projection. This abnormality can usually be differentiated from generalized bulging of the disk with an intact annulus, which uncommonly causes neural compression per se. The bulging disk with an intact annulus tends to produce a rounded, bilateral, symmetric defect (although it may be more pronounced on one side) (Figs 17–48, 17–49). The latter does not, as a rule, extend above or below the interspace and is not accentuated in the oblique projection.

3. COMPRESSION OF THE THECAL SAC.—This type of defect (Fig 17–50) is due to a central herniation through an annular tear or to a central bulge with an intact annulus. The defect is variable in prominence, depending upon the size of the midline protrusion and the distance of the anterior surface of the subarachnoid space from the posterior margin of the vertebral bodies. A small central herniation or bulge may produce no deformity of the contrast column in the frontal view. However, it can be visualized in the lateral projection as an indentation on the anterior aspect of the contrast column, at the level of the interspace (if the contrast column is not remote from the posterior vertebral surface). Slightly larger midline protrusions or herniations produce a larger defect on the anterior aspect of the contrast column in the lateral view. Such protrusions or herniations may also pro-

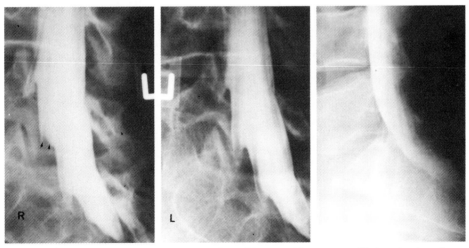

Fig 17–38.—Metrizamide myelogram in a 36-year-old woman with low back pain radiating down the right leg. It was difficult clinically to determine whether the lesion was at L4-5 or L5-S1. The films clearly show widening and compression of the S-1 root on the right *(arrowheads).* Both the right and left oblique projections are presented with the same orientation to facilitate comparison.

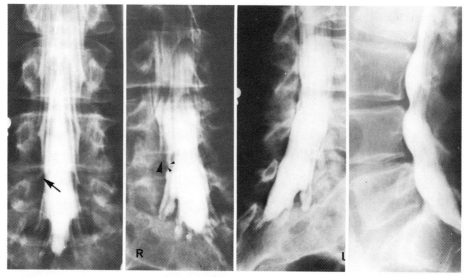

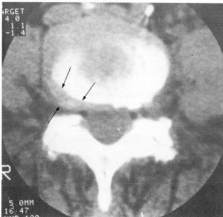

Fig 17–39.—Top, frontal, oblique, and lateral films taken during metrizamide myelography in a 64-year-old woman, showing elevation of the L-5 root on the AP projection *(thick arrow),* widening and flaring of the root *(thick arrowhead),* and minimal compression of the lateral aspect of the thecal sac *(thin arrowheads)* on the oblique projection. **Bottom,** axial CT scan at L4-5, showing a lateral disk herniation on the right side *(arrows)* with displacement and some obliteration of the fat in the intervertebral foramen.

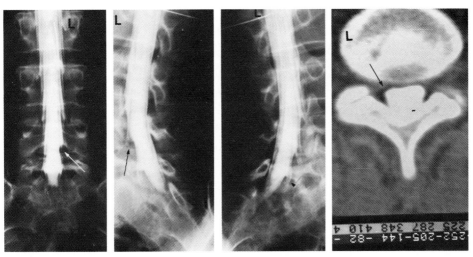

Fig 17–40.—Metrizamide myelogram and axial metrizamide CT study in a 29-year-old man with pain radiating to the right buttocks and leg. There is flaring of the left L-5 root and slight compression of the thecal sac at L4-5 on the left due to a herniated disk.

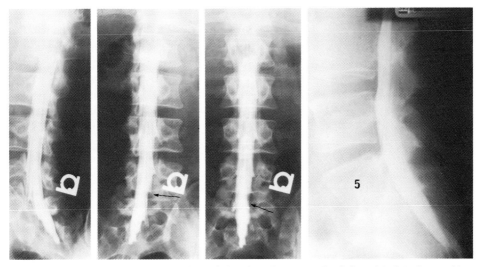

Fig 17–41.—Minimal compression of the thecal sac on the left at L5-S1 along with a cutoff of the S-1 root *(arrows)* in a 35-year-old male.

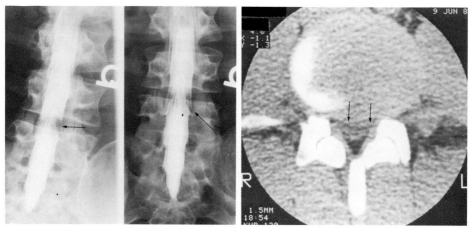

Fig 17–42.—Metrizamide myelogram and axial CT in a 33-year-old male with left-sided sciatica. Note the compression of both the nerve root and the thecal sac on the left side at L4-5 by a large left anterolateral disk herniation.

duce a midline oval or round radiolucency in the contrast column in the frontal projection at the disk level.

For many years, I have also taken erect shoot-through films in extension and flexion, in addition to the prone recumbent lateral shoot-through radiograph. In the erect position, there is usually a decrease in thickness of the anterior epidural space due to emptying out of the valveless vertebral venous plexus. It is common to find shallow indentations on the anterior aspect of the opacified theca at the level of the interspaces due to normal slight bulging of the disks. The bulging is accentuated by extension, which compresses the disks, and diminished in flexion when the compressive force on the nucleus is reduced (Fig 17–50,B). This normal physiologic phenomenon is accentuated in a patient with a bulging disk and a thinned-out, intact annulus. On the other hand, a disk fragment which herniates through a tear in the annulus rarely re-enters the disk proper. Hence, the defect it produces on the anterior aspect of the opacified theca tends to be unchanged in flexion and extension. This maneuver has helped me at times in differentiating a bulging from a herniated disk. The usefulness of the maneuver has also been commented upon by Pilling.

Extruded Disk Fragments

When there is a tear in the posterior longitudinal ligament with expulsion of a free nuclear fragment into the extradural space, the fragment may come to rest some distance above or below the intervertebral disk level (Figs 17–51 to 17–54). In my experience, superior migration of the extruded fragment is more common than inferior migration. In some patients, combined superior and inferior migration occurs. In such instances, there may be compression of two spinal nerves, i.e., the L-4 and L-5 nerves or the L-5 and S-1 nerves. Under such circumstances, particularly in the presence of a complete block, differential diagnosis from an extradural tumor may not always be possible from the myelographic findings alone. Although partial block is not infrequent, complete obstruction is an uncommon sequel of disk

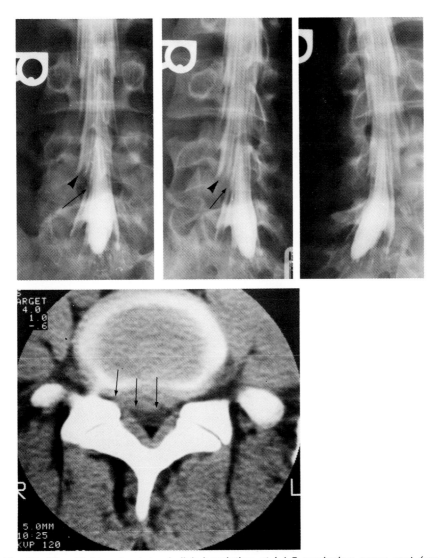

Fig 17–43.—Right anterolateral disk herniation at L4-5 producing nerve root *(arrowhead)* and thecal *(arrows)* compression shown both by metrizamide myelography **(top)** and CT **(bottom).** Both the L-4 and the L-5 roots are compressed on the right side.

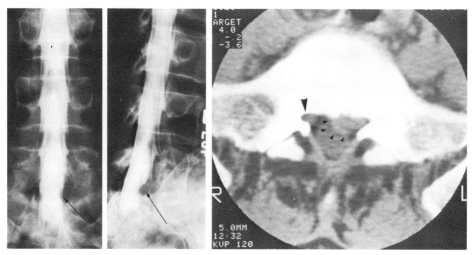

Fig 17–44.—Large left lumbosacral disk herniation producing a combined nerve root–thecal defect on the myelogram *(arrow)*. Note that the CT demonstrates the large size of the herniation and the neural compression more completely *(small arrowheads)*. Note also the normal right S-1 root *(large arrowhead)*.

herniation. When present, it is usually associated with a large nuclear protrusion and a high cerebrospinal fluid protein. This is most common at the L4-5 interspace. A few ancillary findings may be helpful in establishing the correct myelographic diagnosis in the presence of a complete obstruction. The presence of a sharply defined cap defect suggests an intradural lesion (Fig 17–55). Although the myelographic appearance of complete obstruction by extradural tumor and herniated disk may be quite similar, tenting of the ventral surface of the dura at the level of the interspace in association with narrowing of the interspace suggests disk herniation. The obstructed contrast column frequently has a serrated outline, presumably due to nerve root edema from pressure (see Fig 17–30, *top*). The distal end of the column may have an upward-directed convexity, a transverse or an oblique cutoff.

Recurrent disk herniation in a patient with a previous laminectomy constitutes a challenge for the myelographer. If a classic herniated disk defect is present on the postoperative myelogram (1) at a different interspace from the original lesion or (2) at the same interspace on the opposite, unexplored side, the diagnosis of a recurrent herniation can be made with confidence. If, however, the defect is found at the site of the original exploration, the problem is considerably more difficult. I have found CT metrizamide myelography to be helpful in this situation. It is important to differentiate recurrent disk herniation (Figs 17–56, 17–57) from (1) a postoperative fibrotic mass (Fig 17–58), (2) a retractile scar, and (3) arachnoiditis (Fig 17–59). Arachnoiditis can be recognized from agglutination of the nerve roots. Localized scarring usually manifests itself by retraction of the theca toward the operative side. The real problem arises in trying to distinguish a recurrent disk herniation from a postoperative fibrous or fibroadipose mass, i.e., where the nerve root had been wrapped in fat at the original operation and a mass of fibrous tissue had enveloped it. Both lesions present as space-occupying masses displacing the thecal sac. At times, the higher attenuation number of the disk herniation may help

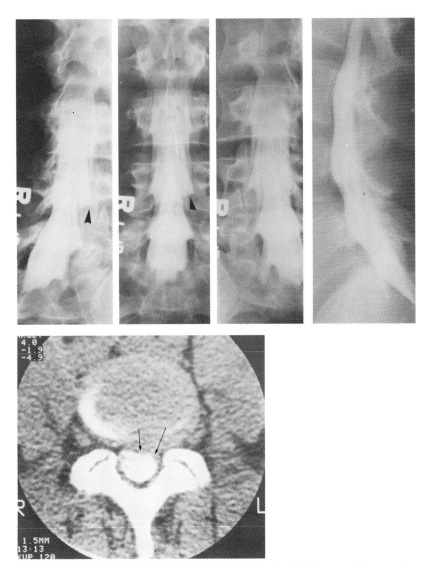

Fig 17–45.—Metrizamide myelogram **(top)** followed by CT **(bottom)** in a 26-year-old man with left sciatic pain. Note the minor myelographic defect, i.e., slight elevation of the left L-4 root. Contrast this with the fairly large left anterolateral herniation at L4-5 demonstrated by CT. The latter clearly shows the thecal and nerve root compression *(arrows)*.

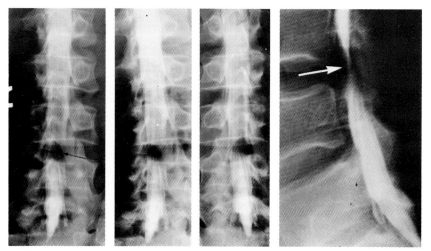

Fig 17–46.—Pronounced thecal and nerve root deformity due to a large left-sided disk herniation at L3-4. Note the marked defect in the lateral view *(arrow)*.

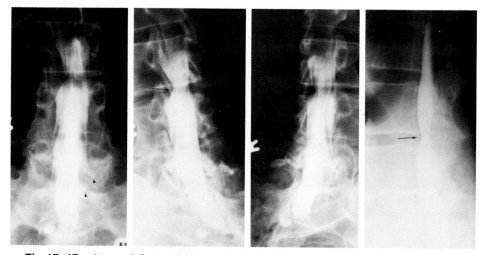

Fig 17–47.—Large defect at L3-4 on the right with compression of the nerve root and theca *(arrow)* in a 26-year-old woman. Note the conjoint nerve roots at L5-S1 on the left *(arrowheads)*.

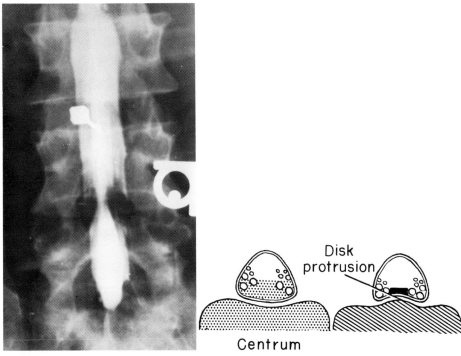

Fig 17–48.—Left, generalized bulging of the L4-5 disk with an intact annulus (proved at surgery). Note the fairly symmetric bilateral defect, slightly larger on the left, confined to the interspace. **Right,** cross-sectional diagram opposite the vertebral body showing, *left,* a normal disk; *right,* a midline protrusion separating the nerve roots into two lateral bundles with a shallow, Pantopaque-filled gutter between. (After Begg, Falconer, and McGeorge.)

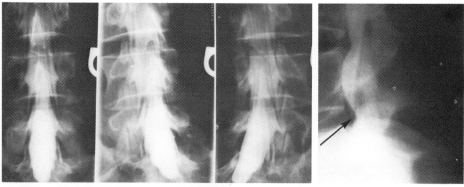

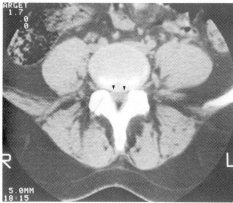

Fig 17–49.—Mild symmetric bulging of the L4-5 disk with an intact annulus demonstrated by metrizamide myelography **(top)** and CT **(bottom)** in a 36-year-old female with negative neurologic findings. The defect *(arrow)* is best appreciated in the lateral projection.

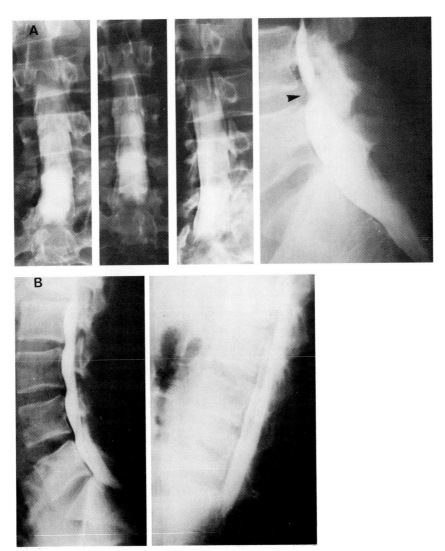

Fig 17–50.—A, midline disk herniation at L4-5 in a 33-year-old male with severe low back pain radiating down both legs. Note the thecal deformity in the lateral projection *(arrowhead).* **B,** lateral films during metrizamide lumbar myelography showing elongation of the thecal tube in flexion *(right)* and shortening in extension *(left).* Note also the diminution of the slight bulging of the disks and the dura in flexion.

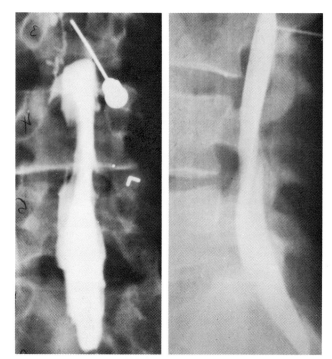

Fig 17–51.—The patient was a 30-year-old male complaining of low back pain for 1 year. Recently, the pain began to radiate into the right leg. Sensation in the L-4 dermatome was diminished, but the motor function was intact. Myelography shows a large irregular extradural defect compressing both the right lateral aspect of the thecal sac and the adjacent nerve roots. The defect extends from the L4-5 interspace inferiorly up to the midbody of L-4. At operation, a large extruded disk fragment from the L4-5 interspace had migrated superiorly. The preoperative diagnosis was extradural tumor.

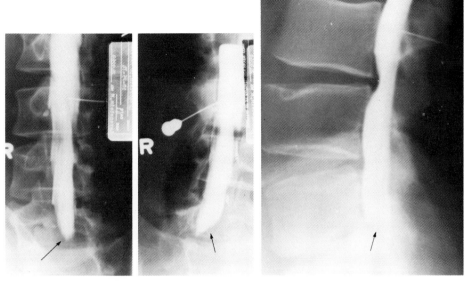

Fig 17–52.—Upright films from a Pantopaque myelogram showing a complete cutoff of the contrast column at L5-S1 *(arrow)*. Surgery revealed a large free disk fragment which had extruded from the lumbosacral interspace. The patient was a 41-year-old physician with acute severe low back pain radiating into both lower extremities.

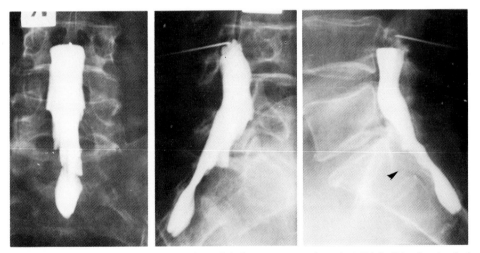

Fig 17–53.—At surgery, a large free disk fragment was found at S1-2; it had extruded from the lumbosacral interspace and migrated caudad. The scalloping of the posterior surface of the sacrum is a normal variant *(arrowhead)*. (Courtesy of D.J. McIntyre.)

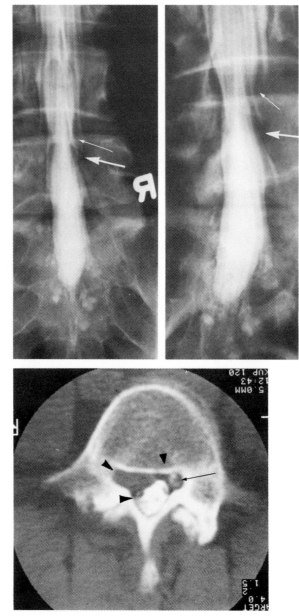

Fig 17–54.—Metrizamide myelogram **(top)** and CT **(bottom)** in a 59-year-old female with left-sided sciatica. At operation, a large free disk fragment was found at the level of the lateral recess which had been extruded from the L4-5 interspace and had migrated downward. The myelogram demonstrates flaring and compression of the L-4 root *(thin arrow)* at the level of the interspace and compression of the L-5 root by the free fragment *(large arrow)*. The CT elegantly shows the large free fragment at the level of the lateral recess compressing the right anterolateral aspect of the thecal sac *(arrowheads)*. Note the normal nerve root on the left side *(arrow)*.

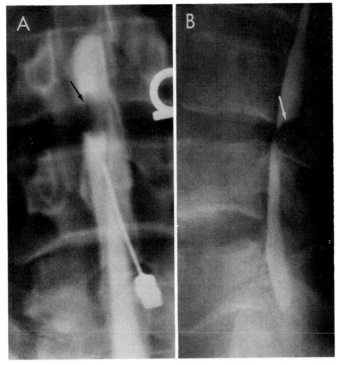

Fig 17–55.—**A,** intradural neurilemoma at L3-4 producing an incomplete obstruction *(arrow).* **B,** note the sharply defined defect on the posterior aspect of the Pantopaque column in the lateral projection, which serves to differentiate this lesion from a herniated disk *(arrow).*

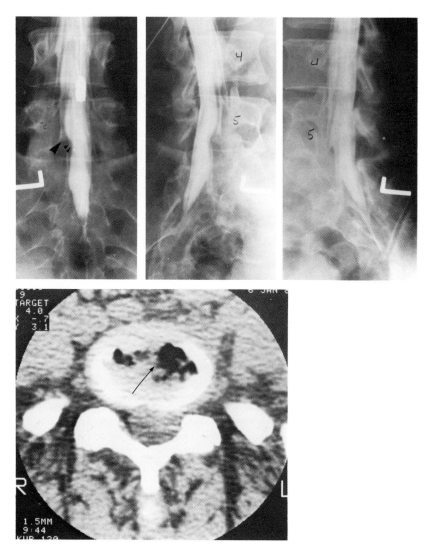

Fig 17–56.—The patient, a 46-year-old female, had undergone a previous operation at L5-S1 on the left. During the past several months, she developed recurrent left-sided sciatica. The myelogram **(top)** shows a well-defined extradural defect at L5-S1 on the left, characterized by elevation and flaring of the S-1 root *(large arrowhead)* and a slight indentation on the left anterolateral aspect of the thecal sac *(small arrowheads)* at the same level. The myelographic findings strongly suggest a recurrent disk herniation. The CT findings **(bottom)** are indeterminate. They show a vacuum disk *(arrow)* absence of the epidural fat and ligamentum flavum on the left side at the site of the previous operation, and slight overall bulging of the disk more marked on the left side. In this case, myelography was much more helpful than CT. At operation, a recurrent disk herniation was found.

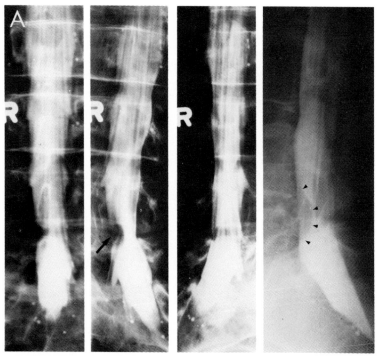

Fig 17–57.—**A,** metrizamide myelogram in a 58-year-old female who had a herniated disk removed at L4-5 on the left side after a positive Pantopaque myelogram. The right side was not explored at that time. The patient was symptom-free until 6 months before admission, when she developed persistent severe right-sided sciatica. The myelogram shows a typical extradural defect at L4-5 on the right *(arrow)* with displacement of the nerve root and thecal sac suggestive of a herniated disk. At operation, a herniated disk was removed corresponding to the myelographic defect. **B** (p. 466), the patient, a 50-year-old male, came in complaining of low back pain radiating down both legs. He had had a previous myelogram on March 4, 1981 **(p. 466)** which demonstrated a bilateral defect limited to the L4-5 interspace, slightly more marked on the right side. This is strongly suggestive of diffuse bulging of the disk with an intact annulus. At operation, a central bulging disk with an intact annulus was removed. The patient was free of pain for 6 months postoperatively. He then developed right-sided sciatica. Repeat myelography on September 9, 1981 **(p. 466)** shows a defect on the right side at L4-5 compatible with disk herniation. However, it is difficult to exclude a postoperative scar on the basis of the myelogram. A metrizamide CT scan clearly demonstrated a disk herniation on the right side with posterior displacement of the thecal sac *(arrows)*. This was confirmed at surgery.

Continued.

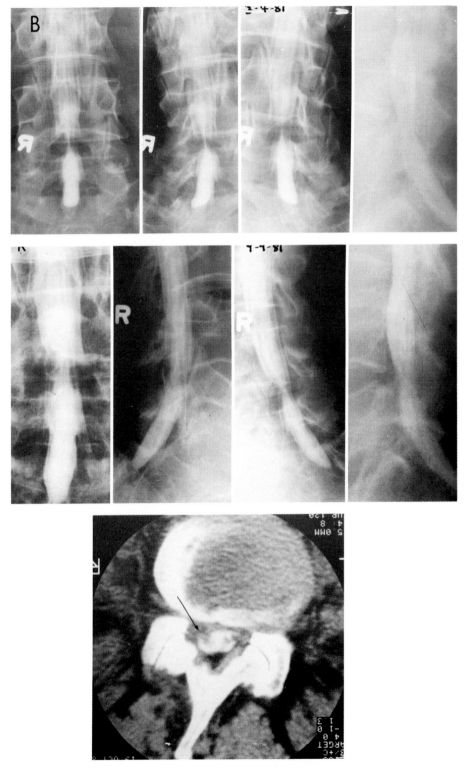

Fig 17–57 (cont.).

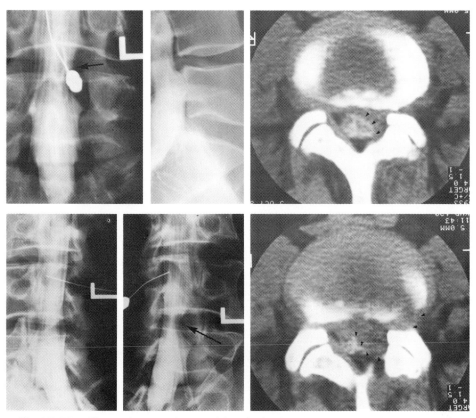

Fig 17–58.—The patient, a 53-year-old male, had undergone a previous laminectomy and disk removal at L4-5 on the left side. He developed recurrent symptoms at the same time. Metrizamide myelography showed a prominent extradural defect at L4-5 on the left consistent with a recurrent disk herniation *(arrow)*. A metrizamide CT study showed a large extradural mass on the left side compressing the thecal sac, with disk bulging into the intervertebral foramen *(arrowheads)*. At operation, there was a prominent mass of fibrous tissue with some fat in it. (The nerve had been wrapped in fat at the previous operation). The mass was compressing the thecal sac and nerve. There was very little recurrent disk herniation.

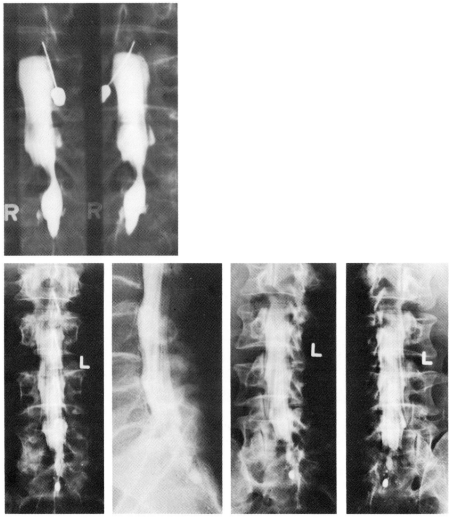

Fig 17–59.—This 54-year-old man had a Pantopaque myelogram on June 21, 1977 **(top),** which revealed an extradural defect at L5-S1 on the right, characteristic of a herniated disk. The latter was removed and the patient remained well for approximately 18 months. He then developed recurrent right sciatica. This prompted a second myelogram with metrizamide **(bottom)** on June 19,1979. The findings are those of arachnoiditis and scarring of the distal caudal sac. At operation, in addition to the above, there was also a large recurrent disk fragment at L5-S1 on the right displacing the S-1 root craniad. There is no way in which the recurrent herniated disk could be diagnosed by myelography in the presence of the extensive scarring. Unfortunately, metrizamide CT was not performed.

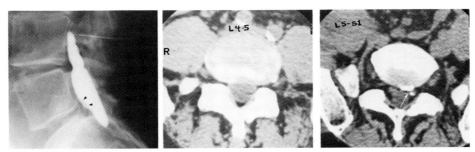

Fig 17–60.—This 52-year-old man was hospitalized because of left sciatic pain. The lateral radiograph made in hyperextension in the course of a Pantopaque myelogram performed on the outside accentuates a minimal defect on the anterior aspect of the oil column at L4-5. There is a double density at L5-S1 *(arrowheads),* suggesting unilateral pressure. The myelogram is not diagnostic. However, the CT scan shows minimal bulging of the disk at L4-5 and posterior displacement and compression of the left S-1 nerve by an osteophyte arising from the posterior aspect of the body of L-5 *(arrow).* There is a drop of Pantopaque in the sleeve surrounding the left S-1 nerve.

in differential diagnosis, but this is not always clear-cut. Schubiger and Valavanis have suggested that CT scanning before and after the intravenous injection of contrast material is helpful in this regard. According to these authors, scar tissue shows definite contrast enhancement while disk herniations do not. This has been confirmed by Teplick and Haskin.

An extradural defect at the level of the intervertebral disk space resembling that of a herniated disk can also be produced by localized scar, bony spurs (Fig 17–60), trauma, and tumor. Correct differential diagnosis may not always be possible, but there are a few findings that may be helpful. Postoperative localized arachnoiditis may present a somewhat elongated, scalloped, shallow defect at the level of the vertebral body (Fig 17–61). Dilated pial veins frequently accompany other lesions, such as tumor or disk prolapse, occurring at or slightly below the level of the lesion, probably due to interference with venous drainage. Fracture of a vertebral pedicle may also produce a unilateral extradural defect in the contrast column, but careful clinical examination and inspection of the plain radiographs of the lumbar spine should help to establish the correct diagnosis. In general, extradural tumors have no particular tendency to localize at an interspace, whereas most herniated disks occur at the latter site. Tumors may, however, occur at the interspace level, whereas free-lying disk fragments can lie above or below the interspace. In the presence of a complete block at the level of the intervertebral disk space, it may be impossible to differentiate preoperatively between an extradural tumor and a free-lying herniated disk. When tenting of the anterior aspect of the contrast column is seen on the lateral prone radiograph, it is highly suggestive of a herniated disk.

Beatty et al. have reported an interesting case of protrusion of the posterior longitudinal ligament simulating a herniated lumbar disk. Plain films showed narrowing of the involved interspace and intervertebral foramen, with overriding of the facets and shingling of the laminae. At operation, the bulging posterior longitudinal ligament compressed a nerve root. The scanty nuclear material in the disk space was nonprotruding.

McNab reviewed a series of 842 patients who underwent surgical exploration of

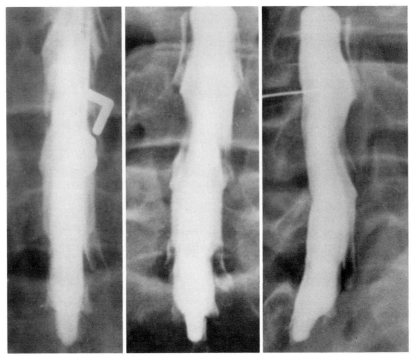

Fig 17–61.—Left, indeterminate myelogram in a patient with a herniated disk at L4-5 on the right side at operation; **right,** a repeat myelogram 9 months later demonstrated an elongated, scalloped defect on the right between the attachment of the L-4 and L-5 nerve roots. A second laminectomy revealed only adhesions.

the lumbar spine because of persistent nerve root irritation. In this group, there were 68 patients in whom no disk herniation was found. More extensive exploration of the nerve root revealed one of the following conditions in 50 of the latter cases: (1) migration of a disk fragment into the intervertebral foramen, which cannot be visualized by myelography but can be diagnosed by CT; (2) extraforaminal lateral disk herniation, which likewise cannot be diagnosed by Pantopaque or gas myelography but can be diagnosed by CT; (3) central spinal stenosis, which should be evident from plain films, tomography, myelography and CT; (4) articular process (facet) hypertrophy with impingement on a nerve root, which can best be diagnosed by CT; (5) nerve root kinking by a pedicle, i.e., secondary to advanced degeneration and narrowing of the lateral recess along with some descent of the upper vertebral body. The ipsilateral pedicle, which descends with the body, kinks the emerging nerve root, particularly if the latter courses transversely. The myelogram in these patients may be negative or show a nonspecific defect.

In a series of 1,986 laminectomies performed at Karolinska Sjukhuset for suspected lumbar disk herniation, the preoperative diagnosis was confirmed in 74%, a negative exploration was encountered in 14%, and other significant pathologic findings were noted in 12% (i.e., osteophytes, disk protrusion without involvement of nerve root, extradural varix). It is interesting that the neurologic findings agreed with the operative findings in only 46% of the cases, whereas the myelographic findings agreed with the operative findings in 83% of the cases. More than two thirds of the herniated disks found at operation after negative myelography were located at L5-S1.

My personal experience with Pantopaque myelography indicates an accuracy of approximately 90% at the L4-5 interspace and 80% at the lumbosacral interspace. Although I have no precise statistics, it is my impression that metrizamide has improved these figures slightly, i.e., approximately 5%, due largely to visualization of nerve root compression. Irrespective of the contrast medium used, myelography has the following intrinsic handicaps: (1) the lateral half of the lateral recess cannot be evaluated by myelography, (2) a herniated disk fragment in the intervertebral foramen cannot be visualized by myelography, (3) the herniated central lumbosacral disk cannot be visualized by myelography in a patient with a capacious anterior epidural space where the disk fragment does not come into contact with the anterior surface of the opacified theca, (4) an obstruction at L4-5 precludes evaluation of the lumbosacral disk by myelography, (5) the presence of arachnoiditis makes it difficult to evaluate the thecal sac for disk herniation.

Raskin and Keating studied a small series of 106 patients who had been examined by both myelography and CT within a period of 6 weeks. In the subgroup with no previous back surgery, the major discrepancy rate between the two techniques was 1%. Haughton et al. have also shown that high resolution CT scanning compares favorably with myelography in the recognition of lumbar disk disease. In my opinion, high-resolution CT scanning will soon replace myelography in patients who present de novo with a classic clinical picture of a herniated lumbar disk.

THORACIC

Clinically significant herniated disks in the thoracic region are rare, although asymptomatic protrusions are commonly found at necropsy. Love and Kiefer have estimated the incidence of symptomatic thoracic protrusions to be 2–3 per 1,000 cases of herniated disk. Apparently there is no particular age or sex predilection. Although the role of trauma has been denied by some, in Arseni and Nash's series, seven of nine patients developed symptoms immediately following trauma. Thoracic herniations have been reported at every level, but they are more common in the lower thoracic spine, where there is greater mobility.

The symptoms may be variable and not particularly characteristic. Because of the vague symptoms and the paucity of neurologic findings in some patients, the lesion may be overlooked. This is enhanced by a tendency to discount the significance of a minor filling defect in the thoracic segment of the contrast column at myelography. The patients who do present with objective neurologic findings have been divided into three groups by Abbott and Retter (Fig 17–62).

1. Lateral protrusions presenting a clear-cut syndrome of radicular pain. These patients are often considered to have visceral disease because of a lack of familiarity with this lesion.

2. Central herniation in the upper and midthoracic spine. These patients usually have long-tract signs as well as sensory changes, principally pain and anesthesia.

3. T-11 and T-12 protrusions that compress the conus medullaris and cauda equina. These patients have thoracolumbar pain referred to the legs, sphincter disturbances, and a complete or dissociated sensorimotor cauda equina syndrome.

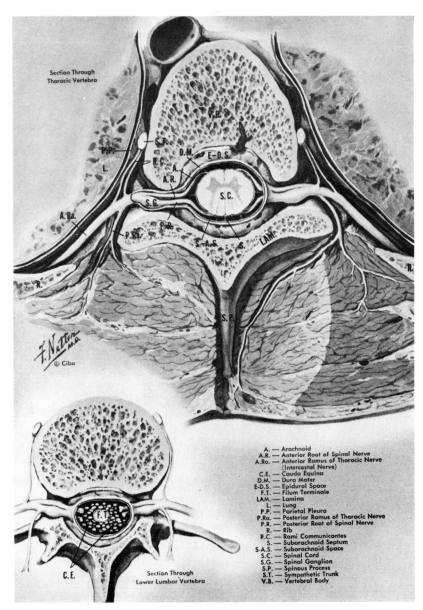

Fig 17–62.—Artist's rendition of a cross-section through a thoracic vertebra, **above,** and a lower lumbar vertebra, **below,** illustrating the anatomical relationships. (From the Ciba Collection of Medical Illustrations by Frank H. Netter, M.D. Copyright Ciba.)

Conventional radiography may reveal a calcified nucleus pulposus. Such calcification, however, commonly occurs in the absence of symptomatic disk protrusion and actually may be present in a patient with a herniated thoracic disk at another level. On the other hand, calcification within the vertebral canal at the level of the interspace is significant (Fig 17–63). When such calcification is found together with narrowing of the corresponding intervertebral disk space, the diagnosis of a herniated thoracic disk is extremely likely (Fig 17–64). In addition to narrowing of the intervertebral disk space, there may be evidence of kyphosis dorsalis juvenilis. Myelography plays a significant role in establishing the diagnosis of a thoracic disk herniation. The characteristic deformity is an oval or round defect on the anterior or anterolateral (Figs 17–65, 17–66) aspect of the contrast column at the level of the disk protrusion. It must be emphasized, however, that defects may occur in patients without clinical evidence of symptomatic thoracic disk herniation (Fig 17–67). This is more common with Pantopaque and not so striking with metrizamide. Consequently, the significance of such a defect must be evaluated in terms of the entire clinical picture. The importance of the lateral prone projection with the horizontal beam cannot be overemphasized. A 2-or-more-millimeter posterior displacement of the contrast column at the level of a narrowed disk space must be viewed with considerable suspicion. At times, one may also see a double contour defect when the disk protrusion is situated to one side of the midline. When there is a partial or complete block with a characteristic oval extradural defect at the interspace, the diagnosis is relatively easy. In the presence of a high-grade obstruction, the head of the contrast column may have the appearance of a U or an inverted U, depending on whether the contrast is introduced via the lumbar or the C1-2 route, respectively. Differentiation from a meningioma usually is possible because the latter commonly demonstrates the typical "cap" defect of an extramedullary intradural lesion and does not produce anterior tenting of the dura. In the absence of calcification or changes in the intervertebral disk space, differentiation of a herniated thoracic disk from a ventral-lying extradural tumor at the level of the interspace may be impossible.

CERVICAL

In 1928, 15 years after Elsberg's description of lumbar extradural chondroma, Stookey published his observations on seven cases of spinal cord compression due to "ventral extradural cervical chondromas." It was not until 1940, however, that Stookey realized that the so-called chondromas were not true neoplasms but protrusions of the nucleus pulposus. In 1943, Semmes and Murphy published their classic paper on lateral cervical disk protrusions that produced radicular arm pain and simulated coronary artery and other visceral disease. As a result of the widespread publicity that the latter publication received, the syndrome of rupture of a cervical intervertebral disk has become established as a well-defined entity.

Although the cervical disk is much smaller than its lumbar counterpart, the spinal cord in the cervical region fills the bony canal more completely than in any other area. Consequently, an extradural mass such as a ruptured disk may readily produce cord compression. The disks in the cervical region commonly protrude posterolaterally and tend to calcify in children. The etiology of the latter calcifications is not known. They may or may not be symptomatic and have been known to

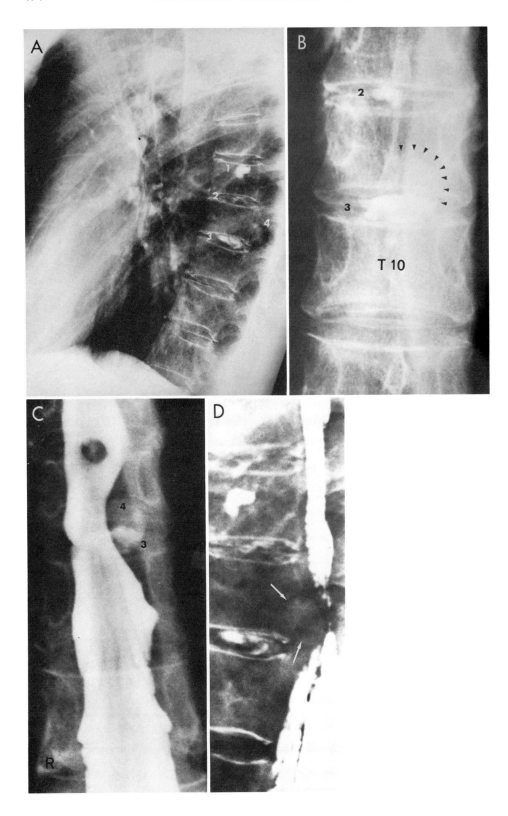

disappear spontaneously. Not infrequently, osteophytes project from the margins of the adjacent vertebrae, thereby constricting the bony canal. According to Spurling, approximately 95% of all cervical disk herniations occur at either the C5-6 or the C6-7 interspace. Of these, about 70% are found at the C6-7 interspace. The remaining protrusions are divided between the C7-T1 interspace (4%) and the C4-5 interspace. Like herniated lumbar disks, this lesion is also much more common in males. A clear-cut history of trauma can be elicited in approximately 25–40% of the patients.

The clinical picture may be divided into the three basic syndromes originally described by Stookey, depending on the location of the protrusion in the spinal canal.

Lateral Protrusions

By far the most common type, lateral protrusions spare the spinal cord but compress one or more cervical nerve roots, producing radicular pain and other sensory disturbances (Fig 17–68). The radicular pain varies in intensity and is characteristically subject to exacerbations and remissions. In addition to the radicular pain, the patient may complain of neck pain and/or a scalenus anticus syndrome. The pain is often accentuated by cervical motion, coughing, straining, or sneezing.

Physical examination reveals relative fixation of the cervical spine, with loss of the normal cervical lordosis. The patient's pain may be reproduced or reinforced by downward or lateral flexion of the neck. There also may be unilateral local tenderness in the neck and axilla when the brachial plexus is subjected to pressure. Sensory changes such as hypesthesia or hyperesthesia in the affected dermatome, alteration of tendon reflexes, and, more rarely, muscle atrophy may be present also.

Because of the individual variation in segmental motor and sensory distribution, as well as sensory overlap between adjacent segments, clinical localization of the level of the disk protrusion is not always reliable. In general, C4-5 protrusion with compression of the fifth cervical nerve may be associated with a depressed or absent biceps tendon reflex, weakness of the deltoid or biceps muscles, occasional hypesthesia over the deltoid distribution, and pain involving the base of the neck, tip of the shoulder, and arm down to the elbow. Herniation at the C5-6 interspace with compression of the sixth cervical nerve also produces depression of the biceps tendon reflex and weakness or atrophy of the biceps muscle. Sensory changes include

---

Fig 17–63.—Herniated thoracic disk at T9-10 with a calcified large free fragment in the canal. The patient was a 57-year-old woman who complained of radicular pain in the distribution of the left ninth thoracic nerve. In **A**, the lateral chest radiograph, a number of calcifications can be seen: *1*, a calcified Ghon lesion in the superior segment of the left lower lobe; *2*, asymptomatic calcification of the intervertebral disk between T-8 and T-9; *3*, more extensive calcification of the nucleus pulposus at T9-10; and *4*, the calcified free fragment in the spinal canal above the T9-10 interspace. In the anteroposterior spot radiograph of the thoracic spine, **B**, the disk calcifications are again demonstrated. The periphery of the faintly calcified free fragment is outlined by arrowheads. The frontal spot film, **C**, made during myelography shows an elongated defect on the left side of the Pantopaque column at T9-10 due to the herniated disk. Note the small round defect at T8-9 due to bulging of an asymptomatic calcified disk (slightly retouched). **D**, the lateral spot film at myelography demonstrates thinning and posterior displacement of the oil column at T9-10 by the calcified free disk fragment *(arrows)* (slightly retouched).

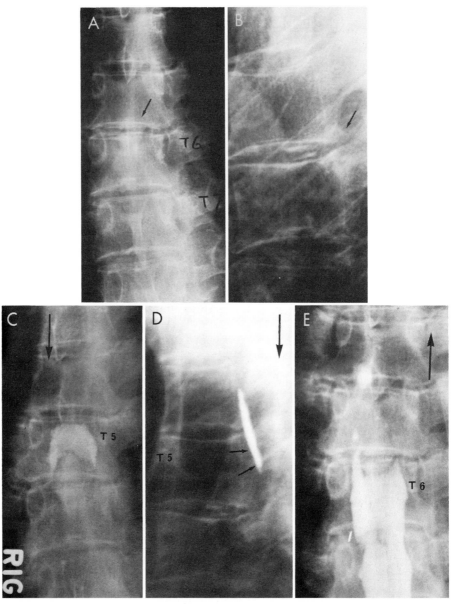

Fig 17–64.—Herniated thoracic disk at T5-6 in a 46-year-old male who complained of impotence, increasing ataxia, and sphincter disturbance of 4–5 months' duration. He presented a clinical picture of tabes dorsalis. The plain radiographs, **A** and **B,** demonstrate the calcification in the intervertebral disk (*arrow* in AP film) and also a small, rounded calcification within the spinal canal (*arrow* in lateral film). Note the narrowing of the involved intervertebral disk space. Cisternal myelography, **C** and **D,** demonstrates a complete obstruction at T5-6 with an inverted U-shaped or pincer-like deformity of the Pantopaque column. Note also the posterior displacement of the dura and cord as a unit *(arrows).* **E,** lumbar myelography shows a similar defect. At operation, a very large disk fragment (only a small portion of which was calcified) invaginated the dura so that the latter had to be opened in order to remove the fragment.

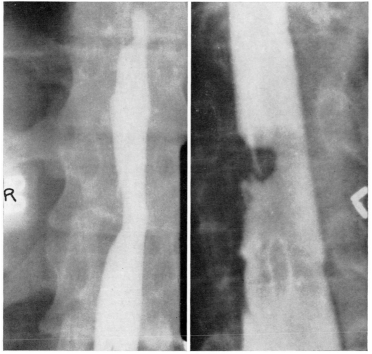

Fig 17–65.—Two patients with herniated thoracic disks demonstrating a typical extra-dural defect on the right anterolateral aspect of the Pantopaque column at the level of the interspace. The herniation on the left is at T11-12 and the one on the right at T9-10. Both patients presented with radicular pain and originally were considered to have visceral disease.

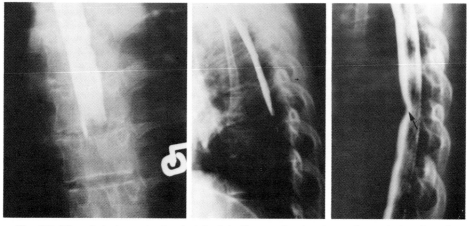

Fig 17–66.—Anterior extradural defect in the contrast column *(arrow)* due to a her-niated disk at T8-9 producing a high-grade obstruction in a 49-year-old female. The con-trast medium seen in the frontal and first lateral view was introduced by a C1-2 puncture. In the lateral projection on the far right, contrast was also introduced from below.

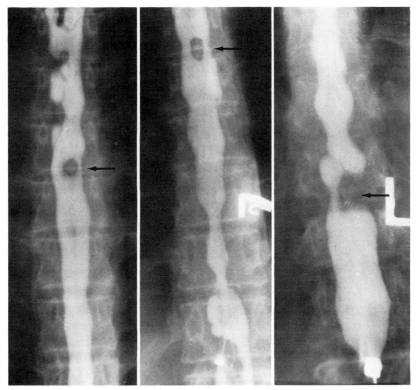

Fig 17–67.—Myelographic montage in three asymptomatic patients showing central defects in two patients produced by bulging of the disk and a lateral defect in the third *(arrows)*. Because this type of defect is common, it must be interpreted in the light of the clinical findings.

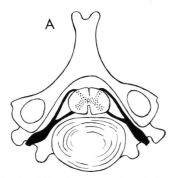 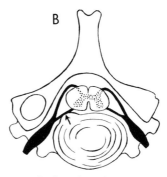

Fig 17–68.—Cross-sectional diagrams of the lower cervical region demonstrating, **A,** normal disk, **B,** lateral protrusion with radicular compression.

pain, hypesthesia, numbness, and tingling along the dorsolateral surface of the thumb and radial surface of the hand. Herniation at the C6-7 interspace with compression of the seventh cervical nerve may result in depression or absence of the triceps tendon reflex and weakness or atrophy of the deltoid, biceps, and triceps muscles. Hypesthesia, pain, numbness, and tingling involve the index and the dorsum of the hand. Protrusion at the C7-T1 level with compression of the eighth cervical nerve is not associated with abnormal tendon reflexes, although there may be weakness or atrophy of the triceps muscle and the intrinsic musculature of the hand. The sensory changes are characterized by hypesthesia, numbness, and tingling in the fifth and ulnar half of the fourth digit and pain in the ulnar distribution, i.e., along the medial inferior surface of the arm, forearm, and hand.

Bilateral Ventral Pressure

In these patients, the disk protrusion, midline in location, compresses the entire ventral surface of the spinal cord (Fig 17–69). The clinical picture depends on whether the cord compression is acute or chronic. Acute compression is relatively rare and exhibits the signs and symptoms of an intraspinal neoplasm. Chronic midline disk protrusions with bilateral ventral cord pressure have a variable symptomatology. Many of these patients have minimal neck pain and limitation of motion. Motor symptoms in the arms also may be minimal, although some patients exhibit muscle atrophy, paresis, or even flaccid paralysis of the upper extremities. The

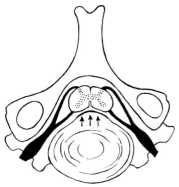

Fig 17–69.—Cross-sectional diagram of the lower cervical spine, showing a midline disk herniation producing compression of the ventral aspect of the spinal cord.

major findings are those due to pyramidal tract compression, that is, hyperactive reflexes, loss of abdominal reflexes, positive Babinski sign, and ankle clonus. Muscle weakness varies in severity but may be minimal. Sensory disturbances also vary in severity. Many patients complain of paresthesia of one or more extremities. Commonly, pain and temperature sensation are affected because of pressure on the spinothalamic tract. Some diminution in tactile sensation may be present also; but the posterior column modalities, that is, position sense, bone, joint, and vibratory sensation, are relatively spared.

From the varying symptomatology that these patients exhibit, it is easy to understand why many of them are erroneously considered to have a cord tumor or degenerative spinal cord disease. It is important to realize that all of the clinical syndromes produced by herniated cervical disks can also be produced by osteophytic spurs.

Kahn has pointed out the important role that the dentate ligaments play in the presence of anterior extradural spinal compression, that is, from midline disk bulging with an intact annulus, midline disk protrusion through a tear of the annulus, osteophytic spurs with or without nuclear protrusion (Fig 17–70). Since the spinal cord is more or less fixed in the bony canal by the paired nerve roots and by the dentate ligaments laterally, it cannot be readily displaced dorsally by extradural ventral pressure. With chronic pressure, the pyramidal tracts, because of the larger size of their fibers and greater stress exerted on them, exhibit a more profound disturbance of conductivity than the pain fibers of the spinothalamic tracts even though the latter are closer to the compressing mass. Touch is preserved because sufficient sensation remains in the more protected posterior columns, in spite of

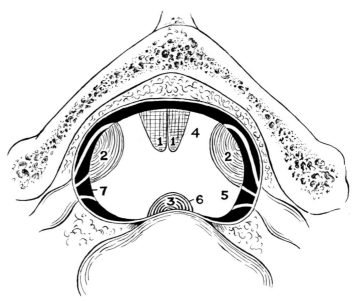

Fig 17–70.—Cross-sectional diagram at C6-7 demonstrating some of the important spinal tracts, the dentate ligaments, and the lines of stress in the presence of a midline disk herniation. (Modified from Kahn.) Symbols: *1,* posterior columns. *2 and 3,* lines of stress. *4,* pyramidal tracts. *5,* lateral spinothalamic tract. *6,* ventral spinothalamic tract. *7,* dentate ligament.

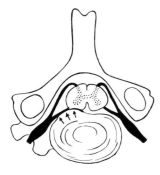

Fig 17–71.—Cross-sectional diagram of the lower cervical spine, showing a disk herniation compressing the ipsilateral root and ventral surface of the spinal cord.

the inability of the ventral spinothalamic tracts to conduct. Since the hand area is medial and the leg area lateral in the pyramidal tracts, the upper extremities usually suffer less disability than the lower extremities. The syndrome, therefore, consists of a spastic motor disturbance of the lower extremities in the absence of definite sensory changes and simulates lateral sclerosis. Surgical division of the dentate ligaments permits the cord to move dorsally in the dural sac, thereby decreasing its compression from a ventral mass.

Unilateral Ventral Pressure

Unilateral pressure on the ventral surface of the spinal cord rarely occurs alone. Usually it is associated with root compression secondary to a relatively large disk protrusion through a posterolateral tear in the annulus (Fig 17–71). These patients

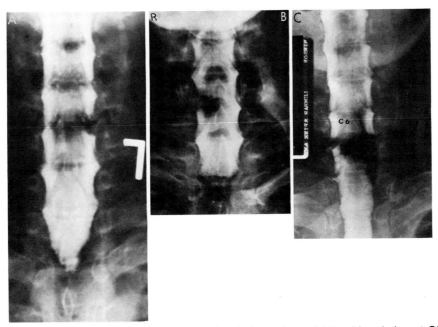

Fig 17–72.—Various-sized cervical disk herniations. A small lateral herniation at C5-6 on the left side **(A).** A slightly larger disk herniation on the right at C6-7 **(B).** A large herniation extending across the midline at C6-7 on the left **(C).**

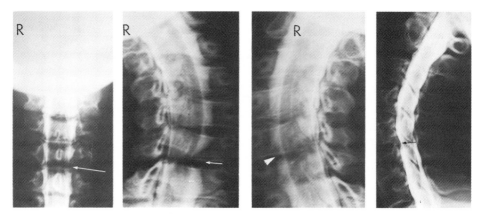

Fig 17–73.—Metrizamide cervical myelogram in a 41-year-old woman, demonstrating a herniated disk on the left side at C5-6 *(arrow)*. Some bony spurring is also present on the right side *(arrowhead)*.

have varying degrees of cervical pain and stiffness. The characteristic neurologic deficit is an incomplete Brown-Séquard syndrome, that is, ipsilateral motor signs due to pyramidal tract compression and contralateral sensory changes resulting from pressure on the spinothalamic tract. The patients, therefore, demonstrate muscle weakness and atrophy of the lower motor neuron type in the upper extremity and spasticity and other pyramidal tract signs of the upper motor neuron type in the lower extremity on the side of the lesion. They also exhibit changes in pain and temperature sensation on the side opposite the lesion. Tactile sensation usually is only slightly affected on the side opposite the lesion because this modality is carried in the posterior columns as well as in the lateral spinothalamic tract. Since the posterior columns are relatively remote from the compression, kinesthetic and vibratory sensations are not compromised.

Radiographic examination of the cervical spine is an integral part of the study of diskogenic disease and spondylosis. Conventional films of the cervical spine should include an anteroposterior view, lateral views in the neutral position, flexion and extension, and right and left oblique views. The plain films may demonstrate loss of the normal cervical lordosis, localized immobility at one level, narrowing of the intervertebral disk space or localized osteophyte formation. These findings are more significant with respect to the diagnosis of a herniated cervical disk if they are localized to one interspace. When multiple interspaces are involved, such findings are more likely to reflect generalized spondylosis.

The defect seen at myelography depends on the location of the protrusion. Small protrusions lying laterally produce a shallow, well-defined semilunar indentation on the lateral aspect of the contrast column at the level of the intervertebral disk space. The corresponding nerve root may be widened due to edema and the axillary pouch may or may not be obliterated (Figs 17–72 to 17–74). The indentation may be demonstrable only in the frontal or oblique projections. It may be absent on the lateral prone radiograph because of obscuration by the contrast medium in the normal half of the subarachnoid space. Larger lateral protrusions produce more striking rounded or wedge-shaped, irregular defects, which may extend toward the midline to a varying degree. Herniations of this size almost uniformly obliterate the

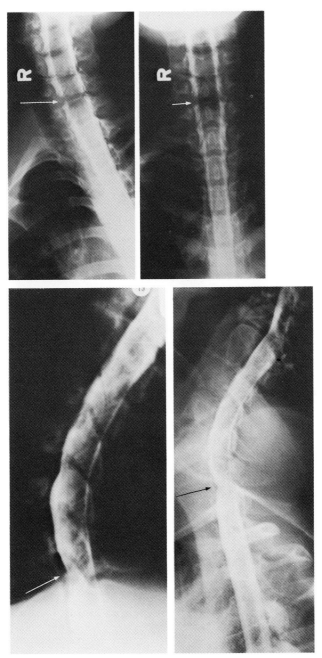

Fig 17–74.—Herniated disk at C6-7 on right in a 24-year-old woman, showing a characteristic extradural defect at metrizamide myelography. The latter was performed via the lumbar route.

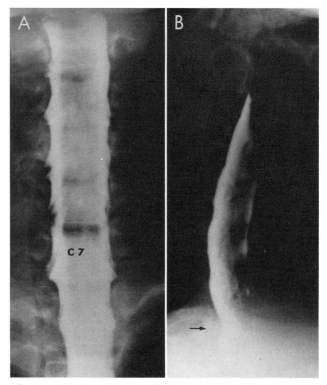

Fig 17–75.—Central disk herniation at C6-7 seen best in **B,** the lateral projection *(arrow).* There is minimal asymmetry at C6-7 in **A,** the frontal projection on the right side, but the patient had no radicular pain.

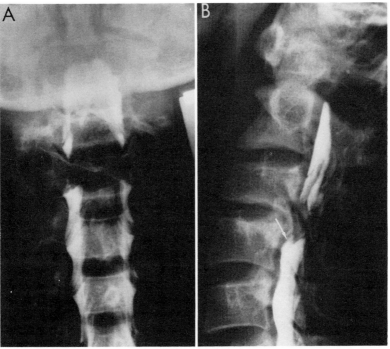

Fig 17–76.—The patient had undergone a pneumoencephalogram several days previously. A second lumbar puncture for myelography because of a suspected C3-4 lesion was unsuccessful. Therefore, a lateral C1-2 puncture was carried out. The prone myelographic film after the injection of Pantopaque shows apparent localized widening of the cord at C3-4 **(A).** The lateral cross-table radiograph **(B)** clearly demonstrates the extradural nature of the lesion, with elevation of the anterior theca *(arrow)* due to a large midline herniated disk.

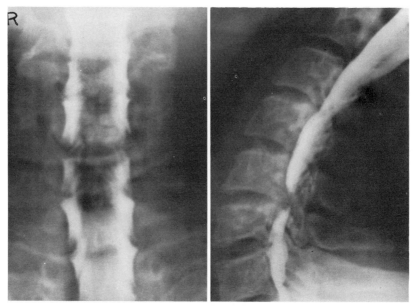

Fig 17–77.—Midline defect at C5-6 produced by osseous spurs arising from the posterior surfaces of C-5 and C-6 without a disk herniation.

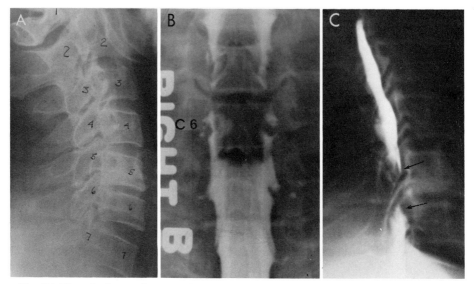

Fig 17–78.—A, the patient, a 43-year-old man, shows some narrowing of the C5-6 interspace, with posterior spur formation on the plain radiograph of the cervical spine. **B,** the frontal spot film during myelography demonstrates suggestive widening of the cord extending over two vertebral segments. **C,** the prone lateral view, however, demonstrates the anterior extradural location of the lesion. Note the tenting of the anterior dura on either side of the interspace *(arrows).* The apparent widening of the cord is due to flattening in the anteroposterior diameter. At operation, a midline disk herniation plus osteophytic ridging was found.

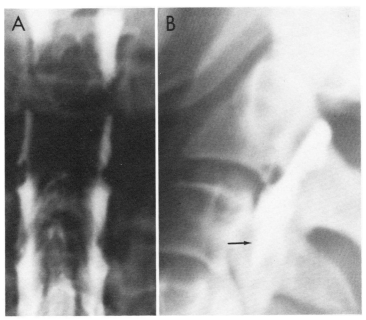

Fig 17-79.—The patient, a 50-year-old male, gave a 6-month history of neck pain and bilateral arm dysesthesia followed by mild weakness in the arms and legs for 3 months prior to admission. Physical examination revealed a mild spastic quadriparesis with distal sensory and mild posterior column loss. The Pantopaque, introduced by lumbar puncture, shows apparent localized widening of the cord at C3-4 **(A),** with a partial block at this interspace and anterior elevation of the theca **(B)** *(arrow)* due to a herniated disk. Following the myelogram, no effort was made to remove the Pantopaque because of the partial obstruction in the presence of a substantial neurologic deficit. Nonetheless, the patient became totally quadriplegic within an hour after myelography and required emergency laminectomy. He ultimately recovered function. This emphasizes the need for close observation of patients with a significant neurologic deficit who demonstrate a high-grade obstruction at myelography.

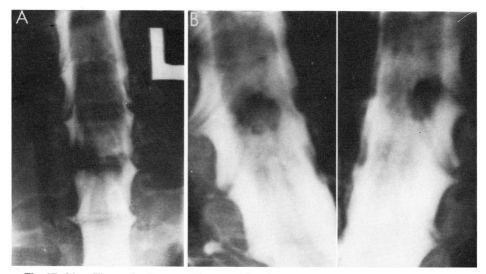

Fig 17–80.—The patient was a 59-year-old male with atrophy of the right interosseous muscles and hypalgesia in the C7-8 distribution on the right. The AP myelogram **(A)** shows a localized defect at C7-T1 on the right suggestive of a herniated disk. The oblique films **(B)** demonstrate the margins of the defect to be fairly well defined. At operation, the disk fragment had penetrated through the dura and was adherent to its inner surface.

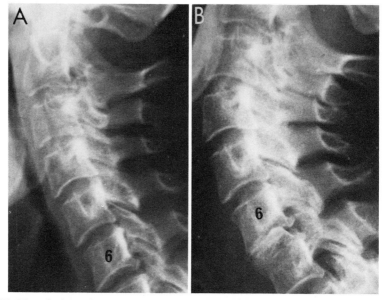

Fig 17–81.—**A,** lateral preoperative radiograph of the cervical spine in a 23-year-old female with a classic C6-7 disk herniation. Note the slight narrowing of the C6-7 interspace and the corresponding posterior spur formation. The film made 4 days postoperatively **(B)** demonstrates the bone plug in the C6-7 interspace.

axillary pouch and may displace the cord laterally. A localized osteophytic spur at the medial margin of the intervertebral foramen can produce a similar defect. A localized spur and a herniated disk are often concurrent findings. Midline herniations result in a central defect at the level of the intervertebral disk space (Figs 17–75, 17–76). Such defects, which vary considerably in size, may also be the result of ridging of the posterior surface of the vertebral body and of a midline bulge of the nucleus with an intact annulus (Fig 17–77). Usually when these defects occur at multiple levels, they are due to diffuse degenerative disease of the cervical spine (spondylosis). In the lateral prone film, a characteristic corrugated, washboard pattern is present in these patients due to multiple indentations on the ventral surface of the contrast column at the interspaces. Occasionally, a large midline protrusion may cause a partial or complete subarachnoid obstruction with an L- or U-shaped deformity of the head of the contrast column at the interspace. The appearance in the frontal projection may be indistinguishable from that seen in intramedullary tumor, but the lateral film with the horizontal beam should establish the correct diagnosis, since the herniated disk indents the anterior aspect of the contrast column (Figs 17–78, 17–79). Rarely, a herniated disk fragment may erode through the dura to present intradurally (Fig 17–80).

One should be familiar with the radiographic appearance following anterior fusion for cervical disk herniation. Successful fusion results in obliteration of the disk space 6–12 months postoperatively (Fig 17–81).

BIBLIOGRAPHY

Abbott K.H., Retter R.H.: Protrusions of thoracic intervertebral discs. *Neurology* 6:1, 1956.

Alajouanine R., Petit-Dutaillis D.: Le nodule fibrocartilagineux de la face postérieure des disques intervertébraux. *Presse Méd.* 38:1657, 1749, 1930.

Andrae R.: Über Knorpelknötchen am hinteren Ende der Wirbelbandscheiben im Bereich des Spinalkanals. *Beitr. Path. Anat.* 82:464, 1929.

Arbuckle R.K., Shelden C.H., Pudenz R.H.: Pantopaque myelography: Correlation of roentgenologic and neurologic findings. *Radiology* 45:356, 1945.

Armstrong J.R.: *Lumbar Disc Lesions.* Baltimore, Williams & Wilkins Co., 1958.

Aronson H.A., Dunsmore R.H.: Herniated upper lumbar discs. *J. Bone Joint Surg.* 45A:311, 1963.

Arseni C., Nash F.: Thoracic intervertebral disc protrusion. *J. Neurosurg.* 17:418, 1960.

Baker A.H.: Lesion of the intervertebral disk caused by lumbar puncture. *Br. J. Surg.* 34:385, 1947.

Bardeen C.R.: The development of the thoracic vertebrae in man. *Am. J. Anat.* 4:163, 1904–1905.

Barr J.S., Hampton A.O., Mixter W.J.: Pain low in the back and "sciatica" due to lesions of the intervertebral disc. *J.A.M.A.* 109:1265, 1937.

Barr J.S., Mixter W.J.: Rupture of the intervertebral disc with involvement of the spinal cord. *N. Engl. J. Med.* 211:210, 1934.

Beadle O.A.: *The Intervertebral Discs.* Med. Res. Council, Special Report Series, No. 161. London, H. M. Stationery Office, 1931.

Beatty R.A., Sugar O., Fox T.F.: Protrusion of the posterior longitudinal ligaments simulating herniated lumbar intervertebral disc. *J. Neurol., Neurosurg. Psychiatr.* 31:61, 1968.

Begg A.C., Falconer M.A., McGeorge M.: Myelography in lumbar intervertebral disk lesions: Correlation with operative findings. *Br. J. Surg.* 34:141, 1946.

Berg A.: Clinical and myelographic studies of conservatively treated cases of lumbar intervertebral disk protrusion. *Acta Chir. Scandinav.* 104:124, 1952.

Boult G.F., Kiernan M.K., Childe A.E.: The importance of minor myelographic deformities in the diagnosis of posterior protrusion of the lumbar intervertebral disc. *Am. J. Roentgenol.* 66:752, 1951.

Bradford F.K., Spurling R.G.: *The Intervertebral Disc*. Springfield, Ill., Charles C Thomas, Publisher, 1945.

Bücker J.: Air myelography in prolapse of the vertebral disk. *Fortschr. Geb. Röntgenstrahlen* 72:493, 1950.

Caffey J.: Achondroplasia of pelvis and lumbar spine. *Am. J. Roentgenol.* 80:448, 1958.

Calvé J., Galland H.: Intervertebral nucleus pulposus. Its anatomy, its physiology, its pathology. *J. Bone Joint Surg.* 12:555, 1930.

Camp J.D.: The roentgenologic diagnosis of intraspinal protrusion of intervertebral discs by means of radio-opaque oil. *J.A.M.A.* 113:2024, 1939.

Camp J.D.: Roentgenologic diagnosis of intraspinal protrusion of intervertebral discs. *Minnesota Med.* 23:688, 1940.

Carson J., Gumpert J., Jefferson A.: Diagnosis and treatment of thoracic intervertebral disc protrusions. *J. Neurol., Neurosurg. Psychiatr.* 34:68, 1971.

Childe A.E.: The role of the x-ray in the diagnosis of posterior herniation of the intervertebral disc. *Can. Med. Assoc. J.* 52:458, 1945.

Cloward R.B.: Anterior herniation of ruptured lumbar disk. Diagnostic value of diskogram. *A.M.A. Arch. Surg.* 64:457, 1952.

Cloward R.B.: Multiple ruptured lumbar disks. *Ann. Surg.* 142:190, 1955.

Compere E.L., Keyes D.C.: Roentgenological studies of the intervertebral disc; discussion of embryology, anatomy, physiology, clinical and experimental pathology. *Am. J. Roentgenol.* 29:774, 1933.

Connell M.C.: Calcification of the intervertebral discs in children. *Clin. Radiol.* 14:87, 1963.

Copleman B.: The roentgenographic diagnosis of the small central protruded intervertebral disc. *Am. J. Roentgenol.* 52:245, 1944.

Cotunio D.: De ischiade nervosa commentorius, 1764. Cited in Armstrong, J.R. *Lumbar Disc Lesions*. Baltimore, Williams & Wilkins Co., 1958.

Craig W.M., et al.: Intraspinal lesions masquerading as protruded lumbar disks. *J.A.M.A.* 149:250, 1952.

Cramer F., Hudson F.: Myelographically demonstrated lesions of the cervical intervertebral discs, coexisting with tumors and other causes of myelopathy. *Acta Radiol.* 46:31, 1956.

Cronqvist S.: The postoperative myelogram. *Acta Radiol.* 52:45, 1959.

Cronqvist S., Fuchs W.: Lumbar myelography in complete obstruction of spinal canal. *Acta Radiol.* 2(n.s.):145, 1964.

Crouzon O., Petit-Dutaillis D., Christophe J.: Sur un cas de compression de la queue de cheval, d'origine traumatique par un nodule fibrocartilagineux du disque intervertébral opération, Guérison. *Rev. Neurol.* 1:612, 1931.

Cyriax J.: Thoracic disk lesions. *St. Thomas's Rep.* 6:171, 1950.

Dandy W.E.: Loose cartilage from intervertebral disk simulating tumor of the spinal cord. *Arch. Surg.* 19:660, 1929.

Dandy W.E.: Concealed ruptured intervertebral disks: Plea for elimination of contrast medium in diagnosis. *J.A.M.A.* 117:821, 1941.

Dandy W.E.: Recent advances in diagnosis and treatment of ruptured intervertebral disks. *Ann. Surg.* 115:514, 1942.

Dandy W.E.: Improved localization and treatment of ruptured intervertebral disks. *J.A.M.A.* 120:605, 1942.

Dandy W.E.: Recent advances in the treatment of ruptured (lumbar) intervertebral disks. *Ann. Surg.* 118:639, 1943.

Davies H., Reid R.G., Fulton G.K.: Discussion on myelography. *Proc. Roy. Soc. Med.* 44:881, 1951.

Eaglesham D.C.: Observations on opaque myelography of lumbar disc herniations. *Br. J. Radiol.* 17:343, 1944.

Echlin F.A., Ivie J.M., Fine A.: Pantopaque myelography as an aid in the preoperative diagnosis of protruded intervertebral discs. *Surg., Gynecol. Obstet.* 80:257, 1945.

Echlin F.A., Selverstone B., Scribner W.E.: Bilateral and multiple ruptured discs as one cause of persistent symptoms following operations for herniated disc. *Surg., Gynecol. Obstet.* 83:485, 1946.

Editorial: Roentgenographic visualization of the intervertebral disc. *Am. J. Roentgenol.* 68:291, 1952.

Elsberg C.A.: Experiences in spinal surgery: Observations upon 60 laminectomies for spinal disease. *Surg., Gynecol. Obstet.* 16:117, 1913.

Elsberg C.A.: The extradural ventral chondromas (ecchondroses). Their favorite sites. The spinal cord and root symptoms they produce and their surgical treatment. *Bull. Neurol. Inst., New York* 1:350, 1931.

Epps P.G.: Case of degeneration of intervertebral disk following lumbar puncture. *Proc. Roy. Soc. Med.* 35:2220, 1942.

Epstein B.S.: Complete block of lumbar spinal canal due to herniation of nucleus pulposus. *Am. J. Roentgenol.* 61:775, 1949.

Epstein B.S., Davidoff L.M.: Iodized oil myelography of the cervical spine. *Am. J. Roentgenol.* 52:253, 1944.

Epstein J.A.: The syndrome of herniation of the lower thoracic intervertebral discs with nerve root and spinal cord compression. A presentation of four cases with a review of the literature. Methods of diagnosis and treatment. *J. Neurosurg.* 11:525, 1954.

Erlacher P.R.: Direct contrast roentgenography of nucleus pulposus: Contribution to pathology of intervertebral disk. *Ztschr. Orthop.* 80:40, 1950.

Erlacher P.: Die Ischialgie und ihre Beziehungen zur Diskushernie. *Wien. Klin. Wehnschr.* 63:193, 1951.

Ernsting W.: Use of contrast medium in diagnosis of hernia of nucleus pulposus. *Geneesk. Gids.* 27:303, 1949.

Fahrenkrug A., Gottschalk B., Højgaard K.: Myelography with water-soluble media in lumbago-sciatica after operation for herniated lumbar disk. *Acta Radiol.* 1(n.s.):138, 1964.

Falconer M.A., McGeorge M., Begg A.C.: Surgery of lumbar disk protrusion: Study of principles and results based upon 100 consecutive cases submitted to operation. *Br. J. Surg.* 35:225, 1948.

Finnegan B.E.: *Low Back Pain.* Philadelphia, J.B. Lippincott Co., 1973.

Fischer F.K.: Neue Methoden zur Darstellung von Bandscheibenveränderungen bei Lumbago und Ischias. *Schweiz. Med. Wehnschr.* 79:213, 1949.

Ford L.T., Key J.A.: Postoperative infection of intervertebral disc space. *South. Med. J.* 48:1295, 1955.

Ford L.T., Key J.A.: Evaluation of myelography in diagnosis of intervertebral disk lesions in low back. *J. Bone Joint Surg.* 32A:257, 306, 1950.

Ford L.T., et al.: Analysis of 100 consecutive lumbar myelograms followed by disk operations for relief of low back pain and sciatica. *Surgery* 32:961, 1952.

French J.D., Payne J.T.: Cauda equina compression syndrome with herniated nucleus pulposus; report of 8 cases. *Ann. Surg.* 120:73, 1944.

Friberg S., Hirsch C.: Anatomic and clinical studies on lumbar disc degeneration. *Acta Orthop. Scandinav.* 19:222, 1949.

Friberg S., Hult S.: Comparative study of abrodil myelogram and operative findings in low back pain and sciatica. *Acta Orthop. Scandinav.* 20:303, 1951.

Gill G.G., White H.L.: Mechanism of nerve root compression in backache. Surgical decompression in intervertebral disc condition, spondylolisthesis, spina bifida occulta and transitional fifth lumbar vertebra. *Clin. Orthop.* 5:66, 1955.

Goldthwait J.E.: The lumbosacral articulation. An explanation of many cases of "lumbago," "sciatica" and "paraplegia." *Boston M. & S. J.* 164:365, 1911.

Grant F.C., et al.: A correlation of neurologic, orthopedic and roentgenographic findings in displaced intervertebral discs. *Surg., Gynecol. Obstet.* 87:561, 1948.

Gurdjian E.S., Ostrowski A.Z., Hardy W.G., et al.: Results of operative treatment of protruded and ruptured lumbar discs. *J. Neurosurg.* 18:783, 1961.

Hakelius A., Hindmarsh J.: The comparative reliability of preoperative diagnostic methods in lumbar disc surgery. *Acta Orthop. Scandinav.* 43:234, 1972.

Hakelius A., Hindmarsh J.: The significance of neurological signs and myelographic findings in the diagnosis of lumbar root compression. *Acta Orthop. Scandinav.* 43:239, 1972.

Haley J.C., Perry J.H.: Protrusions of intervertebral discs. A study of their distribution, characteristics and effects on the nervous system. *Am. J. Surg.* 80:394, 1950.

Hampton A.O.: Iodized oil myelography; use in the diagnosis of rupture of the intervertebral disk into the spinal canal. *Arch. Surg.* 40:444, 1940.

Hampton A.O., Robinson J.M.: Roentgenographic demonstration of rupture of the intervertebral disc into the spinal canal after the injection of Lipiodol; with special reference to unilateral lumbar lesions accompanied by low back pain with "sciatic" radiation. *Am. J. Roentgenol.* 36:782, 1936.

Haughton V.M., Eldevik O.P., Magnaes B., Amundsen P.: A prospective comparison of computed tomography and myelography in the diagnosis of herniated lumbar disks. *Radiology* 142:103, 1982.

Hirsch C., Rosencrantz M., Wickbom I.: Lumbar myelography with water-soluble contrast media, with special reference to the appearances of root pockets. *Acta Radiol. (Diagn.)* 8:54, 1969.

Hitselberger W.E., Witten R.M.: Abnormal myelograms in asymptomatic patients. *J. Neurosurg.* 28:204, 1968.

Hoen T.I., Anderson R.K., Clare F.B.: Symposium on neurosurgery: Lesions of intervertebral disks. *Surg. Clin. North Am.* 28:456, 1948.

Holman C.B.: The roentgenologic diagnosis of herniated intervertebral disk. *Radiol. Clin. North Am.* 4:171, 1966.

Holt E.P., Jr.: Fallacy of cervical discography: Report of 50 cases in normal subjects. *J.A.M.A.* 188:799, 1964.

Horwitz N.H., Whitcomb B.B., Reilly F.G.: Ruptured thoracic discs. *Yale J. Biol. & Med.* 28:322, 1956.

Horwitz T.: Lesions of intervertebral disk and ligamentum flavum of lumbar vertebrae; anatomic study of 75 human cadavers. *Surgery* 6:410, 1939.

Horwitz T.: Diagnosis of posterior protrusion of intervertebral disc. *Am. J. Roentgenol.* 49:199, 1943.

Hudgins W.R.: The predictive value of myelography in the diagnosis of ruptured lumbar discs. *J. Neurosurg.* 32:152, 1970.

Hulme A.: The surgical approach to thoracic intervertebral disc protrusions. *J. Neurol., Neurosurg. Psychiatr.* 23:133, 1930.

Hyndman O.R.: Pathologic intervertebral disk and its consequences. Contribution to cause and treatment of chronic pain low in the back and to subject of herniating intervertebral disk. *Arch. Surg.* 53:247, 1946.

Hyndman O.R., Steindler A., Wolkin J.: Herniated intervertebral disk: A study of the iodized oil column: The procaine test in the differential diagnosis from reflected sciatic pain. *J.A.M.A.* 121:390, 1943.

Imler R.L., Sahs A.L.: Disk herniations in thoracic region. *J. Iowa Med. Soc.* 42:151, 1952.

Jeanmart L., Retif J.: Correlation of myelographic examinations with clinical and operative findings in 150 cases of herniated lumbar intervertebral disks. *J. Belge Radiol.* 50:415, 1967.

Johnson H.F.: Herniation of intervertebral disc with referred sciatic symptoms. *J. Bone Joint Surg.* 22:708, 1940.

Kahn E.A.: The role of the dentate ligaments in spinal cord compression and the syndrome of lateral sclerosis. *J. Neurosurg.* 4:191, 1944.

Kaplan A.: Herniated intervertebral discs producing contralateral symptoms and signs. *Bull. Hosp. Joint Dis.* 10:207, 1949.

Kaplan A., Umansky A.L.: Myelographic defects of herniated intervertebral disks simulating cauda equina neoplasm. *Am. J. Surg.* 81:262, 1951.

Kieffer S.A., Sherry R.G., Wellenstein D.E., King R.B.: Bulging lumbar intervertebral disk: Myelographic differentiation from herniated disk with herniated disk with nerve root compression. *A.J.R.* 138:709, 1982.

Kocher T.: Die Verletzungen der Wirbelsäule zugleich als Beitrag zur Physiologie des menschlichen Rückenmarks. *Mitt. Grenzgeb. Med. Chir.* 1:420, 1896.

Kölliker A.: Über die Beziehungen der Chorda dorsalis zur Bildung der Wirbel der Selachier und einiger anderer Fische. *Verhandl. Phys.-Med. Gesellsch. Würzburg* 10:193, 1860.

Kortzeborn A.: Schmorl'sches Knorpelknötchen unter dem Bilde eines Rückenmarkstumors im Bereich des Halsmarks. *Zentralbl. Chir.* 57:2418, 1930.

Laasonen S.M., Alho A., Karaharju E.O., Paovilainen T.: Short term prognosis in sciatica. A prospective study of factors influencing the results with special reference to myelography. *Ann. Chir. Gynaecol.* 66:47, 1977.

Lange J.: Abrodil myelography in protrusion of intervertebral disk. *Acta Chir. Scandinav.* 104:181, 1952.

Lange J., Ødegaard, H.: Abrodil myelography in herniated disk in lumbar region. *Radiology* 57:186, 1951.

Lansche W.E., Ford L.T.: Correlation of the myelogram with clinical and operative findings in lumbar disc lesions. *J. Bone Joint Surg.* 42A:193, 1960.

Leader S.A., Rassell M.J.: Value of Pantopaque myelography in diagnosis of herniation of nucleus pulposus in lumbosacral spine. 500 cases. *Am. J. Roentgenol.* 69:231, 1953.

LeMay M., Jackson D.M.: Intervertebral disc protrusion masquerading as an intramedullary tumor. *Br. J. Radiol.* 37:463, 1964.

Levy L.I.: Lumbar intervertebral disc disease in Africans. *J. Neurosurg.* 26:31, 1967.

Levy R.W., Payzant A.R., Karr H.H.: Pantopaque myelography in ruptured disk: Correlation with operative findings. *New Orleans M. & S. J.* 103:390, 1951.

Lindblom K.: Eine anatomische Studie über lumbale zwischenwirbelscheiben Protrusionen und zwischenwirbelscheiben Brüche in die Foramina intervertebralia hinein. *Acta Radiol.* 22:711, 1941.

Lindblom K.: Protrusion of discs and nerve compression in lumbar region. *Acta Radiol.* 25:195, 1944.

Lindblom K.: Diagnostic puncture of intervertebral disks in sciatica. *Acta Orthop. Scandinav.* 17:231, 1948.

Lindblom K.: Backache and its relation to ruptures of intervertebral disks. *Radiology* 57:710, 1951.

Lindblom K., Hultquist G.T.: Absorption of protruded disc tissue. *J. Bone Joint Surg.* 32A:557, 1950.

Lindblom K., Rexed B.: Spinal nerve injury in dorsolateral protrusions of lumbar discs. *J. Neurosurg.* 5:413, 1948.

Lindgren E.: Über die Röntgendiagnose des Bandscheibenprolapses. *Radiol. Clin.* 10:337, 1941.

Logue V.: Thoracic disk prolapse with spinal cord compression. *J. Neurol., Neurosurg. Psychiatr.* 15:227, 1952.

Lombardi G., Passerini A.: *Spinal Cord Diseases.* Baltimore, Williams & Wilkins Co., 1964, p. 132.

Love J.G.: Protruded intervertebral disks with note regarding hypertrophy of ligamenta flava. *J.A.M.A.* 113:2029, 1939.

Love J.G.: Differential diagnosis of intraspinal tumors and protruded intervertebral disks and their surgical treatment. *J. Neurosurg.* 1:275, 1944.

Love J.G., Kiefer E.J.: Root pain and paraplegia due to protrusions of thoracic intervertebral disks. *J. Neurosurg.* 7:62, 1950.

Love J.G., Schorn V.G.: Thoracic disk protrusions. *J.A.M.A.* 191:627, 1965.

Love J.G., Walsh M.N.: Intraspinal protrusion of intervertebral disks. *Arch. Surg.* 40:454, 1940.

Love J.G., Walsh M.N.: Protruded intervertebral disks. *Surg., Gynecol. Obstet.* 77:497, 1943.

Löwe L.: Zur Kenntnis der Säugetierchorda. *Arch. Mikrosk. Anat.* 16:597, 1879.

Lyons A.E., Wise B.L.: Subarachnoid rupture of intervertebral disc fragment. *J. Neurosurg.* 18:242, 1961.

McCarty W.C., Lane F.W.: Pitfalls of myelography. *Radiology* 65:663, 1955.

McGinnis K.D., Eisenberg A.B.: Diagnostic criteria for distinguishing cervical disk herniation from spondylosis in the neural compression syndrome. *Radiology* 83:63, 1964.

McNab I.: Negative disc exploration. An analysis of the causes of nerve root involvement in sixty-eight patients. *J. Bone Joint Surg.* 52A:891, 1971.

McNab I.: *Backache.* Baltimore, Williams & Wilkins Co., 1977.

McRae D.L.: Asymptomatic intervertebral disc protrusions. *Acta Radiol.* 46:9, 1956.

Middleton G.S., Teacher J.H.: Injury of the spinal cord due to rupture of an intervertebral disc during muscular effort. *Glasgow Med. J.* 76:1, 1911.

Mixter W.J., Ayer J.G.: Herniation or rupture of intervertebral disc into spinal canal. *N. Engl. J. Med.* 213:385, 1935.

Mixter W.J., Barr J.S.: Protrusion of the lower lumbar intervertebral disks. *N. Engl. J. Med.* 223:523, 1940.

Moreton R.D., Ehni G.: Radiographic findings in protruded cervical discs. *South. Med. J.* 44:582, 1951.

Moseley I.: The oil myelogram after operation for lumbar disc lesions. *Clin. Radiol.* 28:267, 1977.

Movin A.: Myelographic appearances of disk protrusions in different positions. *Acta Radiol. (Diagn.)* 6:524, 1967.

Müller R.: Protrusion of cervical intervertebral disks with lesion of the spinal cord. *Acta Med. Scandinav.* 139:85, 1951.

Müller R.: Protrusion of thoracic intervertebral discs with compression of the spinal cord. *Acta Med. Scandinav.* 139:99, 1951.

Murphy F., et al.: Myelography in patients with ruptured cervical intervertebral discs. *Am. J. Roentgenol.* 56:27, 1946.

Murphy J.P.: Lumbar disc protrusion contralateral to side of symptoms and signs; myelographic verification in 2 cases. *Am. J. Roentgenol.* 61:77, 1949.

Naffziger H.C., Inman V.T., Saunders J.B.: Lesions of the intervertebral disc and ligamenta flava. *Surg., Gynecol. Obstet.* 66:288, 1938.

O'Connell J.E.A.: Protrusions of the lumbar intervertebral discs. Clinical review based on 500 cases treated by excision of the protrusion. *J. Bone Joint Surg.* 33B:8, 1951.

Paine K.W.E., Haung P.W.H.: Lumbar disc syndrome. *J. Neurosurg.* 37:75, 1972.

Peterson H.O.: Intervertebral disc diseases and the radiologist. *Am. J. Roentgenol.* 88:11, 1962.

Peterson H.O., Kieffer S.A.: Radiology of intervertebral disk disease. *Semin. Radiol.* 7:260, 1972.

Peyton W.T., Simmons D.R.: Herniated intervertebral disk: Analysis of 90 cases. *Arch. Surg.* 55:271, 1947.

Pilling J.R.: Water-soluble radiculography in the erect posture: A clinico-radiological study. *Clin. Radiol.* 30:665, 1979.

Püschel J.: Der Wassergehalt normaler und degenerierter Zwischenwirbelscheiben. *Beitr. Path. Anat.* 84:123, 1930.

Raaf J.: Some observations regarding 905 patients operated upon for protruded lumbar intervertebral disc. *Am. J. Surg.* 97:388, 1959.

Raskin S.P., Keating J.W.: Recognition of lumbar disk disease: Comparison of myelography and computed tomography. *AJNR* 3:215, 1982.

Rathcke L.: Über Kalkablagerungen in den Zwischenwirbelscheiben. *Fortschr. Geb. Röntgenstrahlen* 45:66, 1932.

Rees S.E., Donley C.E.: Accuracy of Pantopaque studies in diagnosis of herniated intervertebral disk. *Northwest Med.* 48:180, 1949.

Reeves D.L., Brown H.A.: Thoracic intervertebral disc protrusion with spinal cord compression. *J. Neurosurg.* 28:24, 1968.

Remak R.: *Untersuchungen über die Entwickelung der Wirbeltiere.* Berlin, G. Reimer, 1855.

Robin C.: *Mémoire sur l'Evolution de la Notochorde, des Cavités des Disques Intervertebraux et de Leur Contenu Gelatrineux.* Paris, J.B. Baillière et Fils, 1868.

Robinson J.M.: Retropulsion of lumbar intervertebral discs as cause of low back pain with unilateral "sciatic" radiation; roentgenologic diagnosis with special reference to iodolography. *Am. J. Surg.* 49:71, 1940.

Saenger E.L.: Spondylarthritis in children. *Am. J. Roentgenol.* 64:20, 1950.

Saunders J.B. deC.M., Inman V.T.: The intervertebral disc; critical and collective review. *Internat. Abst. Surg.; Surg., Gynecol. Obstet.* 69:14, 1939.

Saunders J.B. deC.M., Inman V.T.: Pathology of intervertebral disk. *Arch. Surg.* 40:389, 1940.

Scherbel A.L., Gardner W.J.: Infections involving the intervertebral disks: Diagnosis and management. *J.A.M.A.* 174:370, 1960.

Schmorl G.: Über Knorpelknötchen an der Hinterfläche der Wirbelbandscheiben. *Fortschr. Geb. Röntgenstrahlen* 40:629, 1929.

Schmorl G.: Beiträge zur pathologischen Anatomie der Wirbelbandscheiben und ihre Beziehungen zu den Wirbelkörpern. *Arch. Orthop. und Unfall-Chir.* 29:389, 1931.

Schneider R.C.: Chronic neurological sequelae of acute trauma to the spine and spinal cord. II. The syndrome of chronic anterior spinal cord injury or compression. Herniated intervertebral discs. *J. Bone Joint Surg.* 41A:449, 1959.

Schnitker M.T., Boothby G.T.: Pantopaque myelography for protruded disks of the lumbar spine. *Radiology* 45:370, 1945.

Schreiber G., Rosenthal A.: Paraplegia from ruptured lumbar discs in achondroplastic dwarfs. *J. Neurosurg.* 9:648, 1952.

Schubiger O., Valavanis A.: CT differentiation between recurrent disc herniation and postoperative scar formation: The value of contrast enhancement. *Neuroradiology* 22:251, 1982.

Schultz E.H., Jr.: Cervical disc disease simulating intramedullary neoplasm by myelography. *Am. J. Roentgenol.* 91:1051, 1964.

Semmes R.E.: Lateral rupture of cervical disc. Incidence and clinical varieties. *Am. J. Surg.* 75:137, 1948.

Semmes R.E., Murphy F.: Syndrome of unilateral rupture of sixth cervical intervertebral disk with compression of seventh cervical nerve root. *J.A.M.A.* 121:1209, 1943.

Sicard J.A.: Les sciatiques; sciatiques par blessures de Guerre: Sciatiques médicale. *Marseille-Méd.* 53:2, 1918.

Silverman F.N.: Calcification of the intervertebral disks in childhood. *Radiology* 62:801, 1954.

Slater R.A., Pineda A., Porter R.W.: Intradural herniation of lumbar intervertebral discs. *Arch. Surg.* 90:266, 1965.

Smith N.R.: The intervertebral disks. *Br. J. Surg.* 18:358, 1930–31.

Soule A., Gross S.W., Irving J.G.: Myelography by use of Pantopaque in the diagnosis of herniations of the intervertebral discs. *Am. J. Roentgenol.* 53:319, 1945.

Spurling R.G.: *Lesions of the Cervical Intervertebral Disc.* Springfield, Ill., Charles C Thomas, Publisher, 1956.

Spurling R.G., Grantham E.G.: Ruptured intervertebral discs in the lower lumbar region. *Am. J. Surg.* 75:140, 1948.

Spurling R.G., Mayfield F.H., Rogers J.B.: Hypertrophy of the ligamenta flava as a cause of low back pain. *J.A.M.A.* 109:928, 1937.

Stephenson T.F.: Metrizamide myelography for disk disease: Continuing need for epidural venography. *A.J.N.R.* 2:255, 1981.

Stern W.E., Crandall P.H.: Inflammatory intervertebral disc disease as a complication of the operative treatment of lumbar herniations. *J. Neurosurg.* 16:261, 1959.

Stookey B.: Compression of the spinal cord due to ventral extradural cervical chondromas. *Arch. Neurol. Psychiatr.* 20:275, 1928.

Stookey B.: Compression of spinal cord and nerve roots by herniation of nucleus pulposus in cervical region. *Arch. Surg.* 40:417, 1940.

Strully K.J., et al.: Progressive spinal cord disease: syndromes associated with herniation of cervical intervertebral discs. *J.A.M.A.* 146:10, 1951.

Svien H.J., Dodge H.W., Jr., Camp J.D.: Importance of spinal fluid analysis and contrast myelography when protruded lumbar disc is suspected. *Surg., Gynecol. Obstet.* 93:643, 1951.

Svien H.J., Karavitis A.L.: Multiple protrusions of the intervertebral disks in the upper thoracic region; report of a case. *Proc. Staff Meet. Mayo Clin.* 29:375, 1954.

Teplick J.E., Haskin M.E.: CT of the postoperative lumbar spine. *Radiol. Clin. North Am.* 21:395, 1983.

Van Landingham J.H.: Herniation of thoracic intervertebral disc with spinal cord compression in kyphosis dorsalis juvenilis (Scheuermann's disease). *J. Neurosurg.* 11:327, 1954.

Verbrugghen A.: Massive extrusions of the lumbar intervertebral discs. *Surg., Gynecol. Obstet.* 81:269, 1945.

Vesalius A.: De Humani Corporis Fabrica Libri Séptem Basileae per J. Opòrinum, p. 71, 1555.

Virchow R.: *Untersuchungen über die Entwickelung des Schädelgrundes im gesunden und krankhaften Zustande und über den Einfluss derselben auf Schädelform, Gesichtsbildung und Gehirnbau.* Berlin, G. Reimer, 1857.

Vogl A., Osborne R.L.: Lesions of spinal cord (transverse myelopathy) in achondroplasia. *Arch. Neurol. Psychiatr.* 61:644, 1949.

von Luschka H.: *Die Halbgelenke des menschlichen Körpers.* Berlin, G. Reimer, 1858.

Walk L.: Slight myelographic deformities in sciatica. *Acta Radiol.* 50:226, 1958.

Whitcomb B.B.: Symposium on problems in postwar medicine: Rupture of the intervertebral disk. *Med. Clin. North Am.* 30:431, 1946.

Williams L.W.: The later development of the notochord in mammals. *Am. J. Anat.* 8:251, 1908.

Wright F.W., Sanders R.C., Steel W.M., O'Connor B.T.: Some observations on the value and techniques of myelography in lumbar disc lesions. The results over a five year period at the Nuffield Orthopaedic Centre, Oxford. *Clin. Radiol.* 22:33, 1971.

Young H.H.: Non-neurological lesions simulating protruded intervertebral disk. *J.A.M.A.* 148:1101, 1952.

Young R.H.: Protrusion of intervertebral discs. *Proc. Roy. Soc. Med.* 40:233, 1947.

Yuhl E.T., et al.: Diagnosis and surgical therapy of chronic midline cervical disk protrusions. *Neurology* 5:494, 1955.

18

The Narrow Spinal Canal

NARROWING of the bony spinal canal may be conveniently divided into two groups: (1) central and (2) lateral, involving the neural canal (lateral recess) or the neural (intervertebral) foramen. The stenosis may affect the entire spine or only one or two levels.

CLASSIFICATION OF SPINAL STENOSIS

1. Congenital—central
2. Idiopathic developmental—central
3. Acquired
    a. Spondylosis
    b. Spondylolisthesis
    c. Postoperative
    d. Posttraumatic
    e. Miscellaneous—Paget's disease, fluorosis, acromegaly, diffuse idiopathic skeletal hyperostosis (DISH), vitamin D–resistant rickets, etc.

Congenital

Although congenital stenosis (Fig 18-1) is usually generalized, i.e., achondroplasia, it may rarely be focal, i.e., congenital lumbar bony ridge, occipital dysplasia with projection of the hypertrophic condyles into the bony canal. Achondroplasia, the most common type of disproportionate short limb dwarfism, is characterized by an abnormality of enchondral bone formation. In the spine, this results in diminished height of the vertebral bodies and premature fusion of the neurocentral synchondroses. The latter produces marked narrowing of all diameters of the bony spinal canal with short, thick pedicles and thick laminae. The constriction of the bony canal tends to be most pronounced at the craniocervical junction and in the lumbar spine. In the latter area, the decreased sagittal diameter is associated with a decreased interpediculate distance proceeding distally from the lower thoracic to the lumbosacral level. Consequently, the spinal cord, cauda equina, and their meningeal investments fill the narrow bony canal. Compression of the medulla or upper

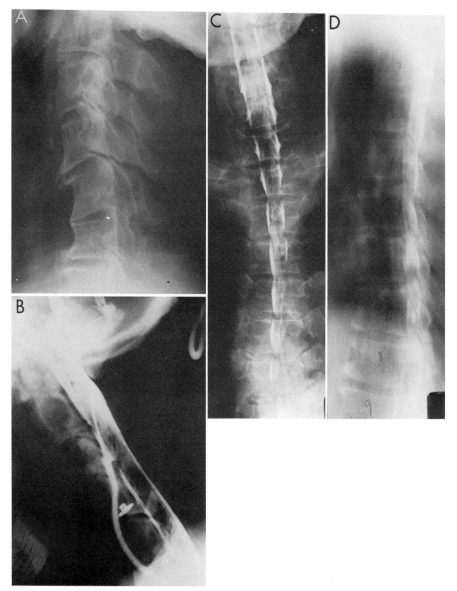

Fig 18–1.—The patient was an adult achondroplastic dwarf who had been gainfully employed until the recent onset of bilateral leg weakness. The plain lateral radiograph of the cervical spine **(A)** shows a marked reduction in the sagittal diameter of the bony canal. Other radiographs of the lumbar spine showed marked narrowing of all diameters of the spinal canal with short thick pedicles and laminae. Myelography was performed via a lateral C1-2 puncture **(B).** The frontal and lateral films of the thoracic cord (**C** and **D**) show multiple indentations of the oil column by the hypertrophic facets and pedicles. The lumbar myelogram demonstrated pronounced narrowing of the oil column at L1-2 and L2-3.

cervical cord due to coarctation of the foramen magnum, or atlantoaxial dislocation is rare in children. Neural compression of the thoracolumbar region is similarly uncommon in childhood and early adult life, even in the presence of a thoracolumbar kyphos. Neural compression begins to manifest itself toward the end of the third decade and in the fourth decade with the onset of disk degeneration. This problem becomes aggravated with the development of progressive spondylotic bone changes and disk degeneration in later decades. Four principal clinical syndromes have been reported in patients with achondroplasia: (1) acute transverse myelopathy usually due to a disk herniation, (2) chronic transverse myelopathy developing slowly over a period of years, particularly in patients with a thoracolumbar gibbus, (3) intermittent cauda equina claudication, (4) nerve root compression.

Idiopathic Developmental

This lesion is the result of a disturbance in vertebral growth of unknown etiology which reaches its peak in adult life, i.e., after the age of 30 years. Patients are frequently asymptomatic until the onset of degenerative disk disease. The characteristic abnormality is a reduction of the sagittal diameter of the cervical, lumbar, or cervicolumbar bony canal.

CERVICAL (Fig 18–2).—The sagittal diameter of the cervical bony canal is measured from a point on the posterior aspect of the vertebral body to a corresponding point on the base of the spinous process. The measurement can be made on a conventional lateral radiograph taken at a 6-foot distance, or from a tomogram. When the canal is narrowed by osteophyte formation, the measurement should be made between the osteophyte on the posteroinferior aspect of the vertebral body

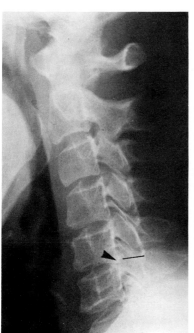

Fig 18–2.—Lateral radiograph of the cervical spine in a 45-year-old female with idiopathic developmental narrowing of the spinal canal (corrected sagittal diameter 9 mm). The patient presented with a myeloradiculopathy due to spondylosis at C5-6. The arrowhead points to the bony spur arising from the posterior inferior margin of C-5, proved to be midline in position by tomography. The straight line extending from the bony spur to the base of the spinous process represents the smallest sagittal diameter of the bony canal.

and the base of the spinous process of the vertebra below. Since the osteophyte visualized on a conventional lateral radiograph may not be in the midline, the measurement is preferably made on a midline sagittal tomogram in the neutral position. Extension can reduce the sagittal diameter by as much as 2 mm, compared with the same measurement in flexion. Spondylotic cord compression is likely to occur in patients with a sagittal diameter of 11 mm or less and unlikely in patients with a sagittal diameter greater than 13 mm.

Lumbar (Fig 18–3).—In 1945, Sarpyener called attention to the narrow lumbar canal in children. In 1949, 1954, and 1955, Verbiest focused attention on spinal stenosis in the adult and pointed out the importance of the diminished sagittal diameter of the bony canal. Verbiest also emphasized the association of idiopathic developmental stenosis with neurogenic claudication of the cauda equina. In 1953, Schlesinger and Taveras published their classic description of the clinical syndrome associated with lumbar spondylosis and a constricted bony canal.

Spondylotic changes rarely produce clinical symptoms in a normal or large canal (Figs 18–4 to 18–6). The uncorrected normal sagittal diameter of the adult lumbar canal on conventional lateral radiographs varies from 22 to 25 mm. The narrow canal has a sagittal diameter of 16 mm or less on the conventional lateral film and a measurement below 13 cm on CT. As in the cervical spine, the measurement is made from the posterior aspect of the vertebral body to the base of the spinous process. Although the latter may be difficult to recognize on conventional radiographs, it can readily be visualized by tomography or by CT. Verbiest has shown

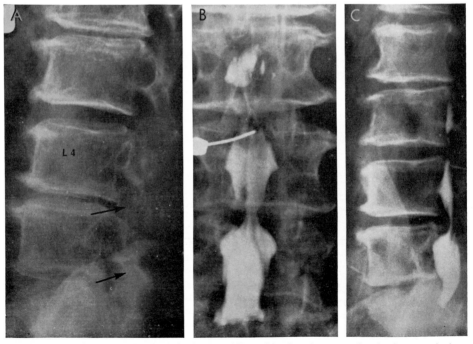

Fig 18–3.—Spondylosis engrafted upon idiopathic developmental spinal stenosis in a 58-year-old man with a narrow sagittal diameter of the lumbar bony canal (11 mm). Note the hypertrophic posterior facets *(arrow),* the vertical alignment of the laminae, the narrowed disk spaces, and osteophyte formation.

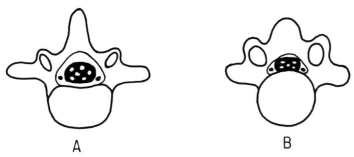

A   B

Fig 18–4.—Coronal diagram of a normal lumbar vertebra **(A)** with an ample bony canal that can accommodate the cauda equina without compression in the presence of moderate spondylosis. **B** illustrates congenital stenosis of the lumbar spinal canal with thick pedicles and laminae, a vertical orientation of the latter, and encroachment on the cauda equina. Obviously, minor degrees of spondylosis can aggravate the impingement on the cauda.

that even the CT measurement is subject to minor error, i.e., the CT measurement may be as much as 1.3 mm larger than the true measurement determined at operation. This is due to angulation of the plane of the transaxial sections, which may not be perpendicular to the anterior wall of the bony canal. Radiographic techniques other than CT cannot adequately evaluate the soft tissue changes which can also contribute to the narrowing of the sagittal diameter of the canal, i,e., disk protrusion, hypertrophy of the ligamentum flavum.

Acquired

The most common cause of acquired spinal stenosis is spondylosis, a disease which may involve the cervical, lumbar, or cervical and lumbar portions of the spine. The disease is extremely rare in the thoracic region. Govoni reported a single case of narrowing of the thoracic spinal canal in a 67-year-old female with marked thickening of the laminae of T-9, resulting in cord compression. In a study of 594 thoracic vertebrae and 11 complete spine specimens, he noted moderate dorsoventral narrowing of the bony canal in four vertebrae, severe narrowing in

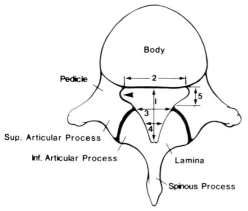

Fig 18–5.—Diagram of a normal lumbar vertebra in the axial projection illustrating various useful measurements. *1,* anteroposterior (sagittal) diameter. *2,* transverse (interpediculate) diameter. *3,* interfacetal diameter. *4,* interlaminar diameter. *5,* height of lateral recess. The lateral recess is identified by an arrowhead.

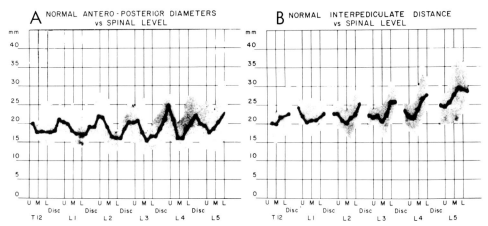

Fig 18–6.—Normal anteroposterior **(A)** and transverse **(B)** diameters at various lumbar levels. The black line represents the mean values and the shaded portion the range of measurements. (Reprinted, with permission, from Ullrich C.G., et al., *Radiology* 134:141, 1980.)

one vertebra, and bony protrusions from the posterior vertebral margins into the spinal canal in two specimens.

The primary lesion in acquired spondylosis is intervertebral disk degeneration. The latter is secondary to dehydration of the nucleus pulposus with subsequent dessication and narrowing. The disk space narrowing results in laxity, bulging, and sometimes tearing of the annulus fibrosus. This, in turn, leads to hypermobility of the intervertebral joint and marginal osteophyte formation. Because the intervertebral disk and the two facet joints represent a tripod joint complex, the narrowed disk space (most marked posteriorly) results in facet joint subluxation in the frontal, sagittal, and axial planes. The added stress on the facet joints produces degenerative changes, i.e., margin erosions, subchondral sclerosis, osteophyte formation. The rotational subluxation usually results in anterior subluxation of the superior articular process. With subluxation of the facet joint and narrowing of the disk space, the passive ligamentum flavum becomes shorter and thicker and is pushed into the intervertebral foramen. The pincer-like effect of the bulging annulus and marginal osteophytes anteriorly, and the subluxed superior facet joint posteriorly, produces neural compression on the narrowed intervertebral foramen (Figs 18–7, 18–8). As the disk narrows, the pedicle may undergo axial displacement with kinking of the nerve root (Fig 18–9).

In some patients, the inferior articular process subluxes into the space between the medial margin of the superior articular process and the superior aspect of the lamina (Figs 18–10, 18–11). The reactive bony sclerosis and hypertrophy at the level of the lateral recess produces entrapment of the nerve root in the recess.

In addition to nerve root compression, spondylosis can also produce a myelopathy due either to direct pressure on the spinal cord or to anterior spinal artery compression with secondary cord ischemia.

Conventional radiography demonstrates a reduction in the sagittal diameter of the bony spinal canal (see Fig 18–24), narrowing of the disk spaces, thickened laminae, hypertrophic facets that protrude into the spinal canal (Fig 18–12), pos-

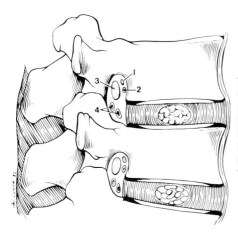

Fig 18–7.—Diagram in the lateral view of the normal lumbar intervertebral foramen and its contents. The normal foramen measures 8–10 mm in height and 4–6 mm in its sagittal diameter. *1,* sinuvertebral nerve. *2,* sinuvertebral artery. *3,* spinal nerve. *4,* radicular vessels. Note that the nerve is situated in the upper half of the foramen above the intervertebral disk level.

terior spurring of the vertebral bodies and of the articular processes forming the zygapophyseal joints. Spinal stenosis is more common in the midlumbar spine, in contrast to herniated lumbar disk disease which has its greatest incidence at L4-5 and L5-S1. The abnormal zygapophyseal joints permit excessive motion that may result in retrolisthesis, i.e., degenerative spondylolisthesis (Figs 18–13, 18–14). The normal inferior facet occupies a plane 90 degrees to the pedicle, making overriding of the facets impossible. In some patients, however, the angle between the facets and the pedicle approximates 180 degrees, which facilitates slipping when degenerative facet joint changes set in. In the lumbar area, retrolisthesis is most common at L4-5, although it may be present at two or more levels. Normally a line drawn through the inferior articular plate of a vertebra in the lateral view intersects the tip of the subjacent superior articular process. With subluxation of the zygapophyseal joints, the line intersects the middle of the superior articular process (see Fig 18–8). As the vertebral bodies come closer together because of disk degeneration, the laminae do likewise. The result is a washboard or shingling effect, with the superior aspect of a lamina lying anterior to the inferior margin of the lamina above it. This accentuates infolding of a normal or thickened ligamentum flavum.

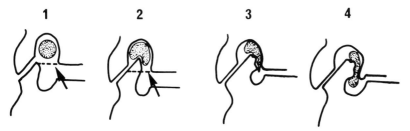

Fig 18–8.—Diagram in the lateral projection of a normal zygapophyseal joint *(1)* and of progressive degenerative changes *(2, 3, 4)* resulting in increasing subluxation of the zygapophyseal joints and neural compression. Note that a line *(arrow)* traversing the inferior articular plate intersects the tip of the superior articular process of the vertebra below in the normal. In posterior joint subluxation, this line crosses the middle of the superior articular process (After MacNab.)

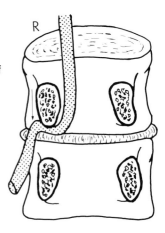

Fig 18–9.—Diagram illustrating kinking of the right L-4 nerve root by the corresponding pedicle due to anterior and caudal slipping of the body of L-4 in a patient with spondylolisthesis at L4-5 (after MacNab). The bony defect was more pronounced on the right side. More commonly, this occurs at L5-S1.

CERVICAL SPONDYLOSIS

Cervical spondylosis is a common disease of the elderly. In Pallis, Jones, and Spillane's study of 50 non-neurologic hospitalized patients, 50% over the age of 50 years and 75% over the age of 75 years had typical radiologic changes of spondylosis. McRae reported a series of 240 patients, with and without symptoms related

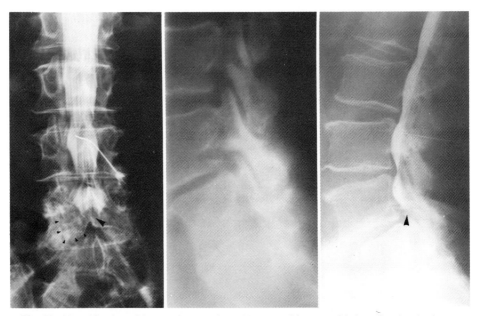

Fig 18–10.—Metrizamide myelogram in a 69-year-old man with localized spinal stenosis and a block *(large arrowhead)* at the level of the body of L-4 due to marked hypertrophy and caudad migration of the inferior articular processes of L-4 *(small arrowheads)*, particularly on the right side. There is also bilateral laminar thickening and subluxation of the superior articular processes of L-5. Note the normal relationship of the superior articular processes of L-2 to the pedicle and transverse process of L-1. At the L4-5 level, the tip of the superior articular process of L-5 abuts the pedicle and base of the transverse process of L-4.

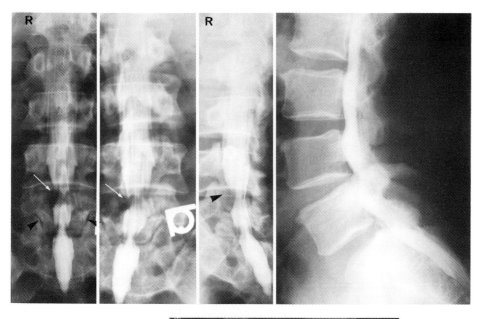

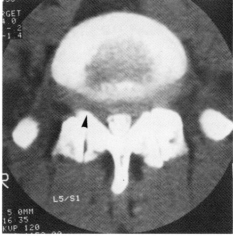

Fig 18–11.—Bilateral hypertrophy of the inferior articular processes of L-5 *(arrowheads)*, producing constriction of the metrizamide column in a 45-year-old man. There is also hypertrophy of the right inferior articular process of L-4 *(arrow)*. The inferior articular process hypertrophy is also seen on the metrizamide CT study at the lumbosacral interspace *(arrowhead)*. The patient also had generalized bulging of the lumbosacral disk with an intact annulus at surgery.

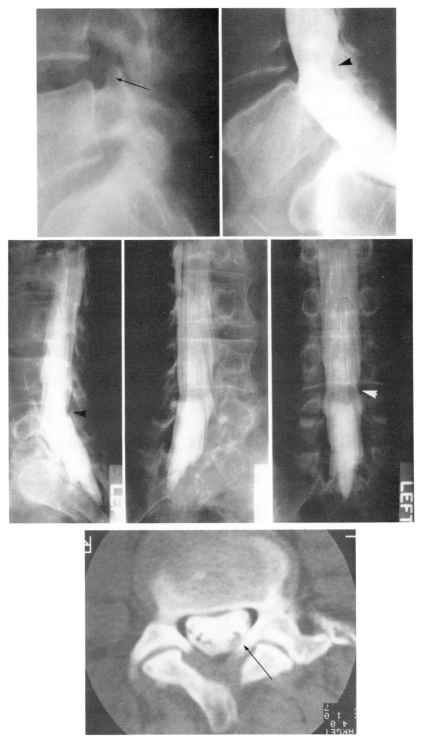

Fig 18–12.—Hypertrophy and sclerosis of the left superior articular process of L-5 *(arrow)*, producing a shallow defect on the left posterolateral aspect of the metrizamide column *(arrowhead)*. This is elegantly portrayed on the metrizamide CT scan *(arrow)*.

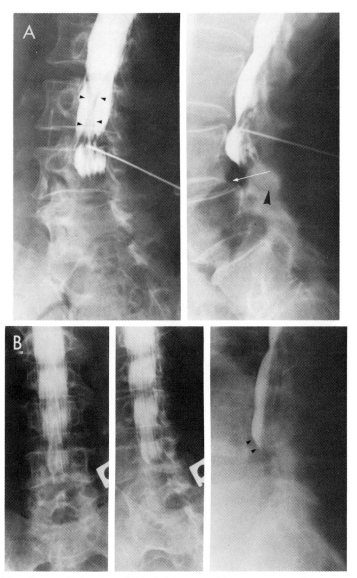

Fig 18–13.—**A,** retrolisthesis at L4-5 *(white arrow)* in a 61-year-old woman with severe spinal stenosis and block. Note the hypertrophy of the posterior elements *(large arrow-head)* and narrowing of the zygapophyseal joints. Note also the redundant nerve roots *(small arrowheads).* **B,** retrolisthesis at L4-5 in a 64-year-old woman with marked localized spinal stenosis at this level. The metrizamide myelogram graphically demonstrates the complete obstruction at the L4-5 interspace, which was present in flexion as well as extension. Note the "lifting up" of the anterior aspect of the thecal sac away from the body of L-4 *(arrowheads).* At operation, a free fragment of herniated disk was found in the spinal canal, along with the bony stenosis.

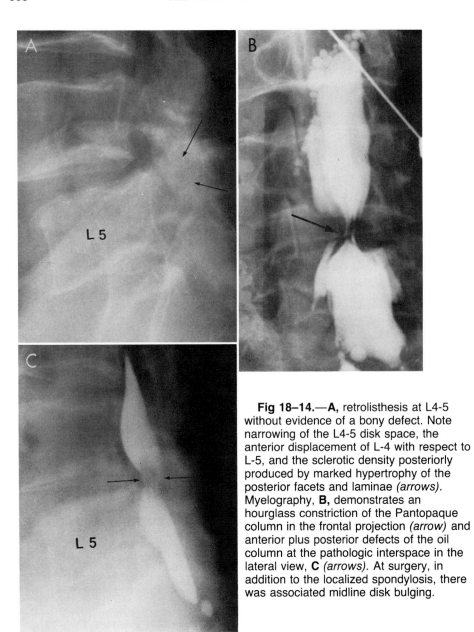

Fig 18–14.—A, retrolisthesis at L4-5 without evidence of a bony defect. Note narrowing of the L4-5 disk space, the anterior displacement of L-4 with respect to L-5, and the sclerotic density posteriorly produced by marked hypertrophy of the posterior facets and laminae *(arrows).* Myelography, **B,** demonstrates an hourglass constriction of the Pantopaque column in the frontal projection *(arrow)* and anterior plus posterior defects of the oil column at the pathologic interspace in the lateral view, **C** *(arrows).* At surgery, in addition to the localized spondylosis, there was associated midline disk bulging.

to the cervical spine or cord. He noted degenerative changes in the upper zyga-pophyseal joints along with disk degeneration and osteophyte formation at C5-6 and/or C6-7 in more than 50% of patients older than 40 years. Consequently, McRae suggested that radiologic findings be considered significant only when they correspond to the clinical neurologic level. I have frequently seen similar radiologic changes in asymptomatic elderly patients. The presence or absence of neurologic findings is probably related to various mechanical factors, i.e., the size of the bony canal, the tautness of the dentate ligaments, the presence or absence of vascular or direct spinal cord compression. In this regard, the sagittal diameter of the cervical bony canal is critical. In general, cord compression is likely if the sagittal diameter measures 10 mm or less with the neck in the neutral position. The smallest sagittal diameter is the distance between the spur on the posterior inferior margin of a vertebral body and the base of the vertebra below (see Fig 18–2). The posterior spur frequently extends across the entire disk space as a bony ridge or bar that indents the anterior surface of the spinal cord. Such bars can produce acute cord damage during a hyperextension injury of the cervical spine.

Thickening and infolding of the ligamentum flavum by hypertrophied laminae also contribute to the reduced space available to the cervical cord. The infolding tends to be most marked in hyperextension as the cord is compressed by the pincer action of the midline posterior vertebral spur in front and the ligamentum flavum and hypertrophied laminae behind (Fig 18–15).

Plain-Film Findings in Cervical Spondylosis

Routine radiography of the cervical spine usually shows disk narrowing (most often at C5-6 and C6-7), osteophytic spurs anteriorly, posteriorly, and posterolater-ally, with constriction of the corresponding intervertebral foramina and narrowing of the zygapophyseal joints, with spur formation. There also may be bony sclerosis

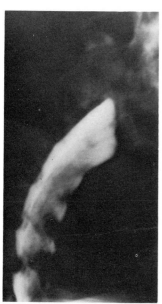

Fig 18–15.—Lateral prone cross-table myelogram in hyperextension showing corrugation of the posterior aspect of the oil column by the ligamentum flavum folded in by the hypertrophic posterior spinal elements. Note also the defects on the anterior aspect of the oil column due to spurring.

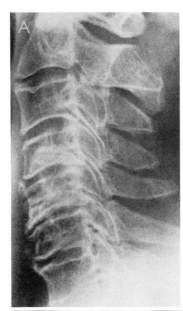

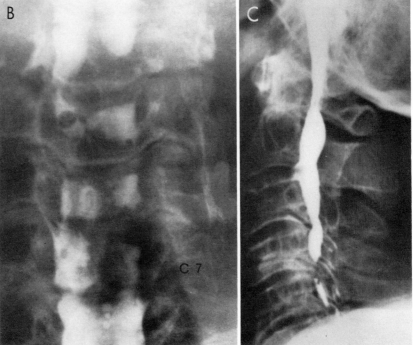

Fig 18–16.—The patient, a 58-year-old man, presented with an 8-month history of pain in the legs and thighs, precipitated by walking, and some difficulty in gait. The peripheral pulses were good. There are extensive degenerative changes at multiple levels seen in **A,** the lateral radiograph of the cervical spine. Myelography shows horizontal ridging of the Pantopaque column at multiple levels, in **B,** and anterior and posterior constriction in the lateral projection, **C.**

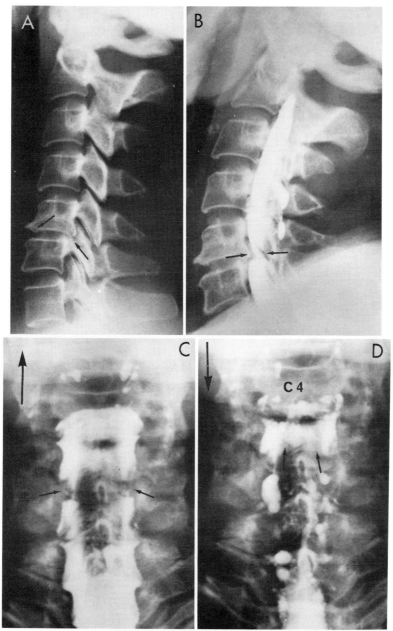

Fig 18–17.—Localized cervical spondylosis at C5-6 in a 40-year-old woman. **A,** the lateral radiograph of the spine demonstrates loss of the normal lordotic cervical curve, narrowing of the C5-6 interspace, and spur formation anteriorly and posteriorly *(arrows).* **B** and **C,** myelography shows localized constriction of the Pantopaque column at C5-6 both anteriorly and posteriorly *(arrows).* The posterior defect is not usually seen in a simple herniated disk and is not necessarily due to hypertrophy of the ligamentum flavum. Often there is folding in of the normal ligamentum flavum by the hypertrophied pedicles and laminae. In **D,** note the hold-up of the Pantopaque by a horizontal ridge of bone at the level of C5-6 *(arrows)* as the oil column is brought down into the lumbar region.

on either side of the narrowed intervertebral disks or zygapophyseal joints. Patients with spondylosis and a Klippel-Feil malformation are likely to show spondylotic changes at the sites of maximal motion, i.e., above and below the nonsegmented vertebrae.

Myelographic Findings in Cervical Spondylosis (Figs 18–16 to 18–22)

Various defects may be observed at myelography: (1) medial displacement of the outer margin of the oil column with or without deformity or obliteration of the nerve root sleeve. This type of defect is due to bony and/or fibrocartilaginous spurring pressing on the lateral aspect of the subarachnoid space and adjacent cord. The defect is often larger, more irregular, and extends more medially than the defect associated with the usual herniated cervical disk. (2) Transverse defects or ridges at one or more interspaces produced by posterior osteophytes extending across the entire width of the disk space (Figs 18–16, 18–17). (3) Defects on the posterior aspect of the Pantopaque column in the lateral projection (often accentuated in extension) due to infolding of the ligamenta flava (Fig 18–15). (4) Spurious widening of the cord in the frontal projection due to compression by the transverse bars (Fig 18–22). The latter should not be confused with true widening of the cord due to an expanding intramedullary lesion. Correct differentiation can readily be made by a lateral shoot-through film, which shows a narrowed sagittal cord diameter in spondylosis and a widened sagittal cord diameter in intramedullary lesions (this is elegantly demonstrated by pneumomyelography). In addition, intramedullary expanding lesions usually extend over several cord segments whereas spurious flattening tends to be limited to one or two segments.

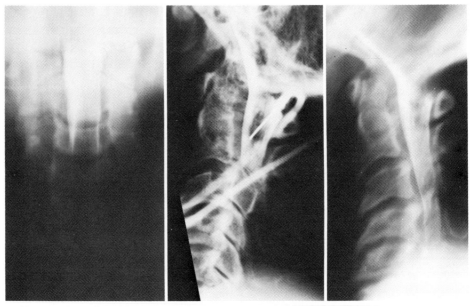

Fig 18–18.—Metrizamide myelogram carried out via a lateral C1-2 puncture in an elderly male with spondylosis. The initial myelographic films suggest a complete block at C2-3. However, delayed tomography demonstrates a narrowed midcervical cord.

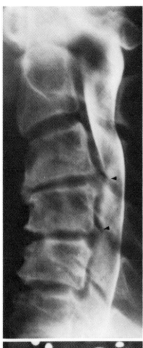

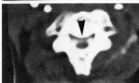

Fig 18–19.—Metrizamide CT myelogram in a 65-year-old man with pronounced cervical spondylosis, showing compression of the anterior subarachnoid space and cord by the spurs *(small arrowheads)*. This is confirmed by CT at the level of C-3 *(large arrowhead)*.

LUMBAR SPONDYLOSIS

Lumbar spondylosis usually occurs in the middle-aged or elderly, without a specific traumatic episode. The common complaints are paresthesias, numbness, and leg weakness, often out of proportion to the leg or back pain. The symptoms frequently appear, or are aggravated, in the standing position or in hyperextension of the spine. The pain is often relieved in the sitting position. Neurologic findings include diminished or absent reflexes and motor weakness in the lower extremities.

Occasionally, patients with spondylosis complain of intermittent claudication due to neural rather than vascular compromise to the legs. It has not been definitely established if the symptoms are due to compression of the microcirculation of the radicular nerves and neural ischemia during the period of increased metabolic neural activity that occurs during exercise. The patient may be incorrectly considered to have Leriche's syndrome. Wilson has pointed out the major features that differentiate the intermittent claudication of aortoiliac disease from that due to cauda equina compression. The pain in the former is usually dull and cramp-like in character, induced by, and limited to, the muscles exercised and relieved by standing still. Neurologic examination is normal and the peripheral pulses usually diminished after exercise. Plain radiography often demonstrates arterial calcification with or without concomitant spondylosis; aortography shows a high-grade or complete

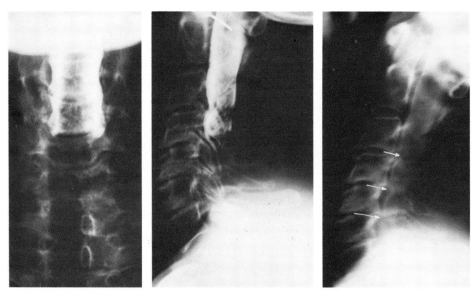

Fig 18–20.—Metrizamide myelogram performed via a lateral C1-2 puncture in a 62-year-old woman with marked cervical spondylosis and a high-grade block at C4-5. A delayed tomogram shows marked impingement on, and flattening of, the cord anteriorly at several levels *(arrows)*.

obstruction at or above the aortic bifurcation. Cauda equina claudication may be either ischemic or postural. If the patient develops symptoms while standing, the cause is likely to be postural, secondary to an exaggerated lumbar lordosis; the symptoms are alleviated when the patient bends forward or squats. However, the discomfort resulting from cauda equina ischemia or arterial insufficiency is unaffected by posture and persists as long as the exercise continues. Patients with an ischemic cauda equina syndrome have variable neurologic findings, with exaggeration of the sensory and motor deficit in the lower extremities after walking. These patients show the characteristic findings of spondylosis by conventional radiography and myelography and no evidence of aortic obstruction by aortography. In the rare patient who has both aortoiliac obstruction and lumbar spondylosis, both aortography and myelography or CT are necessary for correct diagnosis. Some patients have both cervical and lumbar spondylosis (Fig 18–23).

Myelographic Findings in Lumbar Spondylosis (Figs 18–24 to 18–29)

Lumbar puncture frequently is difficult and often reveals a partial or high-grade obstruction, with an elevation of CSF protein. If there is a problem with the puncture in the recumbent position, it should be attempted with the patient erect. In these patients, I make no effort to advance the needle once any flow of CSF is obtained. Since the roots of the cauda equina are tightly packed in a narrowed subarachnoid space, it is reasonable to expect a poor flow of CSF. Myelography confirms the obstruction suggested by lumbar puncture. Not infrequently, a partial obstruction is converted into a complete obstruction when the patient is placed in hyperextension, because of increased protrusion of the intervertebral disks and a

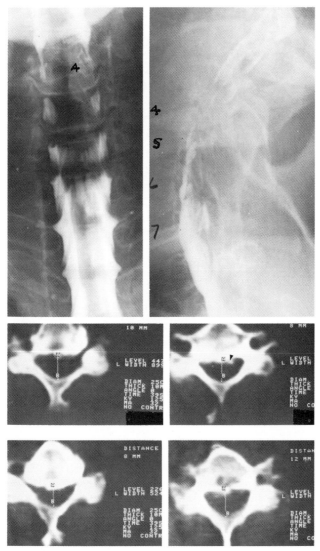

Fig 18–21.—Severe cervical spondylosis in a 64-year-old male with marked posterior osteophyte *(arrowhead)* formation, especially at C-4, constricting the bony canal. This is confirmed by CT, which demonstrates the smallest sagittal diameter of the bony canal at C-4 to be 8 mm.

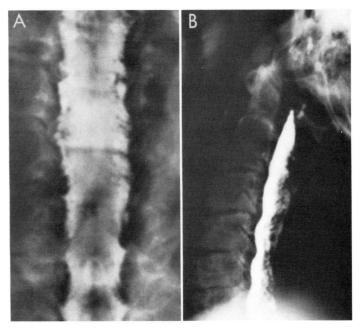

Fig 18–22.—Myelogram in a patient with advanced cervical and lumbar spondylosis. Note the spurious widening of the cervical cord in the frontal projection **(A)** due to compression by transverse bars. The lateral cross-table film **(B)** shows multiple indentations on the anterior surface of the oil column due to the bony spurs, as well as no evidence of enlargement of the sagittal diameter of the cord.

diminution in the sagittal diameter of the spinal canal (Fig 18–26). There are usually multiple, prominent defects (rarely a single defect) on both the anterior and posterior aspects of the oil column. The anterior defects are due to disk degeneration and bony spurring, and the posterior defects to infolding of the thickened ligamenta flava. Because the defects frequently are bilateral, with prominent root shadows, the findings may be confused with arachnoiditis or with an extra-arachnoidal injection.

Sortland et al. have pointed out the usefulness of functional metrizamide myelography in patients with lumbar stenosis (Fig 18–26). With the patient standing or sitting upright, lateral films are made first in flexion, then in the neutral position, and finally in extension. In this way, the involved disks and the degree of spinal stenosis can be accurately evaluated. The severity of the spinal stenosis in some patients may be underestimated by conventional myelography in the neutral position.

Cord compression has also been reported in acromegaly and vitamin D–resistant osteomalacia secondary to the increased bone mass in these conditions.

Localized Postoperative Lumbar Stenosis

Stenosis of the lumbar bony canal is a relatively common finding in symptomatic patients who have undergone a previous posterior spinal fusion or a simple laminectomy for a herniated disk. Quencer et al. reported bony stenosis in 43% of the

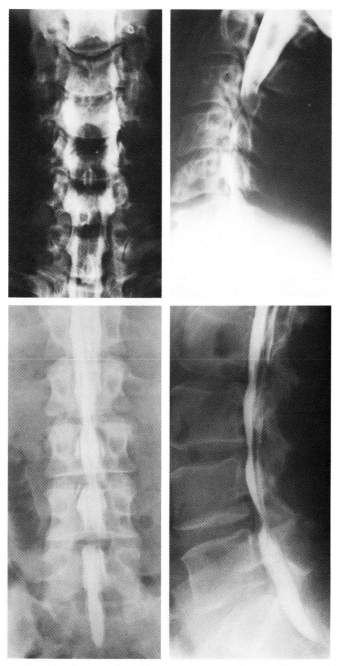

Fig 18–23.—Combined cervical and lumbar spondylosis in a 48-year-old man studied by metrizamide myelography introduced via lumbar puncture at L2-3. The lumbar stenosis is most pronounced at L4-5.

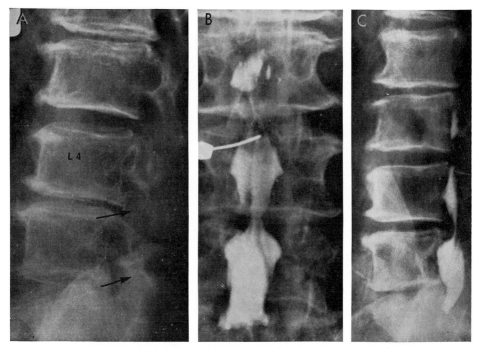

Fig 18–24.—The lateral plain radiograph **(A)** and the frontal myelographic spot film **(B)** demonstrate the narrowed sagittal diameter of the lumbar canal, the hypertrophied posterior facets *(arrows),* and the narrowed zygapophyseal joints along with vertical alignment of the laminae, narrowing of the disk spaces, and spur formation. The patient was a 58-year-old man with spondylosis. The lateral cross-table myelogram **(C)** demonstrates marked indentation on the anterior aspect of the oil column at L4-5.

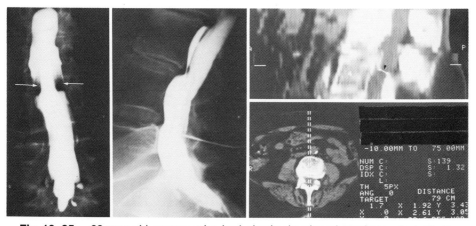

Fig 18–25.—62-year-old woman who had slowly developed weakness in both lower extremities over a period of almost 2 years. This had become accelerated in the second year. The Pantopaque myelogram performed elsewhere had been reported as indeterminate. The patient then saw a neurologist, who suspected spinal stenosis. A review of the myelogram confirmed the diagnosis of spinal stenosis most marked at L3-5. Note the hypertrophic inferior articular processes of L-3 producing the bilateral defects *(arrows).* CT demonstrates the smallest sagittal diameter of the canal *(arrowhead)* to be 7.9 mm.

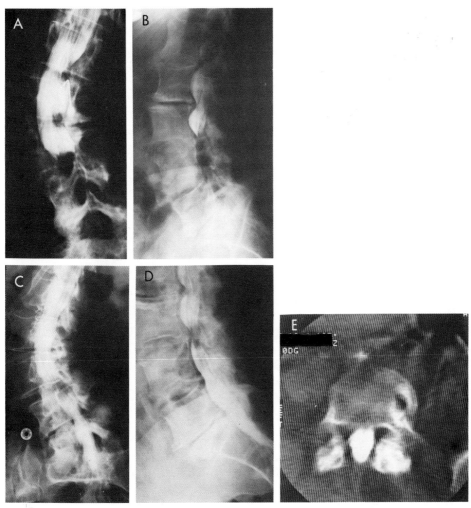

Fig 18–26.—Functional metrizamide myelography in an elderly patient with lumbar sco-liosis and spondylosis. The films made in extension **(A** and **B)** demonstrate a complete block at L3-4. The films made in flexion **(C** and **D)** show passage of the metrizamide caudally into the distal caudal sac. The CT scan at L3-4 **(E)** clearly shows bilateral compression of the thecal sac by the hypertrophic articular processes, which markedly narrow the transverse diameter of the spinal canal.

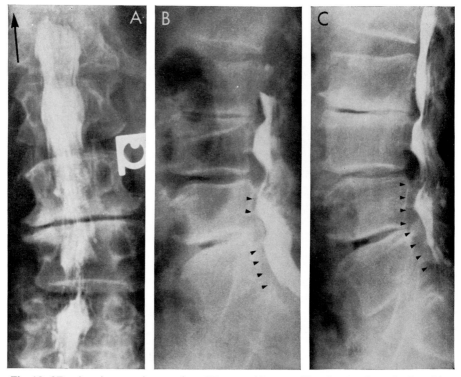

Fig 18–27.—Lumbar myelogram in a 57-year-old man with advanced cervical and lumbar spondylosis. The anteroposterior **(A)** and lateral **(B)** film show marked narrowing, with gas in the degenerated intervertebral disks, spur formation and multiple indentations of the oil column, most marked at L4-5.

former group and 28% of the latter group. The narrowing of the canal is due to thickened laminae, hypertrophic medial protruding articular processes, and osteophytic spurs, as well as soft tissue abnormalities, i.e., scarring, thickening of the dura, hypertrophy of the ligamentum flavum. In patients with only a simple laminectomy and disk removal, secondary degeneration of the facet joints may occur due to increased stress with resultant hypertrophy and subluxation of the articulating facets. The stenosis is best demonstrated by CT. Most of the patients in both groups (91%) were considerably improved after surgical decompression with removal of the hypertrophic bone.

STENOSIS ASSOCIATED WITH SPONDYLOLISTHESIS
(Figs 18–30 to 18–33)

Classification of Spondylolisthesis

1. Isthmic—defect in pars interarticularis.
    a. lytic—separation or dissolution of pars (most common type in patients under 50 years of age).
    b. elongation of pars without a defect.

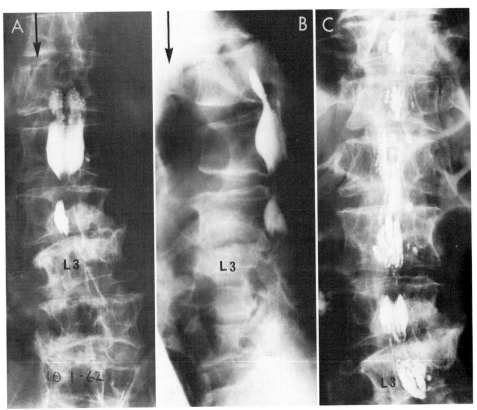

Fig 18–28.—Myelogram in an achondroplastic dwarf of 40 years, demonstrating the marked washboard appearance due to severe lumbar spondylosis. The final effect is exaggerated because of the congenitally narrow spinal canal. **A** and **B,** the original myelogram on November 1, 1962, showed a complete block at L2-3. The oil was left in place. **C,** a repeat film on November 25, 1965, shows Pantopaque below the level of the previous obstruction.

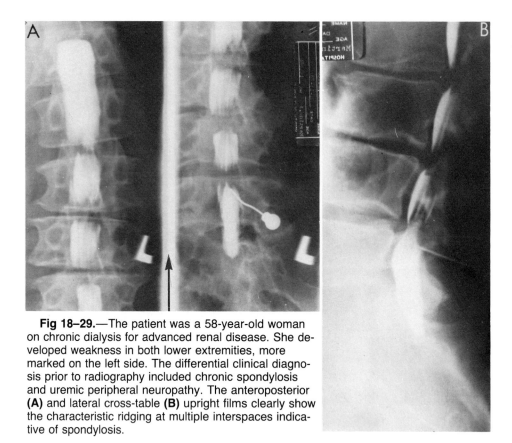

Fig 18–29.—The patient was a 58-year-old woman on chronic dialysis for advanced renal disease. She developed weakness in both lower extremities, more marked on the left side. The differential clinical diagnosis prior to radiography included chronic spondylosis and uremic peripheral neuropathy. The anteroposterior **(A)** and lateral cross-table **(B)** upright films clearly show the characteristic ridging at multiple interspaces indicative of spondylosis.

 c. acquired—in patients at the upper end of a spinal fusion.
 d. pathologic—secondary to localized or generalized bone disease.
 e. acute pars fracture—not always obvious.
 2. Dysplastic—If the superior articular processes of S-1 are underdeveloped and oriented transversely, the inferior articular processes of L-5 can slide forward in the absence of a pars defect or elongation.
 3. Degenerative—secondary to disk degeneration with relaxation of the annulus and remodeling of the articular processes at the level of involvement, most commonly at L4-5.
 4. Pedicular—due to fracture or elongation of the pedicles from generalized bone disease.
Severe spondylolisthesis may produce spinal stenosis due to compression of the cauda equina by the displaced vertebra, hypertrophic bony ridges, and thickening of the posterior neural arch and ligamentum flavum. Neural compression may also occur in less marked cases of spondylolisthesis in the presence of a narrow canal.

LATERAL RECESS SYNDROME (Figs 18–34, 18–35)

Originally described by Ghormley in 1933, this lesion has since been reported by many authors, particularly Epstein and Epstein. The lateral recess or neural

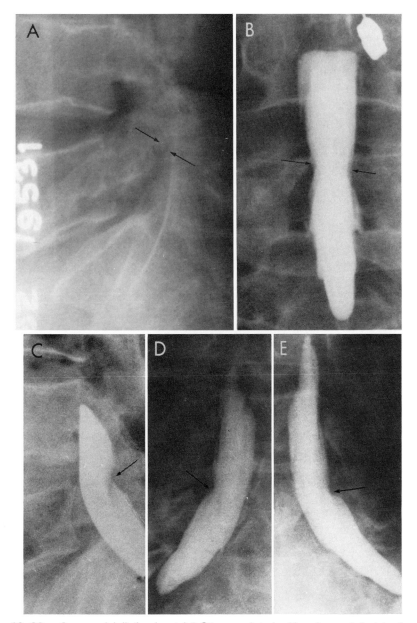

Fig 18–30.—**A,** spondylolisthesis at L5-S1 associated with a bony defect in the pars interarticularis *(arrows).* At myelography, **B–E,** a bilateral defect can be seen on the posterolateral aspect of the Pantopaque column at L4-5 *(arrows).* At surgery, this was found to be due to hypertrophy of the posterior facets; no disk herniation was present.

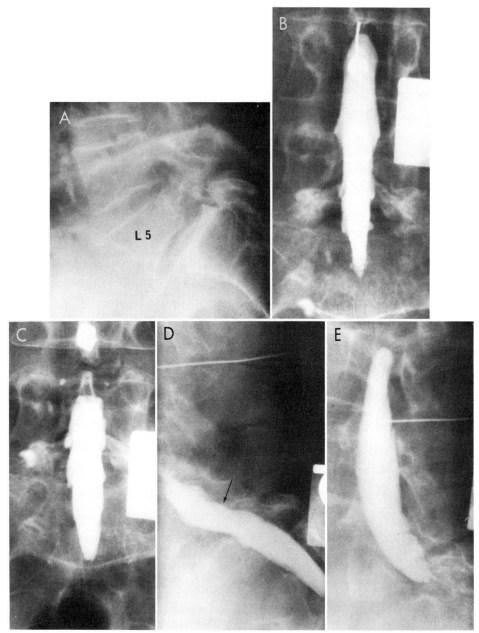

Fig 18–31.—A, marked spondylolisthesis at L5-S1, with an essentially negative myelogram, **B–E.** There is minimal encroachment on the posterior aspect of the oil column at L4-5 *(arrow)* in the lateral view, **D,** due to hypertrophy of the posterior facets.

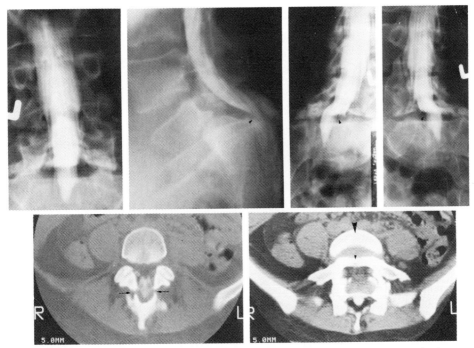

Fig 18–32.—**Top,** metrizamide myelography in a 20-year-old girl with marked spondylolisthesis at L5-S1 due to bilateral defects of the pars interarticularis. The patient had no neurologic findings. Note the intrusion on the thecal sac in the oblique and lateral projections *(arrowheads).* **Bottom,** CT demonstrates the bilateral pars defects *(arrows)* on the scan made through the inferior articular plate of L-4, and the marked anterior displacement of the body of L-5 *(large arrowhead)* with respect to S-1 *(small arrowhead).*

canal is a funnel-shaped extension of the bony canal demarcated anteriorly by the posterolateral surface of the vertebral body, laterally by the pedicle, and posteriorly by the superior articular process. In the upper lumbar spine, the lateral recess is insignificant because of the short intraspinal segment of the corresponding lumbar nerves (Fig 18–35). The latter immediately enters the intervertebral foramen after exiting from the lateral margin of the theca. At L-4, L-5, and S-1, however, the lateral recesses are longer. As the spinal nerve emerges from the thecal envelope, it takes an oblique inferolateral course through the lateral recess, passes medial and inferior to the pedicle, and exits through the intervertebral foramen (Fig 18–36). Hypertrophy of the superior articular facet can readily compress the nerve root at the level of the superior border of the pedicle where the lateral recess is narrowest. Similar neural compression may also be caused by an osteophyte projecting from the posterolateral aspect of the vertebral body (Fig 18–37) and by a lateral disk herniation (Figs 18–36, 18–38).

Although conventional radiography may occasionally suggest the correct diagnosis, lateral tomography accurately defines the depth of the lateral recess between the most anterior aspect of the superior articular process and the posterior border of the vertebral body at the level of the superior margin of the pedicle. However, high-resolution magnification CT with multiple thin slices (1.5 mm) provides the most accurate measurement of the depth of the lateral recess. The depth of the

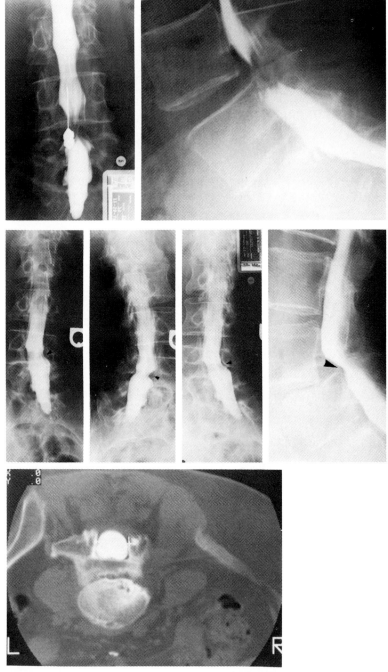

Fig 18–33.—This 59-year-old woman had a Pantopaque myelogram on November 29, 1978, for chronic backache **(top).** The plain films demonstrated a bilateral defect of the pars interarticularis. The original myelogram shows a bilateral symmetric defect in the oil column of L4-5 with a pronounced posterior defect due to articular process and laminar hypertrophy. Approximately 4 years later, she had a metrizamide myelogram **(middle),** followed by CT **(bottom)** because of progressive weakness of both lower extremities. The lateral myelogram shows a pronounced anterior slipping of L-4 on L-5 with considerable pressure of the posterior aspect of L-5 on the anterior theca *(large arrowhead).* CT demonstrates the hypertrophic posterior elements compressing the thecal sac. All of the symptoms due to the marked spinal stenosis were relieved by surgical intervention.

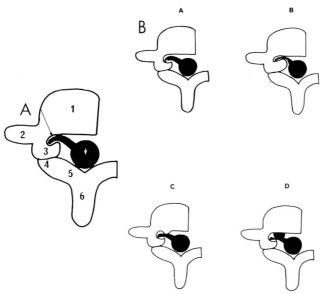

Fig 18–34.—A, diagrammatic schema in the axial projection of the normal relationship of the lumbar nerve at L-4 to the lateral recess *(black arrow)* and the thecal sac *(white arrow). 1,* body of vertebra. *2,* transverse process. *3,* superior articular process. *4,* inferior articular process of L-4. *5,* lamina. *6,* spinous process. **B,** *A,* normal. *B,* hypertrophy of superior articular process. *C,* posterolateral osteophyte. *D,* posterolateral disk herniation.

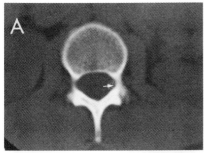

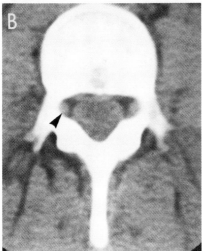

Fig 18–35.—Axial CT slice thru pedicles at level of L-1 **(A)** shows an insignificant lateral recess *(arrow).* A similar section at L-4 **(B)** demonstates a fairly capacious lateral recess with the L-4 nerve root in it *(arrowhead).*

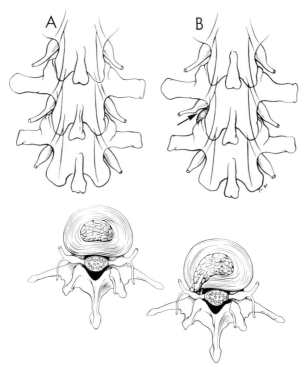

Fig 18–36.—Artist's rendition of the frontal and axial projections of a normal *(arrowhead)* metrizamide myelogram **(A),** showing the nerve exiting from the lateral margin of the thecal sac and traversing the neural canal and neural foramen, respectively. Neural displacement *(arrow)* by a lateral-lying disk herniation is demonstrated in **B.**

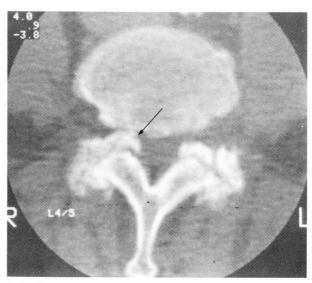

Fig 18–37.—Axial CT scan at L4-5, demonstrating bilateral marked disease of the facet joints. In addition, note the stenosis of the right lateral recess due to osteophyte formation arising from the superior articular process *(arrow).*

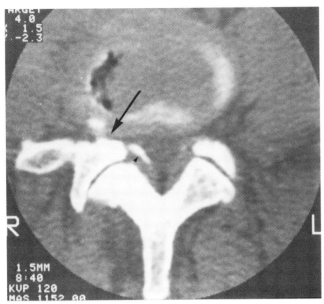

Fig 18–38.—Axial scan at L4-5, demonstrating a herniated disk in the right lateral recess and intervertebral foramen *(arrow)*. Note the calcification of the ligamentum flavum *(arrowhead)* and the vacuum disk.

lateral recess diminishes as one proceeds caudally from L-1 to L-5. The normal lateral recess has a depth greater than 5 mm. A recess that measures less than 3 mm in depth is definitely stenotic. Recesses with a depth of 3–5 mm are problematic and should be correlated with the clinical findings before a diagnosis of stenosis is made.

The myelographic findings are variable in patients with the lateral recess syndrome. Metrizamide, because of its lesser viscosity, penetrates the nerve root sheath for a greater distance than Pantopaque. Hence, it is more useful than Pantopaque in this condition. Pantopaque usually demonstrates amputation of the nerve root sheath at the level of the superior border of the abnormal lateral recess. Metrizamide may show the thickened arachnoidal and dural sleeves overlying the compressed nerve roots (secondary to irritation). It may also show flattening of the nerve root beneath the abnormal superior facet.

In generalized spondylosis, both contrast media commonly demonstrate a shallow or pronounced unilateral or bilateral extradural defect with or without some evidence of block. The most important role of myelography in these patients is the exclusion of other concomitant lesions, i.e., herniated disk, etc.

OSSIFICATION OF THE POSTERIOR LONGITUDINAL LIGAMENTS

Various Japanese authors have described numerous patients with cervical radiculomyopathy due to calcification or ossification of the posterior longitudinal ligaments. Minagi and Gronner reported two similar cases in Caucasians in the United States in 1969. Bakay, Cares, and Smith published seven additional case reports

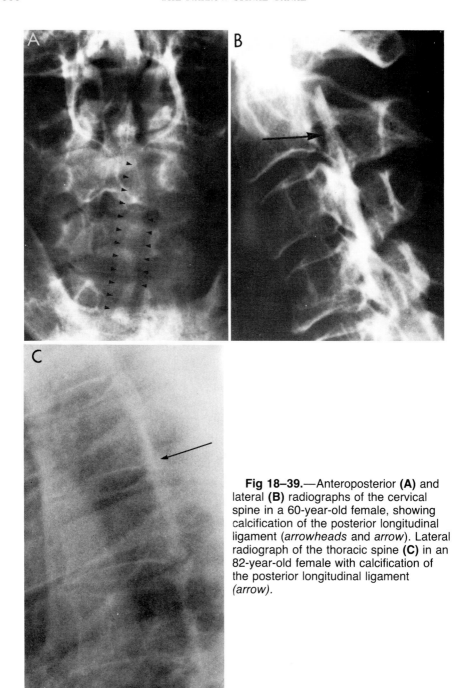

Fig 18–39.—Anteroposterior **(A)** and lateral **(B)** radiographs of the cervical spine in a 60-year-old female, showing calcification of the posterior longitudinal ligament (*arrowheads* and *arrow*). Lateral radiograph of the thoracic spine **(C)** in an 82-year-old female with calcification of the posterior longitudinal ligament (*arrow).*

from the United States in 1970. This entity appears to be more common in Japanese for reasons presently not known. The plain films demonstrate calcification or ossification in the posterior longitudinal ligament, with or without concomitant spondylosis (Figs 18–39, 18–40). According to Takahashi et al., the ossification can occur at any cervical level as short bands or longitudinal streaks on (or 1–3 mm behind) the posterior surfaces of the vertebral bodies. Similar ossifications have been reported in the thoracic (see Fig 18–39,C) and/or lumbar spine. The disease is more common in males, with a peak incidence from 40 to 70 years. The neurologic findings are those of a segmental radiculopathy involving one or more cervical roots and/or myelopathy due to cord compression. The latter is more likely to occur in patients with a narrow sagittal diameter of the bony canal.

Calcification and ossification of the posterior longitudinal ligament have also been reported in 50% of 74 patients with diffuse idiopathic skeletal hyperostosis (DISH). Recently, Alenghat et al. reported cord compression in a 68-year-old man with DISH due to prominent posterior osteophyte formation at C5-6.

Yoshikawa et al. discribed three adult siblings with untreated familial hypophosphatemic vitamin D–resistant rickets. Two of the patients who developed tetraplegia (ages 43 and 48 years) had cervical cord compression and ossification of the posterior longitudinal ligament. The same authors reported two additional cases of untreated adult rickets (without calcification of the posterior longitudinal ligament) with cord compression by exuberant osteoid formation at T-1 and T-4 respectively. Cord compression has also been reported in rare cases of acromegaly secondary to the increased bony mass in these patients.

Weiss and Spencer reported a single interesting case of ossification of the lumbar interspinous ligament between L-4 and L-5 resulting in compression of the cauda equina.

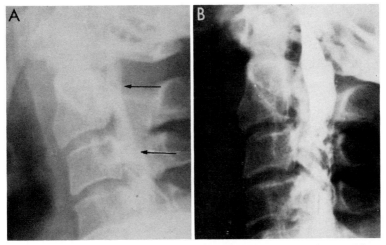

Fig 18–40.—A, ossification of the posterior longitudinal ligament *(arrows)* in a 60-year-old woman with a 1-year history of difficulty in walking. Six weeks prior to hospitalization, her gait became worse and she began to have severe neck pain, paresthesia, and weakness in both arms. At myelography **(B)** there was a marked delay in passage of the Pantopaque beyond C2-4 due to encroachment of the bony bar on the spinal canal. (Reprinted, with permission, from Bakay L., et al., *J. Neurol., Neurosurg. Psychiatr.* 33:263, 1970.)

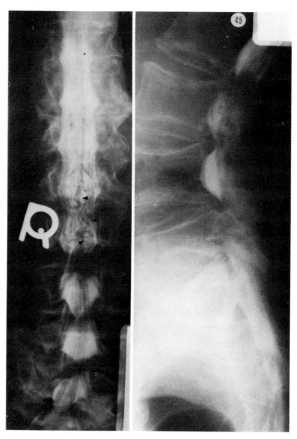

Fig 18–41.—74-year-old woman with marked lumbar spinal stenosis secondary to spondylosis. Note the redundant nerve roots *(arrowheads).*

Since the introduction of high-resolution CT scanning, calcification of the ligamentum flavum is commonly seen (see Fig 18–38).

REDUNDANT NERVE ROOTS

In 1968, Cressman and Pawl, and Schut and Graff each described a single case of a redundant lumbar nerve root. Cressman and Pawl's patient was a 63-year-old male with a 2½-year history of progressive paraparesis and intermittent sciatic pain. Four years previously, he suffered low back pain and weakness of the left leg that resolved spontaneously, only to return 1 year later. At operation, a small, taut caudal sac was found with a large stenotic osteoarthritic bar at L4-5. In addition, there was a markedly redundant nerve root coiled on itself over the cauda at L3-4.

Schut and Graff's patient was a 47-year-old male whose original complaint was low back pain after a fall. He had previously undergone an unsuccessful myelogram followed by laminectomy, at which time the surgeon reputedly found "nerves caught in scar tissue" but no herniated disk. Six months later, the patient presented with a sensory and motor deficit in the lower extremities and sphincter involvement. Myelography performed via lumbar puncture at L1-2 revealed a complete extradural block. At operation, the dura was tense and nonpulsatile. On opening

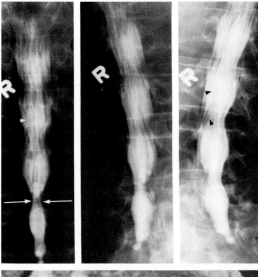

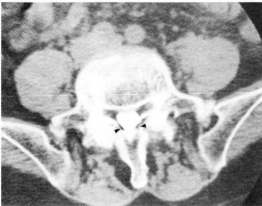

Fig 18–42.—The patient, a 74-year-old female, demonstrates central spinal stenosis at L4-5 due to bilateral laminar hypertrophy. Note the lateral defects at the L4-5 interspace *(arrows)* and the arachnoiditis in the distal cauda sac probably secondary to a previous Pantopaque myelogram. Note also the redundant nerve roots *(arrowhead).* The metrizamide CT section graphically demonstrates the bilateral laminar hypertrophy *(arrowheads)* compressing the lateral margins of the thecal sac.

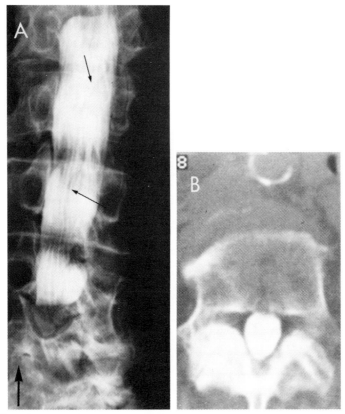

Fig 18–43.—A, serpentine nerve roots *(arrows)* in a 75-year-old woman with a bilateral foot drop. The spondylosis and spinal stenosis are most marked at L4-5, where there is a high-grade obstruction. **B,** axial CT scan at the upper aspect of the body of L-5 showing the stenosis of the bony canal.

the dura, there was immediate herniation of three large nerve roots with normal vascularity. The roots each measured 3 mm in diameter and were 10, 10.5, and 12 cm long, respectively, from the dural sleeve to their entrance into the cauda, where they regained a normal configuration. The remainder of the nerve roots and the filum terminale were normal.

The serpentine filling defect in the contrast column at myelography in each instance mimicked the appearance of a vascular malformation.

Further experience with this entity indicates that it usually occurs in the presence of significant stenosis of the bony spinal canal. The stenosis may be developmental, i.e., achondroplasia, or acquired; it may be localized to one or two segments or involve the entire spine. The serpentine defect is commonly found just proximal to the area of stenosis. There may be a 2–3-mm-wide single, tortuous defect within the contrast column or multiple serpentine defects that preserve their individuality (Figs 18–41 to 18–43). Occasionally, the defect may be quite prominent and present as an irregular mass with interspersed contrast droplets. As the normal nerve roots are displaced craniad due to the spinal stenosis, they become elongated and tortuous because of the decreased space available to them. Hacker

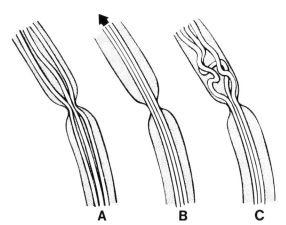

Fig 18–44.—Schematic diagram demonstrating the mechanism of development of redundant lumbar nerve roots in spinal stenosis. A high-grade extradural obstruction can
produce a pincer-like compression of the nerve roots as they pass through **(A).** As the
nerve roots are pulled craniad by positional changes, i.e., flexion, they are trapped at the
site of constriction and cannot slide through **(B).** This repeated stretching results in elongation of the nerve roots proximal to the block. Reverse positional changes, i.e., extension, relieve the craniad traction on the nerve roots and permit the elongated segments to
relax and pile up in redundant loops proximal to the obstruction **(C).** The "slack" cannot
freely slide through the constriction into the caudal sac. It is important to recognize the
entity of elongated nerve roots and not to confuse it with spinal arteriovenous malformation. (Reprinted, with permission, from Hacker D.A., et al., *Radiology* 143:461, 1982.)

et al. have suggested a very plausible mechanism to explain the development of
redundant nerve roots (Fig 18–44).

BIBLIOGRAPHY

Alenghat J.P., Hallett M., Kido K.K.: Spinal cord compression in diffuse idiopathic hyper-
ostosis. *Radiology* 142:119, 1982.
Alexander E., Jr.: Significance of the small lumbar spinal canal: Cauda equina compression
syndromes due to spondylosis. V. Achondroplasia. *J. Neurosurg.* 31:513, 1969.
Arnoldi C.C., Brodsky A.E., Cauchoix J., et al.: Lumbar spinal stenosis and nerve root
entrapment syndromes. Definition and classification. *Clin. Orthop.* 115:4, 1976.
Badgley C.E.: The articular facets in relation to low back pain and sciatic radiation. *J. Bone
Joint Surg.* 23:481, 1941.
Bailey P., Casamajor L.: Osteoarthritis of the spine as a cause of compression of the spinal
cord and its roots: With reports of 5 cases. *J. Nerv. Ment. Dis.* 38:588, 1911.
Bakay L., Cares H.L., Smith R.J.: Ossification in the region of the posterior longitudinal
ligament as a cause of cervical myelopathy. *J. Neurol. Neurosurg. Psychiatr.* 33:263, 1970.
Beatty R.A., Sugar O., Fox T.F.: Protrusion of the posterior longitudinal ligament simulating
herniated lumbar intervertebral disc. *J. Neurol. Neurosurg. Psychiatr.* 31:61, 1968.
Bechar M., Front D., Bornstein B., Matz S.: Cervical myelopathy caused by narrowing of
the cervical spinal canal. The value of x-ray examination of the cervical spinal column in
extension. *Clin. Radiol.* 22:63, 1971.
Becker D.H., Conely F.K., Anderson M.E.: Quadriplegia associated with narrow cervical
canal, ligamentous calcification and ankylosing hyperostosis. *Surg. Neurol.* 11:17, 1979.
Bergmark G.: Intermittent spinal claudication. *Acta Med. Scandinav.* (Suppl.) 264:30, 1950.
Bradley W.G., Banna M.: The cervical dural canal. A study of the "tight dural canal" and of
syringomyelia by prone and supine myelography, *Br. J. Radiol.* 41:608, 1968.
Brain W.R., Wilkinson M.: *Cervical Spondylosis and Other Disorders of the Cervical Spine.*
Philadelphia, W.B. Saunders Co., 1967.

Brish A., Lerner M.A., Braham J.: Intermittent claudication from compression of cauda equina by a narrowed spinal canal. *J. Neurosurg.* 21:207, 1964.

Brodksy A.G.: Postlaminectomy and postfusion stenosis of the lumbar spine. *Clin. Orthop.* 115:130, 1976.

Burrows E.H.: The sagittal diameter of the spinal canal in cervical spondylosis. *Clin. Radiol.* 14:77, 1963.

Caffey J.: Achondroplasia of pelvis and lumbosacral spine. Some roentgenographic features. *Am. J. Roentgenol.* 80:449, 1958.

Cauchoix J., Benoist M., Chassaing V.: Degenerative spondylolisthesis. *Clin. Orthop.* 115:122, 1976.

Chin W.S., Oon C.L.: Ossification of the posterior longitudinal ligament of the spine. *Br. J. Radiol.* 52:865, 1979.

Choudbury A.R., Taylor J.C.: Occult lumbar spinal stenosis. *J. Neurol. Neurosurg. Psychiatr.* 40:506, 1977.

Clark K.: Significance of the small lumbar spinal canal: Cauda equina compression syndromes due to spondylosis. II. Clinical and surgical significance. *J. Neurosurg.* 31:495, 1969.

Crandall P.H., Hanafee W.N.: Cervical spondylotic myelopathy studied by air myelography. *Am. J. Roentgenol.* 92:1260, 1964.

Cressman M.R., Pawl R.P.: Serpentine myelographic defect caused by a redundant nerve root. *J. Neurosurg.* 28: 1968.

Cronqvist S., Thulen C.A.: Significance of tortuous filling defects at lumbar myelography. *Acta Radiol. (Diagn.)* 20:561, 1979.

Donath J., Vogl A.: Untersuchungen über den chondrodystrophischen Zwerguwuchs. Das verhalten der wirbelsäule beim chondrodystrophischen zwerg, Wien. *Arch. Inn. Med.* 10:1, 1925.

Duncan A.W., Kudo D.K.: Serpentine cauda equina nerve roots. *Radiology* 139:109, 1981.

Duvoisin R.C., Yahr M.D.: Compressive spinal cord and root syndromes in achondroplastic dwarfs. *Neurology* 12:202, 1962.

Efird T., Genant H.K., Wilson C.B.: Pituitary gigantism with cervical spinal stenosis. *A.J.R.* 134:171, 1980.

Ehni G.: Significance of the small lumbar spinal canal: Cauda equina compression syndromes due to spondylosis. I. Introduction. *J. Neurosurg.* 31:490, 1969.

Ehni G.: Significance of the small lumbar spinal canal: Cauda equina compression syndromes due to spondylosis. IV. Acute compression artificially induced during operation. *J. Neurosurg.* 31:507, 1969.

Ehni G., Moriel R.H., Bragg T.G.: The "redundant" or "knotted" nerve root: A clue to spondylotic cauda equina. Radiculopathy. *J. Neurosurg.* 32:252, 1970.

Eisenstein S.: Measurements of lumbar spinal canal in two racial groups. *Clin. Orthop.* 115:42, 1976.

Epstein B.S., Epstein J.A., Jones M.D.: Lumbar spinal stenosis. *Radiol. Clin. North Am.* 15:227, 1977.

Epstein B.S., Epstein J.A., Jones M.D.: Anatomico-radiological correlations in cervical spine discal disease and stenosis. *Clin. Neurosurg.* 25:148, 1978.

Epstein B.S., Epstein J.A., Lavine L.: Effect of anatomic variations in lumbar vertebrae and spinal canal on cauda equina and nerve root syndromes. *Am. J. Roentgenol.* 91:1055, 1964.

Epstein J.A.: Diagnosis and treatment of painful neurological disorders caused by spondylosis of lumbar spine. *J. Neurosurg.* 17:991, 1960.

Epstein J.A., Epstein B.S.: Neurological and radiological manifestations associated with spondylosis of the cervical and lumbar spine. *Bull. New York Acad. Med.* 35:370, 1959.

Epstein J.A., Epstein B.S., Lavine L.: Nerve root compression associated with narrowing of the lumbar spinal canal. *J. Neurol., Neurosurg. Psychiatr.* 25:165, 1962.

Epstein J.A., Epstein B.S., Lavine L.S.: Cervical spondylotic myelopathy. The syndrome of the narrow canal treated by laminectomy, foramenotomy and the removal of osteophytes. *Arch. Neurol.* 8:307, 1963.

Epstein J.A., Epstein B.S., Lavine L.S., et al.: Degenerative lumbar spondylolisthesis with an intact neural arch (pseudospondylolisthesis). *J. Neurosurg.* 44:139, 1976.

Epstein J.A., Epstein B.S., Rosenthal A., et al.: Sciatica caused by nerve root entrapment in the lateral recess: The superior facet syndrome. *J. Neurosurg.* 36:584, 1972.

Epstein J.A., Malis L.I.: Compression of spinal cord and cauda equina in achondroplastic dwarfs. *Neurology* 5:875, 1955.

Evans J.G.: Neurogenic intermittent claudication. *Br. Med. J.* 2:985, 1964.

Forcer P., Horsey W.J.: Calcification of the posterior longitudinal ligament at the thoracolumbar junction. *J. Neurosurg.* 32:684, 1970.

Forcies P., Horsey W.J.: Calcification of posterior longitudinal ligament at the thoracolumbar junction. *J. Neurosurg.* 32:684, 1970.

Friedman E.: Narrowing of spinal canal due to thickened lamina. A cause of low back pain and sciatica. *Clin. Orthop.* 21:190, 1961.

Galanski M., Herrmann R., Knoche U.: Neurological complications and myelographic features of achondroplasia. *Neuroradiology* 17:59, 1978.

Gannon W.E.: The radiologic diagnosis of lumbar spondylosis. *Radiol. Clin. North Am.* 4:159, 1966.

Geindre M., Crouzet G., Coulomb M.: Radiologic study of the cervical myelogram in the presence of a narrowed spinal canal. *J. Radiol. et Électrol.* 51:92, 1970.

Gelman M.I.: Cauda equina compression in acromegaly. *Radiology* 112:357, 1974.

Ghormley R.K.: Low back pain: With special reference to the articular facets, with presentation of an operative procedure. *J.A.M.A.* 101:1773, 1933.

Goto K., Takahashi M., Kawanami H.: Ossification of the thoracic and lumbar posterior longitudinal ligament—report of 3 cases. *Clin. Neurol.* 10:329, 1970.

Govoni, A.F.: Developmental stenosis of a thoracic vertebra resulting in narrowing of the spinal canal. *Am. J. Roentgenol.* 112:401, 1971.

Hacker D.A., Latchaw R.E., Yock D.H., Jr., et al.: Redundant lumbar nerve root syndrome: Myelographic features. *Radiology* 143:457, 1982.

Hadley L.A.: *Anatomico-Roentgenographic Studies of the Spine.* Springfield, Ill., Charles C Thomas, Publisher, 1964.

Hancock D.O., Philips D.G.: Spinal compression in achondroplasia. *Paraplegia* 3:23, 1965.

Hayashi K., Tabuchi K., Yabuki T., et al.: The position of the superior articular process of the cervical spine. Its relationship to cervical spondylotic radiculopathy. *Radiology* 124:501, 1977.

Highman J.H.: Complete myelographic block in lumbar degenerative disease. *Clin. Radiol.* 16:106, 1965.

Highman J.H., Sanderson P.H., Sutcliffe M.M.: Vitamin D resistant osteomalacia as a cause of cord compression. *Q. J. Med.* 39:529, 1970.

Hinck V.C., Gordy P.D., Storino H.E.: Developmental stenosis of the cervical spinal canal: Radiological considerations. *Neurology* 14:865, 1964.

Hinck V.C., Hopkins C.E., Clark W.M.: Sagittal diameter of the lumbar spinal canal in children and adults. *Radiology* 85:929, 1965.

Hinck V.C., Sachdev N.S.: Developmental stenosis of the cervical spinal canal. *Brain* 89:27, 1966.

Horntein S., Hambrook G., Eyerman E.: Spinal cord compression by vertebral acromegaly. *Trans. Am. Neurol. Assoc.* 96:254, 1972.

Joffe R., Appleby A., Arjona V.: Intermittent ischaemia of the cauda equina due to stenosis of the lumbar canal. *J. Neurol., Neurosurg. Psychiatr.* 29:315, 1966.

Kavanaugh G.J., Svien H.J., Holman C.B., Johnson R.M.: "Pseudoclaudication" syndrome produced by compression of the cauda equina. *J.A.M.A.* 206:2477, 1968.

Kennedy F., Elsberg C.A., Lambert C.J.: A peculiar and undescribed disease of the nerves of the cauda equina. *Am. J. Med. Sci.* 147:645, 1914.

MacNab I.: Spondylolisthesis with an intact neural arch—the so-called pseudospondylolisthesis. *J. Bone Joint Surg.* 32B:325, 1950.

MacNab I.: Negative disc exploration. An analysis of the causes of nerve root involvement in 68 patients. *J. Bone Joint Surg.* 53A:891, 1971.

McIvor G.W.D., Kirkaldy-Willis W.H.: Pathological and myelographic changes in the major types of lumbar spinal stenosis. *Clin. Orthop.* 115:72, 1976.

McRae D.I.: Asymptomatic intervertebral disc protrusions. *Acta Radiol.* 46:9, 1956.

Mikhael M.A., Ciric I., Tarkington J.A., Vick N.A.: Neuroradiological evaluation of lateral recess syndrome. *Radiology* 140:97, 1981.

Minagi H., Gronner A.T.: Calcification of the posterior longitudinal ligament: A cause of cervical myelopathy. *Am. J. Roentgenol.* 105:365, 1969.

Miyaska K., Kanedo K., Ito T. et al.: Ossification of spinal ligaments causing thoracic radiculomyelopathy. *Radiology* 143:463, 1982.

Moiel R., Ehni G.: Cauda equina compression due to spondylolisthesis with intact neural arch. *J. Neurosurg.* 28:262, 1968.

Moiel R.H., Ehni G., Anderson M.S.: Nodule of the ligamentum flavum as a cause of nerve root compression. Case report. *J. Neurosurg.* 27:456, 1967.

Mooney V., Robertson J.: The facet syndrome. *Clin. Orthop.* 115:149, 1976.

Morris L.: Water soluble contrast myelography in spinal canal stenosis and nerve entrapment. *Clin. Orthop.* 115:49, 1976.

Nakanishi T., Toyokura Y., Mannen T., et al.: Osteosis of cervical posterior ligament–clinical findings and radiological features. *Clin. Neurol.* 7:607, 1967.

Newman P.H.: Stenosis of the lumbar spine in spondylolisthesis. *Clin. Orthop.* 115:116, 1976.

Onji Y., Akiyama H., Shimomura Y., et al.: Posterior paravertebral ossification causing cervical myelopathy. A report of 18 cases. *J. Bone Joint Surg.* 49A:13, 1967.

Ono M., Russell W.J., Kudo S., et al.: Ossification of the thoracic posterior longitudinal ligament in a fixed population. *Radiology* 143:649, 1982.

Palacios E., Brackett C.E., Leary D.J.: Ossification of the posterior longitudinal ligament associated with a herniated intervertebral disk. *Radiology* 100:313, 1971.

Pallis C.A., Jones A.M., Spillane J.D.: Cervical spondylosis. *Brain* 77:274, 1954.

Parker H.L., Adson A.W.: Compression of the spinal cord and its roots by hypertrophic osteoarthritis. Diagnosis and treatment. *Surg. Gynecol. Obstet.* 41:1, 1925.

Pau A., Sehrbundt Viale E., Turtas S., Viale G.L.: Redundant nerve roots of the cauda equina. *Surg. Neurol.* 16:245, 1981.

Payne E.C., Spillane J.D.: Cervical spine; anatomico-pathological study of 70 specimens (using a special technique) with particular reference to problem of cervical spondylosis. *Brain* 80:571, 1957.

Quencer R.M., Murtagh F.R., Post M.J.D., et al.: Postoperative bony stenosis of the lumbar spinal canal: Evaluation of 164 symptomatic patients with axial radiography. *A.J.R.* 131:1059, 1978.

Rask M.R.: Anomalous lumbosacral nerve roots associated with spondylolisthesis. *Surg. Neurol.* 8:139, 1977.

Rengachary S.S., McGregor D.H., Watanabe J., et al.: Suggested pathological basis of "redundant nerve root syndrome" of the cauda equina. *Neurosurgery* 7:400, 1980.

Resnick D., Guerra J., Jr., Robinson C.A., Vint V.C.: Association of diffuse idiopathic skeletal hyperostosis (DISH) and calcification of the posterior longitudinal ligament. *A.J.R.* 131:1049, 1978.

Richter H.P.: Similar myelographic patterns of different origins (spinal angioma and redundant nerve roots of the cauda equina). *Acta Neurochir.* (Wien) 54:283, 1980.

Roberson G.H., Llewellyn H.J., Taveras J.M.: The narrow lumbar spinal canal syndrome. *Radiology* 107:89, 1973.

Ruge D., Wiltse L.L.: *Spinal Disorders.* Philadelphia, Lea & Febiger, 1977.

Sachs B., Fraenkel J.: Progressive ankylotic rigidity of the spine (spondylose rhizomélique). *J. Nerv. Ment. Dis.* 27:1, 1900.

Sarpyener M.A.: Congenital stricture of the spinal canal. *J. Bone Joint Surg.* 27:70, 1945.

Schatzker J., Fennal G.F.: Spinal stenosis, a cause of cauda equina compression. *J. Bone Joint Surg.* 50B:606, 1968.

Schlesinger E.B., Taveras J.M.: Factors in the production of "cauda equina" syndrome in lumbar discs. *Trans. Am. Neurol. Assoc.* 78:263, 1953.

Schnitker M.T., Curzwiler F.C., Jr.: Hypertrophic osteosclerosis (bony spur) of the lumbar spine producing the syndrome of protruded intervertebral disc with sciatic pain. *J. Neurosurg.* 14:121, 1957.

Schubiger O., Valavanis A.: CT differentiation between recurrent disc herniation and postoperative scar formation: The value of contrast enhancement. *Neuroradiology* 22: 251, 1982.

Schut L., Graff R.A.: Redundant nerve roots as a cause of complete myelographic block. Case report. *J. Neurosurg.* 28:394, 1968.

Shibasaki H., Nagamatsu K.: Calcification of the posterior longitudinal ligament—its relation with cervical spondylosis. *Clin. Neurol.* 8:22, 1968.

Sorensen B.F., Wirthlin A.J.: Redundant nerve roots of the cauda equina. *Surg. Neurol.* 3:177, 1975.

Sortland O., Magnaes B., Hauge T.: Functional myelography with metrizamide in the diagnosis of lumbar spinal stenosis. *Acta Radiol.* (Suppl.) 355:42, 1977.

Spanos N.C., Andrew J.: Intermittent claudication and lateral lumbar disc protrusion. *J. Neurol., Neurosurg. Psychiatr.* 29:273, 1966.

Takahashi M., Kawanami H., Tomonaga M., Kitamura K.: Ossification of the posterior longitudinal ligament. *Acta Radiol. (Diagn)* 13:25, 1972.

Teng P.: Spondylosis of the cervical spine with compression of the spinal cord and nerve roots. *J. Bone Joint Surg.* 42A:392, 1960.

Teng P., Papatheodorou C.: Lumbar spondylosis with compression of cauda equina. *Arch. Neurol.* 8:221, 1963.

Teng P., Papatheodorou C.: Myelographic findings in spondylosis of lumbar spine. *Br. J. Radiol.* 36:122, 1963.

Towne E.B., Reichert F.L.: Compression of the lumbosacral roots of the spinal cord by thickened ligamenta flava. *Ann. Surg.* 94:327, 1931.

Ullrich C.G., Binet E.F., Sanecki M.G., Kieffer S.A.: Quantitative assessment of the lumbar spinal canal by computed tomography. *Radiology* 134:137, 1980.

Verbiest H.: Radicular syndrome from developmental narrowing of the lumbar vertebral canal. *J. Bone Joint Surg.* 36B:230, 1954.

Verbiest H.: Further experiences on the pathological influence of developmental narrowness of the bony lumbar vertebral canal. *J. Bone Joint Surg.* 37B:576, 1955.

Verbiest H.: Sur certaines formes rares de compression de la queue de cheval, in *Hommage á Clovis Vincent.* Paris, Maloine, 1979, p. 161.

Vogl A.: The fate of the achondroplastic dwarf (neurologic complications of achondroplasia). *Exper. Med. Surg.* 20:108, 1962.

Vogl A., Osborne R.L.: Lesions of the spinal cord (transverse myelopathy) in achondroplasia. *Arch. Neurol. Psychiatr.* 61:644, 1949.

Waltz T.A.: Physical factors in the production of the myelopathy of cervical spondylosis. *Brain* 90:395, Part II, 1967.

Wassmann H., Hollbach K.H., Bonatelli A.P.: Stenosis of the spinal canal in case of chondrodystrophy. *Nervenarzt* 48:342, 1977.

Weiss M.H., Spencer G.E.: Ossification of a lumbar interspinous ligament with compression of the cauda equina. *J. Bone Joint Surg.* 52A:165, 1970.

Wilkinson H.A., LeMay M.L., Ferris E.J.: Roentgenographic correlations in cervical spondylosis. *Am. J. Roentgenol.* 105:370, 1969.

Wilkinson M.: *Cervical Spondylosis.* London, William Clowes & Sons, Ltd., 1971.

Wilson C.B.: Significance of the small lumbar spinal canal: Cauda equina compression syndromes due to spondylosis. III. Intermittent claudication. *J. Neurosurg.* 31:499, 1969.

Yamada H., Ohya M., Okada T., Shizawa Z.: Intermittent cauda equina compression due to narrow spinal canal. *J. Neurosurg.* 37:83, 1972.

Yanagi T., Yamamura Y., Ando K., Sobue I.: Ossification of the posterior longitudinal ligament of cervical spine—analysis of 37 cases. *Clin. Neurol.* 7:727, 1967.

Yoshida H., et al.: Paraplegia caused by ossification of the ligamentum flavum—a case study. *Jpn. J. Clin. Med.* 34:3085, 1976.

Yoshikawa S., Shiba M., Suzuki A.: Spinal cord compression in untreated adult cases of vitamin D-resistant rickets. *J. Bone Joint Surg.* 50A:743, 1968.

19

Miscellaneous Non-Neoplastic Lesions of the Extradural Tissues, Meninges, Spinal Cord, and Cauda Equina

EXTRADURAL LESIONS

VARIOUS NON-NEOPLASTIC, noninflammatory diseases of the vertebrae can compress the spinal cord or cauda equina.

1. *Congenital.* Some congenital lesions, e.g., hemivertebrae, duplication of the posterior vertebral arch (see Fig 12–41) may rarely produce direct pressure on the cord or cauda equina. Hereditary multiple exostoses (diaphyseal aclasis) usually involve the long tubular bones and, to a lesser extent, the flat bones. Rarely, an osteochondroma or exostosis arising from a vertebral neural arch may compress the spinal cord. Of the 19 cases reported in the literature, 15 were in the thoracic or lumbar region and only 4 in the cervical spine. The age span in the cases reported was 13–33 years.

2. *Severe kyphoscoliosis* (idiopathic, associated with neurofibromatosis or Morquio-Brailsford disease) can compress the spinal cord (Figs 19–1 to 19–3). The contrast medium tends to flow along the convex side of the curve, and its craniad progress is frequently retarded at the apex of the maximal deformity (Fig 19–4). These patients are best studied by the full-volume technique recommended by Gold and his co-workers if Pantopaque is used. In patients with severe scoliosis, neurotoxic changes can theoretically be produced by metrizamide lying in contact with a focal segment of spinal cord for a prolonged period of time.

3. *Fracture-dislocation of the spine* may result in deformities of the Pantopaque column, with partial or complete block, as discussed in Chapter 13.

4. *Extramedullary hematopoiesis* has been described in a number of different diseases, principally thalassemia major and myelosclerosis. Large unilateral or bilateral intrathoracic masses are not rare in thalassemia major. The masses usually arise from the vertebral ends of the ribs or the transverse processes and project into the posterior mediastinum. However, neurologic symptoms and signs due to

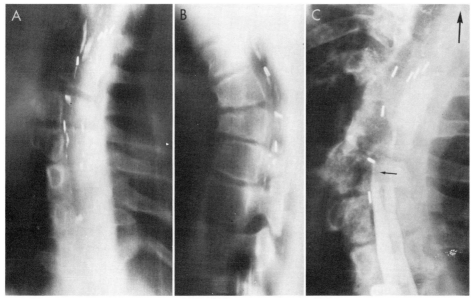

Fig 19–1.—Congenital hemivertebra with severe thoracic kyphoscoliosis in a teenaged male. The anteroposterior, **A,** and lateral, **B,** tomograms made following laminectomy demonstrate the skeletal abnormalities. At myelography, **C,** there was complete obstruction to the craniad flow of Pantopaque at the level of the greatest curvature of the thoracic spine *(arrow).*

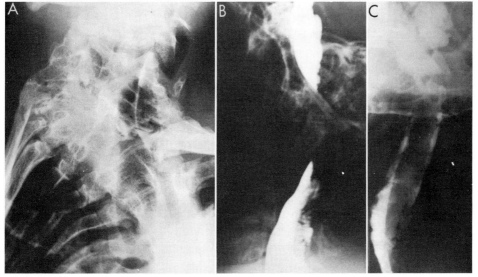

Fig 19–2.—The patient, a 23-year-old man with a congenital skeletal deformity, complained of pain and some numbness in the left upper extremity. The neurologic examination was remarkably normal considering the degree of skeletal deformity. The anteroposterior radiograph **(A)** demonstrates multiple block cervical vertebrae, several thoracic hemivertebrae, and a pronounced scoliosis in the cervicothoracic region. Additional films also showed atlanto-occipital assimilation. At myelography, there was difficulty in keeping the oil column intact in the atlanto-occipital region **(B)** and displacement of the cervicothoracic cord to the left because of the skeletal deformity **(C).**

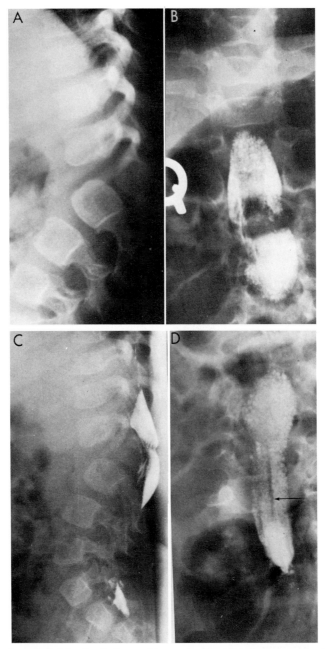

Fig 19–3.—Congenital kyphosis in an 11-month-old child due to marked posterior displacement of L-1 **(A).** The anteroposterior **(B)** and lateral **(C)** myelographic films show a defect in the Pantopaque column due to pressure of the abnormally displaced vertebra. The prone myelographic spot film of the lower lumbar region **(D)** also demonstrates low position of the conus medullaris extending down to the lumbosacral level, as evidenced by the anterior spinal artery *(arrow).*

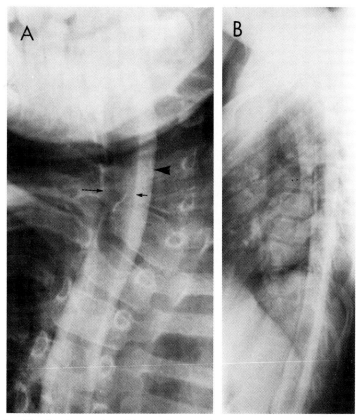

Fig 19–4.—Total-axis metrizamide myelogram (12 ml of contrast; 220 mg I/ml) in a 64-year-old woman with scoliosis secondary to multiple hemivertebrae in the midcervical spine. Note that the spinal cord *(arrow)* hugs the concave side of the curve, while the contrast travels along the convex side *(arrowhead)*.

compression by intraspinal extradural hematopoiesis are quite rare. I have seen two such cases that produced a complete block, one in the midthoracic region and the other at the level of L-1 (Fig 19–5). There are a number of additional cases reported in the literature. In one of the latter cases, the neurologic symptoms improved dramatically following radiation (2,000 rad in 26 days). Simultaneously, a previous complete myelographic obstruction at T9-10 was relieved.

5. *Eosinophilic granuloma.* This lesion of children and young adults commonly presents as a vertebra plana, i.e., collapse of a single vertebra. It may be associated with a paraspinal soft tissue mass, which rarely produces extradural compression of the cord or cauda equina (Fig 19–6).

6. *Gout.* There are two case reports in the literature of paraplegia secondary to the extradural deposition of urate crystals in gout. At operation, each interspace from L-3 through L-5 exhibited large deposits of cheesy calcific material in the ligamentum flavum. These were scooped away. Postoperatively, the 73-year-old patient recovered sufficient function to permit walking with a cane. The single frontal myelographic spot film (Pantopaque instilled via cisternal puncture) showed a

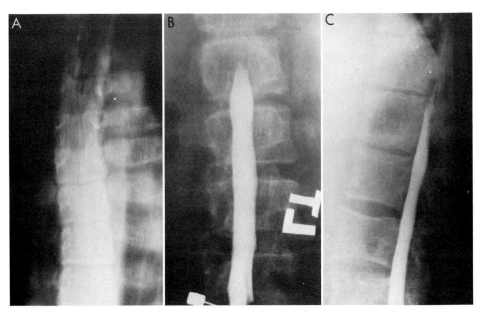

Fig 19–5.—The patient had been known to have thalassemia major for many years. The anteroposterior thoracic tomogram **(A)** shows expansion of the vertebral ends of the ribs due to extramedullary hematopoiesis. The anteroposterior **(B)** and lateral cross-table **(C)** myelographic films show a complete extradural block at L-1 due to extramedullary hematopoiesis.

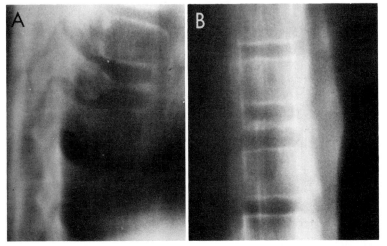

Fig 19–6.—Lateral plain radiograph **(A)** and anteroposterior thoracic tomogram **(B)** in a 9-year-old male showing collapse of T-7 with a left paraspinal mass due to eosinophilic granuloma.

complete extradural block at L-3, with localized, unusual defects at L1-2 and L2-3 produced by the urate deposits.

7. *Paget's disease* is a relatively common lesion that infrequently produces cord compression secondary to bony enlargement of the vertebral body, pedicles, and laminae. There also may be abnormal osteoid tissue in the paravertebral gutter and extradural space. The most common site for neural compression is the upper thoracic spine, where the bony spinal canal has the smallest diameter. Neurologic complications are relatively rare in the cervical region. In the latter area, the bone changes may be misinterpreted because of vertebral collapse and spondylosis. Feldman and Seaman point out that the frequent involvement of the neural arch and the spinous and transverse processes in Paget's disease is helpful in differentiating it from osteolytic or osteoblastic metastases. The myelographic findings are nonspecific, consisting of a partial or a complete block due to extradural compression (Figs 19–7, 19–8). Uncommonly, Paget's disease can undergo sarcomatous degeneration. The malignancies, usually osteoclastic in nature, may be osteosarcoma (most common), chondrosarcoma, or fibrosarcoma (see Fig 17–63).

8. *Lumbar extradural ganglion cyst.* In 1968, Kao et al. reported three cases of extradural ganglion cysts arising from a facet joint at L4-5. In two instances, the cyst projected into the spinal canal, compressing the L-5 nerve root. In the third patient, the cyst projected posteriorly into the paraspinal musculature and was asymptomatic. Four additional cases were reported by Bhushan et al. in 1979. A few scattered individual cases have also been noted in the literature.

It is interesting that the greatest range of motion occurs at L4-5, where the cysts

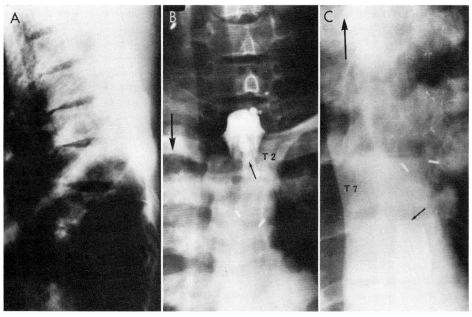

Fig 19–7.—Paget's disease involving the thoracic spine, with extensive sclerotic changes producing a complete obstruction. **A,** lateral radiograph clearly shows the dense overgrowth of bone. **B,** cisternal myelography demonstrates the upper end of the obstruction at T-2 *(arrow),* whereas, **C,** lumbar myelography indicates the lower end of the obstruction at T7-8 *(arrow).*

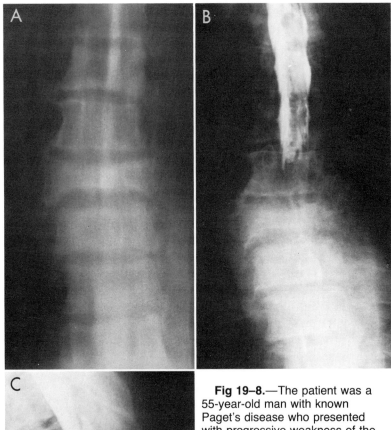

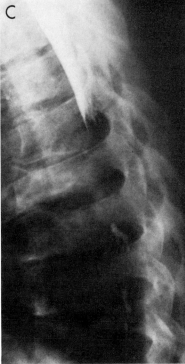

Fig 19–8.—The patient was a 55-year-old man with known Paget's disease who presented with progressive weakness of the lower extremities and no disturbance in sphincter control. The anteroposterior thoracic tomogram **(A)** shows the typical radiographic features of Paget's disease, with a pathologic fracture of T-7 and a right paraspinal mass at T7-8. The anteroposterior **(B)** and lateral **(C)** myelographic films show a complete extradural block at T-6 (the Pantopaque was introduced by a lateral C1-2 puncture). The patient had a decompressive laminectomy from T-7 to T-9. The neurosurgeon noted marked thickening of the pedicles and laminae in this region, with a considerable mass of osteoid tissue on the right side, corresponding to the paraspinal mass seen on the tomogram.

were found. The exact pathogenesis of the cysts is not known. Some authors claim that they represent herniations of the synovial membrane through a tear in the ligamentum flavum, while others suggest that they are due to myxomatous degeneration of connective tissue adjacent to a synovial joint. Microscopically, the cyst has no synovial lining membrane or communication with the joint cavity.

The principal plain radiographic findings are narrowing and sclerosis of the involved facet joint, usually at L4-5. Myelography shows a posterolateral extradural defect adjacent to the abnormal facet joint. Body section radiography may reveal a localized, rounded area or areas of erosion in the pedicle adjacent to the myelographic defect (Figs 19–9, 19–10). Similar changes have been described in ganglion cysts in the vicinity of the joints of long bones. The combination of the tomographic and myelographic findings is highly suggestive of the diagnosis of extradural ganglion cyst. These cysts may, on occasion, rupture spontaneously.

ARACHNOIDITIS OSSIFICANS (SPINAL LITHIASIS).

In a review of 217 unselected autopsies in a general hospital, Knoblich and Olsen demonstrated that calcified and ossified plaques in the spinal arachnoid are relatively common. Plaques were found in 37% of the males and 52% of the females in this series (average patient age was 67.7 years). The plaques varied from a single small focus to multiple large confluent areas encircling the cord. The arachnoidal calcifications, almost invariably dorsal in location, are most common in the lower thoracic and lumbar regions. Although the etiology of the plaques is not definitely known, they probably arise in meningeal cell clusters similar to the cerebral arachnoidal (pacchionian) granulations. Like these, the meningeal clusters have an increased incidence with advancing age. Since the cell clusters have no intrinsic blood supply, they are subject to early degeneration, hyalinization, calcification,

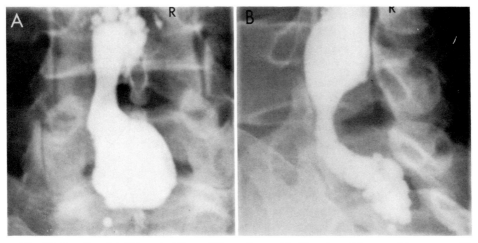

Fig 19–9.—Frontal **(A)** and oblique **(B)** myelographic films in a 52-year-old woman with a lumbar, extradural ganglion cyst arising under the pedicle between L-4 and L-5 on the right. Note the large spherical, extradural posterolateral defect in the oil column on the right at L4-5. (Reprinted, with permission, from Kao C.C., et al., *J. Neurosurg.* 29:168, 1968.)

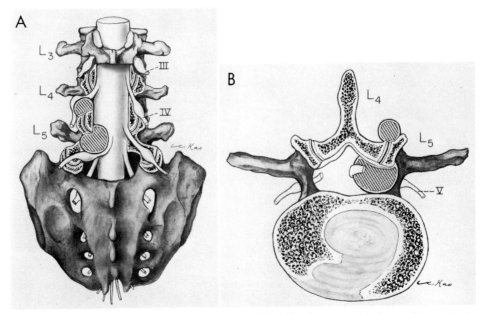

Fig 19–10.—Artist's drawings of the relationship of lumbar extradural ganglion cysts to the synovial joint and nerve roots. **A,** two ganglion cysts growing from the left synovial joint at L4-5. Superior and anterior growth of the cyst will compress the L-4 root, whereas inferior extension compresses the L-5 root **(B).** At the same synovial joint, extraspinal dorsal growth of the cyst may be asymptomatic, whereas intraspinal enlargement will compress the L-5 root. (Reprinted, with permission from Kao C.C., et al., *J. Neurosurg.* 29:168, 1968.)

and actual ossification. The increased number of meningeal cell clusters in the arachnoid on the dorsal surface of the spinal cord, particularly in the lower thoracic region, explains the predilection of calcified plaques in this location.

A review of the literature reveals approximately 20 well-documented cases of arachnoiditis ossificans. In this group, symptoms and neurologic signs were absent in some cases. In others, the clinical findings were not always relieved by surgical intervention. In the majority of cases, the plaques represented an incidental finding associated with a more significant lesion, e.g., meningioma, vascular malformation, arachnoidal cyst, hematoma. In view of this, and because spinal arachnoid plaques are common at autopsy, they probably are not often responsible for symptoms. In the occasional case, however, it is likely that a large, thick plaque can produce cord or root compression (Figs 19–11, 19–12).

HYPERTROPHIC INTERSTITIAL POLYNEURITIS (HYPERTROPHIC NEUROPATHY)

This is a rare disease of unknown etiology with a familial tendency, characterized by thickening and enlargement of the involved nerves due to marked hyperplasia of the nerve sheath. The lesion may involve peripheral nerves, the spinal roots, or the cauda equina. Depending on the nerves involved, the clinical picture may re-

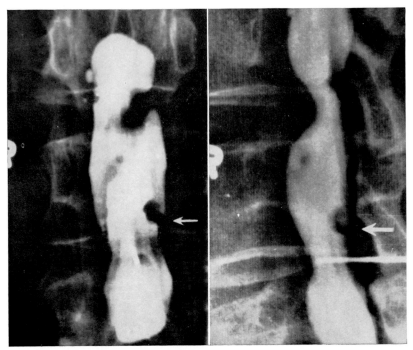

Fig 19–11.—Anteroposterior and oblique myelographic spot films showing multiple defects in the oil column in the lumbar region due to calcareous arachnoidal concretions. (Reprinted, with permission, from Faeth W. H., *J. Neurosurg.* 15:116, 1958.)

semble peripheral polyneuritis or the Charcot-Marie-Tooth type of peroneal atrophy. Cranial nerve involvement also has been described.

Myelography is most valuable in establishing the correct diagnosis. In the seven patients with myelograms described in the literature, the findings were (1) difficulty in obtaining a free flow of CSF because of partial obliteration of the subarachnoid space by the hypertrophic nerve roots; (2) slow flow of the Pantopaque, with partial or complete obstruction (Fig 19–13); (3) vertical, linear, radiolucent streaks in the oil column representing the thickened nerve roots (Fig 19–13); (4) medial displacement of the oil column from the inner aspect of the pedicles by the enlarged roots; (5) transverse bar defects and lateral rounded defects at the intervertebral disk level in the cervical region.

Bellon et al. reported a unique case with bone changes due to vertebral remodeling by the contiguous hypertrophic nerves. The changes were characterized by posterior scalloping of the lumbar vertebral bodies and a unique triangular appearance of the pedicles, with an increased interpediculate distance.

GUILLAIN-BARRÉ SYNDROME (ACUTE INFLAMMATORY POLYRADICULOPATHY)

Hvidsten et al. reported the myelographic findings in seven patients with Guillain-Barré syndrome. Four had normal myelograms, and three exhibited abnormal-

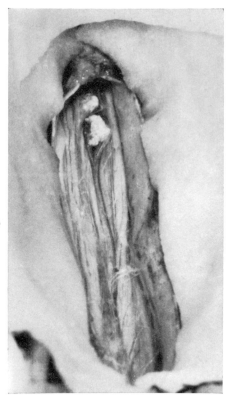

Fig 19–12.—The cauda equina at laminectomy, showing the arachnoidal calcifications. (Reprinted, with permission, from Faeth W.H., *J. Neurosurg.* 15:116, 1958.)

ities, which consisted of uneven widening of lumbar nerve roots with some obliteration of the axillary sleeves. Presumably, the increased diameter of the roots is due to edema and inflammatory infiltration secondary to demyelination.

MULTIPLE SCLEROSIS

A normal-sized spinal cord at myelography is the usual finding. However, cord enlargement as well as a small spinal cord have also been reported in this disease. Edema and reactive inflammatory infiltration secondary to demyelination may uncommonly enlarge the cord. In the later stages of the disease, when gliosis occurs and the cord becomes atrophic, the latter may be recognized at myelography. Haughton et al. described an unusual case with a contracting cord in a 31-year-old woman. During the acute phase of the disease, an enlarged, noncollapsing cervical cord was demonstrated by pneumomyelography. Approximately 6 months later, repeat air myelography revealed a small cord with constant dimensions uninfluenced by changes in the patient's position. At necropsy, the spinal cord was atrophic and exhibited demyelinating lesions characteristic of multiple sclerosis. Haughton has appropriately designated the change in cord size as "the contracting cord sign." This is to be distinguished from "the collapsing cord sign," which refers to changes in cord diameter produced by movement of fluid in and out of a cyst when the patient is tilted into different positions.

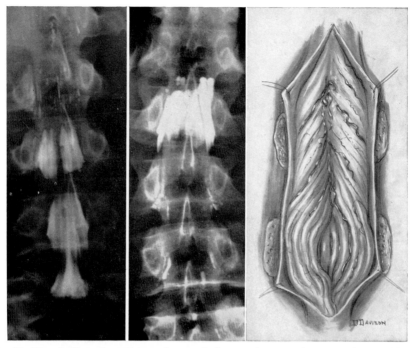

Fig 19–13.—**Left** and **center,** anteroposterior myelograms in two patients with hypertrophic interstitial polyneuritis demonstrating, **left,** the marked increase in size of the roots of the cauda equina associated with a block at L-3 and, **center,** a complete block at L1–2 after cisternal puncture due to the enlarged roots. **Right,** findings at operation. The greatly thickened roots filled the entire spinal canal. (Reprinted, with permission, from Lewtas N.A., Dimant S., *J. Fac. Radiol.* 8:276, 1957.)

MUCOPOLYSACCHARIDOSES

Presently, six different abnormalities of mucopolysaccharide metabolism are recognized. They are all characterized by an absent or defective lysosomal enzyme vital for normal mucopolysaccharide catabolism. As a result of this deficiency, mucopolysaccharides are deposited in the central nervous system or viscera. A variety of bony and ligamentous changes occur, depending on the particular mucopolysaccharide abnormality. These changes consist of a dorsolumbar kyphos and gibbus, dwarfism, rib and bony abnormalities that produce various mechanical deformities (Fig 19–14,*A* and *B*).

Spinal cord compression and myelopathy occur uncommonly in some of these patients. This has usually been due to stenosis of the bony canal or atlantoaxial dislocation secondary to hypoplasia or absence of the dens. In 1977, Sostrin et al. reported two patients with progressive myelopathy due to dural thickening in the cervical region. The myelograms in both instances demonstrated concentric narrowing of the cervical cord and subarachnoid space due to marked thickening of the dura secondary to infiltration with mucopolysaccharides (Fig 19–14,*C* and *D*). The appearance in these patients is similar to that seen in hypertrophic pachymeningitis.

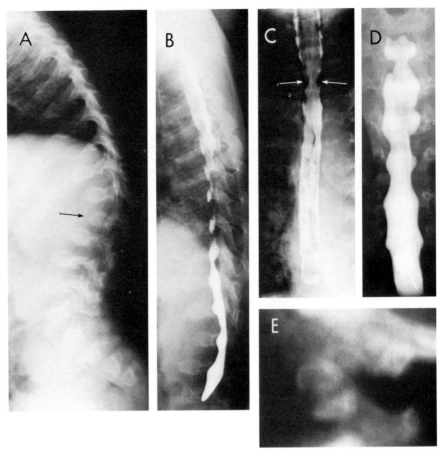

Fig 19–14.—The patient, a 4-year-old boy with Morquio's disease, presented with an extreme left hemiparesis and right-sided spastic weakness as well. The lateral film of the lumbar spine **(A)** demonstrates the abnormalities of the vertebral body with a characteristic kyphos at T12-L1 *(arrow)*. The lateral laminogram of the cervical spine **(E)** shows anterior subluxation of C-1 on C-2. At surgery, there was also stenosis of the foramen magnum. The myelogram shows bilateral extradural compression at T-1 and T-2 **(C)** and in the thoracic and upper lumbar regions **(B and D)** by marked dural thickening due to infiltration with mucopolysaccharides.

SARCOIDOSIS

Although Wiederholt and Siekert state that 3–5% of patients with sarcoidosis exhibit neurologic manifestations, spinal cord involvement is rare. The myelographic findings are nonspecific and depend upon the type and location of the pathologic involvement. Clinical reports include meningeal involvement with arachnoiditis (Fig 19–15), intramedullary granuloma formation, intradural extramedullary granulomas, and granulomas that are entirely extradural. There may or may not be an associated partial or complete obstruction. A few cases of involvement of the cauda equina have been reported with normal myelographic findings, although similar cases have shown beading and focal nodularity of the nerve roots.

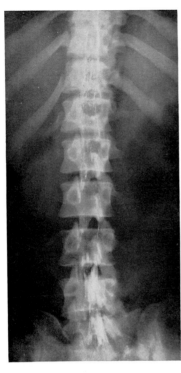

Fig 19–15.—Delayed myelogram made after the cisternal injection of Pantopaque, demonstrating extensive arachnoiditis due to sarcoidosis. (Reprinted, with permission, from Wood E.H., Bream C.A., *Radiology* 73:226, 1959.)

EPIDURAL LIPOMATOSIS

There have been a number of reports of spinal cord or cauda equina compression by epidural fat in patients who developed iatrogenic Cushing's syndrome after prolonged high-dose corticosteroid therapy. Badani and Hinck have also recorded a similar finding in a morbidly obese female without Cushing's syndrome. At operation, these patients had excessive normal epidural fat responsible for the neural compression and deficit.

BIBLIOGRAPHY

EXTRADURAL LESIONS

Congenital
Blaw M.E., Langer L.O.: Spinal cord compression in Morquio-Brailsford's disease. *J. Pediatr.* 74:593, 1969.
Carmel P., Cramer F.J.: Cervical cord compression due to exostosis in a patient with multiple exostoses. Case report. *J. Neurosurg.* 28:500, 1968.
Vinstein A.L., Franken E.A., Jr.: Hereditary multiple exostoses. Report of a case with spinal cord compression. *Am. J. Roentgenol.* 112:405, 1971.

Severe kyphoscoliosis
Curtis B.H., Fisher R.L., Butterfield W.L., Saunders F.P.: Neurofibromatosis with paraplegia. Report of eight cases. *J. Bone Joint Surg.* 51A:843, 1969.
Gold L.A., Leach C.G., Kieffer S.A., et al.: Large-volume myelography: An aid in evaluation of curvatures of the spine. *Radiology* 97:531, 1970.

Extramedullary hematopoiesis
Bree R.L., Neiman H.L., Hodak J.A., Flynn R.E.: Extramedullary hematopoiesis in the spinal epidural space. *J. Can. Assoc. Radiol.* 25:297, 1974.

Layendyk W., Went L., Schaad H.D.G.: Spinal cord compression due to extramedullary hematopoiesis in homozygous thalassemia: Case report. *J. Neurosurg.* 42:212, 1975.

Ross P., Logan W.: Roentgen findings in extramedullary hematopoiesis. *Am. J. Roentgenol.* 106:604, 1969.

Sorsdahl O.S., Taylor P.E., Noyes W.D.: Extramedullary hematopoiesis: Mediastinal masses and spinal cord compression. *J.A.M.A.* 189:343, 1964.

Gout

Koskoff Y.D., Morris L.E., Lubic L.G.: Paraplegia as a complication of gout. *J.A.M.A.* 152:37, 1953.

Litvak J., Briney W.: Extradural spinal depositions of urates producing paraplegia. *J. Neurosurg.* 39:656, 1973.

Paget's disease

Feldman F., Seaman W.B.: The neurologic complications of Paget's disease in the cervical spine. *Am. J. Roentgenol.* 105:375, 1969.

Siegelman S., Levine S.A., Walpin L.: Paget's disease with spinal cord compression. *Clin. Radiol.* 19:421, 1968.

Lumbar extradural ganglion cyst

Bhushan C., Hodges F.J., III, Wityk J.J.: Synovial cyst (ganglion) of the lumbar spine simulating extradural mass. *Neuroradiology* 18:263, 1979.

Brish A., Payan H.M.: Lumbar intraspinal extradural ganglion cyst. *J. Neurol. Neurosurg. Psychiatr.* 35:771, 1972.

Gritzka T.L., Taylor T.K.F.: A ganglion arising from a lumbar articular facet associated with low back pain and sciatica. Report of a case. *J. Bone Joint Surg.* 52B:528, 1970.

Kao C.C., Uihlein A., Bickel W.H., Soule E.H.: Lumbar intraspinal extradural ganglion cyst. *J. Neurosurg.* 29:168, 1968.

Schollner D.: Ganglion an einem Wirbelgelenk. *Ztschr. Orthop.* 102:619, 1966.

Sypert G.W., Leech R.W., Harris A.B.: Posttraumatic lumbar epidural true synovial cyst. *J. Neurosurg.* 39:246, 1973.

ARACHNOIDITIS OSSIFICANS

Bianchi-Maiocchi A.: Uno raro caso di calcificazioni diffuse dell'aracnoide spinale (aracnoide calcarea). *Arch. Ortop.* 68:629, 1955.

Gatzke L.D., Dodge H.W., Dockerty M.B.: Arachnoiditis ossificans: Report of 2 cases. *Proc. Staff Meet. Mayo Clin.* 32:698, 1957.

Herren R.Y.: Occurrence and distribution of calcified plaques in the spinal arachnoid in man. *Arch. Neurol. Psychiatr.* 41:1180, 1939.

Knoblich R., Olsen B.S.: Calcified and ossified plaques of the spinal arachnoid membranes. *J. Neurosurg.* 25:275, 1966.

McKendree C.A., Imboden H.M.: Ossification of the menginges. *Arch. Neurol. Psychiatr.* 6:529, 1921.

Pomerance A.: Spinal arachnoiditis ossificans. *J. Path. Bact.* 87:421, 1964.

Slager V.T.: Arachnoiditis ossificans. *A.M.A. Arch. Pathol.* 70:322, 1960.

Wise B.L., Smith M.: Spinal arachnoiditis ossificans. *Arch. Neurol.* 13:391, 1964.

HYPERTROPHIC INTERSTITIAL POLYNEURITIS

Andermann F., Lloyd-Smith D.L., Mavor H., Mathieson G.: Observations on hypertrophic neuropathy of Dejerine and Sottas. *Neurology* 12:712, 1962.

Bellon E.M., Kaufman B., Tucker M.E.: Hypertrophic neuropathy. Plain film and myelographic changes. *Radiology* 103:319, 1972.

DeBruyn R.S., Stern R.O.: A case of the progressive hypertrophic polyneuritis of Dejerine and Sottas with pathological examination. *Brain* 52:84, 1929.

Hammerschlag S.B., Adelman L.S., Marcus E.M., Wolpert S.M.: Cervical myelographic changes in hypertrophic interstitial polyneuropathy. *Ann. Neurol.* 2:83, 1977.

Hinck V.C., Sachdev N.S.: Myelographic findings in hypertrophic interstitial polyneuritis. *Am. J. Roentgenol.* 95:947, 1965.

Hvidsten K., Larsen J.L., Nyland H.: Myelography in Guillain-Barré syndrome (acute inflammatory polyradiculoneuropathy). *Neuroradiology* 14:235, 1978.

Kremenitzer M., Ager P.T., Zingesser L.H.: Myelographic evidence of nerve root enlargement in a case of Charcot-Marie-Tooth disease. *Neuroradiology* 11:165, 1976.

Lewtas N.A., Dimant S.: The diagnosis of hypertrophic interstitial polyneuritis by myelography. *J. Fac. Radiol.* 8:276, 1957.

Parker J.J., Anderson W.B.: Myelitis simulating spinal cord tumor. *Am. J. Roentgenol.* 95:942, 1965.

Perreau P., Fresneau M., Bouvelot M.: Images of spinal block in acute edematous infectious myelitis. *Presse Méd.* 62:1470, 1954.

Symonds C.P., Blackwood W.: Spinal cord compression in hypertrophic neuritis. *Brain* 85:251, 1962.

MULTIPLE SCLEROSIS

Haughton V.M., Ho K.C., Boedecker R.A.: The contracting cord sign of multiple sclerosis. *Neuroradiology* 17:207, 1979.

McDonald W.I.: Pathophysiology of multiple sclerosis. *Brain* 97:179, 1974.

Vakili H.: *The Spinal Cord.* New York, Intercontinental Medical Book Corp., 1967, p. 316.

Weinig C., Kammerer V.: Myelographic findings in multiple sclerosis in combination with cervical spondylosis. *Radiologe* 15:323, 1975.

MUCOPOLYSACCHARIDOSES

Kennedy P., Swash M., Dean M.F.: Cervical cord compression in mucopolysaccharidosis. *Dev. Med. Child Neurol.* 15:194, 1973.

Sostrin R.D., Hasso A.N., Peterson D.I., Thompson J.R.: Myelographic features of mucopolysaccharidoses: A new sign. *Radiology* 125:421, 1977.

SARCOIDOSIS

Askanazy C.L.: Sarcoidosis of the central nervous system. *J. Neuropathol. Exper. Neurol.* 11:392, 1952.

Banarjee T., Hunt W.E.: Spinal cord sarcoidosis. Case report. *J. Neurosurg.* 36:490, 1972.

Barauh J.K., Glasauer F.E., Sil R., Smith B.H.: Sarcoidosis of the cervical spinal cord: Case report. *Neurosurgery* 3:216, 1978.

Baringer J.R.: Sarcoidosis of the nervous system. *California Med.* 113:61, 1970.

Bernstein J., Rival J.: Case reports: Sarcoidosis of the spinal cord as the presenting manifestation of the disease. *South. Med. J.* 71:1571, 1978.

Brooks B.S., El Gammal T., Hungerford G.D., et al.: Radiological evaluation of neurosarcoidosis: Role of computed tomography. *A.J.N.R.* 3:513, 1982.

Campbell J.N., Black P., Ostrow P.T.: Sarcoid of the cauda equina. Case report. *J. Neurosurg.* 47:109, 1977.

Erickson T.C., Odom G.L., Stern K.: Boeck's disease (sarcoid) of the central nervous system. Report of a case with complete clinical and pathologic study. *Arch. Neurol. Psychiatr.* 48:613, 1942.

Jefferson M.: Sarcoidosis of the nervous system, *Brain* 80:540, 1957.

Kendall B.E., Tatler G.L.V.: Radiological findings in neurosarcoidosis. *Br. J. Radiol.* 51:81, 1978.

Kirks D.R., Newton T.H.: Sarcoidosis: A rare cause of spinal cord widening. *Radiology* 102:643, 1972.

Longcope W.T.: Sarcoidosis or Besnier-Beck-Schauman disease. *J.A.M.A.* 117:1321, 1941.

Mayock R.L., Bertrand P., Morrison C.E., et al.: Manifestations of sarcoidosis: Analysis of 145 patients with a review of nine series selected from the literature. *Am. J. Med.* 35:67, 1963.

Nathan M.P.R., Chase P.H., Elguezabel A., Weinstein M.: Spinal cord sarcoidosis. *N.Y. State J. Med.* 76:748, 1976.

Semins H., Nugent G.R., Chori S.M.: Intramedullary spinal cord sarcoidosis. Case report. *J. Neurosurg.* 37:233, 1972.

Snyder R., Towfighi J., Gonatas N.K.: Sarcoidosis of the spinal cord. Case report. *J. Neurosurg.* 44:740, 1976.

Urich H.: Neurological manifestations of sarcoidosis. *Practitioner* 202:632, 1969.

Whiteley A.M., Hauw J.J., Escourolle R.: A pathological survey of 41 cases of acute intrinsic spinal cord disease. *J. Neurol. Sci.* 42:229, 1979.

Wiederholt W.C., Siekert R.G.: Neurological manifestations of sarcoidosis. *Neurology* 15:1147, 1965.

Wood E.H., Bream C.S.: Spinal sarcoidosis. *Radiology* 73:226, 1959.

EPIDURAL LIPOMATOSIS

Badami J.P., Hinck V.C.: Symptomatic deposition of epidural fat in a morbidly obese woman. *A.J.N.R.* 3:664, 1982.

Butcher D.L., Sahn S.A.: Epidural lipomatosis: A complication of corticosteroid therapy. *Ann. Intern. Med.* 90:60, 1979.

Godeau P., Brunet P., Wechsler B., Fohanno D.L.: Lipomatose extradurale compressive, accident inhabitual de la corticotherapie. *Nouv. Presse Med.* 8:3889, 1979.

Guegan Y., Fardoun R., Lanois B., Pecker, J.: Spinal cord compression by extradural fat after prolonged corticosteroid therapy. *J. Neurosurg.* 56:267, 1982.

Lee M., Lekias J., Gubbay S.S., Hurst P.E.: Spinal cord compression by extradural fat after renal transplantation. *Med. J. Aust.* 1:201, 1975.

Lipson S.J., Naheedy M.H., Kaplan M.M., Bienfang, D.C.: Spinal stenosis caused by epidural lipomatosis in Cushing's syndrome. *N. Engl. J. Med.* 302:36, 1980.

20

Limitations and Complications of Myelography

LIMITATIONS

IT IS IMPORTANT to appreciate the limitations and possible pitfalls of myelography in order to use it intelligently and interpret its results properly. Unfortunately, myelography has been both unfairly maligned and uncritically championed. As is often the case, the truth lies somewhere between these extremes. Given the proper indications, myelography is a very useful method. When the myelographic findings, either positive or negative, are intelligently correlated with the clinical and laboratory data, a high degree of diagnostic accuracy can be expected.

The difficulties encountered can be grouped into two broad categories—technical and anatomical.

Technical Difficulties

To a large extent, these problems have been discussed in the chapters dealing with technique and artifacts. Meticulous care should be taken to perform a non-traumatic midline puncture at a level not under clinical suspicion. Furthermore, sufficient contrast medium should be introduced to fill the subarachnoid space adequately. Inadequate filling may not only produce troublesome artifacts, especially with Pantopaque, but may also result in failure to demonstrate some lesions.

Another case of error is inadequate scope of the examination, particularly in the investigation of suspected herniated lumbar disks. It is well known that sciatic pain can be produced by a lesion as high as T-10. Consequently, in examining a patient with a suspected herniated lumbar disk, it is necessary to observe the flow of the contrast column up to T-10. This is also important in the detection of multiple lesions where a large, more caudally situated lesion may clinically obscure the symptoms of a smaller craniad lesion. Occasionally, it is advisable to remove the needle and examine the patient in the supine position in order to visualize the posterior aspect of the subarachnoid space more adequately. This is particularly true in suspected vascular abnormalities of the spinal cord, which are characteristically located on the dorsal surface of the cord.

Anatomical Difficulties

Various anatomical features in a given patient may reduce or eliminate the possibility of demonstrating some lesions, particularly herniated intervertebral disks.

NARROW SUBARACHNOID SPACE.—When the bony spinal canal is relatively wide and the subarachnoid space conversely narrow from side to side, a laterally placed herniated disk may be present without producing a myelographic deformity, since the disk is remote from the opacified subarachnoid space.

SHALLOW SUBARACHNOID SPACE.—At times, the subarachnoid space may be relatively shallow in the anteroposterior diameter. In addition, the anterior surface of the subarachnoid space may be relatively remote from the posterior margin of the vertebral bodies. It is obvious that slight herniations of intervertebral disks may fail to indent the contrast column under these circumstances and will, therefore, not be diagnosed by myelography. By using the horizontal beam to take a lateral radiograph with the patient erect and the spine hyperextended, it may be possible at times to reveal a midline herniation that otherwise would not be evident. Hyperextension decreases the sagittal diameter of the spinal canal, and the upright position reduces the depth of the anterior extradural space, thus enhancing the chance of demonstrating a small midline protrusion.

CAUDAL SAC ANOMALIES.—There is considerable variability in the level of termination of the caudal sac. Although most caudal sacs end at the S1-2 interspace or at the level of the body of S-2, in some cases the caudal sac may terminate more cephalad or may taper quite sharply from side to side as well as anteroposteriorly. Under these circumstances, a herniated lumbosacral disk may be missed at myelography because the protruded fragment does not come in contact with the contrast column. More often, however, what appears to be a short caudal sac in the anteroposterior projection is an artifact due to angulation because of foreshortening of the end of the theca. This may be readily recognized in the lateral upright projection.

LATERALLY PLACED DISKS.—I have previously discussed (Chap. 17) the difficulty of visualizing disk herniations in the neural canal (lateral recess) by myelography and the impossibility of demonstrating disk herniations in the neural foramen by this technique. CT is the technique of choice in these situations.

DEFECTS DUE TO PREVIOUS PROCEDURE.—Hematoma or localized extravasation of spinal fluid from previous lumbar puncture or myelography may persist for some time. I have found a residual deformity at the site of a previous lumbar puncture as long as 2 weeks after the initial procedure. Whenever possible, therefore, myelography should not be performed earlier than 2 weeks after previous lumbar puncture. Furthermore, residual deformities at the site of a puncture should be evaluated in the light of the above knowledge.

Previous laminectomy may produce defects of various types because of postoperative meningeal thickening and adhesions. This makes it difficult to be certain of the significance of a myelographic defect at the level of an earlier laminectomy in a patient with recurrent symptoms.

ERRONEOUS LOCALIZATION.—Anatomical variations in the number of lumbar vertebrae and anomalies of sacralization of the last lumbar vertebra are common.

Unless the radiologist and the referring clinician have a consistent, mutually acceptable terminology, a misunderstanding of the correct level of a lesion may arise. For many years, I have used the phrase "presacral, non-rib-bearing vertebrae" to describe the vertebrae craniad to the sacrum in the lumbar region. Whenever indicated, the phrase "with unilateral or bilateral sacralization of the transverse processes of the last vertebra" is added. This makes it unnecessary to take roentgenograms of the entire spine. The location of a herniated disk then may be described at the L4-5, L5-6, L6-S1 level, and so on.

Erroneous localization may also occur as a result of progressive tumor growth. An extradural tumor on the dorsal aspect of the cord at the T-11 level may compress and displace the cord ventrally and completely obliterate the ventral subarachnoid space for some distance. The contrast column, therefore, may become arrested by the compressed cord at a point other than the actual location of the tumor.

In view of the above limitations, it is difficult to determine the over-all statistical accuracy of myelography. This difficulty is reflected in the great discrepancy among various reports in the literature dealing with this problem. Thus, at one extreme, Scoville, Moretz, and Hankins reported overall errors in 33% of their cases, whereas others state that the accuracy of myelography should approximate 95%. Such statistics are usually obtained by reviewing the myelographic examination without knowledge of the clinical or operative findings. Yet it is generally acknowledged that it is a poor practice to interpret films in vacuo, that is, without knowledge of all the available clinical and laboratory findings. This applies equally well to myelography because, in the final analysis, the surgeon does not perform a laminectomy on a myelogram but on a patient. It should be obvious from the preceding discussion that a myelographic deformity may be present without any clinical significance. It should be equally patent that under certain conditions a lesion may be present with a negative myelogram. Therefore, the myelographic findings and the clinical and laboratory data should be considered as vitally important complementary information. In my experience, there is a high index of accuracy in diagnosis when the myelographic findings are correlated with the history and the physical and laboratory data, taking into consideration the limitations of myelography in a given case. Moreover, the accuracy of this method depends to a great extent on the skill of the examiner in the performance and interpretation of myelography, particularly with respect to minor deformities.

COMPLICATIONS

Postlumbar-Puncture Headache

Following lumbar puncture, there is an arachnoidal rent with escape of CSF into the extra-arachnoidal space. Hypotension of the CSF ensues when the rate of fluid leakage is greater than the rate of fluid secretion by the choroid plexus. Headache is presumably the result of traction on pain-sensitive anchoring structures. With careful technique, using a 22-gauge needle for metrizamide and a 20-gauge needle for Pantopaque, the incidence and severity of this complication is diminished. When headache does occur, it ordinarily responds to bed rest in the horizontal position, hydration, and analgesics after one to several days. Rarely, the headache may be quite severe and last for a month or longer. In cases with severe, prolonged spinal headache, Glass and Kennedy have suggested treatment with an epidural blood patch. Using strict aseptic technique, 10 ml of venous blood are withdrawn from the patient into a plastic syringe and injected into the epidural space. If possible, lumbar puncture is performed at the original site until the needle enters the epidural space. This can best be checked by injecting 1 mm of metrizamide under fluoroscopic guidance. The syringe is withdrawn, the patient is placed in the supine position for 30 minutes, and is then asked to get up and walk around. The patient should be instructed to avoid straining and to take a laxative for 48 hours following the treatment. This technique should only be used for unremitting, severe headache of prolonged duration and never in the presence of sepsis.

Alemohammad and Bouzarth reported a case of a cerebral subdural hematoma in a 40-year-old patient 4 weeks after a Pantopaque lumbar myelogram with a no. 18 spinal needle. Presumably a persistent cerebrospinal fistula at the site of the lumbar puncture resulted in CSF hypotension with collapse of the cerebral mantle and shearing of the bridging cortex-to-dura veins. Gabriele also reported a patient who became lethargic 5 days after lumbar myelography and diskography and died 3 days later. The patient had multiple punctures of the lumbar theca. At necropsy, a subdural hematoma was found. I am unaware of any other similar cases in the literature.

Postmyelographic Coccygodynia

Miller has reported coccygodynia following myelography, presumably secondary to trauma by the needle or chemical irritation of the sacral nerve roots.

Herniated Intervertebral Disk

Improper technique may cause traumatic perforation of the annulus fibrosus, with subsequent herniation of disk material. This difficulty should not occur if the lumbar puncture is performed cautiously and slowly.

Transection of Nerve Filament

Young and Burney reported a case of transection and withdrawal of a 7-cm length of nerve filament during myelography performed with an end-hole—side-hole needle. Apparently, the filament had passed through the side hole and had been fixed by the stylet against the inner wall of the needle. As the needle was withdrawn, the stylet transected the nerve filament that followed along the needle tract out the lumbar puncture site. Similar accidents have been reported with modifications of the original Cuatico needle. In my opinion, use of this type of needle carries an unwarranted small risk of nerve root avulsion. Therefore, I do not use this type of needle, even though it facilitates Pantopaque removal at the end of the examination.

Iatrogenic Intraspinal Epidermoid

In a review of the literature dealing with intraspinal epidermoids (Fig 20–1), Manno, Uihlein and Kernohan ascribed the etiology of the tumor in 37 cases to

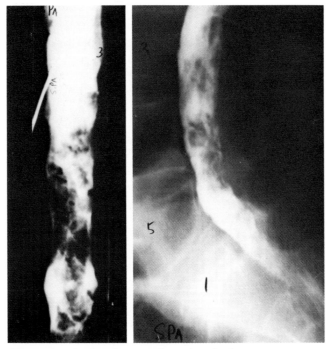

Fig 20–1.—The patient had undergone thoracic spinal surgery many years previously. He was hospitalized because of the recent onset of paraparesis. Myelography demonstrates an intra-arachnoid tumor extending over several segments. The lesion is characterized by multiple varying-sized contiguous filling defects surrounded by contrast medium. At operation, a semiencapsulated, elongated mass of amorphous, cheesy debris intermingled with the roots of the cauda equina was resected. There was no neural invasion. Histologic study revealed an epidermoid sequestration cyst. In all likelihood, this was iatrogenic, secondary to a previous myelogram or the previous surgery.

iatrogenic implantation of epidermal tissue at the time of lumbar puncture, myelography, or disk puncture. Boyd reported a similar intradural tumor at L4-5 documented by myelography before and after formation of the lesion. Pear included Boyd's case in the series of three patients he reported and pointed out that the incubation period varied from 2½ to 23 years following implantation. It is important to do the lumbar puncture and to remove the needle with a well-fitting stylet in place in order to avoid this complication.

Infection

Failure to observe meticulous asepsis may result in the introduction of organisms into the subarachnoid space and adjacent tissues, thereby producing meningitis, osteomyelitis, septic arthritis, or soft tissue abscess. It is of the utmost importance to be uncompromisingly insistent on strict asepsis in the performance of myelography. This means that the ancillary technical assistants must be intimately familiar with aseptic technique. Should there be a break in technique for any reason, it is wise to use a broad-spectrum antibiotic for 5–7 days after examination.

Arachnoiditis

It is my opinion, based on clinical experience and animal experiments, that Pantopaque can produce varying degrees of arachnoiditis. This effect is enhanced by the simultaneous presence of blood in the cerebrospinal fluid. The degree of the inflammatory reaction is relatively mild compared with that produced by Lipiodol. However, whenever feasible, an effort should be made to remove the oil completely at the end of the examination. Because there is some controversy about whether intrathecal methylprednisolone acetate (Depo-Medrol) helps prevent arachnoiditis or causes arachnoiditis itself, I do not use this drug in patients with iatrogenic blood or residual Pantopaque in the CSF.

Tabaddor reported visual loss in a young woman 35 days after a cervical myelogram. During the procedure, some of the oil inadvertently entered the basilar cisternae and was observed around the right optic nerve. Thirty-one days later, she developed pain in the right eye, followed 4 days later by right papillary dilatation, a sluggish response to light, and loss of vision except for light perception. The patient was given prednisone (40 mg daily) because the findings were considered to be due to a chemical arachnoiditis. Vision improved in 2 days and returned to normal by the end of a week.

It is also important to remember that traces of detergent solutions used for cleaning syringes can produce arachnoiditis.

Unusual Sensitivity Reactions

Rarely, an unpredictable reaction may occur due to hypersensitivity of the patient to the iodized oil. The unusual reports by Luce, and by Mason and Raaf have been described in detail in Chapter 2.

Venous Intravasation

The inadvertent injection of Pantopaque into the extradural venous plexus is an uncommon accident. This may occur because of faulty technique, with injection of the oil into the bony skeleton and vertebral vein system (Ginsberg and Skorneck). It may also be due to traumatic perforation of an extradural vein during the introduction or removal of the Pantopaque (Steinbach and Hill). The Pantopaque may actually be observed fluoroscopically to disappear suddenly from the subarachnoid space. A chest film taken at this time will demonstrate many tiny pulmonary oil emboli. In addition to the obvious traumatic cases, the literature contains a small number of reports of nontraumatic venous intravasation which have a different explanation. Evidence from a variety of sources supports the concept of direct absorption of contrast medium via connections between the arachnoid and venous channels. The evidence comes from direct anatomical (Elman, Welch and Pollay, Kido et al.) as well as kinetic studies (Lorenzo et al., Golman, Enzmann et al.).

Cardiac Arrest

Cooper reported an unusual case of cardiac arrest on the myelographic tilt table. The patient, a 43-year-old male with low back pain and left sciatica, was otherwise healthy although apprehensive. Premedication consisted of 100 mg of pentobarbital at 11:30 A.M. and 35 mg of meperidine hydrochloride at 12:30 P.M. At 1:00 P.M., he was placed on the x-ray table in the prone position with a folded pillow under the abdomen. After the table was tilted 35 degrees toward the feet, the patient fainted. The table then was rapidly lowered to the Trendelenburg position and the patient promptly regained consciousness. He was given 20 mg of methoxamine hydrochloride in an effort to prevent orthostatic hypotension and the abdominal pillow was removed. After a 10-minute wait, the table was again slowly and cautiously tilted toward the feet. The patient again lost consciousness and failed to respond to the head-down position. Respiration and heartbeat ceased. Following ineffectual mouth-to-mouth artificial respiration and external cardiac massage, the chest was opened and the heart directly massaged. Restoration of breathing and cardiac action was accomplished and the patient recovered. It is well known that apprehension can produce increased vagal tone. Abdominal compression by the pillow may have impeded venous return to the right side of the heart, while caudad tilting of the table probably resulted in peripheral venous pooling. The cumulative effect of these changes in a patient with an unusually labile circulatory system apparently was sufficient to cause syncope and cardiac arrest.

It probably is wise to check the blood pressure of patients prior to myelography and to inquire about a past history of orthostatic hypotension. In addition, early removal of the abdominal pad may be desirable. Despite having seen mild symptoms of orthostatic hypotension, e.g., sweating, dizziness, light-headedness, nausea, in patients undergoing myelography when the table was tilted into the upright position, I am unaware of any other report similar to Cooper's.

Respiratory Arrest

Benedict and Janower reported a case of fatal respiratory arrest in a 55-year-old female who had undergone a left radical mastectomy for carcinoma of the breast 2 years previously. Pantopaque cervical myelography was performed because of flaccid paralysis of both upper extremities. There were no respiratory signs or symptoms, and no premedication was given. Several minutes after the patient was placed in the prone, head-down position, she became cyanotic and apneic. There was no evidence of hypotension, cardiac arrest, arrhythmia, or hypersensitivity to contrast media. Immediately after endotracheal intubation and the administration of oxygen, the patient regained consciousness. However, she failed to resume spontaneous respiration and died 3 weeks later with bilateral bronchopneumonia. Necropsy revealed an upper mediastinal tumor mass surrounding the phrenic and vagus nerves, the brachial plexus bilaterally, and the superior vena cava. The authors suggest caution in performing myelography in patients with severe muscular or neuromuscular diseases that may interfere with normal respiration. Such patients are presumably at greater risk for respiratory arrest. Prior to myelography, diaphragmatic motion and pulmonary function should be evaluated. Sedation before the myelogram should be avoided. If feasible, the examination should be carried out in the supine and lateral positions to avoid the reduction in thoracic excursion associated with the prone position.

Spinal Shock

The inadvertent injection of aqueous contrast media into the subarachnoid space during diskography may produce spinal shock with paraplegia or ascending paralysis. Mishkin et al. described this complication following aortography or selective visceral arteriography and suggested a therapeutic rationale to treat this potentially catastrophic event. Their approach was based upon the observation that postmortem CSF iodine levels were very high in two patients who died of this complication. Consequently, these authors recommended the following therapeutic regimen for patients who develop spinal shock: (1) immediate rapid withdrawal of CSF in 10-ml increments, replacing the CSF with physiological saline; (2) positioning the patient with the head elevated to promote CSF drainage and removal. In two patients I am aware of with this complication, rapid clinical improvement with no neurologic sequelae followed CSF lavage. Before this regimen was implemented, a patient died of spinal shock. Although Mishkin et al. did not mention the use of corticosteroids, I would be inclined to add intravenous hydrocortisone to this regimen.

Sudeck's Atrophy (Reflex Algodystrophy)

Morretin and Wilson reported two patients who developed severe reflex algodystrophy following myelography. I have never seen this complication and know of no other similar cases in the literature.

The first patient, a healthy 21-year-old girl, suffered a back injury during judo practice. A laminectomy was performed because of clinical diagnosis of a herniated lumbar disk, but no lesion was found. Because of persistent symptoms, a second laminectomy was carried out a month later, with removal of some disk material from the L4-5 and L5-S1 interspaces. Again, there was no relief from symptoms. Three years later, because of a clinical diagnosis of arachnoiditis, Pantopaque myelography was performed, with negative findings. After removal of the oil, 80 mg of methylprednisolone acetate (Depo-Medrol) was instilled into the subarachnoid space. Shortly thereafter, the patient complained of excruciating back pain radiating into the left leg. One week later, edema, redness, and irregular cyanosis of the left foot and ankle appeared; severe pain in the foot discouraged walking. Radiographs of the left foot and ankle 8 weeks later revealed spotty demineralization of the bones. A lumbar sympathectomy was performed 5 months later because of persisting symptoms. This resulted in considerable improvement in the soft tissue dystrophic changes and bone pain, although the radiographic findings remained unchanged. Is this an example of chemical neuritis due to Depo-Medrol?

The second patient had undergone myelography during a work-up for long-standing, severe headache. The myelogram had been reported as negative. The patient stated that she experienced a transient sensation of intense warmness and some pain in the left leg when the needle was first inserted into the subarachnoid space. After completion of the myelogram, the pain increased in severity, with radiation from the low back down the posterior left leg into the toes. Two weeks later, the pain in the left foot had become unbearable, making walking impossible. Examination at that time showed hypesthesia, edema, redness, and blotchy cyanosis of the left leg. Following left lumbar sympathectomy, there was little improvement.

Six months later, although the trophic soft tissue changes in the left leg had disappeared, the intractable pain persisted. Radiography showed diffuse, uniform osteoporosis of the left foot. A chordotomy was carried out because of incapacitating pain. The symptoms and function improved after chordotomy, although the radiographic changes in the bones remained stationary. Presumably this is an example of direct needle trauma to a nerve root (during lumbar puncture) that initiated the onset of a reflex algodystrophy.

BIBLIOGRAPHY

Alemohammad S., Bouzarth W.F.: Intracranial subdural hematoma following lumbar myelography. Case report. *J. Neurosurg.* 52:256, 1980.

Aspelin P., Lester J.: Pantopaque pulmonary embolism following myelography. *Neuroradiology* 14:43, 1977.

Azar I., Betcher A.M.: Epidural blood patch for spinal headache. *Mt. Sinai J. Med.* 47:592, 1980.

Barthelemy C.R.: Arachnoiditis ossificans. *J. Comput. Assist. Tomogr.* 6: 809, 1982.

Bastow M., Godwin-Austen R.B.: Cervical myelopathy after metrizamide myelogram. *Br. Med. J.* 2:1262, 1979.

Benedict K.T., Jr., Janower M.L.: Respiratory arrest. A fatal complication of myelography. *Radiology* 122:729, 1977.

Boyd H.: Iatrogenic intraspinal epidermoid. Report of a case. *J. Neurosurg.* 24:105, 1966.

Brodey P.A., London S.S., Sung M.A.: Nerve root avulsion. A complication of the Chynn needle. *Radiology* 125: 734, 1977.

Chynn K.Y.: Painless myelography; introduction of a new aspiration cannula and review of 541 consecutive cases. *Radiology* 109:361, 1973.

Cooper D.R.: Cardiac arrest on the myelographic tilt table. *J.A.M.A.* 187:674, 1964.

Cuatico W.: Letter. *J. Neurosurg.* 41:406, 1974.

Cuatico W., Gannon W., Samouhos E.: A needle designated for myelography. *J. Neurosurg.* 28:87, 1968.

Deeb Z.L., Rosenbaum A.E.: Opacification of the lumbar epidural venous plexus during myelography. *Surg. Neurol.* 12:259, 1979.

DiChiro G., Wener L.: Angiography of the spinal cord. A review of contemporary techniques and applications. *J. Neurosurg.* 39:1, 1973.

Dripps R.D., Vandam L.D.: Hazards of lumbar puncture. *J.A.M.A.* 147:1118, 1951.

Elman R.: Spinal arachnoid granulations with special reference to the cerebrospinal fluid. *Bull. Johns Hopkins Hosp.* 34:99, 1923.

Enzmann D., Norman D., Newton T.: Computer tomography in cisternography with metrizamide. *Acta Radiol.* (Suppl.) 355:294, 1977.

Epstein B.S., Epstein J.A.: The cineroentgenographic observations of Pantopaque intravasation during myelography. *Am. J. Roentgenol.* 94:576, 1965.

Everett A.D.: Lumbar puncture injuries. *Proc. Roy. Soc. Med.* 35:208, 1942.

Fullenlove T.M.: Venous intravasation during myelography. *Radiology* 53:410, 1949.

Gabriele O.F.: Subdural hematoma and lumbar diskography. *J.A.M.A.* 207:154, 1969 (letter).

Gellman M.: Injury to intervertebral discs during spinal puncture. *J. Bone Joint Surg.* 22:980, 1940.

Ginsberg L.B., Skorneck A.B.: Pantopaque pulmonary embolism. Complication of myelography. *Am. J. Roentgenol.* 73:27, 1951.

Glass P.M., Kennedy W.F., Jr.: Headache following subarachnoid puncture; treatment with the epidural blood patch. *J.A.M.A.* 219:203, 1972.

Golman K.: Absorption of metrizamide from cerebrospinal fluid to blood: Pharmacokinetics in humans. *J. Pharm. Sci.* 64:405, 1974.

Greig J.H., Wignall N.: A case of arachnoiditis associated with "Pantopaque" myelography. *J. Can. Assoc. Radiol.* 17:198, 1966.

Hinck V.C.: The myelography needle: A new cannula for aspiration. *Radiology* 120:731, 1976.

Hinkel C.L.: The entrance of Pantopaque into the venous system during myelography. *Am. J. Roentgenol.* 54:230, 1945.

Hungerford G.D., Powers J.M.: Avulsion of nerve rootlets with the Cuatico needle during Pantopaque removal after myelography. *A.J.R.* 129:485, 1977.

Keats T.E.: Pantopaque pulmonary embolism. *Radiology* 67:748, 1956.

Kennedy F., Effron A.S., Perry G.: The grave spinal cord paralyses caused by spinal anesthesia. *Surg., Gynecol. Obstet.* 91:385, 1950.

Kennedy T.F., Steinfeld J.R.: Nerve root avulsion as a complication of myelography with the Cuatico needle. *Radiology* 119:389, 1976.

Kido K., Gomez D.G., Pavese A.M.: Human spinal arachnoid villi and granulations. *Neuroradiology* 11:221, 1976.

King A.Y., et al.: Intravasation of Pantopaque during myelography. *Surg. Neurol.* 11:3, 1979.

Kwan W.W., Kur N.K., Chye L.E.: Pantopaque pulmonary embolism during myelography. *J. Neurosurg.* 46:391, 1977.

Laasonen E.M., Servo A., Soini J., et al.: Gross deformity of the spine. A lumbar myelographic risk with Conray and Dimer X. *Neuroradiology* 15:175, 1978.

Laasonen E.M., Servo A., Soini J., Laasonen L.: A new relative contraindication for lumbar myelography. *Neuroradiology* 16:367, 1978.

Lee S.H.: Venous intravasation of Pantopaque during myelography. Report of two cases and a review of the literature. *J. Can. Assoc. Radiol.* 27:111, 1976.

Lorenzo A.V., Hammerstadt J.P., Cutler R.W.P.: Cerebrospinal fluid formation and absorption and transport of iodide and sulfate through the spinal subarachnoid space. *J. Neurol. Sci.* 10:247, 1970.

Luce J.C., Leith W., Burrage W.C.: Pantopaque meningitis due to hypersensitivity. *Radiology* 57:878, 1951.

MacCarty W.C., Jr., Lane F.W., Jr.: Pitfalls of myelography. *Radiology* 65:663, 1955.

Mais T.E., Fortin D.: Intravasation of Pantopaque during myelography without associated traumatic tap. *A.J.N.R.* 2:589, 1981.

Maltby G.L., Pendergrass R.C.: Pantopaque myelography. Diagnostic errors and review of cases. *Radiology* 47:35, 1946.

Manno N.J., Uihlein A., Kernohan J.W.: Intraspinal epidermoids. *J. Neurosurg.* 19:754, 1962.

Martin C.M.: Myelography with sodium diatrizoate (Hypaque). Report of a case of inadvertent use complicated by acute renal failure. *California Med.* 115:57, 1971.

Mason M.S., Raaf J.: Complications of Pantopaque myelography. Case report and review. *J. Neurosurg.* 19:302, 1962.

McCulloch G.A.J.: Arachnoidal calcification producing spinal cord compression. *J. Neurol. Neurosurg., Psychiatr.* 38:1059, 1975.

Miller D.S.: Post-myelographic coccygodynia. *Am. J. Proctol.* 18:292, 1967.

Mishkin M.M., Baum S., Ng L., DiChiro G.: Cerebrospinal fluid iodine levels after uncomplicated and complicated angiography (abstract). *Invest. Radiol.* 7:439, 1972.

Morretin L.B., Wilson M.: Severe reflex algodystrophy (Sudek's atrophy) as a complication of myelography: Report of two cases. *Am. J. Roentgenol.* 110:156, 1970.

Nainkin L.: Arachnoiditis ossificans. Report of a case. *Spine* 3:83, 1978.

Pear B.L.: Iatrogenic intraspinal epidermoid sequestration cysts. *Radiology* 92:251, 1969.

Rice J.F., Shields C.B., Morris C.F., Neely B.D.: Spinal subarachnoid hemorrhage during myelography. A case report. *J. Neurosurg.* 48:645, 1978.

Ritter V.: Dangers and misinterpretations of myelography in suspected cases of disk prolapse. *Fortschr. Geb. Röntgenstrahlen* 75:339, 1951.

Schultz E.C., Miller J.H.: Intravasation of opaque media during myelography; 3 cases. *J. Neurosurg.* 18:610, 1961.

Schurr P.H., McLaurin R.L., Ingraham F.D.: Experimental studies on the circulation of the cerebrospinal fluid and methods of producing communicating hydrocephalus in the dog. *J. Neurosurg.* 10:515, 1953.

Scott R.M.: Myelography (letter). *J.A.M.A.* 237:2380, 1977.

Scoville W.B., Moretz W.H., Hankins W.D.: Discrepancies in myelography. Statistical survey of 200 operative cases undergoing Pantopaque myelography. *Surg., Gynecol. Obstet.* 86:559, 1948.

Sehgal A.D., Gardner W.J., Dohn D.F.: Pantopaque meningitis: Treatment with subarachnoid injections of corticosteroids. *Cleveland Clin. Quart.* 29:177, 1962.

Seigel R.S., Williams A.G., Waterman R.E.: Potential complications in myelography. I. Technical considerations. *A.J.R.* 138:705, 1982.

Steinbach H.L., Hill W.B.: Pantopaque pulmonary embolism during myelography, *Radiology* 56:735, 1951.

Tabaddor K.: Unusual complications of iophendylate injection myelography, *Arch. Neurol.* 29:435, 1973.

Todd E.W., Gardner W.J.: Pantopaque intravasation (embolization) during myelography, *J. Neurosurg.* 14:230, 1957.

Tourtellott W.W., Henderson W.G., Tucker R.P., et al.: A randomized, double-blind clinical trial comparing the 22 versus 26 gauge needle in the production of the postlumbar puncture syndrome in normal individuals. *Headache* 12-73-78, 1972.

Trowbridge W.V., French J.D.: "False-positive" lumbar myelogram. *Neurology* 4:339, 1954.

Von Muralt, R.H.: Failures in myelography. *Praxis* 38:587, 1949.

Welch K., Pollay M.: The spinal subarachnoid villi of the monkeys cercopithecus aethrops sabaceus and macace irus. *J. Neurol. Sci.* 10:247, 1970.

Winkelman N.W., Gotten N., Scheibert D.: Localized adhesive spinal arachnoiditis. A study of 25 cases with reference to etiology. *Trans. Am. Neurol. Assoc.* 1953, p. 15.

Worthington M., Hills J., Tally F., Flynn R.: Bacterial meningitis after myelography. *Surg. Neurol.* 14:318, 1980.

Young D.A., Burney R.E., II.: Complication of myelography. Transection and withdrawal of a nerve filament by the needle. *N. Engl. J. Med.* 285:156, 1971.

Zito J.L., Schellinger D.: Nontraumatic intravasation of myelographic contrast medium. *A.J.R.* 132:795, 1979.

21

Pneumomyelography

ARTHUR E. ROSENBAUM, M.D.
RICHARD A. BAKER, M.D.

IN 1919, after viewing the upper cervical spinal cord in a patient who underwent air ventriculography, Dandy predicted a broader use of gas to define abnormalities within the vertebral canal. In 1925, he utilized gas to define a thoracic extradural block. It was then only natural to extend the application of gas to define the entire spinal subarachnoid space.

Air as a contrast medium, although innocuous, is difficult to image. Therefore, pneumomyelography was never very popular in the United States, especially after the introduction of positive-contrast media with much greater radiopacity (first Lipiodol, then Pantopaque). However, gas myelography was widely used in Scandinavia and Czechoslovakia until the introduction recently of nonionic contrast media.

The goal of a contrast medium is to create or enhance differences between structures. When the pathologic object and the contrast material are similar in radiodensity and are juxtaposed, they may be indistinguishable from one another, even confluent. This should prompt the myelographer to choose the contrast medium that best produces differences.

ADVANTAGES AND DISADVANTAGES OF GAS AS A CONTRAST MEDIUM

The present indications for gas myelography are infrequent because of the introduction of nonionic contrast media and computed tomography. A severe hypersensitivity to iodine is the primary reason for selecting gas as the contrast medium. Pneumomyelography has also been helpful in diagnosing a variety of lesions, including tethered spinal cord, diastematomyelia, hydromyelia with collapse, spinal trauma, spinal cord tumor, etc. Examples of these entities (Figs 21–1 to 21–11) demonstrate the elegant detail and information obtainable by this technique.

However, gas myelography has the disadvantages of requiring great technical skill on the part of the physician and the technologist, sophisticated tomographic

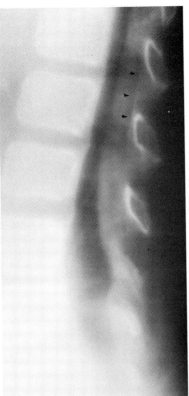

Fig 21–1.—Tethered spinal cord in a 7-year-old who underwent repair of a lumbar lipomyelomeningocele at age 5 months. Tethered cord is a fairly common accompaniment of a repaired myelomeningocele. Here the cord extends at least to the L4–5 level. That it is the spinal cord and not a long extradural defect posterior to the subarachnoid space is denoted by the thin subarachnoid gas lucency coursing between the L1–2 segments *(arrowheads)*.

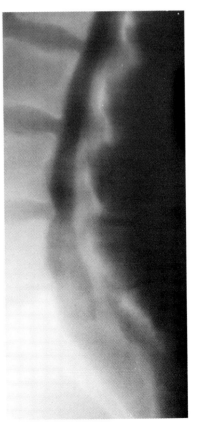

Fig 21–2.—Tethered cord with sacral dermoid in a 28-year-old with 20-year history of urinary and fecal incontinence. The spinal cord reaches the S-2 level. The cord widens to merge with a large, superiorly lobulated sacral soft tissue mass that has expanded the spinal canal and caused an indistinctness of the anterior wall between S-2 and S-3.

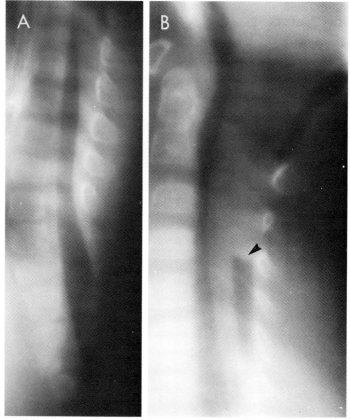

Fig 21–3.—More subtle example of tethered cord. History: 2-year-old repair of meningomyelocele, performed at birth. Recent gait difficulty and deteriorating somatosensory evoked potentials. **A,** the subarachnoid space along its posterior aspect is situated too anteriorly from L-1 to L-3. Whether this thickening is extradural or subarachnoid cannot be determined myelographically. Were gas (or a positive-contrast medium) seen posterior to the thickening, the diagnosis of tethered spinal cord could be made. **B,** images of the cervical region show that the neural axis is thick superiorly down to the C-4 level inferiorly *(arrowhead)*. The "thickening" represents the cerebellar tonsils in this Chiari II malformation.

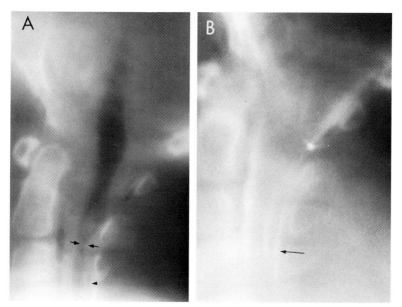

Fig 21–4.—Hydromyelia. **A,** gas myelogram. Note the fourth ventricle situated at the plane of the foramen magnum. Gas extends downward in continuity with a dilated central canal *(arrows)*. Subarachnoid gas is abundant anterior to the cord and appears slit-like posteriorly *(arrowhead)*. These findings are absolutely diagnostic of hydromyelia and are more direct evidence than the "collapsing cord" sign. **B,** metrizamide myelography. This follow-up study, performed months after **A,** allows clinical comparison of the two myelographic methods. The dilated central canal *(arrow)* is now opacified by the positive-contrast medium.

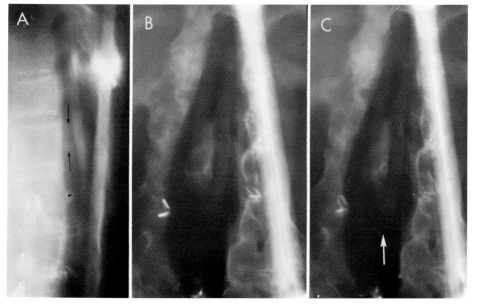

Fig 21–5.—Diastematomyelia. **A,** sagittal section. Harrington rods were inserted to alleviate scoliosis; the latter is responsible for many vertebral elements being out of the tomographic plane of focus. Note the low-lying cord and the peculiar soft tissue projection extending into the subarachnoid space anteriorly *(arrows)*. Immediately inferior are corticated bony septa *(arrowhead)*, which overlie the posteriorly positioned, ectopically low spinal cord. **B,** coronal section. Double spinal cord with corticated bone is juxtaposed to the cord on the reader's side. **C,** coronal section, 2 mm posterior from **B.** The fusion of the split cord (diastematomyelia) below the osseous spur is readily perceived *(arrow)*.

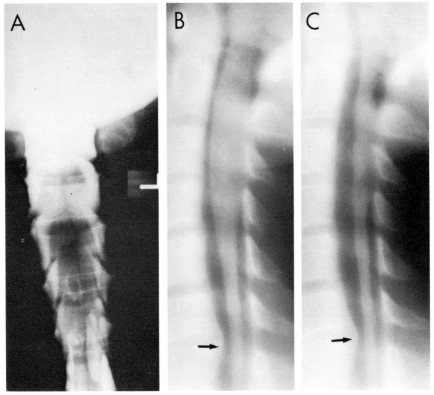

Fig 21–6.—Cord enlargement vs. cord shrinkage. The "collapsing" cord of hydromyelia in a 30-year-old with hand and shoulder weakness. **A,** Pantopaque myelogram. The caliber of the cervical cord is at the upper limits of normal. This orthogonal projection did not clarify the diagnosis. **B,** gas myelogram. Patient's head down −15 degrees. The cord is fusiform and enlarged between C-2 and C-4. Below this level, it is strikingly small. There is a large posterior expansion of the C6-7 intervertebral disk *(arrow).* **C,** gas myelogram. Patient's head up +15 degrees. Note how the spinal cord has contracted in caliber; the intramedullary fluid in the central canal has been displaced to the thoracic cord by tilting the patient. The foramen magnum is not as radiolucent as usual during gas myelography since soft tissue, i.e., the dysplastic cerebellar vermis and tonsils, occupies its subarachnoid space posteriorly. This is characteristic of this condition.

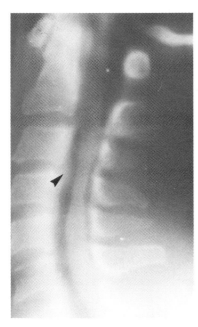

Fig 21–7.—Gas myelography for accurately assessing spinal cord size. This patient with spastic quadriparesis was thought to have multiple sclerosis, often a morphologic diagnosis of exclusion, which new technologies such as NMR may overcome. Gas myelography showed a small spinal cord, especially at the C3-4 level, with the cord more affected anteriorly than posteriorly. Closer scrutiny, however, shows a very large herniated disk (note asymmetry at the interspace) immediately anterior to the shrunken cord *(arrowhead)*.

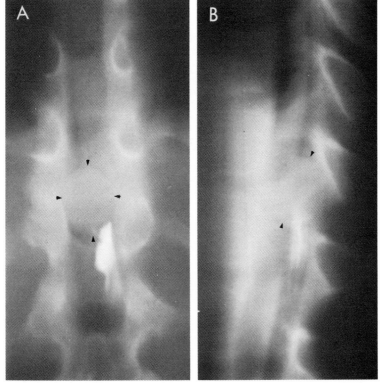

Fig 21–8.—Large intradural-extramedullary mass. **A,** coronal projection. A large, round, smooth mass *(arrowheads)* displaces the spinal cord to the reader's right; since the subarachnoid space on the left is widened rather than narrowed by the mass, an intradural location is confirmed. The upper surface of the mass is distinct from the spinal cord, indicating again that the subarachnoid space is widened unilaterally and confirming the intradural-extramedullary position of the tumor. **B,** the lateral projection shows that the mass lies posterior to the spinal cord, displaces it anteriorly, and expands the subarachnoid space both above and below. A previous 1-ml Pantopaque "test" performed elsewhere obscures the tomographic image of the inferior aspect of the mass. Histopathologic diagnosis: Neurilemoma.

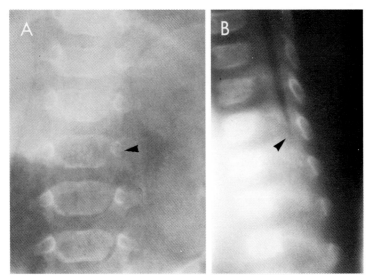

Fig 21–9.—Epidural abscess. **A,** plain film of abdomen. Note the rarefaction of the left L-3 pedicle, especially laterally *(arrowhead)*. **B,** gas myelogram (sagittal section). Gas instilled from the cervical region extends down to the T-11 block *(arrowhead)* (patient tilted head down). The posterior subarachnoid space between T-8 and T-11 can be seen, but it lies excessively anteriorly (i.e., the distance between it and the spinous processes is increased).

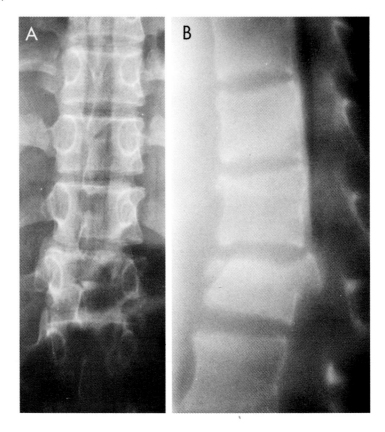

equipment (preferably with image intensification), and complete cooperation of the patient, i.e., the ability to lie on the side in one position for three-quarters to two and one-half hours.

DUAL HYPOBARIC AND HYPERBARIC CONTRAST AGENTS

Another use for gas myelography is the demonstration of the lower border of a complete block that has been identified by a positive-contrast medium. Excellent visualization of both sides of the block can be achieved during one imaging session with the use of dual contrast agents.

In our opinion, a hyperbaric contrast agent (less buoyant or higher specific gravity than CSF) should be used to demonstrate the inferior extent of the block, and a hypobaric (gas) contrast medium (more buoyant than CSF) should be used to visualize the superior extent (Fig 21–12). Although aqueous contrast media are relatively safe, they cannot be fully removed; they ascend into the intracranial subarachnoid space and are eliminated by slow resorption. Gas is less noxious intracranially than either metrizamide or Pantopaque. When large doses of contrast are required, particularly in elderly patients or those with cerebrovascular disease or a shunt, gas myelography may be the procedure of choice in the cervical and thoracic regions.

TECHNIQUE

Lumbar Injection

After slow drainage of all CSF with a 20-gauge needle (22-gauge in children), gas (filtered oxygen, air, nitrous oxide) is instilled over 5–15 minutes until the entire spinal subarachnoid space is filled, if panmyelography is indicated (Fig 21–13). When only the lumbar or lower thoracic region is under investigation, a proportionally smaller quantity of gas is used.

The patient is inclined slightly upright and then tilted into several positions to obtain satisfactory filling. In our experience, a single position, with the patient inclined approximately 15 degrees head down, usually suffices. This position affords excellent control of the gas, thereby obviating unnecessary, untoward intracranial filling. Because the patient is tilted, there is an oblique intraspinal air-fluid level. To see the upper cervical region on slices made from one side of the canal to the

---

Fig 21–10.—Trauma studied by gas myelography. History: A 15-year-old girl in an auto accident was immediately rendered paraplegic with an L-2 sensory level. **A,** frontal projection, nontomogram. Even without tomography (a technique obviously limited by morphology which fails to lie flat within a plane, the lordotic lumbar spine), the subarachnoid gas above the L-1 fracture and the normal spine below it are seen despite the large quantity of bowel gas (ileus). **B,** the L-1 vertebral body is compressed and somewhat wedge-shaped. A large fragment of bone from the superior posterior corner of the vertebral body is avulsed and occupies half of the vertebral canal in this midsagittal tomogram. No gas (introduced cervically) is seen below this level. In fact, the gas column stops just above the bone fragments. Above the fracture, note how the subarachnoid space thins anteriorly due to cord edema. At surgery, a large fragment of bone and extruded disk material were found in the spinal canal.

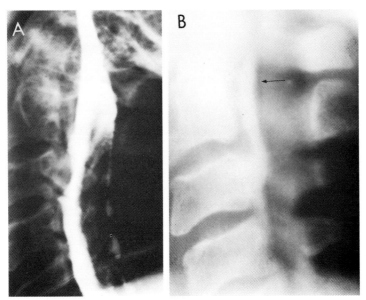

Fig 21–11.—A contrast medium should afford contrast. **A,** Pantopaque myelogram shows a large anterior extradural defect at C1-3 in this 70-year-old man. The cause cannot be determined from this film. **B,** gas myelogram shows a sliver-thin subarachnoid space *(arrow)* immediately behind a densely calcified posterior spinal ligament. The precise relationship of the calcified bulk to the extradural defect is clear when an appropriate contrast medium is used. Pantopaque makes dense calcifications invisible.

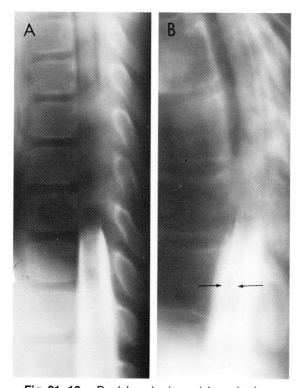

Fig 21–12.—Dual hypobaric and hyperbaric contrast technique. **A,** oxygen, a hypobaric, and metrizamide, a hyperbaric contrast agent, define the upper and lower margins of a three-vertebra-long midthoracic block in a child with lymphoma. Hypocycloidal tomogram; patient position, decubitus and inclined downward 15 degrees. **B,** gas *(above)* and metrizamide *(below)* show a mid-dorsal block caused by metastasis from a bronchogenic carcinoma in an elderly man. Tomography can also be used to screen for regional osseous metastatic deposits. Note subarachnoid seeding *(arrows)*. *Conclusion:* Two contrast agents with different specific gravities and radiopacities may be imaged separately or in combination, as shown here, where a single image clearly shows both sides of a complete block. Both contrast media may also be used in conjunction with CT imaging. The use of two agents is less cumbersome for very ill patients and provides more comprehensive information.

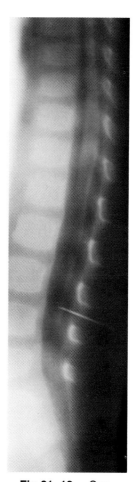

Fig 21–13.—Gas was instilled via lumbar puncture for panmyelography.

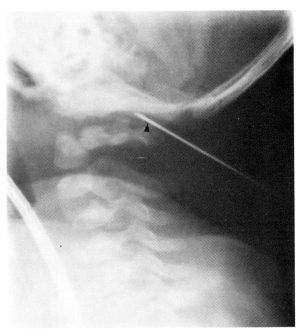

Fig 21–14.—Cisternal puncture. The subarachnoid space is also accessible via the cisternal approach, wherein the puncture is made in the midline just beneath the occiput *(arrow)* with the neck flexed.

other, some basal posterior fossa filling is necessary so that the lower part of the gas-fluid level can reach the foramen magnum. In the alert patient, even prior to intracranial ascent of the gas, headache is more likely to occur from lumbar rather than cervical instillation because cervical or cisternal puncture (Fig 21–14) allows for fractional exchange. When the lumbar route is used, the additional fluid that is retained must be displaced intracranially by adding more gas, thereby increasing CSF pressure. Conversely, an advantage of the lumbar route is the possibility of removing much of the gas after the procedure.

Cervical Injection (Figs 21–15 to 21–24)

The lateral C1-2 puncture (see Fig 21–15) was originally conceived for surgical cordotomy. It soon became the technique of choice for outlining the superior aspect of a complete block. Although this puncture is best performed under image-intensified fluoroscopy, it is possible to place external reference markers on the skin and triangulate a course from the skin to the subarachnoid space (see Fig 21–16).

Optimal needle placement in the lateral posterior C1-2 puncture is made by advancing a spinal needle (20-gauge in adults, 22-gauge in children) perpendicular to the mid-interspace between the spinous processes of C-1 and C-2. The needle is slowly advanced behind the spinal cord by 0.5–1.0-mm increments under fluoroscopic visualization until the posterior extreme of the subarachnoid space is penetrated. When the subarachnoid space is narrow, this progressively anterior course is much safer than less controlled entry.

The patient is inclined slightly (− 15 degrees) head down. The cerebrospinal fluid is removed, and the injected gas (in the absence of spinal block) courses first to the lumbosacral subarachnoid space, the uppermost site. Additional aliquots of gas oc-

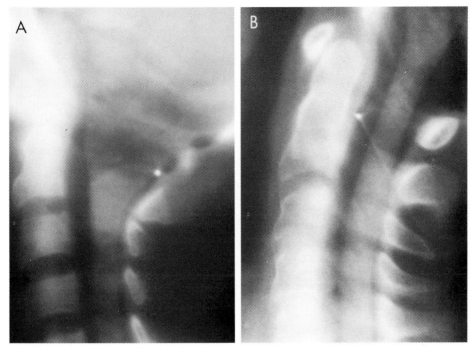

Fig 21–15.—Panmyelography via cervical puncture and CSF-gas exchange. **A,** when lumbar injection is difficult or painful (e.g., in cases of spinal stenosis, postsurgical scarring, repaired meningocele of Chiari II malformation), direct lateral C1-2 puncture may be elected. (In our hands, no complications occurred in over 200 pediatric patients with the Chiari II malformation.) **B,** lateral anterior C1-2 approach, anterior to the spinal cord, may be preferred (rarely our preference). An anterior or posterior puncture is safer than the in-between position (needle tip in the thin subarachnoid space lateral to the cord) because respiration or head movement during positioning may cause the needle to scratch or lacerate the cord.

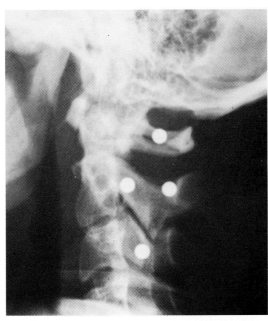

Fig 21–16.—When image-intensified fluoroscopy is not available, we use external reference markers (lead BBs positioned on tape) to identify the puncture site. The needle is inserted perpendicular to the horizontal table and laterally recumbent patient and its advance monitored by sequential films until CSF is successfully withdrawn. A guideline is the "popping" sensation experienced by the operator as the dura is traversed. (This may also indicate that one is too posterior and has traversed the dense-feeling interspinous ligament.) If an epidural vein is punctured (venous blood returns), careful advancement of the needle for 1–2-mm may result in CSF flow and a successful puncture.

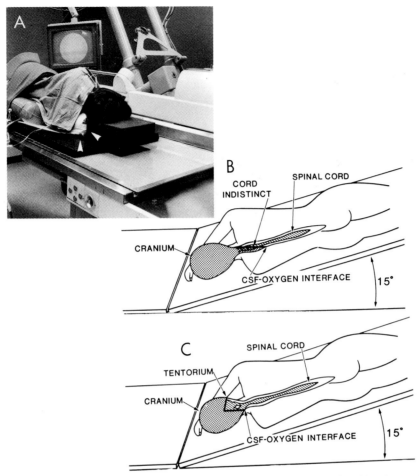

Fig 21–17.—Patient position during lateral C1-2 puncture. **A,** preferably, the patient's back should be toward the technologist and the physician to permit them easier access to the patient. Also, the patient cannot observe the needle in this position. The radiographic system (here, a Universal Polytome Tilt-table) with an image intensifier allows for a fluoroscopically guided puncture and speedy positioning, aided by fluoroscopic centering and fluorotomoscopy.* The spine varies markedly in density. The thin neck can be made more nearly equivalent in radiodensity to the thicker upper thorax and head by placing a 250–500-ml IV infusion bag *(arrowheads)* between the neck and the table-top. The spine's variation in medial-lateral curvature should also be adjusted for, so that adjacent levels are included within the same plane of focus. An airbag is helpful in supporting the sagging lumbar spine. During cervical puncture, the table top is positioned vertically. After the needle enters the subarachnoid space, the patient is tilted 15 degrees head down so that gas fills the lumbosacral space first **(B),** then the thoracic, and finally the cervical region **(C).** Gas can thus be excluded from the intracranial subarachnoid space.

---

*Fluorotomoscopy: Obtaining the slice plane by image-stored overlapping of the fluoroscopically visualized tomographic path. From examining these low-mA images, one can appropriately position the field of interest and select optimal planes for section before generating hard-copy tomograms.

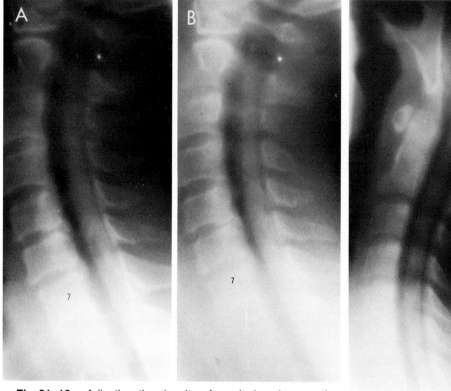

Fig 21–18.—Adjusting the density of cervical and upper thoracic regions for improved visualization. **A,** the film density of the upper thoracic and lower cervical region is excellent, but the upper cervical region is harder to see, since it is excessively dark. **B,** an IV solution bag was used to decrease the density difference between these regions.

Fig 21–19.—Normal cervical myelogram. With proper leveling and density balance, long segments of the spine can be examined successfully. Because it was necessary to visualize the brain stem in this patient, an additional 15-ml aliquot of gas was instilled.

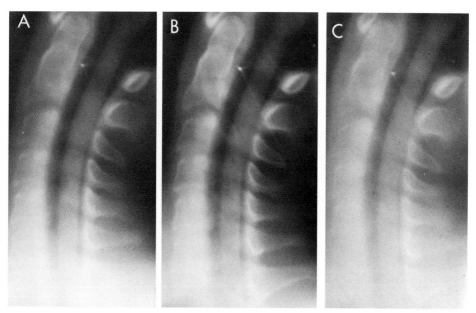

Fig 21–20.—Influences of different kilovoltages and film type on film quality. **A,** relatively high-kilovoltage technique (115 kvp). The spinal cord is seen quite well, but the regional contrast is low and the bony surroundings cannot be optimally imaged, even on a standard contrast film. **B,** lower-kilovoltage technique (90 kvp). The osseous structures, as well as the spinal cord, are well seen with some increased radiation dose. While 80 kvp is adequate for imaging smaller patients, it may be inadequate in large-shouldered patients, particularly when fine (0.3-mm) focal spots are used. This kilovoltage results in sufficient photoelectric effect to allow "shine-through" (incomplete blurring) of the dense, laterally situated apophyseal joints (see C-3 level). **C,** original high-kilovoltage technique (115 kvp) with longer gray scale (less contrast, high-detail film) affords sufficient bone detail and balanced contrast of the spinal cord. Such a combination is optimal for routine cervical gas myelography. (Film, Kodak G; screens, DuPont Hi-Plus; x-ray tube, 0.3 mm, grid-biased.)

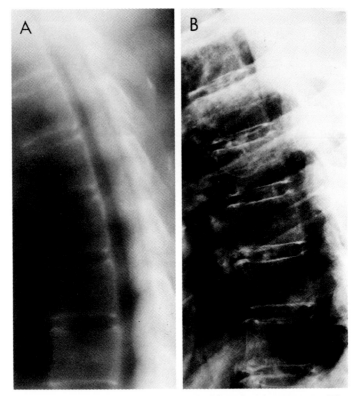

Fig 21–21.—Thoracic cord visualization. **A,** pluridirectional tomogram. The cord is well seen in its usual posterior position. **B,** nongeometric tomogram for comparison. Patient breathing slowly during exposure produces some tomographic effect. However, the gas anterior to the cord is not separated from the gas in the lung, and the posterior aspect of the spinal cord cannot be seen. **C,** same level as **B,** but xerography rather than film-screen imaging used. Patient again breathing slowly to obtain tomographic effect. Note that the edge enhancement of electronic radiography satisfactorily defines the anterior aspect of the cord at most levels. This lesser-detail treatment of the thoracic region, which significantly expedites panmyelography, is a good choice when that area is of low clinical interest.

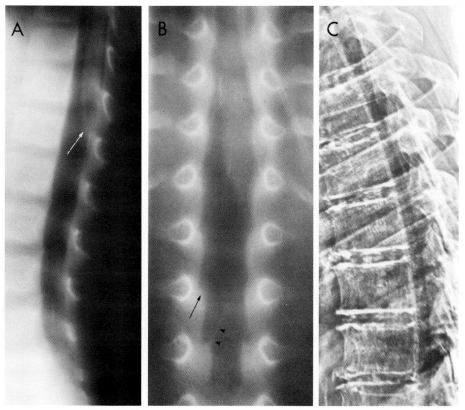

Fig 21–22.—Thoracolumbar, lumbar, and sacral myelography. **A,** midsagittal plane. Note the lower spinal cord *(arrow)* and its termination at T-12. The thecal sac ends at S-2. Subtle posterior bulging of intervertebral disks is seen at several levels. **B,** coronal plane (different patient). The cord's termination is artificially shifted to the left of the midline secondary to CSF removal, analogous to a boat going aground at low tide. Numerous axillary pouches *(arrows)* and a nerve root *(arrowheads)* are well seen on the same single 1-mm-thick image. The spine must, therefore, be quite straight. No gas can be seen below the L3-4 interspace because the spine here curves laterally, and the subarachnoid space lies outside the plane of tomographic focus.

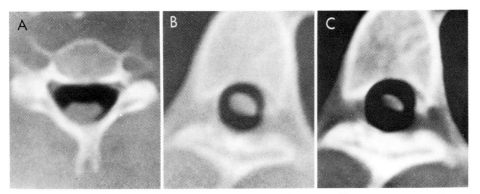

Fig 21–23.—Gas CT myelography. **A,** midcervical region. The atrophic spinal cord (multiple sclerosis) is situated very posteriorly. The gas column anterior to it indicates that no mass either *inside* or *outside* the subarachnoid space is causing this displacement. The effect of the dentate ligaments in establishing a central position for the spinal cord is less apparent. This phenomenon is well demonstrated by axial reconstruction of CT slices. **B,** normal thoracic region. Wide windows: width 4,000, level 1,200. The patient has a slight scoliosis that subtly distorts the spinal cord. The cord is central but slightly ellipsoid, due to the nonperpendicularity of the body. No significant halos mark the interface between the cord and the gas because of the advanced software of high-resolution CT scanners. **C,** spuriously small spinal cord; same slice as **B.** Width 2,000, level 800. Changing the window settings can markedly affect the display of cord size. Windowing to produce cord enlargement is not likely, but false smallness is readily achievable.

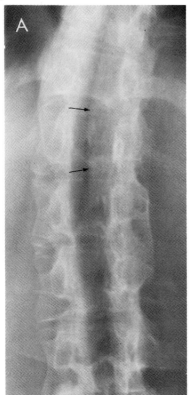

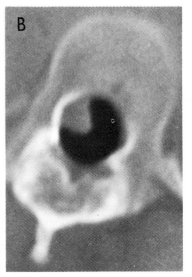

Fig 21–24.—Scoliosis and gas myelography: an uncommon possibility. **A,** simple gas myelography is usually not the preferred technique to study the subarachnoid space and cord in scoliosis; gas is much better visualized by tomography. Thin- or thick-section tomography requires many slices to include the full extent of segments widened by an exaggerated curvature. A nontomographic AP radiograph may occasionally suffice. Here the cord hugs the lesser curvature of the scoliosis *(arrows).* **B,** gas CT myelogram (same patient). Note in axial section (10-mm thickness) how the cord not only lies along one side but also is rotated.

cupy progressively higher levels and ultimately fill the space above the needle. Since the patient is tilted, an additional 10–15 cc of gas are necessary (once no more CSF can be withdrawn from the needle) to visualize the cervicomedullary junction because the needle and the gas occupy the upper, nondependent side. The lower (table-top) side of the circumferential subarachnoid space must also be filled in order to visualize the spinal cord.

BIBLIOGRAPHY

Cook P.L.: Gas myelography in the investigation of occult spinal dysraphism. *Br. J. Radiol.* 49:502, 1976.

Dandy W.E.: Roentgenography of the brain after injection of air into the spinal canal. *Ann. Surg.* 70:397, 1919.

Dandy W.E.: The diagnosis and localization of spinal cord tumors. *Ann. Surg.* 81:223, 1925.

Deeb Z.L., Rosenbaum A.E., Bank W.O., et al.: Reduced morbidity in gas myelography. *Neuroradiology* 16:352, 1978.

Jirout J.: *Pneumomyelography.* Springfield, Ill., Charles C Thomas, Publisher, 1969.

Lindgren E.: On the diagnosis of tumours of the spinal cord by the aid of gas myelography. *Acta Chir. Scand.* 82:303, 1939.

Miyazaki Y.: Selective anterior cervical gas myelography by the lateral approach. *Neuroradiology* 10:151, 1975.

Sicard J.-A., Forestier J.: Méthode radiographique d'exploration de la cavité épidurale par le lipiodol. *Rev. Neurol.* 37:1264, 1921.

Sicard J.-A., Forestier J.: Méthode générale d'exploration radiologique par l'huile iodée (lipiodol). *Bull. Soc. Med. Hôp. Paris* 46:March 17, 1922.

Sicard J.-A., Forestier J.: L'huile iodée en clinique. Applications therapeutiques et diagnostiques. *Bull. Soc. Med. Hôp. Paris* 47: 309, February 23, 1923.

Williams A.L., Haughton V.M.: Improved visualization of the anterior subarachnoid space during cervical gas myelography. *Radiology* 134:257, 1980.

22

Diskography

THE CLASSIC NECROPSY STUDIES by Schmorl form the basis for clinical contrast study of the intervertebral disk. Schmorl originally devised a technique for the postmortem injection of red lead into the intervertebral disks, followed by radiography of the spine. In this way, he was able to define the normal and the pathologic intervertebral disk. Lindblom, in Stockholm, impressed by the limitations of myelography in the diagnosis of ruptured intervertebral disk, applied a modification of Schmorl's technique to the living subject. By injecting Per-Abrodil (Diodrast) directly into the disk through a long, fine needle he succeeded not only in visualizing the internal architecture of the disk but also in correlating pathologic findings with clinical symptoms and signs.

LUMBAR

Indications and Advantages

It is important to realize that diskography is not a substitute for myelography. It is essentially a limited, specialized procedure designed to study the state of the lumbar intervertebral disks. I do not perform diskography as a primary procedure. I have used this technique only after a negative or equivocal myelogram in a patient with a history strongly suggestive of a herniated intervertebral disk with few or no objective neurologic findings or poor neurologic localization (Figs 22–1 to 22–3). This approach has been developed from experience for the following reasons: (1) other lesions, such as tumors, may masquerade clinically as herniated disks; (2) a second intraspinal lesion occasionally may coexist with a disk at a different level; and (3) the abnormal disk may uncommonly be in the thoracic or upper lumbar region.

Diskography has the distinct advantage of providing direct visualization of the intervertebral disk itself. If properly employed in a carefully selected group of patients, it can obviate the necessity for laminectomy in patients with a clinical diagnosis of herniated disk and a normal diskogram. Conversely, it may demonstrate a herniated disk in a patient with meager neurologic findings and a negative myelogram.

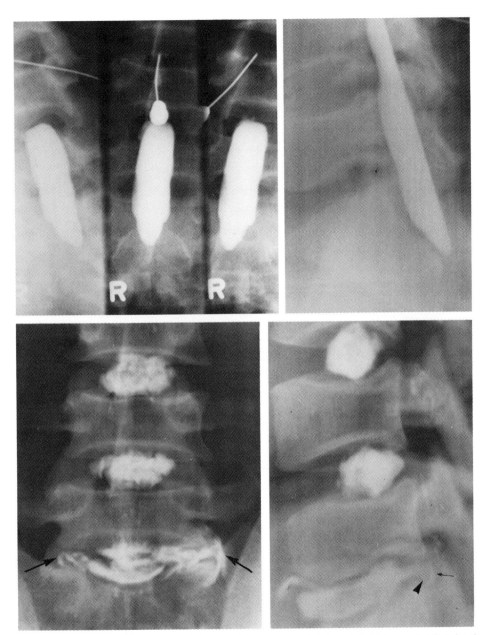

Fig 22–1.—The patient was a 34-year-old man complaining of incapacitating low back pain with bilateral sciatic radiation following an auto accident. He failed to respond to conservative therapy, including traction. The Pantopaque myelogram **(top)** is negative, but the diskogram **(bottom)** clearly shows diffuse degeneration and an annular tear with a disk fragment *(arrowhead)* under the posterior longitudinal ligament *(thin arrow)*. There are also iatrogenic tears of the anterior longitudinal and lateral ligaments *(large arrows)*.

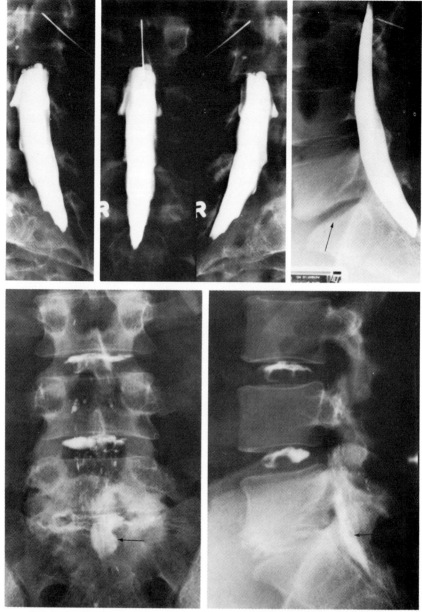

Fig 22–2.—The patient, a 23-year-old policeman, was seen because of severe midline pain in the lower back without radiation. The Pantopaque myelogram **(top)** is unremarkable, but there is narrowing of the lumbosacral disk with a vacuum phenomenon *(arrow)*. Note the significant distance between the anterior aspect of the thecal sac and the back of the L5-S1 interspace. The disk puncture **(bottom)** shows normal disks at L3-4 and L4-5 and diffuse degeneration at L5-S1 without a posterior protrusion or herniation. Note the residual Pantopaque from the previous myelogram *(arrow)*. Ideally, the oil should have been removed prior to the injection of the L5-S1 interspace.

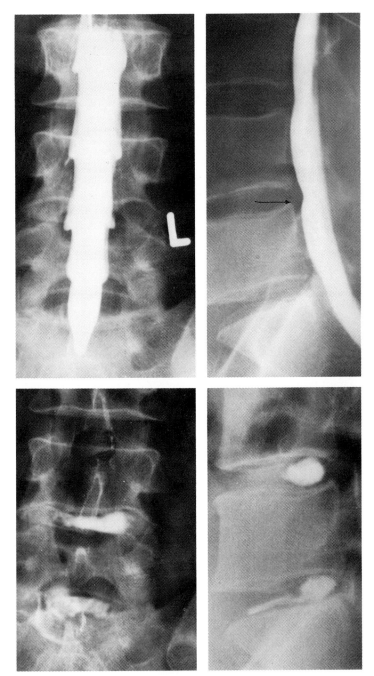

Fig 22–3.—This 27-year-old male had a Pantopaque myelogram because of chronic severe low backache without sciatic radiation. The myelogram shows a slight midline defect on the anterior aspect of the Pantopaque column at L4-5 *(arrow)*. The anterior aspect of the thecal sac at L5-S1 is also fairly remote from the lumbosacral interspace. The disk puncture clearly demonstrates normal disks at L4-5 and L5-S1.

Technique

Three approaches to the intervertebral disk are possible–lateral, posterolateral, and central (Figs 22–4, 22–5). The lateral and posterolateral approaches have the advantage of avoiding a transdural puncture. However, I have often had difficulty in entering the lumbosacral disk with the lateral approach. Hence, I prefer the posterolateral approach. The patient is sedated 1 hour prior to examination and then placed on a fluoroscopic table in the prone position on one or more pillows in order to spread the spinous processes as much as possible. After studying the preliminary anteroposterior and lateral films of the lumbar spine to determine the optimal angle of puncture, appropriate marks are made on the skin under fluoroscopic guidance. The skin is prepared by shaving and cleansing with pHisoHex, Betadine, and alcohol and draped with a fenestration sheet. The skin is infiltrated with 1% lidocaine at the proposed sites of injection.

In the posterolateral technique, the puncture begins lateral to the midline. The needle is angled superiorly and medially toward the disk to be injected. The needle passes lateral to the pedicle of the vertebra below the interspace and enters the disk lateral to the thecal sac. In the transdural midline approach, the needle puncture is made in the midline.

A 21-gauge spinal needle is inserted through the soft tissues to the level of the ligamentum flavum. A 26-gauge long needle is then introduced into the lumen of the 21-gauge needle and advanced into the intervertebral disk. When the needle enters the annulus fibrosus, there is a definite slight resistance followed by a "give" as the nucleus pulposus is punctured. If the needle meets firm resistance and can-

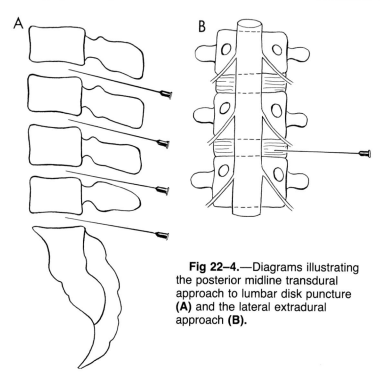

Fig 22–4.—Diagrams illustrating the posterior midline transdural approach to lumbar disk puncture **(A)** and the lateral extradural approach **(B)**.

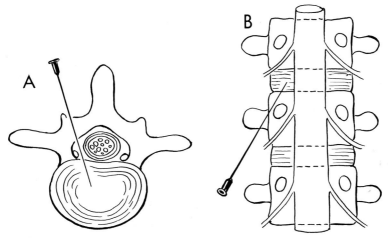

Fig 22–5.—Diagrams illustrating the posterolateral extradural approach to disk puncture.

not be readily advanced, it is in contact with bone and should be withdrawn and repositioned. This procedure is for the L2-3, L3-4, L4-5, and L5-S1 disks. When the examiner believes that the needles are properly placed or when there is difficulty in positioning the needles, a lateral roentgenogram is taken with the horizontal beam. Radiographic confirmation of the position of the inner needle should always be made before injecting contrast material. Appropriate needle adjustment can be made, if necessary, after viewing the roentgenogram. To date, I have used Hypaque (50%) or Renografin (60%) by manual injection (with a 10-ml Luer-Lok syringe and polyethylene tubing) under fluoroscopic control. However, metrizamide is undoubtedly a much safer contrast medium with respect to inadvertent subarachnoid injection. Care should be taken not to inject air along with the contrast medium (Fig 22–6). The normal lumbar disk will accept from 0.5 to 1.0 ml of solution with difficulty. At times, considerable pressure is necessary to force 0.5 ml into a normal disk. In general, one should inject contrast material to the point of mild resistance or reflux. In the absence of resistance or reflux, a maximum of 2–3 ml should be used, which is sufficient to demonstrate degeneration or rupture through a tear in the annulus. Usually, the patient has little or no pain when the normal disk is injected; when considerable pressure is required to inject the disk, there may be some back pain. If one persists in injecting the normal disk in the face of resistance, extravasation will occur. The extravasation may extend under the anterior longitudinal ligament, under the lateral ligaments, or posteriorly along the course of the needle into the extradural space. These overenthusiastic injections into the normal disk are often associated with atypical epigastric or back pain. The artifactual nature of the defects can readily be identified by the sharp, linear tracts surrounding the needle. When the pathologic disk is injected, the patient's clinical pain may be reproduced due to (1) escape of the contrast medium into the extradural space through a tear in the annulus or (2) compression of a nerve root by the ruptured disk as a result of distention of the interspace with contrast material. The needles may either be left in place or removed prior to radiography in the frontal and lateral projections. In addition to these standard views, a posteroanterior film

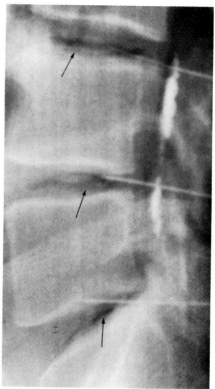

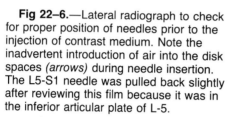

Fig 22–6.—Lateral radiograph to check for proper position of needles prior to the injection of contrast medium. Note the inadvertent introduction of air into the disk spaces *(arrows)* during needle insertion. The L5-S1 needle was pulled back slightly after reviewing this film because it was in the inferior articular plate of L-5.

is made with the tube tilted approximately 20 degrees caudad. In view of the lack of blood supply to the intervertebral disk, it is interesting that the contrast medium is usually absorbed within 30 minutes after injection. After the needles are removed, a sterile dressing is applied and the patient advised to remain recumbent for several hours.

Limitations and Disadvantages

Diskography is definitely more painful than myelography. At times, it may be impossible to puncture an intervertebral disk because of anatomic limitations. It is possible for the contrast medium to dissect posteriorly along the needle tract into the extradural space in the absence of an annular tear (Figs 22–7, 22–8). When this occurs in the presence of a degenerated disk, an erroneous diagnosis of a tear in the annulus with herniation may be made. The occurrence of pain on injection is not reliable. It may be absent in the presence of a frank herniation and present in an asymptomatic degenerated disk—because of this, I have found it difficult to evaluate the significance of pain. Disk degeneration begins at a fairly early age and may be completely asymptomatic. Hence, the use of diskography in patients over 35–40 years of age is probably not warranted.

Potential infection of the disk or interspace is not a contraindication to diskography. The complication of infection is due to a break in sterile technique, which may also occur in improperly performed myelography, with resulting septic arthritis or

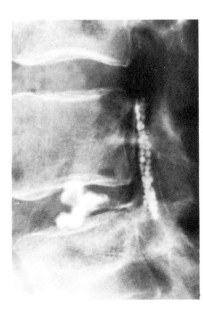

Fig 22–7.—Normal diskogram at L4-5 with posterior tracking of the contrast medium along the needle. There is some Pantopaque in the subarachnoid space from a previous myelogram.

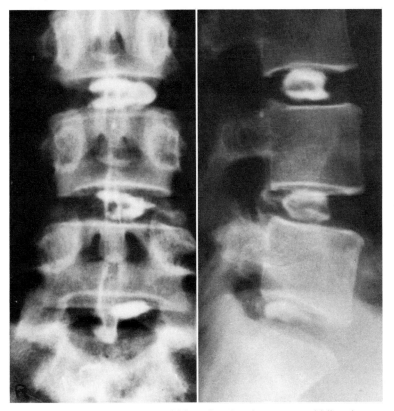

Fig 22–8.—Diskogram in a 25-year-old female, showing a normal bilocular appearance at L3-4 and L4-5. At L5-S1, the contrast was injected into the matrix outside the true cavity of the nucleus pulposus.

meningitis. Although herniation of the nucleus pulposus due to traumatic lumbar puncture has been reported in the literature, this complication has not been seen in experimental animals or humans following carefully performed disk punctures. Severe reactions and death have been described following accidental injection of Hypaque or Renografin into the subarachnoid space because of an error in technique. This can be avoided by taking a preliminary check film to be certain that the tip of each needle is well within the disk prior to injection of the contrast medium.

Kieffer and Peterson have shown that the infantile disk is characterized by a nucleus pulposus containing a clear gel surrounded by a dense annulus fibrosus thicker anteriorly. Disk puncture at this time demonstrates a flattened spheroidal unilocular collection of contrast material. During the first two decades, amorphous collagenous precipitates develop at the periphery of the nucleus, increase in size, and invaginate into the nucleus. Thus, one can consider the adult nucleus pulposus to consist of a central cavity surrounded by a spongy matrix that merges with the annulus. The cavity itself is usually, but not always, bilobar (bilocular) in the craniocaudad direction. Both locules are commonly demonstrated if one locule is injected with sufficient pressure. Quinnell and Stockdale have shown that artifacts can be produced by injecting the nuclear matrix outside the true central nuclear cavity (Figs 22–8, 22–9).

During the next several decades, nuclear involution occurs, with progressive fragmentation and reduction of nuclear material until the disk becomes a mass of

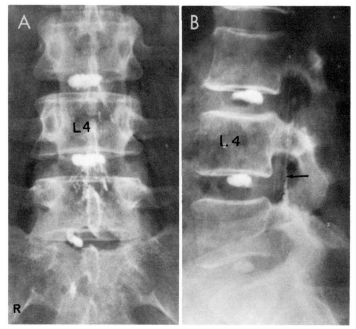

Fig 22–9.—Injection of the upper half of the collar button at L3-4 and L4-5. If slightly more contrast had been injected, the lower half of the nuclear cavity would have been seen to fill at fluoroscopy. The injection at L5-S1 was probably into the nuclear matrix outside the nuclear cavity itself. There is a residual trace of Pantopaque in the lumbar subarachnoid space from a previous myelogram *(arrow).*

fibrous tissue. With further aging, i.e., in the 50s and 60s, multiple fissures occur in the thinned-out, bulging disk. The bulging elevates the periosteum from the vertebral bodies, leading to osteophytic spurring.

The Normal Disk

The young adult nucleus pulposus varies in size from somewhat less than 1.0 to 2.5 cm, with no apparent relationship to body habitus. In general, the smaller nucleus tends to be round or oval in shape, whereas the larger nucleus is usually somewhat more rectangular. At times, the lumbosacral disk may be lozenge shaped (Fig 22–10). Following the injection of contrast medium, the normal nucleus in young patients (<30) may appear as a single transverse, homogeneous density, or as a bilocular density with a radiolucent band passing transversely through its center. The horizontal parallel densities are usually connected posteriorly but may be connected anteriorly as well.

In the lateral view, the normal annulus is frequently deeper anterior to the nucleus than it is posteriorly. Superiorly and inferiorly, the opacified spaces are limited by the vertebral cartilaginous plates. A decrease in vertical height, fissuring of the nucleus, and anterior or bilateral extension confined to the disk space without bulging of the annulus probably indicate early physiologic degeneration but are not regarded as pathologic for clinical purposes. Occasionally, the nucleus may extend

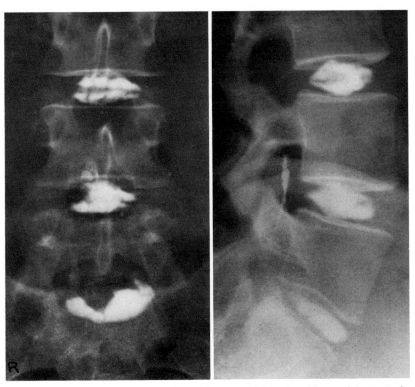

Fig 22–10.—Normal disk puncture in a 30-year-old female with persistent atypical left-sided sciatica. Note the lozenge shape of the lumbosacral disk. An antecedent myelogram (note residual Pantopaque) was entirely normal.

more posteriorly than normal without a bulge or a tear in the annulus (Fig 22–11). This change also probably is not clinically significant.

The Abnormal Disk

Four basic abnormal patterns may exist separately or together in varying combinations.

HERNIATION OF THE NUCLEUS PULPOSUS INTO THE VERTEBRAL BODY (SCHMORL'S NODE).—This most common type of herniation may occur either superiorly or inferiorly through a focal defect in the vertebral cartilaginous plate (Fig 22–12). The defect may be congenital, traumatic, or secondary to acquired infection or degenerative disease. When a Schmorl's node occurs as an isolated finding, it does not produce symptoms and is, therefore, of no clinical significance. At times, however, it may be associated with degenerative changes of the disk, particularly in the lower lumbar spine. The more chronic Schmorl's node is usually demonstrable on the conventional lateral roentgenogram as a defect in the vertebral body with or without marginal sclerosis outlining the periphery of the defect. In more recent herniations of the nucleus into the vertebral body, detectable changes on the plain roentgenogram may be absent. Under these circumstances, the diagnosis can be established only by diskography.

DIFFUSE DEGENERATION OF THE DISK.—The conventional roentgenogram usually demonstrates narrowing of the involved intervertebral disk space with osteophyte formation of the vertebral margins bridging the pathologic interspace. The

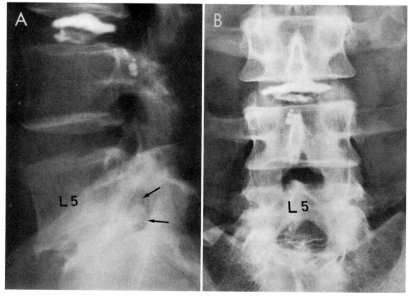

Fig 22–11.—Exaggerated posterior extension of the nucleus at L3-4 without bulging or a tear in the annulus is shown in **A.** This probably should be considered within normal limits for clinical purposes, although it may represent the "prebulging" phase of what eventually will turn out to be a pathologic disk. There is also a grossly pathologic disk at L5-S1, with diffuse degeneration and bulging into the canal posteriorly (arrows) through an annular tear.

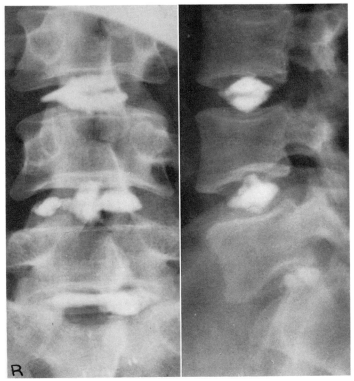

Fig 22–12.—Diskogram demonstrating herniation of the nucleus pulposus into the inferior articular plate of L-4.

diskogram, in turn, shows an irregular, thin distribution of contrast material throughout the entire narrow interspace (Figs 22–13, 22–14). These findings may be associated with significant elevation of the anterior, posterior, or lateral longitudinal ligaments, even with a central needle insertion and the injection of a small volume of contrast material. The changes may be either asymptomatic or associated with back pain; diskography per se cannot differentiate symptomatic from asymptomatic diffuse degeneration.

POSTERIOR BULGING OF THE ANNULUS.—A significant posterior bulge of the annulus without a demonstrable annular tear or extradural extravasation is abnormal (Fig 22–15).

HERNIATIONS ASSOCIATED WITH RUPTURE OF THE ANNULUS FIBROSUS.—This abnormality is characterized by extravasation of the contrast medium into the extradural space. The rent in the annulus may be located posteriorly, posterolaterally, or anteriorly. In extensive posterior tears, the contrast medium may collect beneath the posterior longitudinal ligament due to detachment of the posterior fibers of the annulus fibrosus from the cartilaginous vertebral plate. Posterior or posterolateral tears are the most common variety (Figs 22–15 to 22–21). The latter type is usually associated with sciatic pain whereas the posterior midline herniation is generally associated with low back pain without a radicular component.

In anterior herniation, the contrast material may collect under the anterior lon-

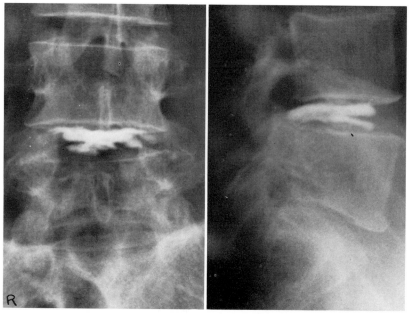

Fig 22–13.—Diskogram demonstrating diffuse degeneration of the disk at L4-5 with posterior bulging.

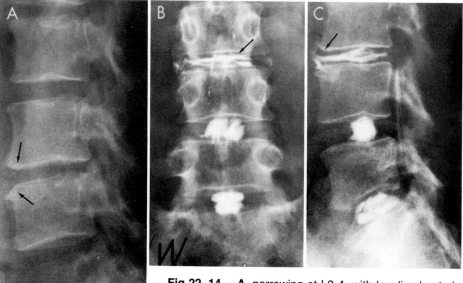

Fig 22–14.—**A,** narrowing at L3-4, with localized anterior spur formation involving the inferior margin of L-3 and the superior margin of L-4 *(arrows)*. Disk puncture **(B** and **C)** clearly demonstrates the diffuse degeneration of the L3-4 disk, with elevation of the anterior longitudinal ligament *(arrow)*. The L4-5 and L5-S1 disks are normal.

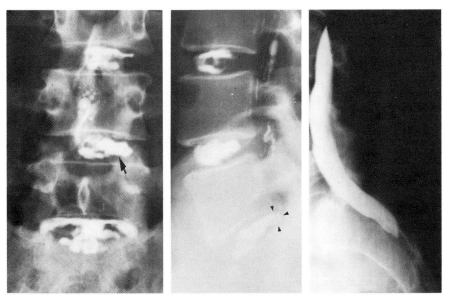

Fig 22–15.—Degeneration of the lumbosacral disk with posterior bulging and an intact annulus *(arrowheads).* The L3-4 disk is normal. The L4-5 disk is also normal, but some of the contrast material has been injected into the matrix outside the central nuclear cavity *(arrow).* The lateral myelographic film is normal.

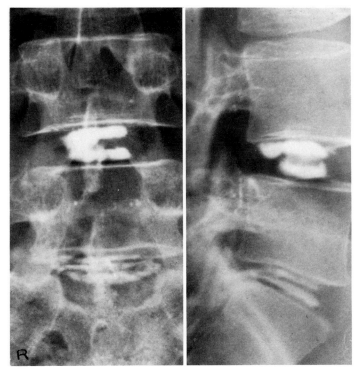

Fig 22–16.—Diskogram showing a right posterolateral tear at L5-S1. The L4-5 disk is normal.

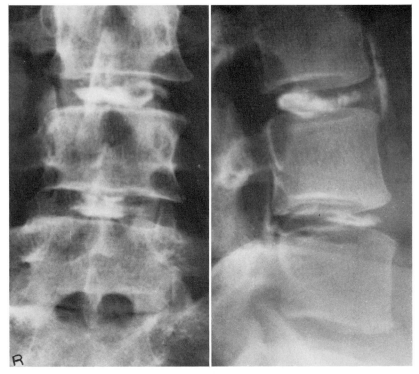

Fig 22–17.—Diskogram showing a posterior tear at L4-5. Note extension of the contrast medium into the extradural space. There is also an anterior tear at L3-4, with dissection of the contrast medium under the anterior longitudinal ligament.

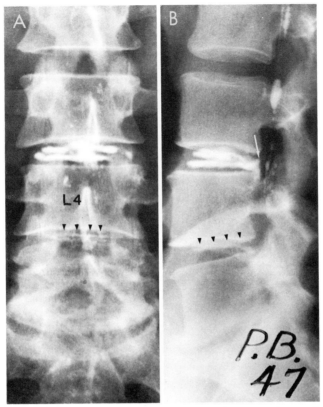

Fig 22–18.—Degenerated disk at L3-4 with a tear of the annulus and dissection of a nuclear fragment under the posterior longitudinal ligament *(arrow)*. The injection at L4-5 *(arrowheads)* was probably made into the inferior articular plate of L-4. Some residual Pantopaque can be seen from a previous myelogram.

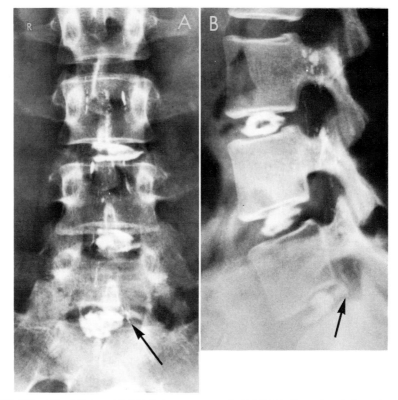

Fig 22–19.—The L3-4 and L4-5 disks are normal. At L5-S1, there is a left posterolateral tear of the annulus, with a corresponding nuclear protrusion *(arrow).*

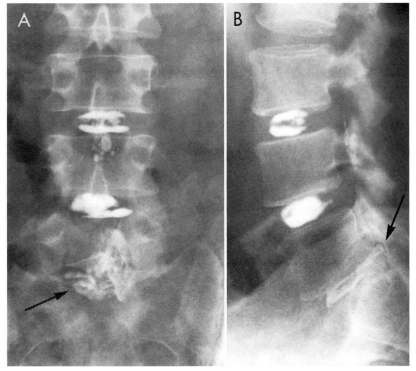

Fig 22–20.—Massive posterior herniation of a disk fragment into the canal *(arrow)* through a tear in the annulus and posterior longitudinal ligament.

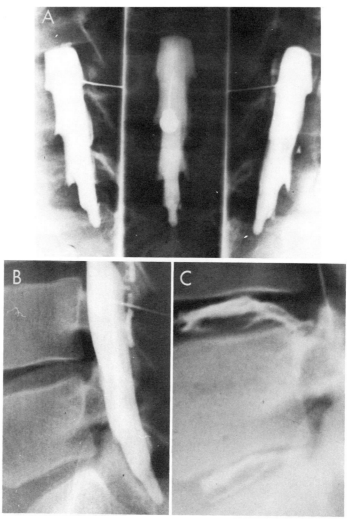

Fig 22–21.—The patient was a 25-year-old male with symptoms and signs of a lumbosacral disk herniation. The frontal and oblique myelographic films **(A)** show a shallow defect and absence of filling of the axillary sleeve at L4-5 on the reader's right. There is also elevation of the axillary sleeve at the lumbosacral interspace on the reader's right. The cross-table lateral film **(B)** shows the anterior aspect of the Pantopaque column to be quite remote from the back of the vertebral bodies. Diskography **(C)** clearly demonstrates disk herniations at both the L4-5 and L5-S1 spaces (confirmed at surgery).

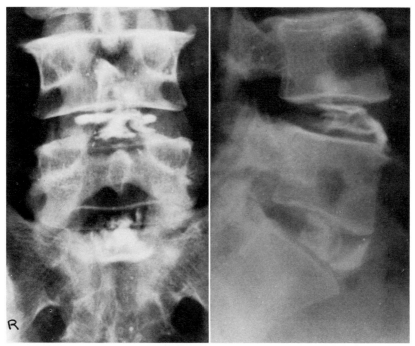

Fig 22–22.—Diskogram demonstrating dissection of contrast medium under the anterior longitudinal ligament at L4-5 and L5-S1. In the absence of other changes of disk degeneration, this is probably iatrogenic.

gitudinal ligament or may extend beyond the ligament (Fig 22–22). In the latter situation, a portion of the disk has become detached. Anterior herniation may occur as an isolated finding, or sometimes it may be associated with a posterior tear and diffuse disk degeneration.

There have been a number of critical studies questioning the reliability of lumbar diskography in the clinical diagnosis of the symptomatic herniated disk (Fernström, Holt). In general, I agree with the limitations described in the literature. However, prior to high-resolution CT, diskography had a definite limited role in the diagnosis of lumbar disk herniations, particularly in younger patients (<35 years of age) in the following circumstances:

1. Atypical findings and a negative myelogram. The demonstration of normal lumbar disks is reassuring and avoids unnecessary laminectomy (see Figs 22–1, 22–2, 22–10).

2. A discrepancy of incomplete correlation between the clinical localization and the myelographic defect (see Fig 22–21).

3. Clinical findings suggestive of L5-S1 herniation and a negative myelogram. Disk puncture may be helpful in demonstrating a significant herniation at the level where Pantopaque has its highest failure rate due to anatomical factors described previously (Figs 22–23; see also Fig 22–3).

4. Recurrent symptoms after laminectomy and removal of a disk herniation. Are the symptoms due to a second herniation at another level (Fig 22–24)?

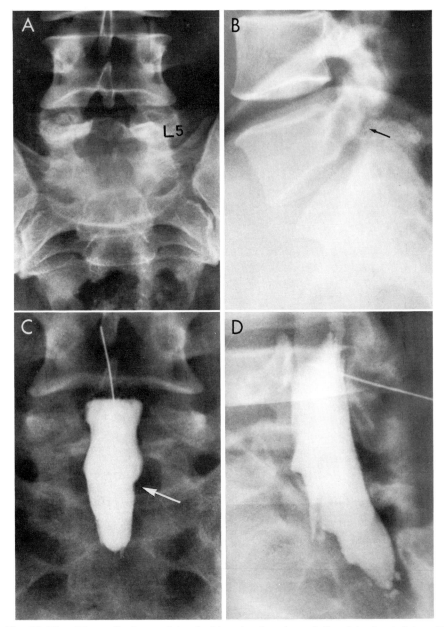

Fig 22–23.—The patient complained of low back pain radiating into the left leg. The plain films demonstrate a spina bifida occulta at L-5 and S-1 **(A)** and spondylolysis at L5-S1 **(B)** *(arrow)*. Myelography **(C–H)** shows minor asymmetry at L5-S1 *(arrow)* with a shallow defect on the left side of the oil column. Disk puncture **(F)** shows a marked posterior herniation of a fragment *(arrow)* into the spinal canal through a massive tear in the annulus and posterior longitudinal ligament (confirmed at surgery).

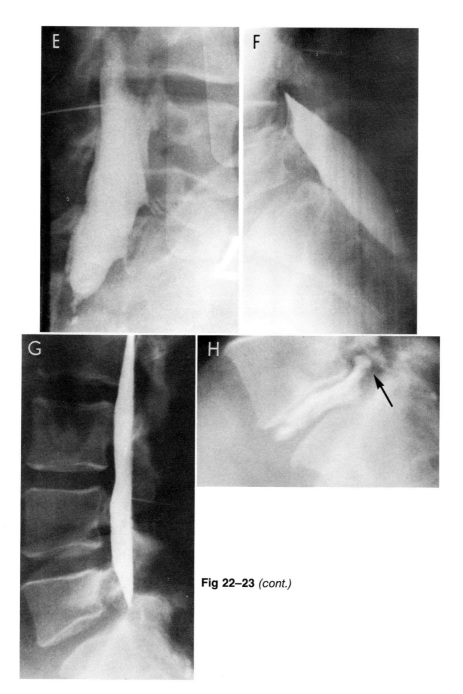

Fig 22–23 *(cont.)*

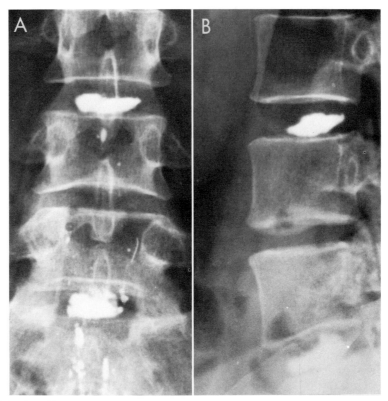

Fig 22–24.—The patient was a 33-year-old female who had a previous laminectomy for a herniated disk at L4-5. Note the slight narrowing and the minimal anterior spurring at this interspace. The patient developed recurrent low back pain a year later suggestive of a lumbosacral disk herniation. Disk puncture at L3-4 and L5-S1 shows normal disks at these interspaces. The L4-5 disk showed diffuse degeneration but no herniation (films not adequate for reproduction).

CERVICAL

Cervical diskography, originally introduced by Smith in 1952, has not gained widespread acceptance.

There are a number of papers in the literature questioning its validity. Holt injected three cervical disk spaces in each of 50 asymptomatic prison volunteers between the ages of 21 and 50 years. Extravasation of contrast medium occurred at two levels in all cases and in 80% of the remaining spaces. A normal configuration of the contrast medium within the nucleus was noted in only 10% of 148 disk spaces injected. Similarly, Sneider reported a total of 121 disks injected in 56 patients with all of the disks normal in only 1 patient. It is important to note that Holt and Sneider both used comparatively large-bore needles (20–22 gauge) instead of the 26-gauge needle recommended. Meyer, using a 25-gauge needle, also reported a series of 32 patients with neck, shoulder, or arm pain syndromes in whom the cervical diskogram was abnormal in every case. Both Sneider and Meyer noted frequent extravasation of contrast medium on the asymptomatic side. Sneider concluded that cervical diskography does not accurately elucidate the nature of cervical and upper-extremity pain and is of little help in determining the cause of symptoms following neck trauma. In view of the questionable validity of the findings in cervical diskography, I do not believe that this technique provides the crucial information in a diagnostic problem. Hence, I do not utilize cervical diskography.

BIBLIOGRAPHY

Butt W.P.: Lumbar discography. *J. Can. Assoc. Radiol.* 14:172, 1963.

Butt W.P.: Discography—some interesting cases. *J. Can. Assoc. Radiol.* 17:167, 1966.

Cloward R.B.: Cervical diskography. *Am. J. Roentgenol.* 79:563, 1958.

Cloward R.B., Buzaid L.L.: Discography; technic, indications and evaluation of normal and abnormal disk. *Am. J. Roentgenol.* 68:552, 1952.

Collis J.S.: *Lumbar Discography.* Springfield, Ill., Charles C Thomas, Publisher, 1963.

Collis J.S., Jr., Gardner W.J.: Lumbar discography; analysis of one thousand cases. *J. Neurosurg.* 19:452, 1962.

Davies J.J., Peirce E.C., II: Discography in diagnosis of herniation of lower lumbar disks. *Illinois Med. J.* 104:118, 1953.

Edholm P., Fernström P., Lindblom K.: Extradural lumbar disc puncture. *Acta Radiol. (Diagn.)* 6:322, 1967.

Erlacher P.: Klinische und diagnostische Bedeutung der Nukleographie. *Ztschr. Orthop.* 79:273, 1950.

Erlacher P.R.: Direkte Kontrastdarstellung des Nucleus Pulposus, zugleich ein Beitrag zur Pathologie der Bandscheibe. *Ztschr. Orthop.* 80:40, 1950.

Erlacher P.R.: Nucleography. *J. Bone Joint Surg.* 34B:204, 1952.

Feinberg S.B.: The place of diskography in radiology as based on 2,320 cases. *Am. J. Roentgenol.* 92:1275, 1964.

Fernström U.: A discographical study of ruptured lumbar intervertebral disc. *Acta Chir. Scandinav.* (Suppl.) 258, 1960.

Friedman J., Goldner M.Z.: Discography in evaluation of lumbar disk lesions. *Radiology* 65:653, 1955.

Gardner W.J., et al.: X-ray visualization of intervertebral disk (by injection of iodopyracet) with consideration of morbidity of disk puncture. *A.M.A. Arch. Surg.* 64:355, 1952.

Greig J.H., Wignell N.: A case of arachnoiditis associated with "Pantopaque" myelography. *J. Can. Assoc. Radiol.* 17:198, 1966.

Hirsch C.: An attempt to diagnose the level of a disk lesion clinically by disk puncture. *Acta Orthop. Scandinav.* 18:132, 1948.

Holt E.P., Jr.: The question of lumbar discography. *J. Bone Joint Surg.* 50A:720, 1968.

Keck C.: Discography: Technique and interpretation. *Arch. Surg.* 80:580, 1960.

Kieffer S.A., Stadlan E.M., Mohandas A., Peterson H.O.: Discographic-anatomical correlation of developmental changes with age in the intervertebral disc. *Acta Radiol. (Diagn.)* 9:733, 1969.

Klafta L.A., Jr., Collis J.S., Jr.: An analysis of cervical discography with surgical verification. *J. Neurosurg.* 30:38, 1969.

Lindblom K.: Discography of dissecting transosseous rupture of disks in lumbar region. *Acta Radiol.* 36:12, 1951.

Martin C.M.: Myelography with sodium diatrizoate (Hypaque). Report of a case of inadvertent use complicated by acute renal failure. *California Med.* 115:57, 1971.

Meyer R.R.: Cervical diskography. A help or hindrance in evaluating neck, shoulder, arm pain? *Am. J. Roentgenol.* 90:1208, 1963.

Morretin L.B., Wilson M.: Severe reflex algodystrophy (Sudeck's atrophy) as a complication of myelography. Report of two cases. *Am. J. Roentgenol.* 110:156, 1970.

Nordlander S., Salén E.F., Unander-Scharin L.: Discography in low back pain and sciatica. Analysis of 73 operated cases. *Acta Orthop. Scandinav.* 28:90, 1958.

Park W.M.: Fissuring of the posterior annulus fibrosus in the lumbar spine. *Br. J. Radiol.* 52:382, 1979.

Perey O.: Contrast medium examination of the intervertebral discs of the lower lumbar spine. *Acta Orthop. Scandinav.* 20:327, 1951.

Quinnell R.C., Stockdale H.R.: An investigation of artefacts in lumbar discography. *Br. J. Radiol.* 53:831, 1980.

Quinnell R.C., Stockdale H.R., Harmon B.: Pressure standardized lumbar discography. *Br. J. Radiol.* 53:1031, 1980.

Simmons E.H., Bhalla S.K.: Anterior cervical discectomy and fusion with a note on discography. Technique and interpretation of results. *J. Bone Joint Surg.* 51B:225, 1963.

Smith G.W.: The normal cervical diskogram. *Am. J. Roentgenol.* 81:1006, 1959.

Smith G.W., Nichols P., Jr.: The technic of cervical discography. *Radiology* 68:718, 1957.

Sneider S.E., Winslow O.P., Jr., Pryor T.H.: Cervical diskography: Is it relevant? *J.A.M.A.* 185:163, 1963.

Stuck R.M.: Roentgen study in cervical discography. *Am. J. Roentgenol.* 86:975, 1961.

Walk L.: *Lumbar Diskography and Its Clinical Evaluation.* Springfield, Ill., Charles C Thomas, Publisher, 1962.

Wilson D.H., MacCarty W.C.: Discography: Its role in the diagnosis of lumbar disc protrusion. *J. Neurosurg.* 31:520, 1969.

Wolkin J., Sachs M.D., Hoke G.H.: Comparative studies of discography and myelography. *Radiology* 64:704, 1955.

Wollin D.G., Lamon C.B., Cawley A.J., Wortzman G.: The neurotoxic effects of water-soluble contrast media in the spinal canal with emphasis on appropriate management. *J. Can. Assoc. Radiol.* 19:296, 1967.

Young D.A., Burney R.E., II: Complication of myelography. Transection and withdrawal of a nerve filament by the needle. *N. Engl. J. Med.* 285:156, 1971.

23

Epidural Venography

In 1951, Anderson visualized the vertebral vein system in a living patient by injecting Diodrast into the femoral vein with compression of the inferior vena cava. Four years later, Helander and Lindblom used the same technique to demonstrate lumbar disk herniation. In the interim, i.e., 1952, Fischgold et al. opacified the vertebral venous plexus by injecting aqueous contrast material into a vertebral spinous process. The latter technique was popularized by Schobinger, Isherwood, and others who employed it to evaluate a variety of extradural lesions, i.e., herniated lumbar disks, extradural metastases. The many disadvantages of the intraosseous approach (severe pain, unpredictable filling of the internal vertebral venous plexus, inadvertent injection into the subarachnoid space) spurred Gargano and Bücheler independently to utilize selective catheterization of the ascending lumbar vein. Since Gargano's and Bücheler's original contributions, many other investigators have published their experience with, and refinement of, this technique.

TECHNIQUE

I commonly perform epidural venography on an outpatient basis. The meal prior to the study is withheld. I do not routinely premedicate the patient, although I do not hesitate to use diazepam (Valium) in a very tense or nervous individual. The patient is told to avoid aspirin and other medication containing aspirin for 24 hours prior to, and after, the study. A femoral vein is catheterized by the Seldinger technique, using a no. 5F or no. 6F end-hole catheter. I usually catheterize the right femoral vein because it is more convenient and comfortable for me to work from the right side. Others recommend the left femoral vein. I do not hesitate to use the left side if I encounter any difficulty on the right. I prefer to place the catheter in the radicular vein (at the appropriate level), the lateral sacral vein, or the ascending lumbar vein on the side in question (Fig 23–1). The left ascending lumbar vein is usually larger than its mate on the right side. I have rarely found it necessary to employ the double catheter technique with bilateral simultaneous injections. Failure to opacify both sides from a unilateral injection can usually be overcome by repositioning the catheter in another vessel (Figs 23–2, 23–3). I use a total of 25 ml of Conray-60 at the rate of 5 ml/sec during abdominal compression and

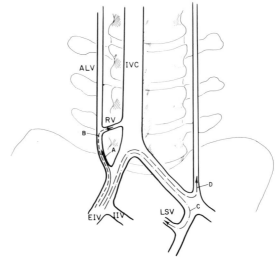

Fig 23–1.—Diagram of various possible catheter positions. *IVC* = inferior vena cava; *ALV* = ascending lumbar vein; *EIV* = external iliac vein; *IIV* = internal iliac vein; *RV* = radicular vein; Position *A* = right ascending lumbar vein; position *B* = right radicular vein at L4-5; position *C* = left lateral sacral vein; position *D* = left ascending lumbar vein.

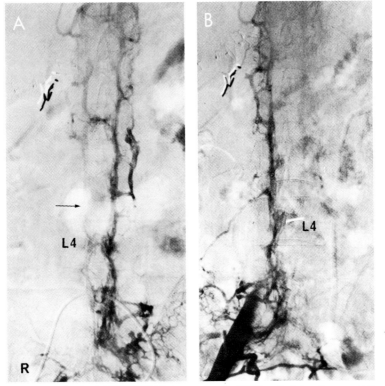

Fig 23–2.—This patient required two injections because adequate bilateral filling of the anterior internal vertebral plexus was not achieved initially. **A,** injection of the left lateral sacral vein results in good filling of the left anterior internal vertebral vein and inadequate filling on the right side at L3-4 *(arrow).* **B,** reinjection into the right ascending lumbar vein fills this vessel at L4-5; note that there is no filling on the left side. The patient's disk puncture at this level was entirely normal.

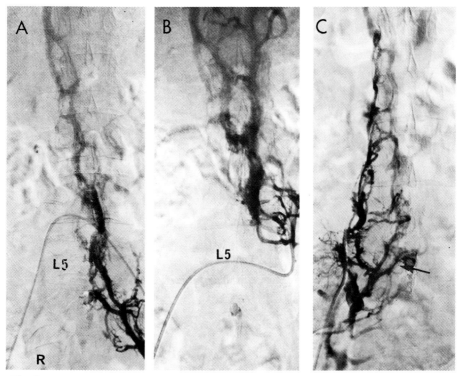

Fig 23–3.—Three separate injections into three different catheter positions were necessary in this patient to complete the examination. **A,** the first injection in the left lateral sacral vein fills the anterior internal vertebral vein (AIVV) on the left at L5-S1 and then crosses over to the right side with no filling on the left above L4-5. **B,** the second injection into the left ascending lumbar vein fills the left AIVV at L4-5 and both AIVV above this level. **C,** the third injection into the right ascending lumbar vein demonstrates obstruction of the right AIVV at L5-S1 *(arrow)*.

the Valsalva maneuver. An injection delay is utilized to obtain one blank film for later subtraction. Filming is carried out in the anteroposterior projection with the patient supine, at the rate of one film per second for ten seconds. At times, additional injections are necessary; rarely, oblique or lateral films are required. Following the procedure, the patient remains in the supine position and is observed for 1 to 2 hours. If there is no bleeding, the patient is discharged on limited activity for the rest of the day.

ANATOMY

The valveless vertebral veins may be divided into external and internal systems, which freely communicate with one another (Figs 23–4, 23–5). The important external vertebral veins in epidural venography are the ascending lumbar and lateral sacral veins. The right and left ascending lumbar veins communicate with the inferior vena cava or with the first and second lumbar veins on either side. The ascending lumbar veins usually arise from the common iliac veins to ascend in the

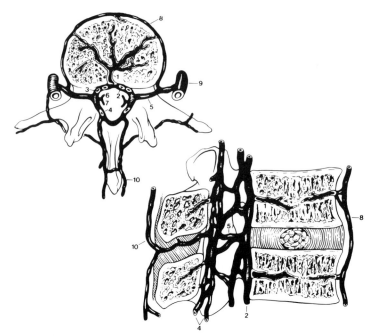

Fig 23–4.—Axial and midsagittal diagrams of the lumbar vertebral plexus. *1,* basivertebral vein. *2,* medial anterior internal vertebral vein (AIVV). *3,* lateral AIVV. *4,* posterior internal vertebral vein. *5,* intervertebral vein. *6,* anterior radicular vein. *7,* posterior radicular vein. *8,* anterior external vertebral vein. *9,* ascending lumbar vein. *10,* posterior external vertebral plexus.

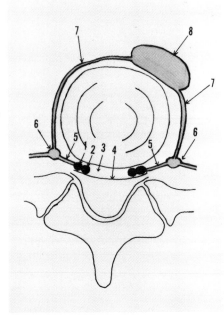

Fig 23–5.—Diagram of an axial section through L3-4 disk demonstrating the anterior internal vertebral (epidural) veins and their communication with the external vertebral plexus. *1,* lateral epidural vein. *2,* medial epidural vein. *3,* anterior epidural fat. *4,* anterior surface of dura. *5,* radicular vein. *6,* ascending lumbar veins. *7,* lumbar veins. *8,* inferior vena cava.

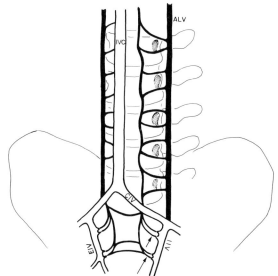

Fig 23–6.—Diagram showing the relationship of the inferior vena cava *(IVC)*, the common *(CIV)*, external *(EIV)*, and internal *(IIV)* veins *(unshaded)* to the ascending lumbar *(ALV)* and epidural veins *(black)*. The lateral sacral veins are designated by arrows.

bony groove at the junction of the vertebral bodies, pedicles, and transverse processes (Fig 23–6). They ultimately drain into the azygos vein on the right side and the hemiazygos vein on the left. A single lateral sacral vein passes through each sacral foramen to connect the external vertebral plexus and the internal vertebral vein (see Fig 23–6).

The important internal vertebral veins in epidural venography are the anterior internal (longitudinal) vertebral veins. The latter usually lie in the anterolateral angle of the spinal canal on either side (Fig 23–7). They are usually in intimate contact with the posterior longitudinal ligament and the intervertebral disk anterior to the thecal sac. Experience with combined CT–epidural venography has, on rare occasion, demonstrated a more posterior position of one or more anterior epidural veins, somewhat remote from a normal disk. Although it has been my impression that there are smaller posterior internal (longitudinal) vertebral veins, Theron de-

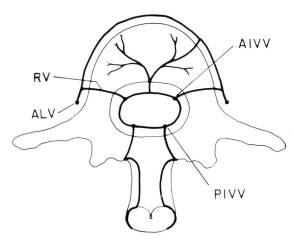

Fig 23–7.—Axial diagram of the vertebral venous plexus.

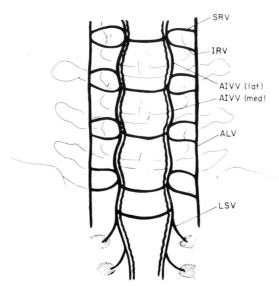

Fig 23–8.—Diagram showing the usual epidural venous anatomy. Note that the veins bend laterally at the level of the disk interspace and medially at the level of the pedicles. *SRV,* superior radicular vein. *IRV,* inferior radicular vein. *AIVV (lat),* lateral anterior internal vertebral veins. *AIVV (med),* medial anterior internal vertebral vein. *ALV,* ascending lumbar vein. *LSV,* lateral sacral vein.

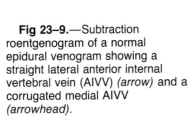

Fig 23–9.—Subtraction roentgenogram of a normal epidural venogram showing a straight lateral anterior internal vertebral vein (AIVV) *(arrow)* and a corrugated medial AIVV *(arrowhead).*

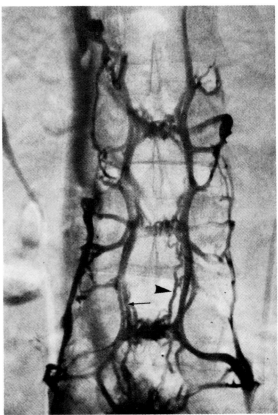

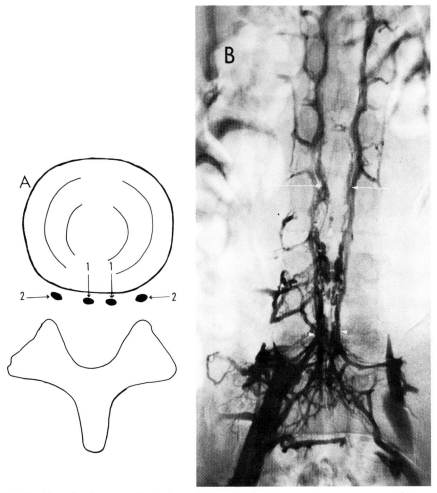

Fig 23–10.—A, diagram of axial section at the lumbosacral interspace demonstrating the medial *(1)* and lateral *(2)* anterior epidural veins forming a horizontal string of beads. According to Theron, there are no posterior internal epidural veins. **B,** subtraction film from a normal epidural venogram demonstrating the closer position of the medial epidural veins at L5-S1 *(arrowheads)* compared with their more lateral position at the more proximal lumbar interspaces *(arrows).*

nies their existence. In any event, they are insignificant even if they do exist because they are remote from the disk.

In the frontal projection, the right and left anterior internal vertebral veins and their connecting transverse veins form a palisade of ovals or hexagons (Fig 23–8). These vessels deviate laterally at each disk level and then medially at the level of the pedicles, where they unite via a connecting vein. Usually there is a lateral anterior epidural vein that tends to be fairly tubular and a more corrugated or undulating medial anterior epidural vein on each side (Fig 23–9). At the lumbar levels other than L5-S1, the lateral and medial epidural veins on each side lie fairly close to one another in the anterolateral angle of the canal. At the lumbosacral interspace, the lateral epidural vein tends to lie more laterally and the medial epidural vein more medially, resembling a string of beads (Fig 23–10). Below the lumbosacral interspace, one frequently is unable to identify four discrete anterior epidural veins. Instead, one commonly finds a series of radicular veins paralleling the corresponding nerve roots as they exit from the anterior sacral foramina.

The connecting transverse veins between the internal and external vertebral systems are (1) anastomosing veins at the level of the pedicles, and (2) the radicular veins, which are usually bilateral paired vessels, above and below the pedicles, traversing the intervertebral foramen at each level. These vessels present a characteristic stepladder appearance on either side. The vein passing below the pedicle is the important vessel because it is intimately associated with the exiting nerve root (see Fig 23–8).

INTERPRETATION OF PATHOLOGIC FINDINGS

This chapter is limited to a consideration of the abnormal findings in lumbar disk herniations. It does not consider epidural metastases, spinal stenosis, and other lesions. A review of the pertinent literature reveals a considerable difference of opinion concerning the accuracy of epidural venography in the diagnosis of lumbar disk herniation. Teal et al. claim that this technique has a 30% incidence of false positive diagnosis, while Gershater indicates a false positive rate as low as 0.3–1%. In my experience, lumbar epidural venography is a reliable, accurate method for the diagnosis of lumbar disk herniation, provided that appropriate technique and "hard-core" criteria for diagnosis are used.

The important vessels to evaluate in the diagnosis of lumbar disk herniation are

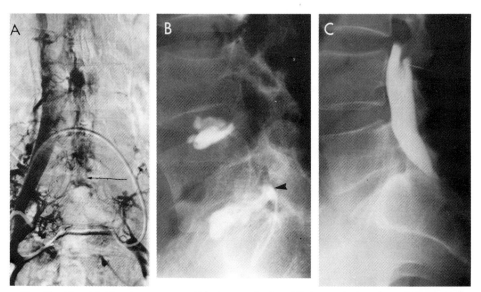

Fig 23–11.—Epidural venogram **(A)** demonstrating bilateral obstruction of the anterior internal vertebral vein (AIVV) at L5-S1 in a 35-year-old man *(arrow)*. Note the posterior herniation of the large free fragment in the canal on the disk puncture *(arrowhead)*, **(B)** and the negative myelogram because of the considerable distance of the anterior thecal sac from the posterior aspect of the disk at the lumbosacral interspace **(C).** Epidural venography and diskography are frequently more accurate than myelography at L5-S1 for this reason.

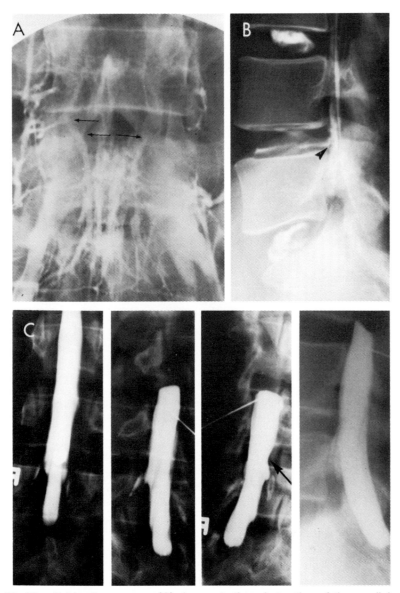

Fig 23–12.—Epidural venogram **(A)** demonstrating obstruction of the medial anterior internal vertebral vein (AIVV) and marked bilateral displacement of the lateral AIVV *(arrows)* at L4-5. The diskogram **(B)** shows a large posterior tear *(arrowhead)* with free extravasation of the contrast into the anterior epidural space *(arrow)*. The myelogram **(C)** shows an extradural defect in the anterolateral aspect of the Pantopaque column at the L4-5 level *(arrow)*.

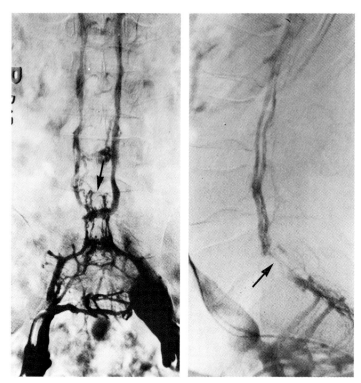

Fig 23–13.—AP and lateral subtraction films from an epidural venogram showing bilateral marked attenuation and a high grade obstruction of the anterior internal vertebral vein (AIVV) *(arrow)* at the lumbosacral interspace due to a large central disk herniation.

the anterior internal vertebral, and the radicular veins. The most dependable signs of a clinically significant disk herniation are (1) compression (narrowing, attenuation) or (2) occlusion (complete interruption) of these veins with good filling above and below the level in question (Figs 23–11 to 23–14). The veins above the pathologic obstructive disk fill by collateral flow. Absence of venous filling at or above the lumbosacral level with satisfactory filling below is usually due to technical factors. In these circumstances, another vein should be catheterized and injected (Fig 23–15). It is not uncommon to find simple venous displacement without compression in patients with asymptomatic bulging of the disk. Hence, this is not a reliable sign per se (Fig 23–16; see also Fig 23–14). In my experience, collateral flow, excessive caudal flow, or localized dilatation of the anterior internal vertebral veins have not proved to be reliable signs of disk herniation in the absence of venous compression or obstruction. The type and degree of venous compression are related to the location and size of the herniated disk. A significant central disk herniation produces bilateral posterolateral displacement and compression or occlusion of both anterior internal vertebral veins. Similar findings are rarely produced by a bulging disk with an intact annulus. A posterolateral disk herniation usually produces unilateral compression or obstruction of the ipsilateral anterior internal vertebral vein or the radicular vein or both. Compression or obstruction of a radicular vein is usually associated with similar changes in the ipsilateral anterior internal vertebral vein.

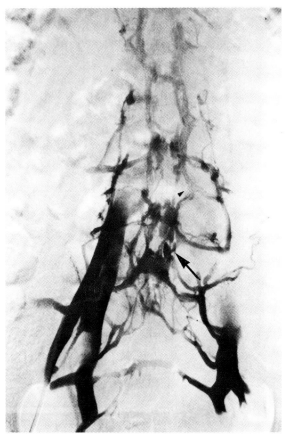

Fig 23–14.—Subtraction roentgenogram showing occlusion of the left anterior internal vertebral vein at L5-S1 *(thick arrow)*—a definite positive finding confirmed at surgery. Note also the slight lateral displacement of the left AIVV at L4-5 *(arrowhead)* due to a slight bulge of the disk with an intact annulus (confirmed at surgery).

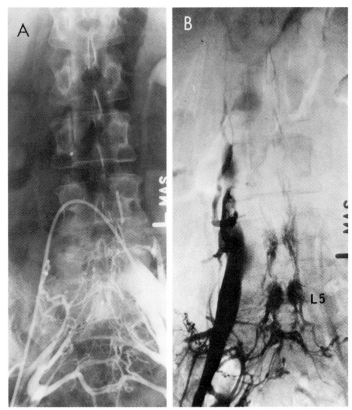

Fig 23–15.—False positive obstruction at L5-S1 due to technical factors on the first injection into the left internal iliac vein. Note the excellent filling below the lumbosacral interspace and the absent filling above this level **(A).** Injection after repositioning of the catheter into the right ascending lumbar vein shows normal filling of the anterior internal vertebral vein at L4-5 and L5-S1 **(B).**

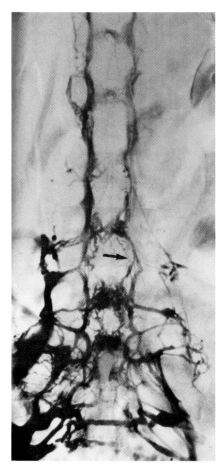

Fig 23–16.—Subtraction film from an epidural venogram showing lateral displacement without compression of the left anterior internal vertebral vein at L4-5 *(arrow)*—a soft finding. Diskography was normal.

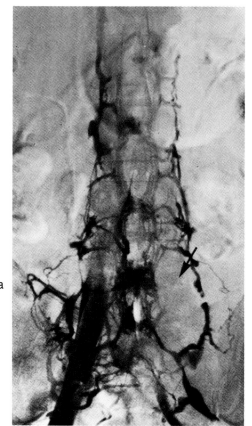

Fig 23–17.—Subtraction film from an epidural venogram showing nonfilling of the left radicular vein at L5-S1 *(arrow)*—a soft finding. Diskography was normal.

Poor or absent filling of a radicular vein per se is not a reliable sign, in my experience (Fig 23–17).

ACKNOWLEDGMENTS.—I would like to thank the editor of *Radiographic Evaluation of the Spine*, Dr. M. Judith Donovan Post, and the publishers, Masson Publishing Co. U.S.A., Inc., for permission to use many of the illustrations that appeared in Chapter 29.

BIBLIOGRAPHY

Anderson R.K.: Diodrast studies of the vertebral and cranial venous system. *J. Neurosurg.* 8:411, 1951.

Arbuckle R.K., Shelden C.H., Pudenz, R.H.: Pantopaque myelography—correlation of roentgenologic and neurologic findings. *Radiology* 45:356, 1945.

Batson O.V.: The function of the vertebral veins and their role in the spread of metastases. *Ann. Surg.* 112:138, 1940.

Begg A.C., Falconer M.A., McGeorge M.: Myelography in lumbar intervertebral disk lesions—correlation with operative findings. *Br. J. Surg.* 34:141, 1946.

Bücheler E., Dux A., Venbrocks H.P.: Die direkte vertebrale Venographie die lumbalen Bandscheibenhernien. *Fortschr. Geb. Röntgenstrahlen* 109:593, 1968.

Camp J.D.: Contrast myelography, past and present. *Radiology* 54:477, 1950.

Epstein B.S.: Low back pain associated with varices of the epidural veins simulating herniation of the nucleus pulposus. *Am. J. Roentgenol.* 57:736, 1947.

Finney L.A., Gargano F.P., Buermann A.: Intraosseous vertebral venography in the diagnosis of lumbar disk disease. *Am. J. Roentgenol.* 92:1282, 1964.

Fischgold H., Adam H., Ecoiffier J., Piequet J.: Opacification des plexus rachidiens et des veines azygos par voie osseuse. *J. Radiol. et Électrol.* 33:37, 1952.

Ford L.T., Key J.A.: Evaluation of myelography in diagnosis of intervertebral disc lesions in low back. *J. Bone Joint Surg.* 32A:257, 1950.

Gargano F.P., Meyer J.D., Sheldon J.J.: Transfemoral ascending lumbar catheterization of the epidural veins in lumbar disk disease. *Radiology* 111:329, 1974.

Gershater R., Holgate R.: Lumbar epidural venography in the diagnosis of disc herniations. *A.J.R.* 126:992, 1976.

Helander C.G., Lindblom A.: Sacrolumbar venography. *Acta Radiol.* 44:410, 1955.

Isherwood I.: Spinal intra-osseous venography. *Clin. Radiol.* 13:73, 1962.

Koch R., Nobbe F.: Die selektive retroperitoneal Venographie in der Diagnostik von lumbalen Diskusprolapsen. *Ztschr. Orthop.* 109:201, 1971.

Larde D.: Le veines epidurales lombosacrees. Étude anatomique et radiologique. Interet de la phlebographie lombaire dans le diagnostic des discopathies. Thesis, Nancy, 1977.

Leader S.A., Rassell M.J.: The value of Pantopaque myelography in the diagnosis of herniation of the nucleus pulposus in the lumbosacral spine. *Am. J. Roentgenol.* 69:231, 1953.

Lessman F.P., Schobinger R., Lasser E.C.: Intraosseous venography. *Acta Radiol.* 44:397, 1955.

Lotz P.R., Seeger J.F., Gabrielsen T.O.: Prospective comparison of epidural venography and iophendylate myelography in the diagnosis of herniated lumbar disks. *Radiology* 134:127, 1980.

Maltby G.L., Pendergrass R.C.: Pantopaque myelography. *Radiology* 47:35, 1946.

Nathan M.H., Blum L.: Evaluation of vertebral venography. *Am. J. Roentgenol.* 83:1027, 1960.

Oberson R., Azam F.: CAT of the spine and spinal cord. *Neuroradiology* 16:369, 1978.

Resjö I.M., Harwood-Nash D.C., Fitz C.R., Chuang S.: Computed tomographic metrizamide myelography in spinal dysraphism in infants and children. *J. Comput. Assist. Tomogr.* 2:549, 1979.

Resjö I.M., Harwood-Nash D.C., Fitz C.R., Chuang S.: Computed tomographic metrizamide myelography in syringohydromyelia. *Radiology* 131:405, 1979.

Resjö I.M., Harwood-Nash D.C., Fitz C.R., Chuang S.: Normal cord in infants and children examined with computed tomographic metrizamide myelography. *Radiology* 130:691, 1979.

Schobinger R.: *Intra-osseous Venography*. New York, Grune & Stratton, 1960.

Schobinger R., Krueger E.F.: Intraosseous epidural venography in the diagnosis of surgical diseases of the lumbar spine. *Acta Radiol.* (Stockh.) 1:763, 1963.

Schobinger R.A., Krueger E.G., Sobel L.: Comparison of intra-osseous vertebral venography and Pantopaque myelography in the diagnosis of surgical condition of the lumbar spine and nerve roots. *Radiology* 77:376, 1961.

Scoville W.B., Moretz W.H., Hankins W.D.: Discrepancies in myelography. *Surg., Gynecol. Obstet.* 86:559, 1948.

Shapiro R.: *Myelography*, ed. 2. Chicago, Year Book Medical Publishers, 1968, p. 392.

Teal J.S., Ahmadi J., Zee C.S.: Inconsistent venous opacification: A pitfall of epidural venography. *A.J.N.R.* 3:157, 1982.

Theron J., Moret J.: Spinal phlebography. Berlin, Springer-Verlag, 1978.

24

Lumbar Epidurography

H. Paul Hatten, Jr., M.D.

THE LUMBAR EPIDURAL SPACE was first visualized radiographically by accident in 1921 by the Frenchmen Sicard and Forestier while they were attempting to inject Lipiodol (an oily iodinated material) for the treatment of "rheumatism." Early radiographic techniques for performing epidurography were described in 1941, using air (Sanford and Doub) and Perabrodil (Knutson), an ionic water-soluble contrast material which was widely used in Europe. Although the term lumbar epidurography most accurately describes the anatomical location of the procedure, other terms such as peridurography and canalography have been used, particularly in Europe.

Several large European series of lumbar epidurograms have been reported in the literature, i.e., Luyendijk and van Voorthiusen from the Netherlands (600 cases), and Lewit from Czechoslovakia (102 cases). The Japanese (Nagamine) have also had some experience with this technique. Dr. C. C. McCormick from Perth, Australia has made an excellent comparison of lumbar epidurography, lumbar discography, and lumbar epidural venography.

However, there is limited experience with lumbar epidurography in the United States. Kido et al. recorded their experience with metrizamide epidurography in dogs; Bromage et al. reported on metrizamide epidurography in both dogs and humans; and Roberson, Hatten, and Hesselink reported a clinical series of lumbar epidurograms from the Massachusetts General Hospital in 1979. This latter series included 53 epidurograms with Dimer-X and iothalamate meglumine (Conray-60) as the contrast media. Both of these media are no longer used because of their toxicity in the event of accidental entry into the subarachnoid space.

Metrizamide is presently the safest contrast material for both the subarachnoid and epidural spaces. The only large clinical series of metrizamide lumbar epidurograms (65 studies) was reported by Hatten in 1980.

ANATOMY

The epidural space extends from the foramen magnum to the sacral notch hiatus. This space is bounded medially by the dura mater and laterally by the periosteum of the vertebral bodies. At the level of the intervertebral foramen, the lateral border of the space is absent, thus permitting lateral flow of contrast material along the nerve root sheaths. The lumbar epidural space contains loose areolar tissue,

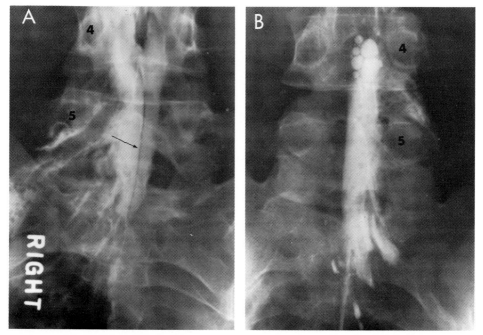

Fig 24–1.—Plica mediana dorsalis seen as median translucency **(A)** *(arrow)* and as a structure totally separating the lumbar epidural space into right and left compartments in another patient in whom only the left side is visualized **(B)**.

adipose tissue, the epidural venous plexus, and the spinal nerve roots with their dural investments.

The plica mediana dorsalis is a very important anatomical structure. On the epidurogram, it is visualized as a thin median translucency that may totally separate the lumbar epidural space into right and left compartments. The presence of the plica stimulated the development of a selective catheter technique to allow consistent visualization of the nerve roots on the side of clinical interest (Hatten).

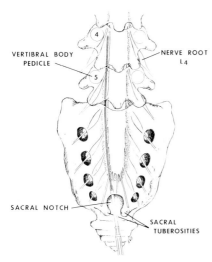

Fig 24–2.—Line drawing with guidewire in epidural space, showing relationship of nerve roots to vertebral body pedicles.

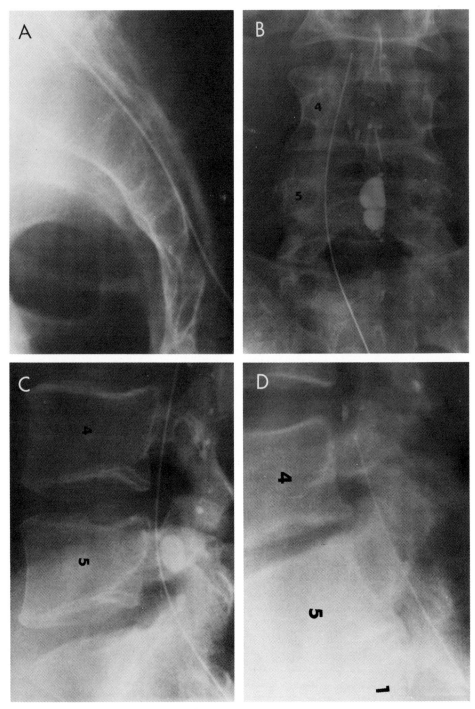

Fig 24–3.—Multiple guidewire positions. Lateral radiograph of normal position guidewire in sacrum **(A).** AP radiograph of normal position guidewire in low lumbar epidural space **(B).** Lateral radiograph of guidewire in ventral epidural space **(C)** and dorsal epidural space **(D).**

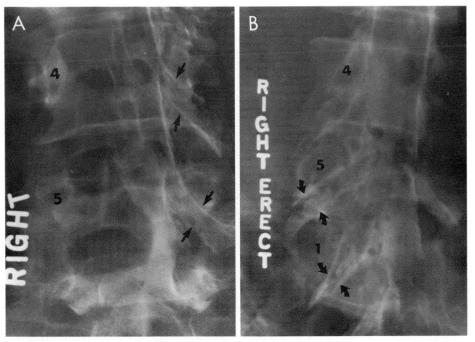

Fig 24–4.—AP **(A)** and oblique **(B)** radiographs with arrows outlining normal nerve root sheath filling. Good example of relationship of nerve root to vertebral body pedicle and the lateral extension of contrast along nerve root sheath.

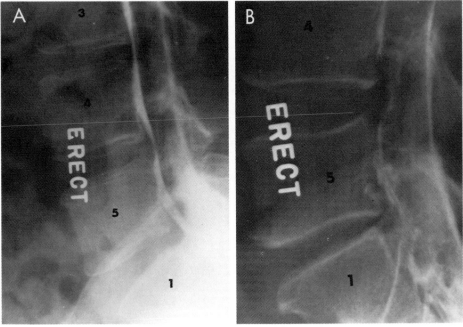

Fig 24–5.—Lateral radiographs in erect position in two different patients. Note ventral layering of contrast and filling of the dorsal lumbar epidural space.

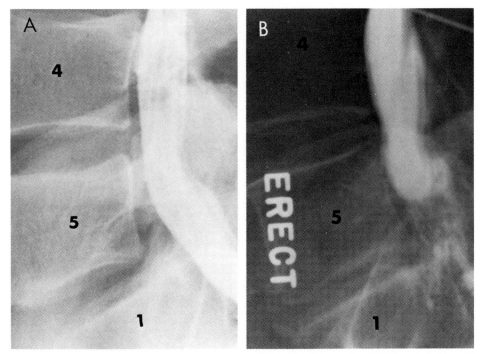

Fig 24–6.—Indications for epidurogram. Lateral film from metrizamide myelogram **(A)** with large ventral epidural space at L5-S1. Lateral film from lumbar myelogram **(B)** with arachnoiditis and scarring of distal thecal sac.

TECHNIQUE

Several radiographic techniques have been employed in lumbar epidurography. Initial efforts in 1941 by both Sanford et al. and by Knutson involved needle puncture of the distal epidural space through the sacral notch followed by injection of contrast medium. The Touhy needle technique used by anesthesiologists for epidural anesthesia (Bromage et al.), and lateral intralaminar puncture of the lumbar epidural space have both been employed for lumbar epidurography. However, a modified Seldinger technique through the sacral notch with selective nerve root injection of metrizamide (Hatten) provides the most reproducible, consistent results. Selective nerve root injection, which is technically easy, is particularly valuable because of the presence of the plica mediana dorsalis.

The patient is placed in the prone position, the sacrum prepped, and the skin over the sacral hiatus liberally anesthetized with 1% lidocaine. The sacral tuberosities are manually palpated and the sacral notch punctured with an 18-gauge, 9-cm-long, beveled needle. Because the sacral notch is covered by the ligamentum flavum, a distinct "pop" is felt when the needle enters the epidural space. If there is difficulty puncturing the sacral notch, the patient should be turned into the true lateral position to visualize this area more clearly by fluoroscopy. After the puncture of the sacral notch, the beveled portion of the needle is directed to the side of clinical interest, and a 0.032-inch guidewire, 80 cm in length with a 5-mm flexible tip, is introduced under fluoroscopic control. The guidewire is directed to the right

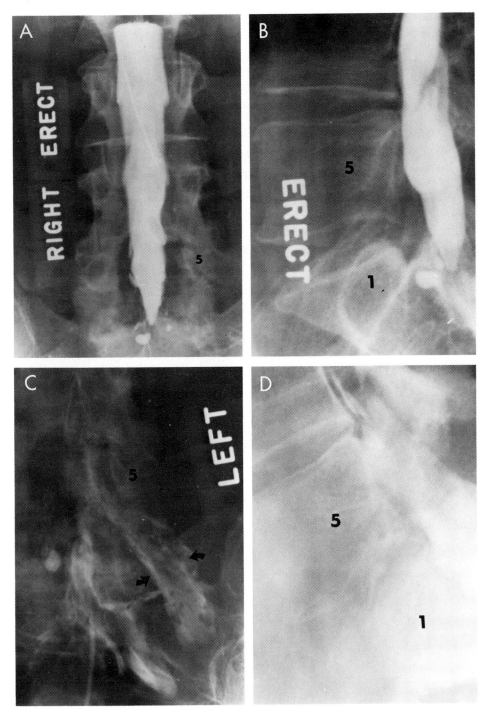

Fig 24–7.—45-year-old female with history of previous back surgery ×2 and currently persistent left-leg pain. Pantopaque lumbar myelogram demonstrates tapering of the thecal sac on AP film **(A)** with a large ventral epidural space at L5-S1 on lateral film **(B)**. Lumbar epidurogram demonstrates clear filling of left L-5 root on AP **(C)** *(arrows)* and filling of ventral epidural space at L5-S1 on lateral film **(D)**.

or left side, the patient is rolled into a lateral decubitus position (taking care to superimpose the femoral heads under fluoroscopy), and the knees flexed to the chest. The guidewire is now further advanced in an effort to pass it into the ventral epidural space. If the guidewire is positioned in the dorsal epidural space, additional contrast must be injected for an adequate examination. With the guidewire correctly positioned, the needle is removed and a 40-cm Teflon, 0.032-inch (0.081 cm) tapered catheter is passed over the guidewire; the guidewire is then removed. Depending on catheter position, 6–12 cc of metrizamide in a concentration of 200 mg I/ml (20%) is injected under fluoroscopic control. It is important to opacify the ventral epidural space with contrast. Additional contrast may have to be injected if the catheter is located in the dorsal epidural space.

After good opacification of the desired nerve roots and ventral epidural space is obtained, the catheter is removed. All of the films are obtained with the spot-film device with the patient in the erect position. It is important to keep the filming technique at 70–75 kvp to take advantage of the K edge of the iodine in the metrizamide. No overhead radiographs are taken. The entire procedure takes 20–40 minutes, and patients may ambulate immediately following the procedure. Lumbar epidurography with metrizamide can be safely performed on outpatients.

INDICATIONS

The role of lumbar epidurography in contemporary neuroradiology is changing with the increased technology available from high-resolution computed tomography (CT) of the lumbar spine. Excellent definition of soft tissue anatomy within the spinal canal (Haughton et al.) is now available from a number of CT manufacturers. There are several crucial requirements for routine CT evaluation of disk herniation. They include (1) a tilting gantry, (2) localizer scan capability, and (3) high-resolution technology.

The growing use of CT evaluation of lumbar disk herniation has reduced but not eliminated the need for lumbar epidurography. CT is less helpful than lumbar epidurography in evaluating the lumbar epidural space and disk herniation in the postoperative patient (Williams et al.). In this situation, the epidural space may be obliterated by postoperative scarring, making CT diagnosis difficult. However, lumbar epidurography is ideal for studying the postoperative patient. Filling of the ventral epidural space and nerve root sheaths in these individuals can obviate unnecessary surgery when a conventional lumbar myelogram shows only arachnoid scarring.

Patients with arachnoiditis can also be satisfactorily evaluated by lumbar epidurography. In these individuals, myelography demonstrates tapering, beading, and constriction of the thecal sac. Droplets of Pantopaque present from earlier myelograms create artifacts which make CT difficult or impossible. Arachnoiditis most commonly occurs following surgery but may be secondary to previous myelography or subarachnoid hemorrhage. In these patients, the purpose of lumbar epidurography is to attempt to identify normal epidural anatomy and nerve root sheaths in an effort to obviate unnecessary surgery.

COMPLICATIONS

The complications of lumbar epidurography with metrizamide are the same as those experienced in myelography with metrizamide. In my series of 65 patients with metrizamide lumbar epidurography, I have encountered headache, back pain, one case of lower-extremity muscle spasm successfully treated with intravenous Valium, and a questionable case of hypersensitivity skin rash. Other potential complications of lumbar epidurography with metrizamide include seizures, which may occur with subarachnoid metrizamide. The same precautions for epidural metrizamide should be observed for subarachnoid metrizamide. Contraindications to lumbar epidurography with metrizamide include: a history of a seizure disorder, neuroleptic analgesics or any phenothiazine-containing drugs within 7 days of the procedure, alcoholism, or hypersensitivity to iodine.

CONCLUSION

The role of lumbar epidurography is changing with the newer technology available from CT scanning of the lumbar spine. As CT resolution continues to improve, the hope exists that a noninvasive method for the primary evaluation of lumbar disk herniation will become a reality. However, there will continue to be patients who require additional diagnostic radiologic studies. For this group of patients, lumbar epidurography may have a useful role.

BIBLIOGRAPHY

Bromage P.R., Bramwell R.S.B., Catchlove R.F.H., et al.: Peridurography with metrizamide: Animal and human studies. *Radiology* 128:123, 1978.

Gonsette R.E.: Metrizamide as contrast medium for myelography and ventriculography. *Acta Radiol.* (Suppl.) 335:346, 1973.

Hatten H.P., Jr.: Lumbar epidurography with metrizamide: Review of 65 cases employing a pure Seldinger technique with caudal approach through the sacral notch and selective nerve root sheath injection. *Radiology* 137:129, 1980.

Hatten H.P., Jr.: Metrizamide lumbar epidurography with Seldinger technique through the sacral notch and selective nerve root injection. *Neuroradiology* 19:19, 1980.

Haughton V.M., Syvertsen A., Williams A.L.: Soft tissue anatomy within the spinal canal as seen on computed tomography. *Radiology* 134:649, 1980.

Kido D.K., Schoene W., Baker R.A., et al.: Metrizamide epidurography in dogs. *Radiology* 128:119, 1978.

Knutson F.: Experiences with epidural contrast investigation of the lumbosacral canal in disc prolapse. *Acta Radiol.* 22:694, 1941.

Lewit K.: The contribution of peridurography to the anatomy of the lumbosacral spinal canal. *Folia Morphol.* (Prague) 24:289, 1976.

Lewit K., Sereghy T.: Lumbar epidurography with special regard to the anatomy of the lumbar peridural space. *Neuroradiology* 8:233, 1975.

Luyendijk W.: Canalography, roentgenological examination of the peridural space in the lumbosacral part of the vertebral canal. *J. Belg. Radiol.* 46:236, 1963.

Luyendijk W.: The plica mediana dorsalis of dura mater and its relation to lumbar peridurography (canalography). *Neuroradiology* 11:147, 1976.

Luyendijk W., van Voorthiusen A.E.: Contrast examination of the spinal and epidural space. *Acta Radiol.* (Diagn.) 5:1051, 1966.

McCormick C.C.: Radiology in low back pain and sciatica. An analysis of the relative efficacy of spinal venography, discography and epidurography in patients with a negative or equivocal myelogram. *Clin. Radiol.* 29:393, 1978.

Nagamine K.: Clinical and biochemical study of accidents in peridurography. *Nagoya J. Med. Sci.* 32:429, 1970.

Roberson G.H., Hatten J.P., Jr., Hesselink J.H.: Epidurography: Selective catheter technique and review of 53 cases. *A.J.R.* 132:787, 1979.

Sanford H., Doub H.P.: Epidurography: A method of roentgenologic visualization of protruded intervertebral disks. *Radiology* 36:712, 1941.

Sicard J.A., Forestier J.: Methode radiographique d'exploration de la cavite epidurale par le Lipiodol. *Rev. Neurol.* 28:1264, 1921.

Williams A.L., Haughton V.M., Syvertsen A.: Computed tomography in the diagnosis of herniated nucleus pulposus. *Radiology* 135:95, 1980.

25

Computed Tomography of the Spine

Victor M. Haughton, M.D.

THE ROLE OF COMPUTED TOMOGRAPHY in diverse types of spinal pathology is still being evaluated. Since 1975, when DiChiro reported the CT demonstration of spinal cord cysts and diastematomyelia, CT has been considered complementary or supplementary to conventional radiographic studies for evaluating spine disorders. With their improved resolution and greater versatility, the newest CT scanners have acquired greater importance in spinal examinations. In recent clinical work, Haughton et al. found that CT equaled or exceeded the accuracy of myelography for demonstrating various common spine lesions such as disk herniations, spondylolysis, and spinal stenosis. Since CT has a number of advantages over myelography—including noninvasiveness, low cost, and axial projections—it is clearly indicated as the primary modality for evaluating the spine in many instances.

To analyze computer tomographic imaging in all types of spine anatomy and pathology requires a book (Haughton and Williams). The aims of a chapter must be more limited and selective. Since this book concerns myelography, this chapter will emphasize how CT has modified the practice of myelography. Therefore, the indications for a primary CT scan and the most significant contributions of CT imaging to the diagnosis of spinal pathology will be emphasized.

ANATOMY

All of the osseous and most of the soft tissues of the spine can be demonstrated effectively with computer tomography. Because the abundant lumbar epidural fat has a low attenuation value easily distinguished in CT images, CT is especially effective in the lumbar region. Within the lumbar epidural fat, CT shows the normal anterior internal vertebral veins, retrovertebral plexuses, root sheaths, ligamentum flavum, and dural sac (Fig 25–1). Normally, contrast medium is not required to demonstrate these structures. When epidural fat is replaced by scar, mass, or degenerative changes, the normal vascular, ligamentous, and neural structures may be obscured. In the thoracic and cervical regions, where the epidural space is small and fat is scarce, individual veins and root sheaths are rarely identified.

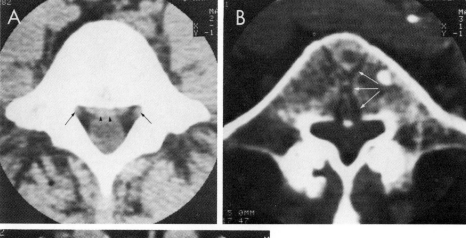

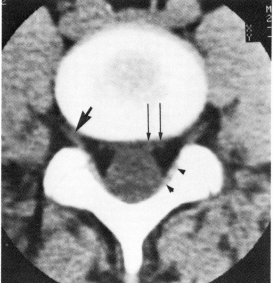

Fig 25–1.—Axial CT sections showing lumbar spine anatomy. In the midportion of L-5 **(A),** CT shows the retrovertebral plexus *(arrowheads),* dural sac, and root sheaths *(arrows).* Epidural fat fills the remainder of the canal. A bone window image near the same level **(B)** shows the basivertebral veins *(arrows).* A section near a lumbar intervertebral disk **(C)** shows the ligamentum flavum *(arrowheads),* spinal nerves in the neural foramen *(short arrow),* and internal vertebral veins *(long arrows).*

Provided optimal techniques are used and the subarachnoid space is not narrowed, CT demonstrates the spinal cord effectively. Therefore, the cervical cord and its normally large subarachnoid space are readily demonstrated (Fig 25–2), while the thoracic cord, surrounded sometimes by a small amount of cerebrospinal fluid, is inconstantly demonstrated (Taylor et al.). Any intramedullary or epidural expanding process that narrows the subarachnoid space decreases the detectability of the spinal cord in CT images. DiChiro and Schellinger found that cord demonstration is improved by enhancing the subarachnoid space with small doses of metrizamide prior to CT imaging (Fig 25–3).

The axial planes are probably the most effective, although at the moment least familiar, for evaluating the intervertebral disks. In axial projection, the contour of the normal intervertebral disk conforms to the shape of the adjacent vertebrae. In the lower lumbar spine, the posterior surface of the intervertebral disk is flat or concave (Fig 25–4).

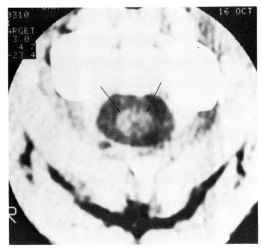

Fig 25–2.—The cervical spine imaged with a prototype 9800 scanner. The cord *(arrows)* and surrounding subarachnoid space are distinguished in the spinal canal. The H-shaped pattern suggests the distribution of gray matter in the cord.

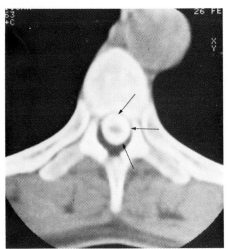

Fig 25–3.—The thoracic spine with intrathecal metrizamide enhancement *(arrows).* Within the contrast medium, the cord is distinguished; surrounding it, the epidural fat.

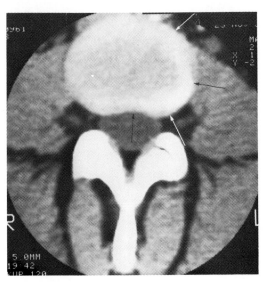

Fig 25–4.—CT section through a normal lumbar intervertebral disk. The disk margin *(arrows)* conforms to the adjacent vertebral end-plate.

In the thoracic region, it is nearly oval; and in the cervical region, it is constricted laterally by the uncinate processes. Although the nucleus pulposus contains amorphous remnants of the primitive notochord, the surrounding annulus fibrosus contains fibrocartilage, while the vertebral end-plate contains hyaline cartilage. These disk components are not discriminated by CT, and the normal disk appears nearly homogeneous in CT images. The periphery of the intervertebral disk may be slightly more dense than the center, either because the vertebral end-plate protrudes slightly into the slice or because the denser outer fibers of the annulus (Sharpey's fibers) have a greater collagen content and density.

TECHNIQUES

For imaging the spine, a CT scanner must have adequate resolution (probably at least 0.8 mm for spatial and 0.5% for contrast resolution). Further essential specifications include a localizer imaging technique, tilting gantry, variable slice thicknesses between 1 and 10 mm, variable photon flux, target or zoom reconstruction, reformatting programs for sagittal and coronal reconstruction, and preferably an extended CT scale of ±2,000 H.U.

Optimal techniques for imaging the spine depend on the structures and lesions to be demonstrated. To image the epidural space, relatively thin slices, an intermediate contrast resolution, and maximal spatial resolution are needed. Therefore, the 5-mm collimation, an intermediate photon flux, and the smallest pixel size (smallest calibration) are usually chosen. To minimize geometric distortion, planes of section perpendicular to the rostral-caudal axis of the spine are desirable. Therefore, the precise levels and planes of imaging (table position and gantry angulation) are best selected from a lateral localizer image of the spine.

Effective imaging of the spinal cord requires maximal contrast resolution, which is obtained by the combination of maximal radiation flux, thickest cuts, and planes of section perpendicular to the rostral-caudal axis. Either intravenous or intrathecal contrast medium improves the definition of the spinal cord with present computer technology.

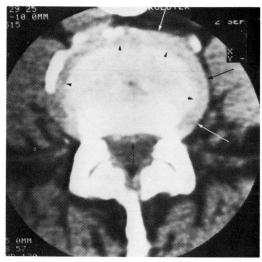

Fig 25–5.—CT demonstration of a bulging intervertebral disk. The disk margins *(arrows)* extend beyond the adjacent vertebral end-plate *(arrowheads)*.

To obtain the best images of the intervertebral disks, axial images precisely in the plane of the disk are required. Therefore, levels and planes of section must be selected from a localizer image, since the orientation of the disks varies from level to level and from patient to patient. Maximal contrast resolution is necessary except where the disk is contiguous to epidural fat. Therefore, high photon flux is mandatory. The CT sections must be thinner than the intervertebral disk space to eliminate partial volume averaging with the adjacent vertebral end-plates. For the normal lumbar intervertebral disks, 5-mm slice thickness is suitable; however, for the cervical and thoracic disks or for pathologically narrowed lumbar disks, thinner sections are needed. To detect nuclear fragments that have migrated some distance from the intervertebral space, a sufficient number of contiguous cuts must be taken. With two or three slices above the plane of the intervertebral disk and one or two below, the important parts of the spinal canal and neural foramina are encompassed by the examination.

INTERVERTEBRAL DISK DISEASE

Normal, degenerated, and herniated intervertebral disks can be distinguished accurately by computed tomography. The most important CT observation is the configuration of the disk margin and secondarily, the attenuation coefficients in its center. If the annulus is bulging, CT shows the entire disk margin extending uniformly and usually symmetrically beyond the adjacent vertebral end-plates (Williams and Haughton). Minor degrees of asymmetry may occur (Fig 25–5). The bulging intervertebral disk narrows the inferior portion of the neural foramen below the nerve root sheath as well as the spinal canal. Therefore, it compresses or displaces the dural sac but usually not the nerve sheaths. When a bulging disk produces radiculopathy, CT shows the disk margin compressing a nerve root. Frequently, CT demonstrates a vacuum phenomenon within a bulging disk, indicating that gas has formed within fissures of the nucleus pulposus.

Lumbar

The CT findings in a lumbar herniated intervertebral disk depend on the location of the nuclear fragments. The most common location of a herniated nucleus pulposus is outside the annulus fibrosus and under the posterior longitudinal ligament (subligamentous herniation). In this location, the herniated nucleus produces a smooth, rounded focal protrusion of the disk margin, which CT demonstrates effectively (Fig 25–6). The protruded margin compresses or displaces the nerve root that is clinically affected (Fig 25–7) and frequently the dural sac, particularly when the herniation is fairly central (Fig 25–8). Where in contact with epidural fat, the protruded disk margin is sharply outlined in the CT image; where in contact with the dural sac, either because of a central location or a narrow spinal canal, or where scar tissue has replaced epidural fat, the disk margin has less contrast (see Fig 25–8). Especially in these situations, high MaS techniques are necessary to demonstrate the herniation.

If the nuclear fragment lies outside the posterior longitudinal ligament (a free or extruded fragment), CT demonstrates different findings. If the fragment lies near

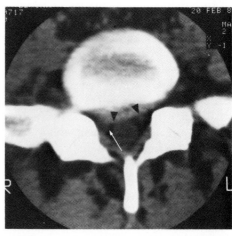

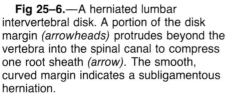

Fig 25–6.—A herniated lumbar intervertebral disk. A portion of the disk margin *(arrowheads)* protrudes beyond the vertebra into the spinal canal to compress one root sheath *(arrow)*. The smooth, curved margin indicates a subligamentous herniation.

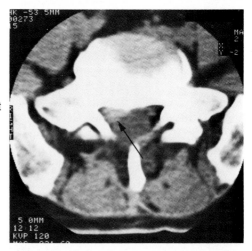

Fig 25–7.—Herniated disk *(arrow)* that displaces and obscures the sheath and nerve clinically affected. The dural sac is deformed as well.

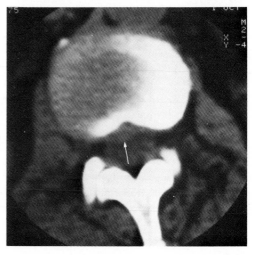

Fig 25–8.—An L2-3 disk herniation. This fairly central herniation *(arrow)*, at a level with little epidural fat, is demonstrated with more difficulty.

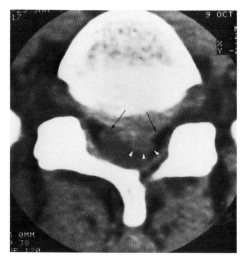

Fig 25–9.—An extruded (free) disk fragment *(arrowheads)* causing an irregular disk margin. A portion of the herniation *(arrows)* is behind the posterior longitudinal ligament.

the disk, the disk margin appears to have an irregular, focally protruded margin (Fig 25–9). If the fragment has migrated into the spinal canal or neural foramen, the disk margin may have a perfectly normal contour and the fragment may appear as a soft tissue mass somewhere within the spinal canal. When the fragment abuts the dural sac or root sheath, the contours of these structures may be obscured. Therefore, when CT shows an apparently asymmetric dural sac or root sheaths, an extruded free fragment of herniated disk must be considered. A free fragment, therefore, may simulate a conjoint root sheath (Fig 25–10). In some cases, density measurements distinguish the free fragment from other processes; in other cases, intrathecal metrizamide must be used to distinguish the free fragments from the unilateral root sheath cyst or abnormality.

A nuclear fragment in the neural foramen (a far-lateral herniation) has specific CT findings. CT shows a tissue with cartilaginous density displacing the fat in the

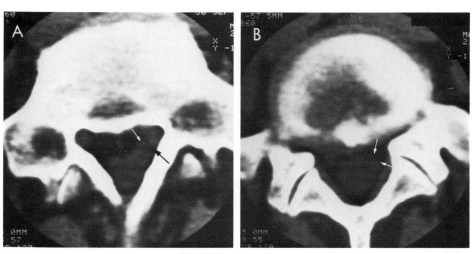

Fig 25–10.—Two contiguous slices **(A** and **B)** through an anomalous dural sac and a conjoint root sheath *(arrows).* A free disk fragment can simulate the shape but not the density of the asymmetric root sheaths.

neural foramen and obscuring the affected spinal nerve (Fig 25–11). Some disk material may even be located lateral to the neural foramen. When a lateral herniation compresses the nerve and root sheath lateral to the sleeve that fills with metrizamide during myelography, myelography is normal. Therefore, a suspected lateral disk herniation is an indication for CT even if myelography is normal.

A central disk herniation deforms the dural sac and displaces some epidural fat but seldom distorts the root sheaths (see Fig 25–8). Central herniations do not ordinarily produce radicular pain. Therefore, a CT study demonstrating a central herniation probably does not explain the etiology of sciatic pain. The margin of a central herniation contrasted with the dural sac may be less sharply delineated than posterolateral or lateral disk herniations outlined by fat.

Calcifications or gas may be found in some herniations. The calcification may result from the degenerative process within the nucleus or from an avulsion fracture of the ring apophysis. A calcified herniated disk fragment may be difficult to distinguish from spondylosis. Gas in a protruded disk is probably due to a vacuum phenomenon developing in the nucleus before it herniates.

Thoracic

Experience with the CT diagnosis of thoracic disk herniations is limited. Less than 1% of intervertebral disk herniations are said to occur in the thoracic region. Since the level of a thoracic disk herniation cannot always be predicted accurately on clinical examination, CT, which is not cost-effective for studying long segments of the spinal axis, is not usually employed.

The CT findings in a thoracic disk herniation depend on the amount of epidural fat and size of the subarachnoid space, both of which vary from patient to patient. CT may show the herniated material as a clearly defined mass in the epidural fat lateral to the dural sac or as an abnormal disk margin indenting the dural sac (Haughton and Williams). Thoracic disk herniations frequently contain some calcium.

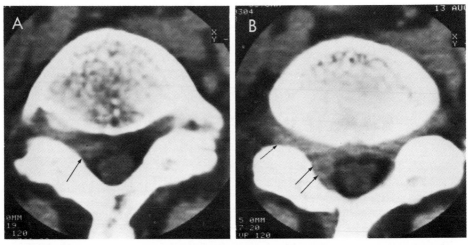

Fig 25–11.—**A** and **B,** a lateral disk herniation *(arrows)* filling the neural foramen but not distorting the dural sac. Myelography is negative in some of these herniations.

Cervical

CT of cervical intervertebral disk herniation has been less completely evaluated because cervical herniations are less common, anatomical correlations are not so readily available, and computer tomographic techniques are more critical. The major problem in studying the intervertebral disks with CT is obtaining suitably thin cuts with adequate contrast resolution. Because of the normally thin cervical disks, thin CT sections are necessary in this region to diagnose herniation. Contrast resolution is, therefore, inferior. Furthermore, because the cervical epidural space contains little fat, CT shows a cervical disk herniation in contrast to dural sac or root sheath. Intrathecal enhancement may be required in some cases, especially when cord compression due to disk disease is to be evaluated (Fig 25–12).

With disk degeneration, the uncinate processes hypertrophy, often compressing root sheaths in the neural foramina. CT is an effective means of demonstrating the hypertrophy and compression. Obliteration of the fat normally surrounding the nerve and sheath is presumptive evidence that the nerve is compressed. Occasionally, when the herniation distorts the epidural venous plexus and intravenous contrast medium is given, an abnormal epidural enhancement that simulates a meningioma may be detected by intravenously enhanced CT.

Diskitis

In diskitis, the CT localizer or a radiograph demonstrates disk space narrowing. The axial computed tomograms demonstrate vertebral end-plate destruction with more reliability than myelography or plain films (Haughton and Williams). Also, according to Haughton et al., degenerated nuclear fragments lying within the neural foramina or spinal canal are shown by CT more effectively than by myelography.

Accuracy of CT in Disk Disease

The accuracy of CT has been compared in a few studies to date (Haughton et al., Gado et al., Glenn et al., Teplick et al.). Detection of herniated disks by CT is excellent. The sensitivity (true positive rate) for CT in herniated disks was 96% in

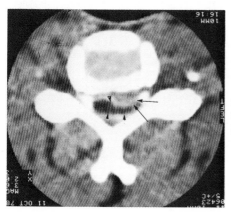

Fig 25–12.—A cervical disk herniation *(arrows)* shown with CT and intrathecal metrizamide enhancement. The cord *(arrowheads)* is deformed.

recent studies, compared to 90–94% for myelography (Haughton et al., Gado et al.). CT is superior to myelography for detecting herniations, especially where epidural fat is plentiful or the dural sac is located at some distance from the vertebral bodies, for example at L5-S1 (Fig 25–13) and where disk herniations are far-lateral (see Fig 25–11). False negative CT interpretations are due to scanning at the wrong level, or to interpreting a disk as bulging that the surgeon subsequently interprets as herniated at operation. The surgical diagnoses used for verification in these studies are probably not 100% reliable. Other potential causes of false negative diagnoses are a conus medullaris tumor or a high lumbar disk herniation that is studied by means of CT cuts through the lower lumbar disks. In postlaminectomy or in spinal stenosis, sensitivity of CT is reduced because of scarce epidural fat.

The specificity (true negative interpretations) of CT also exceeded that of myelography (Haughton et al., Gado et al.). Fewer false positive CT diagnoses of disk herniation were encountered than false positive myelographic diagnoses. One reason for false positive CT diagnosis was interpreting dense, protruding disk margins

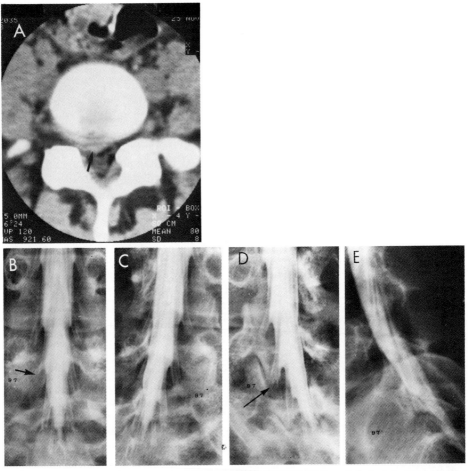

Fig 25–13.—CT **(A)** and myelography **(B–E)** in an L5-S1 herniated disk *(arrow)* in a large epidural space anterior to the dura. The myelogram shows subtle changes in the right S-1 root sheath *(arrowheads)*. (Myelogram shown with patient's right to reader's left.)

as calcified herniations while the surgeon designated them as spurs. Although technically false positives, the CT studies accurately demonstrated the pathologic anatomy. Other potential causes of false positive CT interpretations can be mentioned. In spondylolisthesis, the distorted disk may simulate a herniation. However, slippage of one vertebra with respect to another causes the disk to appear displaced dorsally with respect to one vertebra, but not both. A pars defect will be recognized in cuts 10 mm above the disk. The intraspinal mass of a vertebral metastasis or epidural tumor may simulate a herniation. These malignant processes nearly always produce some bone destruction or hyperostosis. The similarity of a conjoint root sheath and a free fragment of disk herniation has been mentioned (see Fig 25–10).

Because of its safety and accuracy, CT will probably replace most lumbar myelograms. However, when many levels must be studied, myelography is probably more efficient than CT. To exclude a conus lesion or high lumbar disk herniation, myelography may be more cost-effective than CT. To find a thoracic disk herniation or a myelopathy that cannot be well localized clinically, myelography is less time consuming than CT. On the other hand, a negative myelogram does not exclude a lumbar disk herniation as effectively as CT.

CONGENITAL SPINAL ANOMALIES

Until the development of high-resolution spinal CT, demonstration of spinal cord abnormalities required myelography. With computed tomography of sufficient resolution to demonstrate the spinal cord, congenital spinal anomalies can be investigated noninvasively. Except to demonstrate extensive regions of the spinal column, myelography has been replaced by CT as the procedure of choice. CT can be adequately diagnostic without any contrast enhancement if high-resolution techniques are used, or with very low radiation techniques if intrathecal metrizamide is used. Because the indications for CT are less stringent than for myelography, the spectrum of congenital anomalies demonstrated by CT is different.

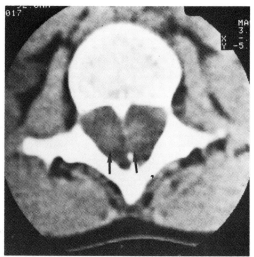

Fig 25–14.—Diastematomyelia. The divided spinal cord *(arrows)* can be demonstrated by CT even if no spur is present.

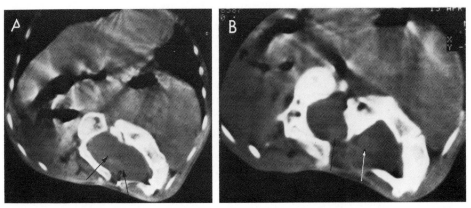

Fig 25–15.—Diastematomyelia with a large spur. In the axial image, the spinal column appears duplicated. Arrows point to spinal cord in **A** and divided cord in **B**.

Diastematomyelia is the most common congenital spine lesion referred for CT imaging (James and Oliff, Lohkamp et al., Wolpert et al.). It can be studied either with unenhanced or intrathecally enhanced techniques. In diastematomyelia, CT shows division of the spinal cord into two hemicords which are often unequal in size and always smaller than normal. Like myelography, CT often demonstrates the cords separated by a fibrous band, an osseous spur (Fig 25–14), or a large osseous structure that gives the impression that the spinal column is duplicated (Fig 25–15). However, a larger number of diastematomyelic cords without a fibrous or bony spur are discovered by CT than by myelography, probably because the indications for study are more flexible (Arrendondo et al., Harwood-Nash and Fitz, Resjo et al.). Low-density regions within one of the hemicords suggesting a small syrinx or possibly lipoma may be seen. Associated abnormalities include meningocele, spina bifida, or filum terminale lipoma, each of which can be demonstrated with CT (Fig 25–16).

A variety of other congenital lesions have been evaluated with CT, including tethered cord, extraspinal and intraspinal meningoceles, neurenteric, teratoid and arachnoid cysts, bone dysplasias, scoliosis, etc. (Harwood-Nash and Fitz). CT shows an unexpectedly high frequency of incidentally discovered tethered cords in adults

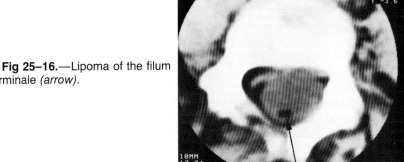

Fig 25–16.—Lipoma of the filum terminale *(arrow)*.

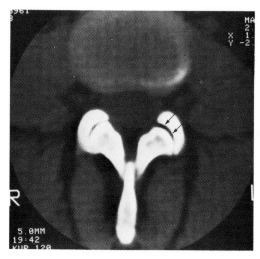

Fig 25–17.—Normal facet joint in a CT image *(arrows)*.

(Kaplan and Quencer). The role of CT in all of these disorders has not been fully evaluated. In many of these conditions, CT obviates the need for myelography.

FACET JOINT DISEASE

Facet joint disease, an underdiagnosed cause of low back and sciatic pain, although not easily detected in conventional radiographic studies, can be effectively demonstrated by computed tomography (Carrera et al.). Clinically, facet joint disease may simulate a herniated disk, either by compressing a nerve root in the neural foramen, or without radiculopathy by referring pain from the involved joint to a sclerotome of the adjacent spinal nerves. The normal facet joint is visualized as a space 2–4 mm wide between the superior and inferior articular surfaces. The latter have smooth, curved, uniform cortical margins. Surrounding the joint is

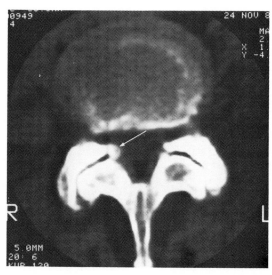

Fig 25–18.—Degenerated facet joints. The space between the superior and inferior articular process is narrowed; the articular cortex is thickened. Gas is present in the joint spaces, especially on the left. The joint capsule is calcified on the right *(arrow).*

a capsule lined by synovium that inserts in shallow grooves on the lamina (Fig 25–17).

Five stages or processes in facet joint disease have been recognized pathologically, including synovitis, joint capsule laxity, articular cartilage destruction, herniation of joint contents through the articular cartilage, and sclerosis of periarticular bone. Each of these stages has characteristic CT findings.

The CT findings of synovitis, although probably absent in most acute cases, are characterized in chronic cases by calcification in the facet capsule medial or lateral to the joint and in the adjacent ligamentum flavum (Fig 25–18). To detect the calcification, bone window images must be inspected. The calcification of the capsule and ligament must be distinguished from osteophytes or from the normal ridge of bone in which the ligamentum flavum inserts. Calcification is most frequently detected in association with other degenerative changes of the facet joint.

In joint capsule laxity, the superior and inferior articular processes may have an abnormal relationship. In many cases, a vacuum joint phenomenon occurs as the superior and inferior articular processes are distracted. The vacuum joint phenomenon in the facet joint is recognized as a tissue of low density (-500 to $-1,000$ H.U.) between the articular surfaces (Fig 25–19). Almost invariably, these vacuum joint phenomena are associated with severe degenerative changes of the facet joint. Rarely, due perhaps to muscular imbalance, the vacuum phenomenon can be seen without significant facet joint degeneration.

With articular cartilage destruction, the space between the superior and inferior articular processes diminishes. CT shows the articular surfaces less than 2 mm from each other. When the facet joint does not have a vertical orientation, measurement of the joint space may be inaccurate. The cartilage destruction is usually accompanied by other degenerative changes, such as erosions and eburnation in adjacent processes, which CT demonstrates effectively (Fig 25–20). The erosions appear as small foci of bone destruction adjacent to the joint space and represent herniation of joint material into the articular bone. The medullary cavity of the articular processes is usually sclerotic. Patients with articular cartilage destruction, articular ero-

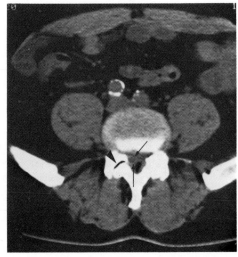

Fig 25–19.—Vacuum phenomenon *(arrowhead)* in a facet joint, possibly secondary to abnormally lax facet capsule and distractive forces. Also note the extradural synovial cyst *(arrows)* secondary to facet degeneration.

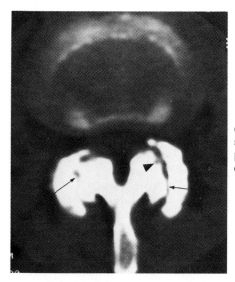

Fig 25–20.—Facet arthropathy. Because of thinned articular cartilage *(arrows),* severe sclerosis is evident in the articular processes. Note the subchondral synovial cyst *(arrowhead).*

sions, and sclerosis respond well to intra-articular injections of steroid and local anesthetic (Carrera et al.).

The final stage of articular degeneration is osteophytes, which narrow either the spinal canal, neural foramen, or both. Facet joint osteophytes are considered in the next section.

SPINAL STENOSIS

Because it shows the spine in an axial projection, CT demonstrates spinal stenosis more effectively than conventional radiographic projections and myelography; because it demonstrates the soft tissues in the spinal canal, it detects spinal stenosis more sensitively than transverse axial tomography. Therefore, computed tomography has improved the accuracy of evaluating spinal stenosis radiographically. Although spinal stenosis generally results from disk and facet joint degeneration, it can be divided arbitrarily into central stenosis (narrowing of the spinal canal) and lateral stenosis (narrowing of the neural foramen or lateral recess). The CT criteria of spinal stenosis, although more accurate, are less familiar than those of conventional myelography and radiography.

Central stenosis cannot be evaluated as effectively by measuring anteroposterior and lateral diameters of the spinal canal with CT or plain films as by measuring the cross-sectional area of the canal. Ullrich et al. report that most patients with lumbar cross-sectional areas less than 1.5 sq cm have symptomatic spinal stenosis. However, measurements of the bony canal disregard the important soft tissue components of spinal stenosis, such as intervertebral disk bulging and ligamentum flavum hypertrophy. In most cases of spinal stenosis, lateral or central, a bulging disk or ligamentum flavum hypertrophy produces some of the narrowing. When the width of the ligamentum flavum exceeds 5 mm, hypertrophy can be diagnosed, although the primary pathologic change in the ligamentum flavum is fibrosis rather than hypertrophy. CT shows these soft tissue components of spinal stenosis as well as the common osseous contributions from osteophytes (Fig 25–21). Narrowing of the

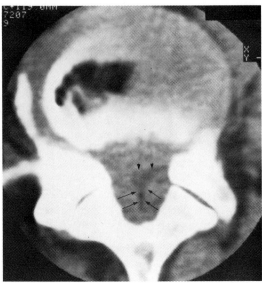

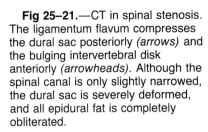

Fig 25–21.—CT in spinal stenosis. The ligamentum flavum compresses the dural sac posteriorly *(arrows)* and the bulging intervertebral disk anteriorly *(arrowheads)*. Although the spinal canal is only slightly narrowed, the dural sac is severely deformed, and all epidural fat is completely obliterated.

spinal canal becomes symptomatic when both the subarachnoid and epidural spaces are obliterated. Where the epidural space is large, as in the lumbar region, the most obvious CT sign of spinal stenosis is obliteration of fat surrounding the dural sac. In lumbar spinal stenosis, except in cases associated with hypertrophic fat (e.g., in Cushing's disease), CT shows complete obliteration of epidural fat that normally surrounds the dural sac.

In regions with a small epidural and large subarachnoid space (e.g., cervical spine), the most obvious finding in stenosis is obliteration of the subarachnoid space. Therefore, to evaluate cervical spinal stenosis, the subarachnoid space must be demonstrated, which necessitates intrathecal metrizamide enhancement. Symp-

Fig 25–22.—Atrophic spinal cord. Note the small, misshapen cord.

tomatic stenosis can be diagnosed when the subarachnoid space is completely obliterated and the spinal cord is compressed.

Lateral spinal stenosis can also be diagnosed effectively by CT. When the lateral recess or neural foramen is narrowed to 3 mm or less, lateral spinal stenosis is common. Although osteophytes from the superior articular facets are usually the most significant factor in lateral stenosis, both hypertrophy of the ligamentum flavum and bulging of the disk may also contribute. When lateral stenosis is symptomatic, CT shows obliteration of the fat that normally surrounds the nerve in the neural foramen.

Both myelography and CT are effective for diagnosing spinal stenosis. When specific levels can be identified for computer tomographic evaluation, as in the usual acquired lumbar stenosis, the diagnosis can be made efficiently with CT. When many levels must be demonstrated, as in congenital conditions like achondroplasia and thoracic cord compression, myelography is often more cost-effective.

CORD DISEASE

The CT diagnosis of cord atrophy (Naidich and Pudlowski), syringomyelia (Bonafe et al., Forbes and Isherwood, Resjo et al.), and possibly multiple sclerosis (Coin and Hucks-Folliss) has been shown. Demonstration of cord gray and white matter and small focal intramedullary demyelinations may be achieved effectively by some scanners.

Since atrophy usually causes shrinkage without a large decrease in attenuation coefficients, atrophic spinal cords in the relatively large surrounding subarachnoid space can be readily recognized in CT images of the spine (Fig 25–22). In multiple sclerosis, demyelination of the cord may result in foci of diminished density, some of which can be demonstrated by high-resolution CT imaging (Fig 25–23). If the cord is largely demyelinated, demonstration of the cord outline may be hampered because contrast between it and the subarachnoid space is diminished.

Although early low-resolution CT had a relatively poor sensitivity for demonstrating spinal cord cysts (Carrera et al., Di Chiro et al.), present high-resolution CT

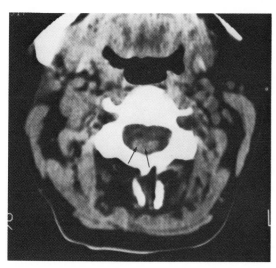

Fig 25–23.—CT of the cervical cord in a patient with multiple sclerosis. The regions of diminished attenuation *(arrows)* may represent demyelinated plaques.

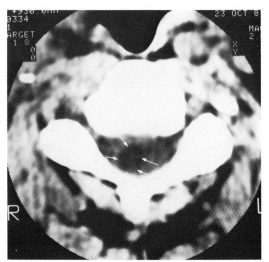

Fig 25–24.—Syringomyelia. CT shows a cyst in the cord *(arrows)*.

demonstrates even tiny cystic spaces (Fig 25–24). In fact, large cysts may be more difficult to diagnose than small ones because the attenuated cord displaced against the spinal column by the enlarging cyst may simulate an empty spinal canal (Fig 25–25). When the normal spinal cord silhouette cannot be identified within the canal, the margins of the canal must be inspected carefully.

Syringomyelia or hydromyelia appears in CT images as a well-defined, homogeneous, low-density region in the cord. Unless the protein concentration in the cyst

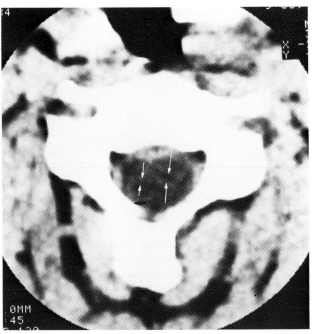

Fig 25–25.—Syringomyelia. The cyst is so large that the cord *(arrows)* is compressed against the spinal canal.

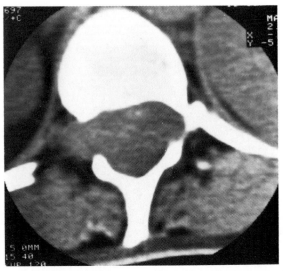

Fig 25–26.—CT of an intradural mass. The tumor (a schwannoma) obliterates the subarachnoid space, erodes the pedicle, and fills the neural foramen.

fluid is high, the density of the cyst approximates that of cerebrospinal fluid. Intrathecal metrizamide may be useful to demonstrate some cases of syringomyelia and to detect a communication with the subarachnoid space. Metrizamide injected into the subarachnoid space enters the syrinx rapidly if it communicates with the subarachnoid space or slowly if no direct communication exists. After intrathecal injection of metrizamide, the intramedullary cyst may be hyperdense, hypodense, or isodense with respect to the spinal cord, depending on the rate of transport of metrizamide into the cyst and the amount of time elapsed between intrathecal injection and scanning. Therefore, both immediate and delayed images after intrathecal injection are useful. In many cases of hydromyelia, the deformed tonsils of an associated Chiari malformation are demonstrated by CT in the upper cervical canal. If the tonsils displace all cerebrospinal fluid from the upper cervical canal, they obscure the cord silhouette.

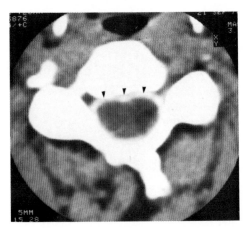

Fig 25–27.—Ependymoma enlarging the cervical cord. The subarachnoid space is enhanced with metrizamide *(arrowheads)*.

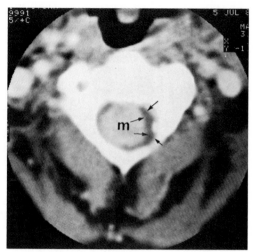

Fig 25–28.—Meningioma. A dense mass *(m)* fills the canal and compresses the spinal cord *(arrows).*

CT and myelography are probably complementary for evaluating intramedullary cysts. CT demonstrates the cyst effectively and more conveniently than positive-contrast or gas myelography; however, myelography provides a more efficient and less tedious means of surveying the entire spinal canal. A collapsing cord, the pathognomonic myelographic sign of syringomyelia or hydromyelia, is not effectively demonstrated with CT. Therefore, movement of fluid within a cyst is better evaluated with myelography than with CT.

SPINAL TUMORS

The disadvantages of CT for demonstrating spinal tumors are (1) often large regions of the canal must be examined because clinical localization may be inaccurate,

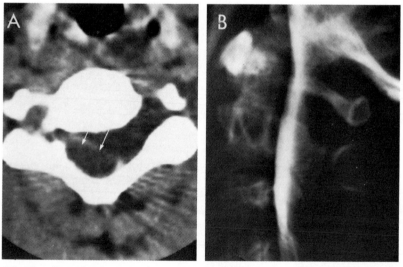

Fig 25–29.—Extradural tumor *(arrowheads)* shown by CT **(A)** and myelography **(B).** The mass displaces the dural sac *(arrows)* and enlarges the left neural foramen. The histologic diagnosis was lymphoma.

(2) intraspinal tissues are more difficult to demonstrate and differentiate if the sub-arachnoid space is narrowed by an expanding process and the cord contrasts less with the cerebrospinal fluid when diminished in density by a tumor or edema (Fig 25–26). Measurements of attenuation coefficients may also be unrelated with CT techniques currently used. In many cases, intrathecal metrizamide is necessary to enhance the subarachnoid space for computer tomographic demonstration of spinal tumors.

The most common intramedullary tumors are ependymoma and astrocytoma, which appear in CT as low attenuation processes enlarging the cord (Fig 25–27). Little or no contrast enhancement is usually demonstrated in these tumors after intravenous contrast medium. No specific patterns have been identified; but enhancement near the center of the cord suggests ependymoma, whereas more peripheral enhancement suggests astrocytoma. Dense, relatively homogeneous enhancement may characterize hemangioblastomas.

Extramedullary neoplasms such as neurofibroma and meningioma often have fairly specific CT findings. A meningioma is usually considerably more dense than

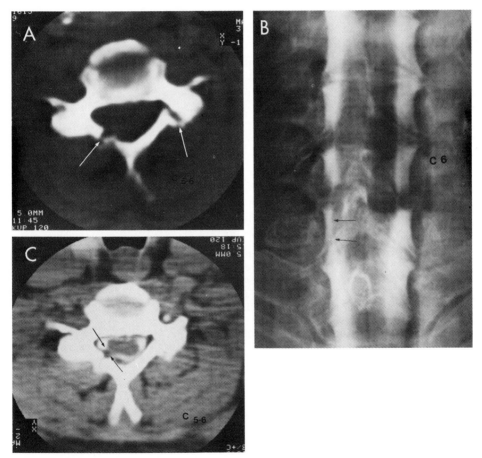

Fig 25–30.—Cord compression secondary to a healing fracture. CT **(A)** demonstrates laminar fractures at C-5 *(arrows)* following an auto accident. Because of posterior column signs, a myelogram **(B)** was done which showed apparent enlargement of the cord *(arrows)*. CT with intrathecal metrizamide **(C)** shows a hematoma and/or callus at one fracture site *(arrows)* compressing the cord.

the spinal cord and frequently associated with dramatic osteoblastic activity effectively demonstrated by CT (Fig 25–28). Although a meningioma enhances after intravenous contrast medium, qualitative attenuation changes may be difficult to detect because of the already high density of the tumor. A neurofibroma seldom produces sclerosis but very often erosion of bone near a neural foramen. The density of neurofibroma is typically slightly more than that of the spinal cord, but less than that of a meningioma. Moderate homogeneous enhancement after intravenous contrast medium is customary. Cystic degeneration or calcification is unusual.

Epidural spinal neoplasms are commonly malignant and include metastases, sarcoma, and lymphoma. In most of these, a soft tissue mass replacing epidural fat and bone destruction or hyperostosis is evident in CT (Fig 25–29). Even in very malignant tumors, the margins of the epidural mass in the CT image may be sharply demarcated and smooth. Contrast enhancement may not be obvious after intravenous contrast medium. Differentiation of epidural tumor types by CT has not yet been described; but lymphoma commonly causes bone sclerosis, whereas carcinoma more often causes destruction.

FRACTURES

Trauma to the spine deserves a short discussion because some spinal injuries warrant CT or myelography, and CT has some significant advantages for evaluating trauma. CT can be used for spinal, head, abdominal, or thoracic injuries (Naidich et al.). CT effectively shows traumatic disk herniations, spinal canal compression (Fig 25–30) (Kramer and Krouth), and possibly hematomas (Brant-Zawadzki). For detecting fractures, especially vertically oriented ones, CT is effective. For supplementing the plain-film diagnosis of fracture, CT is more effective than polytomography. CT, especially if enhanced with small amounts of metrizamide, provides as much or more diagnostic information with less risk. As more experience with CT is obtained in spinal trauma, a greater role can be anticipated.

BIBLIOGRAPHY

Arrendondo F., Haughton V.M., Hemmy D.C., et al.: Computed tomographic appearance of the spinal cord in diastematomyelia. *Radiology* 136:685, 1980.

Aubin M.L., Jardin C., Bar D., Vignard J.: Computerized tomography in 32 cases of intraspinal tumor. *J. Neuroradiologie* 6:81, 1979.

Bonafe A., Ethier R., Melancon D., et al.: High-resolution computed tomography in cervical syringomyelia. *J. Comput. Assist. Tomogr.* 4:42, 1980.

Brant-Zawadzki M., Miller E.R., Federle M.P.: CT in the evaluation of spinal trauma. *A.J.R.* 136:369, 1981.

Carrera G.F., Haughton V.M., Syvertsen A., Williams A.L.: Computed tomography of the lumbar facet joints. *Radiology* 136:145, 1980.

Carrera G.F., Williams A.L., Haughton V.M.: Computed tomography in sciatica. *Radiology* 136:433, 1980.

Coin C.G., Hucks-Folliss A.: Cervical computed tomography in multiple sclerosis with spinal cord involvement. *J. Comput. Assist. Tomogr.* 3:421, 1979.

Colley D.P., Dunsker S.B.: Traumatic narrowing of the dorsolumbar spinal canal demonstrated by computed tomography. *Radiology* 129:95, 1978.

DiChiro G., Axelbaum S.B., Schellinger D., et al.: Computerized tomography in syringomyelia. *N. Engl. J. Med.* 292:13, 1975.

DiChiro G., Schellinger D.: Computed tomography of the spinal cord after lumbar intrathecal introduction of metrizamide (computer-assisted tomography). *Radiology* 120:101, 1976.

Faerber E.W., Wolpert S., Scott R.M., et al.: Computed tomography of spinal fractures. *J. Comput. Assist. Tomogr.* 3:657, 1979.

Forbes W.S.C., Isherwood I.: Computed tomography in syringomyelia and the associated Arnold-Chiari Type I malformation. *Neuroradiology* 15:73, 1978.

Harwood-Nash D.C., Fitz C.R.: Computed tomography and the pediatric spine: Computed tomographic metrizamide myelography in children, in Post M.J.D. (ed.): *Radiographic Evaluation of the Spine: Current Advances With Emphasis on Computed Tomography.* New York, Masson Publishing Co., 1980.

Haughton V.W., Eldevik O.P., Magnaes B., Amundsen P.: A prospective study of CT and myelography in the diagnosis of herniated lumbar disc. *Radiology* 142:103, 1982.

Haughton V.M., Williams A.L.: *Computed Tomography of the Spine.* St. Louis, C. V. Mosby Co., 1982.

James H.E., Oliff M.: Computed tomography in spinal dysraphism. *J. Comput. Assist. Tomogr.* 1:391, 1977.

Kaplan J.O., Quencer R.M.: The occult tethered conus syndrome in the adult. *Radiology* 137:387, 1980.

Kramer L.D., Krouth G.J.: Computerized tomography, an adjunct to early diagnosis in the cauda equina syndrome of ankylosing spondylitis. *Arch. Neurol.* 35:116, 1978.

Lohkamp F., Claussen C., Schumacher A.: CT demonstration of pathologic changes in the spinal cord accompanying spina bifida and diastematomyelia, in Kaufman H.S. (ed.): *Progress in Pediatric Radiology: Skull, Spine and Contents,* part 2, vol. 6. Basel, Karger, 1978.

Meyer G.A., Haughton V.M., Williams A.L., Syvertsen A.: Diagnosis of lumbar herniated disc with computed tomography. *N. Engl. J. Med.* 301:1166, 1979.

Naidich T.P., Pudlowski R.M.: High Resolution CT of the Cervical Spinal Cord, in Caille J.M., Solomon F. (eds.): *Computerized Tomography.* Berlin, Springer-Verlag, 1980.

Naidich T.P., Pudlowski R.M., Moran C.J., et al.: Computed tomography of spinal fractures. *Adv. Neurol.* 22:207, 1979.

Nakagawa H., Huang Y.P., Malis L.I., Wolf B.S.: Computed tomography of intraspinal and paraspinal neoplasms. *J. Comput. Assist. Tomogr.* 1:377, 1977.

Resjo I.M., Harwood-Nash D.C., Fitz C.R., Chuang S.: Computed tomographic metrizamide myelography in spinal dysraphism in infants and children. *J. Comput. Assist. Tomogr.* 2:549, 1978.

Resjo I.M., Harwood-Nash D.C., Fitz C.R., Chuang S.: CT metrizamide myelography for intraspinal and paraspinal neoplasms in infants and children. *A.J.R.* 132:367, 1979.

Resjo I.M., Harwood-Nash D.C., Fitz C.R., Chuang S.: Computed tomographic metrizamide myelography in syringohydromyelia. *Radiology* 131:405, 1979.

Taylor A.J., Haughton V.M., Doust B.: CT imaging of the thoracic spinal cord without intrathecal contrast medium. *J. Comput. Assist. Tomogr.* 4:223, 1980.

Ullrich C.G., Binet E.F., Sanecki M.G., Kieffer S.A.: Quantitative assessment of the lumbar spinal canal by computed tomography. *Radiology* 134:137, 1980.

Williams A.L., Haughton V.M.: CT appearance of bulging annulus. *Radiology* 142:403, 1982.

Williams A.L., Haughton V.M., Syvertsen A.: CT in the diagnosis of herniated nucleus pulposus. *Radiology* 135:95, 1980.

Wolpert S.M., Scott R.M., Carter B.L.: Computed tomography in spinal dysraphism. *Surg. Neurol.* 8:199, 1977.

PRESENTATIONS

Gado M.H., Chandra-Schur B., Patel J., et al.: An Integrated Approach to the Diagnosis of Lumbar Disc Disease by Computed Tomography and Myelography. Presented at the 67th Scientific Assembly and Annual Meeting of the Radiologic Society of North America,

Glenn W.V., Brown B.M., Murphy R.M., et al.: Computed Tomography and Myelography in the Evaluation of Lumbar Disc Disease. Presented at the 67th Scientific Assembly and Annual Meeting of the Radiologic Society of North America,

Teplick J.G., Peyster R.G., Teplick S.K., et al.: Computed Tomography and Lumbar Disc Herniation: A Prospective Study. Presented at the 67th Scientific Assembly and Annual Meeting of the Radiologic Society of North America,

26

Choice of Procedure

THE BROAD ARMAMENTARIUM OF TECHNIQUES available to the radiologist for the diagnosis of spinal disease emphasizes the need for a wise choice. This implies a thorough evaluation of the clinical findings and a review of the plain radiographs (and, where indicated, conventional tomograms) prior to selection of the best technique to solve a given problem. Each examination should be tailored to the individual patient with careful consideration of the risks, the benefits, and the cost to the patient. This chapter discusses the choice of techniques for various major disease categories.

SPINAL CORD COMPRESSION

No Extraspinal Primary Tumor Suspected

The acute onset of symptoms and signs (hyperreflexia and loss of sphincter control, with or without a sensory level) demands prompt surgical intervention to forestall irreversible neurologic damage. This is a bona fide emergency that requires expeditious radiologic study.

Often the plain films are helpful in localizing the diseased segment of the spine; sometimes they are indeterminate or negative. In any event, metrizamide myelography is the procedure of choice. If the lesion is thought to be cervical in location, a C1-2 puncture is best, although an adequate study can also be obtained via lumbar puncture. If a lesion is suspected in the thoracic or lumbar region, the metrizamide should be injected into the lumbar subarachnoid space. If an extradural or intradural extramedullary lesion is found at myelography, no further study is necessary in most instances.

The demonstration of an intramedullary process may require additional study for more specific diagnosis. CT is the procedure of choice for differentiating a cystic from a solid lesion of the spinal cord. Similar information can also be provided by pneumomyelography. Since tumors may also have cystic components, the CT demonstration of a cystic lesion with penetration of metrizamide into the cystic cavity, or the pneumomyelographic demonstration of a collapsing cord does not entirely exclude neoplasm. In this situation, careful correlation of the myelographic and CT findings is important with particular reference to the presence of irregular defects in the contrast column suggestive of tumor.

If the primary problem is differentiation of a nonsurgical (demyelinating process) from a surgical lesion with multiple areas of compression, total axis metrizamide myelography is the procedure of choice. In my experience, this is best carried out via lumbar puncture.

Spinal arteriography is indicated when the myelographic findings suggest the presence of an arteriovenous malformation. This technique is also helpful when hemangioblastoma of the cord is a serious consideration.

Extraspinal Primary Tumor Present

This problem can be satisfactorily studied in several ways. Metrizamide introduced by lumbar puncture is an excellent choice in the patient suspected of having a single metastatic lesion. If a complete block is found, the proximal margin of the obstruction can be delineated either (1) by injecting a small volume of metrizamide via C1-2 puncture or (2) by injecting air via C1-2 puncture with the patient in the decubitus head-down position. The latter technique makes it possible to demonstrate the proximal and distal margins of the obstructing lesion on a single film.

An equally satisfactory technique first involves the injection of 1–2 ml of Pantopaque by lumbar puncture. If a high-grade block is encountered, a similar aliquot of Pantopaque is injected via a C1-2 puncture to define the lower and upper ends of the obstruction. The oil is not removed. This method has the advantage of permitting radiographic postoperative or postirradiation follow-up. If no obstruction is present, a metrizamide myelogram is carried out via the lumbar puncture needle.

If multiple metastatic lesions are suspected clinically, Pantopaque is the contrast medium of choice. I begin by injecting 2–3 ml by lumbar puncture to exclude a complete block. If a total obstruction is not found, additional oil (18–36 ml) is added, as required, to delineate the entire spinal axis. Supine and lateral decubitus films with the horizontal beam are taken when indicated. I usually leave sufficient Pantopaque (8–12 ml) behind to permit radiographic postirradiation follow-up.

Patients with widespread metastatic disease on chemotherapy are often immunologically or hematologically compromised. Hence, they are especially prone to infection or bleeding. Therefore, the presence of an epidural compressive lesion in such a patient may represent abscess or hematoma rather than metastasis.

RADICULAR COMPRESSIVE SYNDROME

Herniation of the Nucleus Pulposus

This is the most common cause of nerve root compression and radicular pain. It is most prevalent in the lower lumbar spine, less common in the lower cervical region, and rare in the thoracic spine. In my own personal experience and the experience of others (Haughton et al., Anand and Lee, Raskin et al.), high-resolution CT is the primary procedure of choice for the diagnosis of suspected lumbar disk herniation in the previously unoperated spine. CT eliminates the morbidity associated with myelography and increases the diagnostic accuracy in patients in whom myelography has inherent handicaps, i.e., lateral herniations, large lumbosacral anterior epidural space. If CT is unsatisfactory or indeterminate, and there is strong clinical suspicion of radicular compression, metrizamide myelography is carried out.

One can choose a transaxial, nonangulated beam CT technique beginning at the level of the upper pedicle of L-3 and extending 2 cm caudal to the posterior margin of the superior aspect of S-1. Contiguous 5-mm slices are cut from L-3 down to and including S-1. A few additional slices are cut through the L1-2 disk and L2-3 disk spaces for completeness. Coronal and sagittal reconstruction is optional. This usually requires 30–35 slices.

Another satisfactory technique involves gantry angulation. A cursor is used on the lateral localizer to determine the planes of the intervertebral disks. Appropriate table positions and gantry tilts are selected to obtain the best CT image in the planes of the L3-4, L4-5, and L5-S1 disks. When the plane of a particular disk cannot be satisfactorily traversed (within the 20-degree tilting limit of the gantry after building up the patient's hips and thorax to decrease the lumbosacral lordosis), the closest angle is approximated, with the sections passing through the posterior disk margin. Occasionally, overlapping sections are necessary. In addition to the sections through the disks, three additional contiguous sections are cut above the disk and one below the disk to detect displaced free fragments. The technique utilizes 5-mm slice thickness, 768 mAs (400 mA/and 120 kvp) to reduce tube cooling time. The total scanning takes 35–45 minutes for the average patient. The radiation skin dose is 4–5 rad (0.04–0.05 Gy) per slice. I use soft tissue targeting (target factor 4.0) with a 42-cm field of view prospectively reconstructed to 10 cm. The soft tissue algorithm produces a magnified image without loss of resolution superior to that obtained with the smaller reconstruction circle. The images are also photographed with a bone window setting to determine the margins of the bony spinal canal, to detect facet disease, and to exclude bony overgrowth as the cause for a lateral recess syndrome.

The rare patient still suspected clinically of having neural compression after an indeterminate metrizamide myelogram or CT study can have the suspicion confirmed or excluded by disk puncture, epidural venography, or epidurography.

Because cervical disks are small and the cervicothoracic junction may be obscured by artifacts, I believe that the procedure of choice, at the present time, is myelography. I use metrizamide on inpatients and Pantopaque if the procedure must be done on an outpatient basis.

The rare herniated thoracic disk can occasionally be detected on the plain spine roentgenogram when it calcifies. In the latter instance, CT is an excellent technique. In noncalcified thoracic disk herniation where examination of a large segment of spine is required, I prefer metrizamide myelography via lumbar puncture. Gas myelography is a satisfactory alternate technique.

The postoperative patient with persistent or recurrent sciatic pain constitutes a much more difficult problem. There are a number of options available. One can perform metrizamide myelography followed by CT scanning 4–6 hours later or choose primary metrizamide CT. If a disk herniation is demonstrated at a level other than the operative interspace or on the unexplored side at the operative level, the diagnosis can be made with great confidence. An extradural defect at the operative site poses a greater problem. Differentiation of recurrent disk herniation from a postoperative fibrotic mass may be difficult. The intravenous enhancement technique recommended by Schubiger and Valavanis seems to be quite useful. Usually, a postoperative fibrotic scar will enhance sufficiently after intravenous contrast injection to permit differentiation from a recurrent disk herniation. Where differentiation is problematic, epidurography may be helpful in ruling out nerve root compression. I believe it is important to be certain about the presence of neural compression before a patient is subjected to another operative procedure.

Spinal Stenosis

Metrizamide myelography and CT are the most helpful techniques for evaluating suspected spinal stenosis as a cause of radicular compression. Indeed, metrizamide myelography followed by delayed CT is the technique I prefer wherever possible. The myelogram delineates the multiple levels of involvement and the CT defines the nature of the compressive lesions. It is most important to correlate the patient's neurologic findings with the many radiographic defects to determine which of the latter are clinically significant. In this way, unnecessary extensive bone surgery leading to an unstable spine can be avoided. Patients with significant lumbar spondylosis or kyphosis who require metrizamide cervical myelography are best studied by a C1-2 puncture. If the contrast medium is injected into the lumbar subarachnoid space in such patients, the study is often inadequate because of dilution by the time the metrizamide arrives in the cervical region.

MARKED SPINAL DEFORMITY

The most common mechanical deformity producing spinal cord compression is acquired scoliosis. Metrizamide myelography (with or without polytomography) is a very satisfactory technique in most cases. However, in patients with a very pronounced scoliosis, the dependent segment of spinal cord in the area of maximal deformity may be bathed by the contrast medium for a relatively prolonged period of time. This raises the theoretical possibility of a local neurotoxic effect on the aforementioned cord segment, which can be avoided by using Pantopaque or air instead of metrizamide. In my experience, full-volume Pantopaque myelography is a good method for studying many of these patients because of the absence of acute neurotoxicity associated with the oil. This technique has the disadvantage of requiring complete removal of the Pantopaque, which usually poses no great problem. In some cases, however, with a high-grade incomplete obstruction, total removal of the oil is not possible.

Pneumomyelography is completely nontoxic. However, it requires meticulous technique and experience. Furthermore, polytomography in these patients is more difficult and demanding, even for the experienced examiner.

Patients with congenital spinal deformities may have associated lesions, e.g., meningomyelocele, congenital benign tumors, large spinal canal and subarachnoid space. In these circumstances, the metrizamide may become too dilute to be visualized adequately by conventional radiography. Polytomography and/or CT are most helpful in such cases.

TRAUMA

Experience at the Yale Spinal Cord Trauma Center has led to the following practices.

Fractures Without Laminographic Evidence of Dislocation

Metrizamide myelography is carried out only in those patients with an incomplete neurologic deficit who show no improvement. Patients with a complete neurologic deficit, i.e., transection of the cord, do not benefit from myelography.

Fractures With Dislocation

Metrizamide myelography is performed in patients who show no neurologic improvement after complete reduction of the dislocation. Metrizamide myelography is also performed in patients with incomplete reduction of the dislocation if more than a third of the diameter of the bony spinal canal is compromised. Patients who have less than one third of the bony spinal canal do not need myelography.

SPINAL INFECTION

Plain films and radionuclide bone scans frequently indicate the involved area in patients with, or suspected of having, acute spinal infection. CT is most helpful in demonstrating the extent of the bone destruction and the associated paraspinal mass, if present. Needle aspiration under CT guidance to culture the organism is also useful. Myelography may not add any significant additional information in this group of patients. If precise localization of the lesion cannot be made by the above methods, metrizamide myelography is the technique of choice. The puncture should never be performed in an area where there is clinical suspicion of involvement because of the risk of seeding organisms from an acute epidural abscess into the subarachnoid space.

Patients suspected of having a compressive chronic epidural granuloma are best examined by metrizamide myelography. Again, the puncture should be performed at a site remote from the clinical area of suspicion.

BIBLIOGRAPHY

Anand A.K., Lee B.C.P.: Plain and metrizamide CT of lumbar disk disease: Comparison with myelography. *A.J.N.R.* 3:567, 1982.

Haughton V.M., Eldevik O.P., Magnaes B., Amundsen P.: A prospective comparison of computed tomography and myelography in the diagnosis of herniated lumbar disks. *Radiology* 142:103, 1983.

Raskin S.P., Keating J.W.: Recognition of lumbar disk disease: Comparison of myelography and computed tomography. *A.J.N.R.* 3:215, 1982.

Schubiger O., Valvanis A.: CT differentiation between recurrent disc herniation and postoperative scar formation: The value of contrast enhancement. *Neuroradiology* 22:251, 1980.

Teplick J.G., Haskin M.E.: Computed tomography of the postoperative lumbar spine. *A.J.R.* 141:865, 1983.

Index